Sickness and Health
in America

# SICKNESS AND HEALTH IN AMERICA

*Readings in the*
*History of Medicine and*
*Public Health*

Second Edition, Revised

*Edited by*
JUDITH WALZER LEAVITT
*and*
RONALD L. NUMBERS

*The University of Wisconsin Press*

The University of Wisconsin Press
114 North Murray Street
Madison, Wisconsin 53715

3 Henrietta Street
London WC2E 8LU, England

10    9    8    7    6    5    4    3    2

Printed in the United States of America

Library of Congress Cataloging-in-Publication Data
Main entry under title:
Sickness and health in America.
    Reprinted from various sources.
    Bibliography: pp. 525–534.
    Includes index.
    1. Medicine—United States—History—Addresses,
essays, lectures. 2. Public health—United States—
History—Addresses, essays, lectures. I. Leavitt,
Judith Walzer. II. Numbers, Ronald L. [DNLM: 1. History
of Medicine, Modern—United States—collected works.
2. Public Health—history—United States—collected
works. WZ 70 AA1 S48]
R151.S5        1985        362.1′0973        85-40370
ISBN 0-299-10270-X
ISBN 0-299-10274-2 (pbk.)

*To Our Students*
*Past, Present, and Future*

# CONTENTS

# Preface to the Second Edition

The history of American medicine and public health is a rapidly expanding field. Because historians are continually publishing new work, revising old conclusions, and charting new territory, we feel that an updating of our 1978 reader is necessary. This second edition recognizes some of the newer scholarship by adding 18 new essays, including entirely new sections on Race and Medicine, Women and Medicine, and the Art and Science of Medicine. To do this, we had to delete a number of excellent articles that appeared in the first edition. While it is rewarding to recognize new work, we are sad to let some of our old favorites go. We hope this edition follows in the tradition of the first in reflecting the dynamic state of scholarship in the history of American medicine and public health.

Sickness and Health
in America

# Sickness and Health in America:
## An Overview

The history of health care in America is much more than the accomplishments of a few prominent physicians. It encompasses all efforts to cure and prevent illness — lay as well as professional, the failures as well as the successes. In recognition of this diversity, we have included in this collection essays ranging from physicians to patent medicines, from masturbation to smallpox, from birthing to bacteriology. Food and filth often play as important roles as doctors and hospitals. Although, for example, we recognize the skill of surgeons who extended a few lives by dramatically transplanting human hearts, their historical significance pales in comparison with their contemporaries who organized comprehensive health centers in the rural South, markedly reducing infant mortality through unglamorous improvements in diet, sanitation, and preventive medicine.

When we look at the broad picture of sickness and health in America, two trends immediately capture our attention: the conspicuous decline in mortality and the corresponding increase in life expectancy for all ages. Although health records before 1900 are fragmentary and precision is illusory, there is little doubt that average Americans today live more than twice as long as their colonial forebears, whose life expectancy at birth was under 30 years and half of whose children died before their tenth birthdays (see Fig. 1). Unfortunately, not all Americans have benefitted equally from these changes. Women live increasingly longer than men, while whites continue to outlive nonwhites (see Figs. 1 and 2).

The changing disease pattern in America presents several problems for the historian. Health statistics before 1933, when the United States adopted uniform registration procedures for reporting diseases, must be used with caution. They are seldom complete and often inconsistent in clas-sifying diseases. Many of today's clinical distinctions did not exist in the past, and those that did were frequently blurred by practitioners with little diagnostic sophistication. To compound our difficulties, disease patterns varied widely from city to city and state to state, so that what was typical of one region may have been rare in another. Nevertheless, we should not let these problems deter us from attempting qualified generalizations.

Early settlers in America often suffered from malnutrition, which increased their vulnerability to infectious diseases. These maladies, transmitted from one person to another, can be either *endemic*, that is, always present, or *epidemic*, appearing from time to time with great intensity. The gravest threats to life and health were malaria and dysentery in summer and respiratory ailments, like influenza and pneumonia, in winter. Sporadic outbreaks of smallpox, yellow fever, and diphtheria created widespread panic, but over the long run they took far fewer lives than the more familiar scourges.

As living conditions improved during the 18th and early 19th centuries, so apparently did the health of Americans. But with increasing urbanization and industrialization the situation in the cities soon deteriorated. In Boston, New York, Philadelphia, and New Orleans, for example, the death rate per 1,000 rose from 28.1 for the quarter century 1815–1839 to 30.2 for the following 25 years.[1] By mid-century some American cities were scarcely better off than the notorious industrial centers of Europe. Lemuel Shattuck of Massachusetts sadly reported in 1850 that "London, with its imperfect supply of water, — its narrow, crowded streets, — its foul cesspools, — its hopeless pauperism — its crowded grave-yards, — and its other monstrous sanitary evils, is as healthy a city as Boston, and in some respects more so."[2]

3

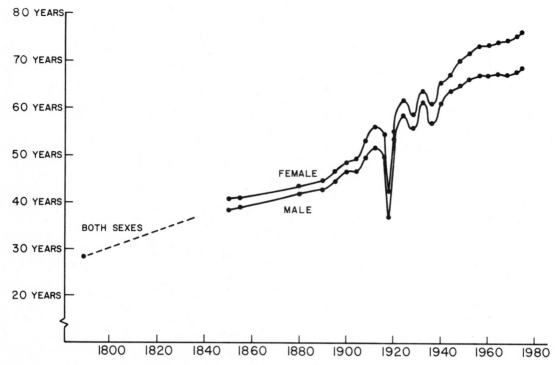

Fig. 1: Life expectancy at birth, 1789–1974, United States. Sources: Frederick L. Hoffman, "American mortality progress during the last half century," in *A Half Century of Public Health*, ed. Mazyck P. Ravenel (New York: American Public Health Association, 1921), p. 98; U.S. Bureau of the Census, *Historical Statistics of the United States: Colonial Times to 1970* (Washington, D.C.: Government Printing Office, 1975), Part 1, pp. 55–56; U.S. Bureau of the Census, *Statistical Abstract of the United States, 1976* (Washington, D.C.: Government Printing Office, 1976), p. 60. Note: The figure for 1789 is for Massachusetts and New Hampshire only, and the data between 1850 and 1900 are for Massachusetts only. The decrease in life expectancy in 1918–1919 is largely attributable to a severe influenza epidemic.

The mid-century increases in urban mortality resulted primarily from the numerous infectious diseases that attacked the nation's increasingly dense population centers. Besides intermittent epidemics of yellow fever, cholera, and smallpox, which caused more fear than mortality, there were the ever-present influenza and pneumonia, typhus, typhoid fever, diphtheria, scarlet fever, measles, whooping cough, dysentery, and—above all—tuberculosis. Tuberculosis, sometimes called consumption or phthisis, was the greatest killer of 19th-century Americans. Although present in America since the settling of Jamestown, it did not acquire its deadly reputation until it attacked heavily crowded cities. As early as the 1810s Boston, for example, experienced a tuberculosis mortality rate of 472 per 100,000 inhabitants. By the close of the century this rate had fallen by more than half, and in the mid-1970s tuberculosis killed fewer than two Americans out of every 100,000 (see Fig. 3).

The American health picture began to improve by the late 19th century, as evidenced by the declining urban death rate. The cities of Boston, New York, Philadelphia, and New Orleans, which had suffered under a death rate of 30.2 per 100,000 between 1840 and 1864, saw this figure drop to 25.7 between 1865 and 1889 and down to 18.9 between 1890 and 1914.[3] Even more dramatic was the precipitous fall of infant mortality rates. During the first three decades of the 20th century infant mor-

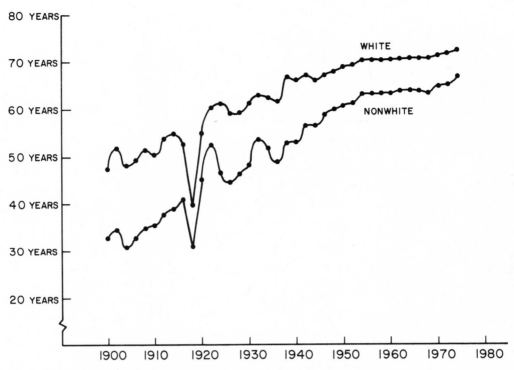

Fig. 2: Racial differences in life expectancy, 1900–1974, United States. Sources: U.S. Bureau of the Census, *Historical Statistics of the United States: Colonial Times to 1970* (Washington, D.C.: Government Printing Office, 1975), Part 1, p. 55; U.S. Bureau of the Census, *Statistical Abstract of the United States, 1976* (Washington, D.C.: Government Printing Office, 1976), p. 60.

tality decreased by more than 50 percent, and fell at an even greater rate during the next 20 years (see Fig. 4). But despite these improvements, the United States continued to lag behind many other industrialized nations in reducing infant deaths, a symbolic indicator of national health standards.

As the familiar infectious diseases of the 19th century diminished in virulence, a host of chronic, degenerative diseases appeared to take their place (see Figs. 5 and 6). By the mid-1970s tuberculosis, gastritis, and diphtheria no longer ranked among the nation's top ten killers, but heart problems, cancer, and cerebrovascular disorders (e.g., strokes), all typical of an older population, headed the list.

Given the available evidence, it is not easy to find an explanation for the decline of infectious diseases and the increase in life expectancy. But the three most likely candidates are medical prac-

tice, public health measures, and improvements in diet, housing, and personal hygiene.

Popularizers of medical history like to glorify the intrepid "doctors on horseback" and the marvelous "magic bullets" of white-coated medical scientists in explaining the miracles of the past hundred years. The historical record, however, suggests a different interpretation. Clearly, the brief improvement of health conditions in the 18th century owed little to the efforts of physicians, who probably did their patients more harm than good. Dr. William Douglass, a prominent Boston physician, observed at mid-century that "more die of the practitioner than of the natural course of the disease."[4] If this was true of the 18th century, it was probably even more so in the early 19th century during the heyday of "heroic" medicine, when regular physicians intemperately bled, purged, and puked their patients. Until the latter part of the century doctors

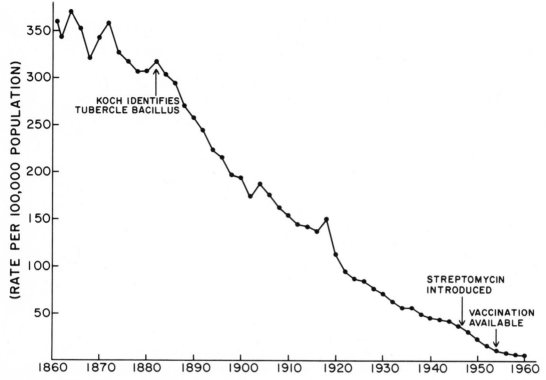

Fig. 3: Death rate for tuberculosis, 1860–1960, United States. Source: U.S. Bureau of the Census, *Historical Statistics of the United States: Colonial Times to 1970* (Wash- ington, D.C.: Government Printing Office, 1975), Part 1, pp. 58, 63. Note: Data between 1860 and 1900 are for Massachusetts only.

possessed few specific remedies besides quinine for malaria, digitalis for dropsy, and lime juice for scurvy.

America's experience with three diseases—tuberculosis, diphtheria, and smallpox—further illustrates the limitations of 19th-century medicine. Tuberculosis, the most deadly of the three in Victorian America, declined for almost a century before physicians discovered an effective way to treat or prevent it (see Fig. 3). By the time streptomycin was introduced in 1947, the death rate from tuberculosis had already dropped to 33.5 per 100,000. The use of chemotherapy markedly accelerated the rate of decline, from 44.9 percent during the 1940s to 69.7 percent in the 1950s, but even without this therapy, it seems likely that the death rate would have continued its decline.

For diphtheria, the story is somewhat different.

Although the death rate from this disease dropped dramatically after antitoxin became available in 1894 (see Fig. 7), it is debatable how much of the decline is attributable to this measure. First, the national death rate for diphtheria had been fluctuating downward for almost two decades prior to the introduction of antitoxin; second, antitoxin was neither systematically nor consistently used throughout the country. Thus it is probable that other nonmedical factors also contributed to the downfall of diphtheria in the 1890s.

In the case of smallpox, medicine *did* offer a means of protection, as early as the 1720s, when Cotton Mather introduced inoculation (variolation). This method gave treated persons a mild case of smallpox, which provided lifetime immunity. Although inoculation often spread the disease, it also appears to have lessened mortality in

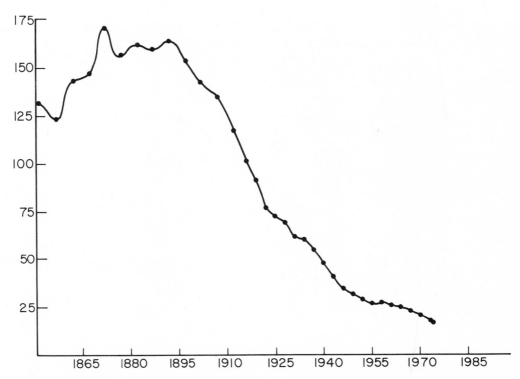

Fig. 4: Infant mortality rate per 1,000 live births, 1851–1974, United States. Sources: U.S. Bureau of the Census, *Historical Statistics of the United States: Colonial Times to 1970* (Washington, D.C.: Government Printing Office, 1975), Part 1, p. 57; U.S. Bureau of the Census, *Statistical Abstract of the United States, 1976* (Washington, D.C.: Government Printing Office, 1976), p. 64. Note: Data between 1851 and 1913 are for Massachusetts only.

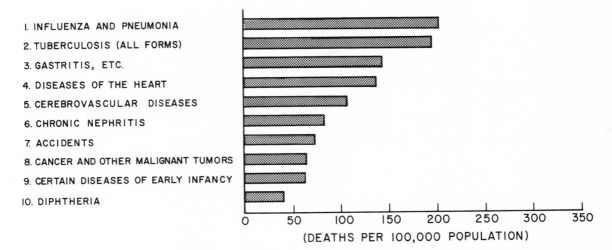

Fig. 5: Leading causes of death in the United States, 1900. Source: Monroe Lerner and Odin W. Anderson, *Health Progress in the United States: 1900–1960* (Chicago: Univ. of Chicago Press, 1963), p. 16.

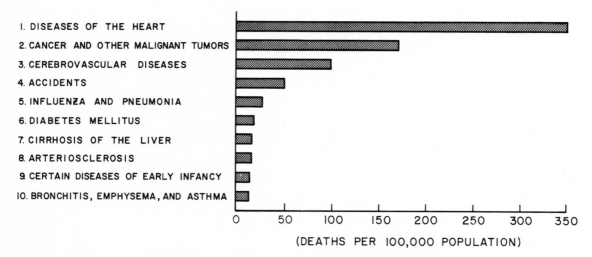

Fig. 6: Leading causes of death in the United States, 1974. Source: U.S. Bureau of the Census, *Statistical Abstract of the United States, 1976* (Washington, D.C.: Government Printing Office, 1976), p. 66.

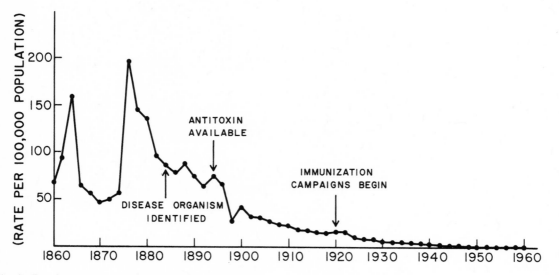

Fig. 7: Death rate for diphtheria, 1860–1960, United States. Source: U.S. Bureau of the Census, *Historical Statistics of the United States: Colonial Times to 1970* (Washington, D.C.: Government Printing Office, 1975), Part 1, pp. 58, 63. Note: Data between 1860 and 1900 are for Massachusetts only.

the 18th century. At the turn of the 19th century vaccination with cowpox virus, an even safer method, became available. But despite these measures, smallpox continued to plague Americans until the 20th century (see Fig. 8), primarily because many chose to ignore the protection medicine offered them.

If we can generalize from these three examples, it seems that medicine contributed little to the initial decline of infectious diseases in the United States, but sometimes played a crucial role in the 20th century. The discovery in the 1930s and 1940s of powerful new drugs, like the sulphonamides and antibiotics, finally gave physi-

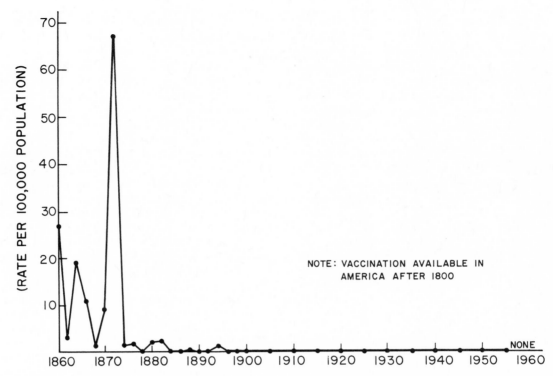

Fig 8: Death rate for smallpox, 1860–1960, Massachusetts. Source: U.S. Bureau of the Census, *Historical Statistics of the United States: Colonial Times to 1970* (Washington, D.C.: Government Printing Office, 1975), Part 1, p. 63.

cians effective weapons with which to fight infection.

The public health movement proved more effective than medicine in combatting communicable diseases during the 19th century. It reduced exposure to infectious diseases by cleaning up the physical environment and improving living conditions, and it helped to lower the incidence of waterborne infections like cholera and dysentery by regulating urban water sources and sewerage.

Filth was the premier public health problem in the 19th century. Most physicians thought that dirt caused disease and that cleaning up the cities was the best preventative to high mortality. But as traditional methods of keeping cities clean broke down in the wake of massive population increases, those responsible for public health faced unprecedented problems. Festering piles of garbage littered urban streets, dead animals lay where they fell,

privies and cesspools overran into drainless, unpaved streets. Horses defecated indiscriminately. Municipal employees spent countless hours trying to staunch the seemingly endless flow of waste products, and, to varying degrees, they were successful. They removed garbage, emptied privies, drained stagnant pools, improved and extended water and sewer systems, and slowly created an environment in which it was possible to walk down the street without dragging one's skirt in the filth or having to hold a handkerchief over one's nose. Health departments also regulated food and housing, at least minimally. Undoubtedly these efforts, to the extent they were successful, significantly reduced the spread of infectious diseases that thrived in unhygienic, congested environments. Their precise impact cannot be measured, because conditions at the local level varied so greatly. But it hardly seems coincidental that mortality from communicable diseases declined at the very time American cities were waging vigorous sanitation campaigns.

Improved water supplies and sewerage provided additional protection against infectious diseases. As more and more American cities installed municipal water systems, urbanites no longer had to consume water from contaminated wells and polluted rivers. The construction of sewers, which carried off tons of septic waste products each day, eliminated another source of infection. All of these public health measures, plus the isolation of the sick during times of epidemics and the regulation of foodstuffs, helped to turn mortality rates downward.

It also seems likely that living conditions — diet, housing, and personal hygiene — contributed to reducing mortality. Recent studies, for example, have demonstrated a high correlation between malnutrition and susceptibility to infectious diseases. Unfortunately, historical data regarding the way people lived are so scarce, we must rely more on inference than hard evidence.

Seventeenth-century colonists frequently suffered from severe food shortages and consequent malnutrition. As one pioneer observed in 1628, "for want of wholesome Diet and convenient Lodgings, many die of Scurvys and other Distempers."[5] These shortages largely disappeared as agricultural production stabilized in the 18th century, but the staple American diet of corn and pork, though ample in quantity, hardly provided a balanced diet.

It was not until the coming of railroads in the 1840s and 1850s and the development of the canning industry after 1860 that products like milk, fruit, and vegetables became readily available year-round, especially to urban dwellers. It is impossible to tell exactly how much the availability of these products increased the consumption of them, but we do know that one early 19th-century family spent 9.7 percent of its food budget on milk, fruit, and vegetables, while a century later another family spent 40.8 percent.[6] This revolution in American eating habits, suggests one historian, "may have contributed as fully to the development of a healthful, vigorous manhood as major measures of sanitary reform and preventive medicine."[7] Certainly it was an important factor.

In the 20th century diet continued to influence the nation's health, though its effect was often negative. As affluent Americans ate more fats and sugar and less fruit, vegetables, and grain products, they fell victim to a form of malnutrition that some authorities predicted might be "as profoundly damaging to the Nation's health as the widespread contagious diseases of the early part of the century." By the mid-1970s six of the ten leading causes of death — heart disease, cancer, cerebrovascular disease, diabetes, arteriosclerosis, and cirrhosis of the liver — could be tied to dietary habits like the overconsumption of saturated fats, cholesterol, sugar, salt, and alcohol.[8] Such evidence clearly demonstrates that to understand sickness and health in America we must study not only medicine, but public health and life-style as well.[9]

## NOTES

1   Frederick L. Hoffman, "American mortality progress during the last half century," in *A Half Century of Public Health*, ed. Mazyck P. Ravenel (New York: American Public Health Association, 1921), p. 101.

2   *Report of the Sanitary Commission of Massachusetts* (Boston: Dutton and Wentworth, 1850), p. 281.

3   Hoffman, "American mortality progress," p. 101.

4   Quoted in John Duffy, *Epidemics in Colonial America* (Baton Rouge: Louisiana State Univ. Press, 1971), p. 4.

5   Quoted *ibid.*, p. 11.

6   Chase Going Woodhouse, "The standard of living at the professional level, 1816–17 and 1926–27," *J. Polit. Econ.*, 1929, *37*: 565–567.

7   Richard Osborn Cummings, *The American and His Food: A History of Food Habits in the United States* (Chicago: Univ. of Chicago Press, 1941), p. 52.

8   U.S. Senate Select Committee on Nutrition and Human Needs, *Dietary Goals for the United States* (Washington, D.C.: Government Printing Office, 1977), p. 9.

9   Thomas McKeown's provocative *The Modern Rise of Population* (New York: Academic Press, 1976) inspired this essay.

# Theory

Ideas, like individuals and institutions, have their own histories, and concepts of sickness and health are no exception. What one generation of Americans may have considered an illness, another regarded as perfectly normal. As both Tristram Engelhardt and Barbara Sicherman show, the existence of disease entities may relate as much to the needs of doctors and patients as to objective phenomena.

The history of masturbation, described by Engelhardt, illustrates a common progression from sin to sickness to normal, healthy behavior. Prior to the 19th century Americans widely regarded "self-abuse" as a bad habit, condemned by Scripture and society. During the Victorian age, however, this practice partially escaped its immoral past and metamorphosed into a disease, with distinctive etiology and therapy. Still later, it dropped its pathological connotation and emerged as an acceptable, if not quite respectable, activity. Other practices once attributed to character defects have undergone similar transformations. Today alcoholism, drug addiction, and obesity all seem to be winning recognition as legitimate illnesses, freeing their sufferers from moral blame. At times the change of label from sin to sickness appears arbitrary, as when the Supreme Court in 1962 declared drug addiction to be a disease rather than a crime, and when psychiatrists in 1973 decided that homosexuality was not a form of mental illness.

Sicherman's study provides still another example of changing disease concepts. Neurasthenia, once "the national disease," quietly disappeared in the 20th century, when it no longer served the purpose for which it had been invented a half-century earlier. Americans continued to suffer and die from nervous exhaustion, but physicians, aided by new diagnostic techniques, now interpreted exhaustion as a mere symptom of other diseases. Benjamin Rush's theory of the unity of disease experienced a similar fate. Rush, the foremost physician and medical educator of the early Republic, assured his students in 1796 that "there is but one disease in the world," the essence of which was vascular tension. Within a short time, however, diagnostic sophistication and a new philosophy of medicine had reduced vascular tension to the status of a symptom.

Because illness is a departure from the normal, the more familiar a condition, the less likely it is to be labeled a disease. Malaria, for example, was so common in the Midwest during the mid-19th century, one medical historian, Erwin Ackerknecht, has argued that it briefly lost its identity as a disease. Views of childbirth likewise changed over time. During most of the 18th and 19th centuries, women, who bore many children at home without the aid of a physician, regarded delivery as a normal—if risky—part of life. But when women began having fewer children, and having them in hospitals attended by physicians, the event took on the characteristics of an illness.

11

# 1

## The Disease of Masturbation: Values and the Concept of Disease

### H. TRISTRAM ENGELHARDT, JR.

Masturbation in the 18th and especially in the 19th century was widely believed to produce a spectrum of serious signs and symptoms, and was held to be a dangerous disease entity. Explanation of this phenomenon entails a basic reexamination of the concept of disease. It presupposes that one think of disease neither as an objective entity in the world nor as a concept that admits of a single universal definition: there is not, nor need there be, one concept of disease.[1] Rather, one chooses concepts for certain purposes, depending on values and hopes concerning the world.[2] The disease of masturbation is an eloquent example of the value-laden nature of science in general and of medicine in particular. In explaining the world, one judges what is to be significant or insignificant. For example, mathematical formulae are chosen in terms of elegance and simplicity, though elegance and simplicity are not attributes to be found in the world as such. The problem is even more involved in the case of medicine which judges what the human organism should be (i.e., what counts as "health") and is thus involved in the entire range of human values. This paper will sketch the nature of the model of the disease of masturbation in the 19th century, particularly in America, and indicate the scope of this "disease entity" and the therapies it evoked. The goal will be to outline some of the interrelations between evaluation and explanation.

The moral offense of masturbation was transformed into a disease with somatic not just psy-

H. TRISTRAM ENGELHARDT, JR., is Professor in the Departments of Medicine and Community Medicine, and Member of the Center for Ethics, Medicine, and Public Issues at Baylor College of Medicine, Houston, Texas.

Reprinted with permission from the *Bulletin of the History of Medicine*, 1974, *48*: 234–248.

chological dimensions. Though sexual overindulgence generally was considered debilitating since at least the time of Hippocrates,[3] masturbation was not widely accepted as a disease until a book by the title *Onania* appeared anonymously in Holland in 1700 and met with great success.[4] This success was reinforced by the appearance of S. A. Tissot's book on onanism.[5] Tissot held that all sexual activity was potentially debilitating and that the debilitation was merely more exaggerated in the case of masturbation. The primary basis for the debilitation was, according to Tissot, loss of seminal fluid, 1 ounce being equivalent to the loss of 40 ounces of blood.[6] When this loss of fluid took place in another than recumbent position (which Tissot held often to be the case with masturbation), this exaggerated the ill effects.[7] In attempting to document his contention, Tissot provided a comprehensive monograph on masturbation, synthesizing and appropriating the views of classical authors who had been suspicious of the effects of sexual overindulgence. He focused these suspicions clearly on masturbation. In this he was very successful, for Tissot's book appears to have widely established the medical opinion that masturbation was associated with serious physical and mental maladies.[8]

There appears to have been some disagreement whether the effect of frequent intercourse was in any respect different from that of masturbation. The presupposition that masturbation was not in accordance with the dictates of nature suggested that it would tend to be more subversive of the constitution than excessive sexual intercourse. Accounts of this difference in terms of the differential effect of the excitation involved are for the most part obscure. It was, though, advanced that "during sexual intercourse the expenditure of nerve force is compensated by the magnetism of the partner."[9] Tissot suggested that a beautiful sexual partner was of particular benefit or was at least less exhausting.[10] In any event, masturbation was held to be potentially more deleterious since it was unnatural, and, therefore, less satisfying and more likely to lead to a disturbance or disordering of nerve tone.

At first, the wide range of illnesses attributed to masturbation was striking. Masturbation was held to be the cause of dyspepsia,[11] constrictions of the urethra,[12] epilepsy,[13] blindness,[14] vertigo, loss of hearing,[15] headache, impotency, loss of memory, "irregular action of the heart," general loss of health and strength,[16] rickets,[17] leucorrhea in women,[18] and chronic catarrhal conjunctivitis.[19] Nymphomania was found to arise from masturbation, occurring more commonly in blondes than in brunettes.[20] Further, changes in the external genitalia were attributed to masturbation: elongation of the clitoris, reddening and congestion of the labia majora, elongation of the labia minora,[21] and a thinning and decrease in size of the penis.[22] Chronic masturbation was held to lead to the development of a particular type, including enlargement of the superficial veins of the hands and feet, moist and clammy hands, stooped shoulders, pale sallow face with heavy dark circles around the eyes, a "draggy" gait, and acne.[23] Careful case studies were published establishing masturbation as a cause of insanity,[24] and evidence indicated that it was a cause of hereditary insanity as well.[25] Masturbation was held also to cause an hereditary predisposition to consumption.[26] Finally, masturbation was believed to lead to general debility. "From health and vigor, and intelligence and loveliness of character, they became thin and pale and cadaverous; their amiability and loveliness departed, and in their stead irritability, moroseness and anger were prominent characteristics. . . . The child loses its flesh and becomes pale and weak."[27] The natural history was one of progressive loss of vigor, both physical and mental.

In short, a broad and heterogeneous class of signs and symptoms was recognized in the 19th century as a part of what was tantamount to a syndrome, if not a disease: masturbation. If one thinks of a syndrome as the concurrence or running together of signs and symptoms into a recognizable pattern, surely masturbation was such a pattern.

It was more, though, in that a cause was attributed to the syndrome providing an etiological framework for a disease entity. That is, if one views the development of disease concepts as the progression from the mere collection of signs and symptoms to their interrelation in terms of a recognized causal mechanism, the disease of masturbation was fairly well evolved. A strikingly heterogeneous set of signs and symptoms was unified and comprehended under one causal mechanism. One could thus move from mere observation and description to explanation.

Since the signs and symptoms brought within the concept of masturbation were of a serious order associated with marked debility, it is not unexpected that there would be occasional deaths. The annual reports of the Charity Hospital of Louisiana in New Orleans which show hospitalizations for masturbation over an 86-year period indicate that, indeed, two masturbators were recorded as having died in the hospital. In 1872, the reports show that there were two masturbators hospitalized, one of whom was discharged, the other one having died.[28] The records of 1887 show that of the five masturbators hospitalized that year two improved, two were unimproved and one died.[29] The records of the hospital give no evidence concerning the patient who died in 1872. The records for 1887, however, name the patient, showing him to have been hospitalized on Tuesday, January 6, 1887, for masturbation. A 45-year-old native of Indiana, a resident of New Orleans for the previous 35 years, single, and a laborer, he died in the hospital on April 8, 1887.[30] There is no indication of the course of the illness. It is interesting to note, though, that in 1888 there was a death from anemia associated with masturbation, the cause of death being recorded under anemia. The records indicate that the patient was hospitalized on August 17, 1887, and died on February 11, 1888, was a lifelong resident of New Orleans, and was likewise a laborer and single.[31] His case suggests something concerning the two deaths recorded under masturbation: that they, too, suffered from a debilitating disease whose signs and symptoms were referred to masturbation as the underlying cause. In short, the concept of masturbation as a disease probably acted as a schema for organizing various signs and symptoms which we would now gather under different nosological categories.

As with all diseases, there was a struggle to develop a workable nosology. This is reflected in the reports of the Charity Hospital of Louisiana (in New Orleans) where over the years the disease was placed under various categories and numerous nomenclatures were employed. In 1848, for example, the first entry was given as "masturbation," in 1853 "onanism" was substituted, and in 1857 this was changed to "onanysmus."[32] Later, as the records began to classify the diseases under general headings, a place had to be found for masturbation. Initially in 1874, the disease "masturbation" was placed under the heading "Male Diseases of Generative Organs." In 1877 this was changed to "Diseases of the Nervous System," and finally in 1884 the disease of "onanism" was classified as a "Cerebral-Spinal Disease." In 1890 it was reclassified under the heading "Diseases of the Nervous System," and remained classified as such until 1906 when it was placed as "masturbation" under the title of "Genito-Urinary System, Diseases of (Functional Disturbances of Male Sexual Organs)." It remained classified as a functional disturbance until the last entry in 1933. The vacillation in the use of headings probably indicates hesitation on the part of the recorders as to the nature of the disease. On the one hand, it is understandable why a disease, which was held to have such grossly physical components, would itself be considered to have some variety of physical basis. On the other hand, the recorders appear to have been drawn by the obviously psychological aspects of the phenomenon of masturbation to classify it in the end as a functional disturbance.

As mentioned, the concept of the disease of masturbation developed on the basis of a general suspicion that sexual activity was debilitating.[33] This development is not really unexpected: if one examines the world with a tacit presupposition of a parallelism between what is good for one's soul and what is good for one's health, then one would expect to find disease correlates for immoral sexual behavior.[34] Also, this was influenced by a concurrent inclination to translate a moral issue into medical terms and relieve it of the associated moral opprobrium in a fashion similar to the translation of alcoholism from a moral into a medical problem.[35] Further, disease as a departure from a state of stability due to excess or under-excitation offered the skeleton of a psychosomatic theory of the somatic alterations attributed to the excitation associated with masturbation.[36] The categories of over- and under-excitation suggest cogent, basic categories of medical explanation: over- and under-excitation, each examples of excess, imply deleterious influences on the stability of the organism. Jonathan Hutchinson succinctly described the etiological mechanism in this fashion, holding that "the habit in question is very injurious to the nerve-tone, and that it frequently originates and keeps up maladies which but for it might have been avoided or cured."[37] This schema of causality presents the signs and symptoms attendant to masturbation as due to "the nerveshock attending the substitute for the venereal act, or the act itself, which, either in onanism or copulation frequently indulged, breaks men down."[38] "The excitement incident to the habitual and frequent indulgence of the unnatural practice of masturbation leads to the most serious constitutional effects. . . ."[39] The effects were held to be magnified during youth when such "shocks" undermined normal development.[40]

Similarly, Freud remarks in a draft of a paper to Wilhelm Fliess dated February 8, 1893, that "Sexual exhaustion can by itself alone provoke neurasthenia. If it fails to achieve this by itself, it has such an effect on the disposition of the nervous system that physical illness, depressive affects and overwork (toxic influences) can no longer be tolerated without [leading to] neurasthenia. . . . *neurasthenia in males* is acquired at puberty and becomes manifest in the patient's twenties. Its source is masturbation, the frequency of which runs completely parallel with the frequency of male neurasthenia."[41] And Freud later stated, "It is the prolonged and intense action of this pernicious sexual satisfaction which is enough on its own account to provoke a neurasthenic neurosis. . . ."[42] Again, it is a model of excessive stimulation of a certain quality leading to specific disabilities. This position of the theoreticians of masturbation in the 19th century is not dissimilar to positions currently held concerning other diseases. For example, the first Diagnostic and Statistical Manual of the American Psychiatric Association says with regard to "psychophysiologic autonomic and visceral disorders" that "The symptoms are due to a chronic and exaggerated state of the normal physiological expression of emotion, with the feeling, or subjective part, repressed.

Such long continued visceral states may eventually lead to structural changes."[43] This theoretical formulation is one that would have been compatible with theories concerning masturbation in the 19th century.

Other models of etiology were employed besides those based upon excess stimulation. They, for the most part, accounted for the signs and symptoms on the basis of the guilt associated with the act of masturbation. These more liberal positions developed during a time of reaction against the more drastic therapies such as Baker Brown's use of clitoridectomy.[44] These alternative models can be distinguished according to whether the guilt was held to be essential or adventitious. Those who held that masturbation was an unnatural act were likely to hold that the associated guilt feelings and anxiety were natural, unavoidable consequences of performing an unnatural act. Though not phrased in the more ethically neutral terms of excess stimulation, still the explanation was in terms of a pathophysiological state involving a departure from biological norms. "The masturbator feels that his act degrades his manhood, while the man who indulges in legitimate intercourse is satisfied that he has fulfilled one of his principal natural functions. There is a healthy instinctive expression of passion in one case, an illegitimate perversion of function in the other."[45] The operative assumption was that when sexual activity failed to produce an "exhilaration of spirits and clearness of intellect" and when associated with anxiety or guilt it would lead to deleterious effects.[46] This analysis suggested that it was guilt, not excitation, which led to the phenomena associated with masturbation. "Now it happens in a large number of cases, that these young masturbators sooner or later become alarmed at their practices, in consequence of some information they receive. Often this latter is of a most mischievous character. Occasionally too, the religious element is predominant, and the mental condition of these young men becomes truly pitiable. . . . The facts are nearly these: Masturbation is not a crime nor a sin, but a vice."[47] Others appreciated the evil and guilt primarily in terms of the solitary and egoistic nature of the act.[48]

Such positions concerning etiology graded over into models in which masturbation's untoward signs and symptoms were viewed as merely the result of guilt and anxiety felt because of particular cultural norms, which norms had no essential basis in biology. "Whatever may be abnormal, there is nothing unnatural."[49] In short, there was also a model of interpretation which saw the phenomena associated with masturbation as merely adventitious, as due to a particular culture's condemnation of the act. This last interpretation implied that no more was required than to realize that there was nothing essentially wrong with masturbation. "Our wisest course is to recognize the inevitableness of the vice of masturbation under the perpetual restraints of civilized life, and, while avoiding any attitude of indifference, to avoid also an attitude of excessive horror, for that would only lead to the facts being effectually veiled from our sight, and serve to manufacture artificially a greater evil than that which we seek to combat."[50] This last point of view appears to have gained prominence in the development of thought concerning masturbation as reflected in the shift from the employment of mechanical and surgical therapy in the late 19th century to the use of more progressive means (i.e., including education that guilt and anxiety were merely relative to certain cultural norms) by the end of the century and the first half of the 20th century.[51]

To recapitulate, 19th-century reflection on the etiology of masturbation led to the development of an authentic disease of masturbation: excessive sexual stimulation was seen to produce particular and discrete pathophysiological changes.[52] First, there were strict approaches in terms of disordered nerve-tone due to excess and/or unnatural sexual excitation. Over-excitation was seen to lead to significant and serious physical alterations in the patient, and in this vein a somewhat refined causal model of the disease was developed. Second, there were those who saw the signs and symptoms as arising from the unavoidable guilt and anxiety associated with the performance of an unnatural act. Third, there were a few who appreciated masturbation's sequelae as merely the response of a person in a culture which condemned the activity.

Those who held the disease of masturbation to be more than a culturally dependent phenomenon often employed somewhat drastic therapies. Restraining devices were devised,[53] infibulation or placing a ring in the prepuce was used to make masturbation painful,[54] and no one less than Jonathan Hutchinson held that circumcision acted as a preventive.[55] Acid burns or thermoelectrocautery[56] were utilized to make masturbation painful and, therefore, to discourage it. The alleged seriousness of this disease in females led, as Professor John Duffy has shown, to the employment of the rather radical treatment of clitoridectomy.[57] The classic monograph recommending clitoridectomy, written by the British surgeon Baker Brown, advocated the procedure to terminate the "long continued peripheral excitement, causing frequent and increasing losses of nerve force. . . ."[58] Brown recommended that "the patient having been placed completely under the influence of chloroform, the clitoris [be] freely excised either by scissors or knive—I always prefer the scissors."[59] The supposed sequelae of female masturbation, such as sterility, paresis, hysteria, dysmenorrhea, idiocy, and insanity, were also held to be remedied by the operation.

Male masturbation was likewise treated by means of surgical procedures. Some recommended vasectomy[60] while others found this procedure ineffective and employed castration.[61] One illustrative case involved the castration of a physician who had been confined as insane for seven years and who subsequently was able to return to practice.[62] Another case involved the castration of a 22-year-old epileptic "at the request of the county judge, and with the consent of his father . . . the father saying he would be perfectly satisfied if the masturbation could be stopped, so that he could take him home, without having his family continually humiliated and disgusted by his loathsome habit."[63] The patient was described as facing the operation morosely, "like a coon in a hollow."[64] Following the operation, masturbation ceased and the frequency of fits decreased. An editor of the *Texas Medical Practitioner*, J. B. Shelmire, added a remark to the article: "Were this procedure oftener adopted for the cure of these desperate cases, many, who are sent to insane asylums, soon to succumb to the effects of this habit, would live to become useful citizens."[65] Though such approaches met with ridicule from some quarters,[66] still various novel treatments were devised in order to remedy the alleged sequelae of chronic masturbation such as spermatorrhea and impotency. These included acupuncture of the prostate in which "needles from two to three inches in length are passed through the perineum into the prostate gland and the neck

of the bladder. . . . Some surgeons recommend the introduction of needles into the testicles and spermatic cord for the same purpose."[67] Insertion of electrodes into the bladder and rectum and cauterization of the prostatic urethra were also utilized.[68] Thus, a wide range of rather heroic methods was devised to treat masturbation and a near fascination developed on the part of some for the employment of mechanical and electrical means of restoring "health."

There were, though, more tolerant approaches, ranging from hard work and simple diet[69] to suggestions that "If the masturbator is totally continent, sexual intercourse is advisable."[70] This latter approach to therapy led some physicians to recommend that masturbators cure their disease by frequenting houses of prostitution,[71] or acquiring a mistress.[72] Though these treatments would appear ad hoc, more theoretically sound proposals were made by many physicians in terms of the model of excitability. They suggested that the disease and its sequelae could be adequately controlled by treating the excitation and debility consequent upon masturbation. Towards this end, "active tonics" and the use of cold baths at night just before bedtime were suggested.[73] Much more in a "Brownian" mode was the proposal that treatment with opium would be effective. An initial treatment with 1/12 of a grain of morphine sulfate daily by injection was followed after ten days by a dose of 1/16 of a grain. This dose was continued for three weeks and gradually diminished to 1/30 of a grain a day. At the end of a month the patient was dismissed from treatment "the picture of health, having fattened very much, and lost every trace of anaemia and mental imbecility."[74] The author, after his researches with opium and masturbation, concluded, "*We may find in opium a new and important aid in the treatment of the victims of the habit of masturbation by means of which their moral and physical forces may be so increased that they may be enabled to enter the true physiological path.*"[75] This last example eloquently collects the elements of the concept of the disease of masturbation as a pathophysiological entity: excitation leads to physical debilitation requiring a physical remedy. Masturbation as a pathophysiological entity was thus incorporated within an acceptable medical model of diagnosis and therapy.

In summary, in the 19th century, biomedical

scientists attempted to correlate a vast number of signs and symptoms with a disapproved activity found in many patients afflicted with various maladies. Given an inviting theoretical framework, it was very conducive to think of this range of signs and symptoms as having one cause. The theoretical framework, though, as has been indicated, was not value free but structured by the values and expectations of the times. In the 19th century, one was pleased to think that not "one bride in a hundred, of delicate, educated, sensitive women, accepts matrimony from any desire of sexual gratification: when she thinks of this at all, it is with shrinking, or even with horror, rather than with desire."[76] In contrast, in the 20th century, articles are published for the instruction of women in the use of masturbation to overcome the disease of frigidity or orgasmic dysfunction.[77] In both cases, expectations concerning what should be significant structure the appreciation of reality by medicine. The variations are not due to mere fallacies of scientific method,[78] but involve a basic dependence of the logic of scientific discovery and explanation upon prior evaluations of reality.[79] A sought-for coincidence of morality and nature gives goals to explanation and therapy.[80] Values influence the purpose and direction of investigations and treatment. Moreover, the disease of masturbation has other analogues. In the 19th century, there were such diseases in the South as "Drapetomania, the disease causing slaves to run away," and the disease "Dysaesthesia Aethiopis or hebetude of mind and obtuse sensibility of body—a disease peculiar to negroes—called by overseers 'rascality'."[81] In Europe, there was the disease of *morbus democritus*.[82] Some would hold that current analogues exist in diseases such as alcoholism and drug abuse.[83] In short, the disease of masturbation indicates that evaluations play a role in the development of explanatory models and that this may not be an isolated phenomenon.

This analysis, then, suggests the following conclusion: although vice and virtue are not equivalent to disease and health, they bear a direct relation to these concepts. Insofar as a vice is taken to be a deviation from an ideal of human perfection, or "well-being," it can be translated into disease language. In shifting to disease language, one no longer speaks in moralistic terms (e.g., "You are evil"), but one speaks in terms of a deviation from a norm which implies a degree of imperfection (e.g., "You are a deviant"). The shift is from an explicitly ethical language to a language of natural teleology. To be ill is to fail to realize the perfection of an ideal type; to be sick is to be defective rather than to be evil. The concern is no longer with what is naturally, morally good, but what is naturally beautiful. Medicine turns to what has been judged to be naturally ugly or deviant, and then develops etiological accounts in order to explain and treat in a coherent fashion a manifold of displeasing signs and symptoms. The notion of the "deviant" structures the concept of disease providing a purpose and direction for explanation and for action, that is, for diagnosis and prognosis, and for therapy. A "disease entity" operates as a conceptual form organizing phenomena in a fashion deemed useful for certain goals. The goals, though, involve choice by man and are not objective facts, data "given" by nature. They are ideals imputed to nature. The disease of masturbation is an eloquent example of the role of evaluation in explanation and the structure values give to our picture of reality.

## NOTES

Read at the 46th annual meeting of the American Association for the History of Medicine, Cincinnati, Ohio, May 5, 1973. I am grateful for the suggestions of Professor John Duffy, and the kind assistance of Louanna K. Bennett and Robert S. Baxter, Jr.

1   Alvan R. Feinstein, "Taxonomy and logic in clinical data," *Ann. N.Y. Acad. Sci.,* 1969, *161*: 450–459.

2   Horacio Fabrega, Jr., "Concepts of disease: logical features and social implications," *Perspect. Biol. & Med.,* 1972, *15*: 583–616.

3   For example, Hippocrates correlated gout with sexual intercourse, *Aphorisms*, VI, 30. Numerous passages in the *Corpus* recommended the avoidance of overindulgence especially during certain illnesses.

4   René A. Spitz, "Authority and masturbation. Some remarks on a bibliographical investigation," *Yearbook of Psychoanalysis,* 1953, *9*: 116. Also, Robert H. MacDonald, "The frightful consequences of onanism: notes on the history of a delusion," *J. Hist. Ideas,* 1967, *28*: 423–431.

5   Simon-André Tissot, *Tentamen de Morbis ex Manu-*

*strupatione* (Lausanne: M. M. Bousquet, 1758). An anonymous American translation appeared in the early 19th century: *Onanism* (New York: Collins & Hannay, 1832). Interestingly, the copy of Tissot's book held by the New York Academy of Medicine was given by Austin Flint. Austin Flint in turn was quoted as an authority on the effects of masturbation: see Joseph W. Howe's *Excessive Venery, Masturbation and Continence* (New York: Bermingham, 1884), p. 97. Also the American edition of Tissot's book, to show its concurrence with an American authority, added in a footnote a reference to Benjamin Rush's opinion concerning the pernicious consequences of masturbation. See Tissot, *Onanism*, p. 19, and Benjamin Rush's *Medical Inquiries and Observations Upon the Diseases of the Mind* (Philadelphia: Kimber and Richardson, 1812), pp. 348–349; also Tissot, *Onanism*, p. 21.

6   Simon-André Tissot, *Onanism* (New York: Collins & Hannay, 1832), p. 5.

7   *Ibid.,* p. 50.

8   E. H. Hare, "Masturbatory insanity: the history of an idea," *J. Mental Sci.*, 1962, *108*: 2–3. It is worth noting that Tissot, as others, at times appears to have grouped together female masturbation and female homosexuality. See Vern L. Bullough and Martha Voght, "Homosexuality and its confusion with the 'secret sin' in pre-Freudian America," *J. Hist. Med.*, 1973, *28*: 143–155.

9   Howe, *Excessive Venery*, pp. 76–77.

10   Tissot, *Onanism*, p. 51.

11   J. A. Mayes, "Spermatorrhoea, treated by the lately invented rings," *Charleston Med. J. & Rev.*, 1854, *9*: 352.

12   Allen W. Hagenbach, "Masturbation as a cause of insanity," *J. Nerv. & Ment. Dis.*, 1879, *6*: 609.

13   Baker Brown, *On the Curability of Certain Forms of Insanity, Epilepsy, Catalepsy, and Hysteria in Females* (London: Hardwicke, 1866). Brown phrased the cause discreetly in terms of "peripheral irritation, arising originally in some branches of the pudic nerve, more particularly the incident nerve supplying the clitoris. . . ." (p. 7)

14   F. A. Burdem, "Self pollution in children," *Mass. Med. J.,* 1896, *16*:340.

15   Weber Liel, "The influence of sexual irritation upon the diseases of the ear," *New Orleans Med. & Surg. J.,* 1884, *11*: 786–788.

16   Joseph Jones, "Diseases of the nervous system," *Tr. La. St. Med. Soc.* (New Orleans: L. Graham & Son, 1889), p. 170.

17   Howe, *Excessive Venery*, p. 93.

18   J. Castellanos, "Influence of sewing machines upon the health and morality of the females using them," *Southern J. Med. Sci.*, 1866–1867, *1*: 495–496.

19   Comment, "Masturbation and ophthalmia," *New Orleans Med. & Surg. J.*, 1881–1882, *9*: 67.

20   Howe, *Excessive Venery*, pp. 108–111.

21   *Ibid.*, pp. 41, 72.

22   *Ibid.*, p. 68.

23   *Ibid.*, p. 73.

24   Hagenbach, "Masturbation as a cause of insanity," pp. 603–612.

25   Jones, "Diseases of the nervous system," p. 170.

26   Howe, *Excessive Venery*, p. 95.

27   Burdem, "Self pollution," pp. 339, 341.

28   *Report of the Board of Administrators of the Charity Hospital to the General Assembly of Louisiana* (for 1872) (New Orleans: The Republican Office, 1873), p. 30.

29   *Report of the Board of Administrators of the Charity Hospital to the General Assembly of Louisiana* (for 1887) (New Orleans: A. W. Hyatt, 1888), p. 53.

30   Record Archives of the Charity Hospital of Louisiana [in New Orleans] MS, "Admission Book #41 from December 1, 1885 to March 31, 1888 Charity Hospital," p. 198. I am indebted to Mrs. Eddie Cooksy for access to the record archives.

31   *Ibid.*, p. 287.

32   This and the following information concerning entries is taken from a review of the *Report of the Board of Administrators of the Charity Hospital*, New Orleans, Louisiana, from 1848 to 1933. The reports were not available for the years 1850–1851, 1854–1855, 1862–1863, and 1865.

33   Even Boerhaave remarked that "an excessive discharge of semen causes fatigue, weakness, decrease in activity, convulsions, emaciation, dehydration, heat and pains in the membranes of the brain, a loss in the acuity of the senses, particularly of vision, *tabes dorsalis*, simplemindedness, and various similar disorders." My translation of Hermanno Boerhaave's *Institutiones Medicae* (Vienna: J. T. Trattner, 1775), p. 315, paragraph 776.

34   "We have seen that masturbation is more pernicious than excessive intercourse with females. Those who believe in a special providence, account for it by a special ordinance of the Deity to punish this crime." Tissot, *Onanism*, p. 45.

35   ". . . the best remedy was not to tell the poor children that they were damning their souls, but to tell them that they might seriously hurt their bodies, and to explain to them the nature and purport of the functions they were abusing." Lawson Tait, "Masturbation. A clinical lecture," *Med. News, N.Y.*, 1888, *53*: 2.

36   Though it has not been possible to trace a direct influence by John Brown's system of medicine upon the development of accounts of the disease of masturbation, yet a connection is suggestive. Brown had left a mark on the minds of many in the 18th and

19th centuries, and given greater currency to the use of concepts of over and under excitation in the explanation of the etiology of disease. Guenter B. Risse, "The quest for certainty in medicine: John Brown's system of medicine in France," *Bull. Hist. Med.*, 1971, *45*: 1–12.

37  Jonathan Hutchinson, "On circumcision as preventive of masturbation," *Arch. Surg.*, 1890–1891, *2*: 268.

38  Theophilus Parvin, "The hygiene of the sexual functions," *New Orleans Med. & Surg. J.*, 1884, *11*: 606.

39  Jones, "Diseases of the nervous system," p. 170. It is interesting to note that documentation for the constitutional effects of masturbation was sought even from post-mortem examination. A report from Birmingham, England, concerning an autopsy on a dead masturbator, concluded that masturbation ". . . seems to have acted upon the cord in the same manner as repeated small haemorrhages affect the brain, slowly sapping its energies, until it succumbed soon after the last application of the exhausting influence, probably through the instrumentality of an atrophic process previously induced, as evidenced by the diseased state of the minute vessels" ([James] Russell, "Cases illustrating the influence of exhaustion of the spinal cord in inducing paraplegia," *Med. Times & Gaz., Lond.*, 1863, *2*: 456). The examination included microscopic inspection of material to demonstrate pathological changes. Again, the explanation of the phenomena turned on the supposed intense excitement attendant to masturbation. "In this fatal vice the venereal passion is carried at each indulgence to the state of highest tension by the aid of the mind, and on each occasion the cord is subjected to the strongest excitement which sensation and imagination in combination can produce, for we cannot regard the mere secretion of the seminal fluid as constituting the chief drain upon the energies of the cord, but rather as being the exponent of the nervous stimulation by which it has been ejaculated" (*ibid.*, p. 456). The model was one of mental tension and excitement "exhausting" the nervous system by "excessive functional activity" leading to consequent "weakening" of the nervous system. Baker Brown listed eight stages in the progress of the disease in females: hysteria, spinal irritation, hysterical epilepsy, cataleptic fits, epileptic fits, idiocy, mania and finally death; Brown, *Curability*, p. 7.

40  "Any shock to this growth and development, and especially that of masturbation, must for a time suspend the process of nutrition; and a succession of such shocks will blast both body and mind, and terminate in perpetual vacuity." Burdem, "Self pollution," p. 339. In this regard, not only adolescent but childhood masturbation was the concern of

19th-century practitioners; e.g., Russell, "Influence of exhaustion," p. 456.

41  Sigmund Freud, *The Standard Edition of the Complete Psychological Works of Sigmund Freud*, I (London: The Hogarth Press, 1971), 180.

42  *Ibid.*, III, Heredity and the Aetiology of the Neuroses," p. 150.

43  *Diagnostic and Statistical Manual: Mental Disorders* (Washington, D.C.: American Psychiatric Association, 1952), p. 29.

44  "Mr. Baker Brown was not a very accurate observer, nor a logical reasoner. He found that a number of semi-demented epileptics were habitual masturbators, and that the masturbation was, in women, chiefly effected by excitement of the mucous membrane on and around the clitoris. Jumping over two grave omissions in the syllogism, and putting the cart altogether before the horse, he arrived at the conclusion that removal of the clitoris would stop the pernicious habit, and therefore cure the epilepsy." Tait, "Masturbation," p. 2.

45  Howe, *Excessive Venery*, p. 77.

46  *Ibid.*, p. 77.

47  James Nevins Hyde, "On the masturbation, spermatorrhoea and impotence of adolescence," *Chicago, Med. J. & Exam.*, 1879, *38*: 451–452.

48  "There can be no doubt that the habit is, temporarily at least, morally degrading; but if we bear in mind the selfish, solitary nature of the act, the entire absence in it of aught akin to love or sympathy, the innate repulsiveness of intense selfishness or egoism of any kind, we may see how it may be morally degrading, while its effect on the physical and mental organism is practically nil." A. C. McClanahan, "An investigation into the effects of masturbation," *N.Y. Med. J.*, 1897, *66*: 502.

49  *Ibid.*, p. 500.

50  Augustin J. Himel, "Some minor studies in psychology, with special reference to masturbation," *New Orleans Med. & Surg. J.*, 1907, *60*: 452.

51  Spitz, "Authority and masturbation," esp. p. 119.

52  That is, masturbation as a disease was more than a mere collection of signs and symptoms usually "running together" in a syndrome. It became a legitimate disease entity, a causally related set of signs and symptoms.

53  C. D. W. Colby, "Mechanical restraint of masturbation in a young girl," *Med. Rec. in N.Y.*, 1897, *52*: 206.

54  Louis Bauer, "Infibulation as a remedy for epilepsy and seminal losses," *St. Louis Clin. Rec.*, 1879, *6*: 163–165. See also Gerhart S. Schwarz, "Infibulation, population control, and the medical profession," *Bull. N.Y. Acad. Med.*, 1970, *46*: 979, 990.

55  Hutchinson, "Circumcision," pp. 267–269.

56  William J. Robinson, "Masturbation and its treatment," *Am. J. Clin. Med.*, 1907, *14*: 349.

57  John Duffy, "Masturbation and clitoridectomy: a nineteenth-century view," *J.A.M.A.*, 1963, *186*: 246–248.

58  Brown, "Curability," p. 11.

59  *Ibid.*, p. 17.

60  Timothy Haynes, "Surgical treatment of hopeless cases of masturbation and nocturnal emissions," *Boston Med. & Surg. J.*, 1883, *109*: 130.

61  J. H. Marshall, "Insanity cured by castration," *Med. & Surg. Reptr.*, 1865, *13*: 363–64.

62  "The patient soon evinced marked evidences of being a changed man, becoming quiet, kind, and docile." *Ibid.*, p. 363.

63  R. D. Potts, "Castration for masturbation, with report of a case," *Texas Med. Practitioner*, 1898, *11*: 8.

64  *Ibid.*, p. 8.

65  *Ibid.*, p. 9.

66  Editorial, "Castration for the relief of epilepsy," *Boston Med. & Surg. J.*, 1859, *60*: 163.

67  Howe, *Excessive Venery*, p. 260.

68  *Ibid.*, pp. 254–255, 258–260.

69  Editorial, "Review of European legislation for the control of prostitution," *New Orleans Med. & Surg. J.*, 1854–1855, *11*: 704.

70  Robinson, "Masturbation and its treatment," p. 350.

71  Parvin, "Hygiene," p. 606.

72  Mayes, "Spermatorrhoea," p. 352.

73  Haynes, "Surgical treatment," p. 130.

74  B. A. Pope, "Opium as a tonic and alternative; with remarks upon the hypodermic use of the sulfate of morphia, and its use in the debility and amorosis consequent upon onanism," *New Orleans Med. & Surg. J.*, 1879, *6*: 725.

75  *Ibid.*, p. 727.

76  Parvin, "Hygiene," p. 607.

77  Joseph LoPiccolo and W. Charles Lobitz, "The role of masturbation in the treatment of orgasmic dysfunction," *Arch. Sexual Behavior*, 1972, *2*: 163–171.

78  E. Hare, "Masturbatory insanity," pp. 15–19.

79  Norwood Hanson, *Patterns of Discovery* (London: Cambridge Univ. Press, 1965).

80  Tissot, *Onanism*, p. 45. As Immanuel Kant, a contemporary of S.-A. Tissot remarked, "Also, in all probability, it was through this moral interest [in the moral law governing the world] that attentiveness to beauty and the ends of nature was first aroused." (*Kants Werke*, Vol. 5, *Kritik der Urtheilskraft* [Berlin: Walter de Gruyter & Co., 1968], p. 459, A 439. My translation.) That is, moral values influence the search for goals in nature, and direct attention to what will be considered natural, normal, and nondeviant. This would also imply a relationship between the aesthetic, especially what was judged to be naturally beautiful, and what was held to be the goals of nature.

81  Samuel A. Cartwright, "Report on the diseases and physical peculiarities of the negro race," *New Orleans Med. & Surg. J.*, 1850–1851, *7*: 707–709. An interesting examination of these diseases is given by Thomas S. Szasz, "The sane slave," *Am. J. Psychoth.*, 1971, *25*: 228–239.

82  Heinz Hartmann, "Towards a concept of mental health," *Brit. J. Med. Psychol.*, 1960, *33*: 248.

83  Thomas S. Szasz, "Bad habits are not diseases: a refutation of the claim that alcoholism is a disease," *Lancet*, 1972, *2*: 83–84; and Szasz, "The ethics of addiction," *Am. J. Psychiatry*, 1971, *128*: 541–546.

# 2

# The Uses of a Diagnosis: Doctors, Patients, and Neurasthenia

## BARBARA SICHERMAN

In 1869 George M. Beard suggested a common origin and the designation "neurasthenia" for a staggering variety of symptoms that had long taxed the ingenuity and the patience of physicians. A pioneer specialist in neurology, Beard made his reputation in New York City by treating the functional nervous disorders, that is, those for which no gross pathology could be found.[1] Neurasthenia was one of these, a disease characterized by profound physical and mental exhaustion. It was also a protean condition that might attack any organ or function. Its characteristic symptoms included sick headache, noises in the ear, atonic voice, deficient mental control, bad dreams, insomnia, nervous dyspepsia, heaviness of the loin and limb, flushing and fidgetiness, palpitations, vague pains and flying neuralgia, spinal irritation, uterine irritability, impotence, hopelessness, and such morbid fears as claustrophobia and dread of contamination.[2]

To a modern observer, as to a contemporary critic, Beard appears to have "greatly overloaded his subject."[3] But by suggesting a common pathology, prognosis, history, and treatment for such varied behavioral attributes, Beard was attempting to bring order to the chaotic field of the functional nervous disorders. In the absence of clear anatomical changes, or hard and fast tests, such conditions not only tested the physician's diagnostic skills, but invited the disbelief of friends and relatives. Beard acknowledged that neurasthenia was subjective, its symptoms "slippery, fleeting, and vague." But he insisted that it was as real a disease, with as genuinely somatic a course, as

smallpox or cholera. "In strictness," he wrote, "nothing in disease can be imaginary. If I bring on a pain by worrying, by dwelling on myself, that pain is as real as though it were brought on by an objective influence."[4]

Beard had not discovered a new disease, as even he acknowledged. But until his premature death in 1883, he labored to secure for neurasthenia an honored place in the medical lexicon. Motivated in part by personal need—he had wrestled with the symptoms of the disease in his youth—Beard was able to transform his own struggles into a disease syndrome that struck a responsive chord among his contemporaries. By interpreting diverse physical and mental symptoms as the common consequence of an excessive expenditure of nervous energy, he brilliantly blended scientific theories about the nature of the nervous impulse, the conservation of energy, and biological evolution into a plausible disease entity.

Beard defined neurasthenia as an "impoverishment of nervous force. . . . 'Nervousness' is really nervelessness." Physicians in the late 19th century believed that each individual possessed a fixed amount of nervous energy, determined mainly by heredity, which acted as a messenger between various parts of the body. Neurasthenia resulted when demand exceeded supply; even a tiny excess could cause the entire system to break down. Immoderate toil or worry, lack of food or rest, could induce an acute attack or even a chronic condition. The exhaustion of any one bodily system—the brain, for instance—could by the principle of reflex irritation spread to the reproductive and digestive systems, causing a total breakdown. Two popular metaphors—the overloaded electrical circuit and the overdrawn bank account—graphically illustrated the process for layman and physician alike.[5]

BARBARA SICHERMAN is Kenan Professor of American Institutions and Values at Trinity College, Hartford, Connecticut.

Reprinted with permission from the *Journal of the History of Medicine and Allied Sciences*, 1977, *32*: 33–54.

Just as physicians considered nervous energy limited, they believed that contemporary society placed inordinate demands on that supply. The dynamism of the Gilded Age, so welcome in other respects, thus became a source of social and psychological as well as physical stress. Beard drew on evolutionary theory to support his belief that nervousness was peculiarly an American phenomenon. In his long list of causes, he gave special attention to the periodical press, steampower, the telegraph, the sciences, and the increased mental activity of women. By encouraging men and women to experience life more fully, these five characteristic features of the 19th-century civilization—most advanced in America—placed too many demands on their limited supplies of nervous energy. Civilized society also demanded repression of the emotions, a refinement from which savages were exempt, and thus additionally drained human energies.[6]

Beard thought his work had initially been ignored, but by 1880 he contended that the subject "after long standing and waiting at the doors of science, has, at last, gained admission." A large popular and technical literature supported his claim. A tract by S. Weir Mitchell, the Philadelphia neurologist who developed the rest cure for neurasthenia, choicely titled *Wear and Tear*, sold out in ten days and went through five editions between 1871 and 1881; his *Fat and Blood* did even better. In the late 1880s a *Journal of Nervous Exhaustion* appeared briefly. And in the 1890s, two Shattuck lecturers, charged with enlightening members of the Massachusetts Medical Society on diseases prevalent in the Commonwealth, chose neurasthenia as their subject. When Beard's one-time partner, A. D. Rockwell, brought out a new edition of Beard's treatise for physicians in 1901, he noted that "neurasthenia is now almost a household word." Whether accurate or not, he continued, the diagnosis proved "often as satisfactory to the patient as it is easy to the physician."[7]

Even as Rockwell wrote, Beard's classic formulation of neurasthenia as a syndrome characterized by a deficiency of energy had begun to break down. The diagnosis had become so widespread, its use so imprecise, that many physicians believed it had outlived its usefulness. One called it the newest garbage can of medicine.[8] No longer able to provide a coherent explanation for the symptoms it had

once readily encompassed, neurasthenia lost ground in the first two decades of the 20th century both to demonstrably organic ills and to conditions increasingly assumed to be of psychological origin. New diagnostic tests made it possible to distinguish a number of conditions characterized by exhaustion, among them anemia, pulmonary tuberculosis, incipient paresis, lead poisoning, and Addison's disease together with other endocrine disorders.[9] Just as the diagnosis fever had earlier given way to more precise formulations, so exhaustion came to be viewed less as an essence than as a symptom.

A preference for psychological interpretations of the psychoneuroses was also apparent by 1900, a consequence mainly of the discovery of unconscious mental states. Pioneer psychopathologists like Pierre Janet and Sigmund Freud proposed psychodynamic interpretations of many physical and psychological symptoms formerly assumed to be of somatic origin. Thus Janet substituted the term *psychasthenia* for neuroses in which obsessions and phobias predominated. He attributed these to reduced psychic energy and discarded neurasthenia because he found no evidence of any physiological etiology. Freud retained the term, but wished to limit it to the relatively infrequent cases of physical exhaustion brought on by masturbation or noctural emissions. He considered it an actual neurosis as distinct from the more common psychoneuroses that psychoanalysis did so much to elucidate.[10] American physicians debated these concepts and, although some still accorded neurasthenia a limited place, Beard's earlier synthesis was effectively demolished by 1920.[11]

In retrospect it is clear that what was called neurasthenia actually comprehended a range of conditions that included depressive, obsessive, and phobic states later classified as psychoneuroses; mildly psychotic and borderline states; palpable physical ills that could not then be adequately diagnosed; and a host of symptoms that are today considered psychophysiological. Leonard Woolf was quite correct when he called neurasthenia "a name, a label, like neuralgia or rheumatism, which covered a multitude of sins, symptoms, and miseries."[12]

This modern diagnostic nemesis has recently attracted the attention of historians precisely because it so neatly illustrates the interplay of scientific theory and cultural values in the fashioning of a disease entity. Concentrating on physicians' generalizations about the disease, scholars for the most part have considered neurasthenia within the framework of intellectual history. The best of these studies securely anchors Beard's work in the medical and social structures of the Gilded Age, taking seriously his now dated explanatory model as a measure of the intellectual temper of the time.[13] Others, unable to see past the colorful etiology of the disease, have claimed that the term *neurasthenia* "stood for conflicting . . . ideologies," and, on the patient's part, was "a reservoir of class prejudices, status desires, urban arrogance, repressed sexuality, and indulgent self-centeredness."[14]

However imprecise the label *neurasthenia* now appears, it is surely unfair to doctors and especially to patients to view illness purely as an intellectual construct. To ignore the clinical context in which disease is identified is to miss the distinguishing feature of medical practice. For it is in the consulting room, the hospital clinic, and at the bedside that the daily drama of diagnosis and treatment takes place. There the patient offers up the symptoms that have already caused sufficient distress to prompt the encounter. As a psychoanalyst reminds us: "For the patient illness is always an uncanny experience. He feels something has gone wrong with him, something that might, or certainly will, do him harm unless dealt with properly and swiftly. What 'it' is, is difficult to know."[15]

In what is frequently a highly charged atmosphere, the physician's primary task is to identify "it," to transform the diffuse symptoms of his patient into a condition that can be rationally understood and treated. To such an encounter each party brings his own preconceptions about illness, expectations of the other, and more or less enduring personality traits, shaped by class and social position as well as individual need. If the physician fails to make sense of the patient's troubles — or to relieve them — neither he nor his patient will retain much confidence in his skill. If the interpretation is unacceptable, the patient may take his business elsewhere.

In the late 19th century, neurasthenia proved a satisfactory label to doctors and patients alike. By incorporating into a disease picture a host of behavioral symptoms, many of which would otherwise have been deemed self-willed and thus devi-

ant, the diagnosis legitimized new roles for physicians and their patients. For patients, it provided the most respectable label for distressing, but not life-threatening, complaints, one that conferred many of the benefits — and fewest of the liabilities — associated with illness. Certainly it was preferable to its nearest alternatives — hypochondria, hysteria and insanity, not to mention malingering.

At a time when psychiatry was limited to the institutional care of psychotic patients, those who specialized in the functional nervous disorders were actually providing psychiatric services for many patients. Thoughtful clinicians understood that deep-rooted personality needs often influenced the onset of an illness, and that the relationship between doctor and patient affected the patient's capacity to recover. Although their suspicion of psychology kept them from exploring this relationship fully, physicians sometimes acknowledged that they ministered to the soul as well as the body. As confessors, they concerned themselves with all aspects of the patient's behavior. Neurasthenia was thus an important chapter in the expansion of the medical sphere that has characterized modern American society.

As a diagnosis on the borderland of medicine and psychiatry, neurasthenia augmented therapeutic approaches in both fields. Medicine had reached an ambiguous stage when the disparity between actual achievement and future promise was especially great. Scientists, by correlating clinical and pathological data, had identified the basic diseases in modern form by mid-century. As typhus and malaria replaced the symptomatic designation fever, it became possible to search for pathogenic microorganisms. The first such organism was identified in 1876, but two decades elapsed before the great medical discoveries yielded practical results. In the meantime, death rates remained high and the art of therapeutics perilously low. Recognizing that there were few specific remedies, medical leaders repudiated many traditional therapies as unavailing or positively harmful. This therapeutic nihilism, although an advance over the heavy drugging of the past, left the practitioner in a peculiarly vulnerable position. For, as the authors of guides for aspiring physicians noted, patients expected medicines and even specific courses of treatment. If they did not receive them from members of the regular profession, they might patronize adherents of medical sects who still offered a holistic view of disease, or one of the numerous vendors of patent medicines.[16]

The laboratory cast of mind of professional leaders at the end of the century further highlighted the practitioner's impotence. In this era of extreme somaticism, a respectable disease required a specific and identifiable etiology, pathology, and therapy. The discovery that microorganisms caused specific diseases contributed to this outlook. So did insistence on a localized pathology exemplified in Rudolf Virchow's famous dictum: "There are no general diseases . . . only diseases of organs and cells." In their efforts to make medicine an exact science the most prominent physicians often overlooked—and certainly underrated—the importance of clinical medicine. Their emphasis on basic research in chemistry, bacteriology, and anatomy, so productive in other respects, did little to help either the ambitious practitioner or the anxious patient in their mutual quest.[17]

Neurasthenia offered the practitioner a way out of this therapeutic dilemma. The new label, with its implied precision, emphasized what physicians could do for their patients rather than their impotence. At a time when physicians felt comfortable only with clearly organic disorders, a diagnosis of neurasthenia permitted some to address themselves to less tangible clinical issues and to provide an essentially psychological therapy under a somatic label. The diagnosis and its treatment helped physicians to justify a traditional role, threatened by the one-sided emphasis on science, of providing advice and comfort to patients and their families. In view of the impoverished state of medical therapeutics in the late 19th century, this was by no means an insignificant achievement.[18]

Conditions of weakness had long been known to physicians by a variety of names, among them debility. But the emphasis on weakness of the nerves coincided with the rise of neurology as a medical specialty in the years after the Civil War. Knowledge of the brain and nervous system advanced rapidly in Europe after 1860 as experimental physiologists demonstrated that fixed parts of the brain controlled specific motor activities. Important clinical advances, especially J. Hughlings Jackson's work on epilepsy and Jean-Martin Charcot's delineations of several classic neurological disorders, followed. By the late 1860s, important teaching and hospital positions in neurology had been established in England, France, and the German-speaking world, a sign that the specialty had come of age.[19]

Beard and Mitchell belonged to the pioneer generation of physicians who established neurology on a firm professional footing in the United States. Concentrated in large cities on the eastern seaboard and Chicago, they began in the 1870s to found the journals and societies that constitute the core of a professional identity. In their bid for recognition, the neurologists encountered resistance from general practitioners opposed to specialization of any kind, and outright hostility from the medical superintendents of asylums for the insane who sincthe 1840s had claimed exclusive authority over the care of the mentally ill. At a time when all experts considered insanity a disease of the brain, neurologists legitimately claimed competence in the field of mental as well as neurological disorders. But because the two fields had developed separately in the United States, ambitious young specialists like Beard found it necessary to challenge what amounted to the superintendents' monopoly in caring for the mentally ill. Rivalry between competing specialists was particularly intense during the 1870s and 1880s. In the struggle for professional status and monetary rewards, neurasthenia helped the neurologists build up their clienteles. Since the organic nervous disorders were relatively rare, specialists welcomed patients with less tangible ills who crowded their waiting rooms. Some earned sizable fees for this work; Weir Mitchell reputedly made $70,000 in a good year, much of it in consulting fees.[20]

Professional needs help to explain the advantage of a new diagnosis. But to discern how and why neurasthenia was used, one must turn from the institutional to the clinical setting. The typical neurasthenic patient presented the physician with a rich variety of symptoms. A diagnosis by exclusion, neurasthenia could be established only after a thorough physical examination and appraisal of the patient's actual, as distinct from stated, discomfort had ruled out any other condition. (Beard once listed 48 ailments with which it might be confounded.[21]) Once satisfied that the patient had no organic disease, the physician must decide what label to attach to the condition.

Neurasthenia had most often to be distinguished from hysteria and hypochondria, the other major functional nervous disorders. Hysteria, long the most frequent nervous disease of women, had become in Weir Mitchell's view, "the nosological limbo of all unnamed female maladies. It were as well called mysteria." The typical hysteric manifested bizarre symptoms — convulsive fits, trances, choking, tearing the hair, and rapid fluctuations of mood. Where languor characterized the neurasthenic, Beard considered "acuteness, violence, activity, and severity" the essence of hysteria. Moral considerations as well as the physician's empathy for particular patients undoubtedly influenced diagnostic decisions in ambiguous cases. Where neurasthenics seemed deeply concerned about their condition and eager to cooperate, hysterics were accused of evasiveness — *la belle indifférence* — and even intentional deception. Physicians sometimes contrasted the hysteric's lack of moral sense with the neurasthenic's refined and unselfish nature. "The sense of moral obligation [in the hysteric] is so generally defective as to render it difficult to determine whether the patient is mad or simply bad." By contrast, patients suffering from "impaired vitality" were "of good position in society . . . just the kind of women one likes to meet with — sensible, not over sensitive or emotional, exhibiting a proper amount of illness . . . and a willingness to perform their share of work quietly and to the best of their ability."[22]

Hypochondria had been the most common diagnosis for men with ill-defined complaints. Once a medically respectable disease, by the 1870s hypochondriasis had acquired the connotation of an imaginary illness. Neurasthenics and hypochondriacs both displayed inordinate interest in the vagaries of their bodies, but physicians considered the former more often the victims of circumstances, or lack of prudence, while the difficulties of the latter, if not dismissed entirely, appeared to be distinctly self-induced.[23]

Although 19th-century physicians and historians alike have written at length about women's ill health, the subject of illness in men has been neglected.[24] Yet neurasthenia seems to have been a particularly useful label for men. If women were sometimes expected, and perhaps even encour-

aged, to be weak and sickly, an ethos of fortitude made it difficult for men to exhibit weakness of any kind. Illness, in all its presumed objectivity, was one of the permissible exceptions. It is significant, therefore, that several physicians — mistakenly — considered neurasthenia a male disease, a striking assertion at a time when the profession rarely lost an opportunity to decry the ill-health of American women.[25] While acknowledging that neurasthenia afflicted women more often than men, Beard was especially eager to legitimize it as a diagnosis for men. He insisted that hypochondria, which he defined as "groundless fear of disease," was extremely rare; the label too often covered the diagnostician's failure to detect the real trouble.[26]

Neurasthenia then was the diagnosis of choice for men and women whose diffuse symptoms might otherwise have been dismissed as hypochondria or hysteria. As a new diagnosis, neurasthenia escaped the pejorative connotations associated with its nearest alternatives. Doctors had often suffered from neurasthenia themselves — Beard estimated that physicians constituted one-tenth of his clientele — and empathized with similarly distressed patients.[27] Certainly many of its putative causes — overwork or the too solicitous care of sick relatives — resulted from an excess of essentially admirable traits.

Neurasthenia was also preferable to a diagnosis of insanity, then considered an incurable disease. Despite their rivalry, American neurologists and superintendents agreed with Beard that neurasthenia was "the door that opens into so many phases of mental disease." It was a warning signal, which, if unheeded, might lead from a temporary physical breakdown to a permanent state of melancholia. Edward Cowles, the influential superintendent of McLean Asylum, went so far as to suggest in his Shattuck lecture of 1891 that "all people of previously sound health and constitutions, who become insane with ordinary functional mental disorders, have their psychoses dependent upon neurasthenic conditions of the organism."[28]

Neurasthenics suffered from many of the symptoms of those hospitalized for insanity, including loss of mental control, depression, morbid fears, and obsessions. Presumably the persistence and severity of these symptoms helped to separate the insane from the neurasthenic, but diagnostic criteria were by no means clear. Class considerations, the tolerance of physicians for particular symptoms, and the ability of family members to care for patients undoubtedly influenced diagnostic decisions, then as now. Like Virginia Woolf, an upper-class patient suffering from hallucinations and severe feeding disorders might frequently be diagnosed as neurasthenic.[29] An individual with similar problems, but fewer financial resources and less loyal family and friends, might have been declared insane and placed in an asylum. Given the importance of the therapist's expectations on the patient's chances of recovery, the more optimistic diagnosis may have kept some individuals who would today be considered schizophrenic or borderline from long hospital stays and possible deterioration.[30]

Class prejudice undoubedly influenced the attitudes of upper- and middle-class patients and their physicians toward the asylums, as the rhetorical query of one neurologist suggests: "Should the psychical symptoms of instability, distrust, and confusion of mind be used as an excuse for, and can such a condition be most effectively combated by, sending such a delicate, sensitive, nervous invalid to an insane asylum? We think not." But at a time when public hospitals suffered from overcrowding, understaffing, and low recovery rates, treatment at home or in one of the new nerve retreats was the rational choice for those who could afford it. Such individuals could also escape the stigmatizing label of insanity. For even after recovery, formerly hospitalized patients often continued to be reminded that they had been "crazy a number of years ago."[31]

Many late 19th-century physicians accepted Beard's generalization that neurasthenia was principally a disease of the "comfortable classes." Like Beard, their patients were probably drawn largely from the business and professional classes in large cities. Those with diverse clienteles reached other conclusions. In 1869, the year Beard published his first article on the subject, a superintendent in Michigan independently discovered neurasthenia —and so labeled it—in the hardworking farm women near his hospital. To his surprise, Weir Mitchell diagnosed it in such unlikely victims as working-class male clinic patients. By the early years of the 20th century, neurasthenia had become the most frequent diagnosis of the working-class patients who attended the neurological outpatient clinics at Boston City and Massachusetts General hospitals. The deficient energy syndrome could be applied to the most varied individuals, and was not just a euphemism for serious mental illness in middle-class patients.[32]

It would appear that age and marital status had more to do with the disease, or at least with the diagnosis, than either class or sex. Many neurasthenic patients were young and single. In one study of 333 neurasthenics, two-thirds were between the ages of 20 and 40, with the incidence highest among those 20 to 30 and the average age 33.3. Almost one-third of the women and over two-fifths of the men were single, a figure no doubt partly related to their age.[33] Observing the relationship between neurasthenia and young adulthood, Beard noted that the "dark valley of nervous depression" often disappeared between the ages of 25 and 35. Once cured, the former sufferer went on to a "healthy and happy maturity."[34]

Beard spoke from personal experience. Between the ages of 17, when he completed his preparatory course at Phillips Andover Academy, and 23, when he graduated from Yale, Beard suffered from ringing in the ears, pains in the side, acute dyspepsia, nervousness, morbid fears, and "lack of vitality." His journal reveals a young man beset by religious and vocational indecision. Reared in an austere and religious family that rejected drinking and smoking and warned its children of the snares of worldly success, Beard chastized himself for his coldness and "hanging back" in religious matters. Health and joy finally came with his decision to become a physician (which was equally a rejection of the ministry, the occupation of his father and two brothers). Beard entered medicine with a passionate commitment to medical and hygienic reform. By this time, too, he had begun to enjoy the worldly pleasures of champagne and Turkish tobacco, and soon after became engaged. His recovery seems to have been permanent. A minister who knew Beard in later life described him as a man who "put courage, hope, strength into one's heart, and his atmosphere was always healthy. He did not gush with over-warmth, or freeze with over-cold."[35]

In conjunction with other case materials, Beard's experience suggests that for many middle-class men and women neurasthenia incorporated elements of today's fashionable identity crisis. Clearly individuals reaching maturity in the second half of the 19th century had no monopoly on the trials of establishing a satisfactory adult identity. But cultural imperatives may have made the task particularly problematic. Intellectuals who struggled to emancipate themselves from the introspective and gloomy religious teachings of their childhood often suffered acutely from the loss of faith that accompanied Darwinism, higher criticism of the Bible, and the growing authority of Science. In a society of changing and often conflicting values, the decline of spiritual certitude intensified feelings of isolation. Educated women struggled to reconcile their desire for independence with still potent family expectations that they would live out traditional female roles. For men, longer professional training and the desire to achieve a higher standard of living necessitated later marriages; prescriptions for "masculinity" often meant disavowing "feminine" emotional impulses. Both men and women encountered a sexual code that demanded purity in thought as well as in deed, restraint within marriage as well as abstinence outside it. But men were sometimes also expected to be rough and ready.[36]

William James is a good example of a Victorian incapacitated by psychosomatic ills, mental anguish, indecision, and an inability to believe. As a young man he developed digestive and eye troubles, weakness of the back, and a "feeling of loneliness and intellectual and moral deadness." He feared being alone in the dark, had morbid obsessions, and for a time felt continually on the verge of committing suicide. His family considered his condition hypochondriacal, but James claimed he was "a victim of neurasthenia, and of the sense of hollowness and unreality that goes with it." Relief first came with his decision to believe in free will. Of the same generation as Beard, James tried to reconcile science and religion, resisted determinism in both, and struggled to find a genuine vocation. He successively tried art, natural history, medicine, and psychology and did not commit himself to philosophy, his first love, until the age of 57. It has recently been suggested that James's intense relationship with his domineering Swedenborgian father complicated this struggle, and that his illness gave him a psychic moratorium and a legitimate reason for disobeying parental wishes. His symptoms subsided following his first professional position (at 30) and marriage (at 36).[37]

If men sometimes found it difficult to choose the right profession, educated women faced a dilemma merely by wanting to have a vocation. Those who chose to defy convention as well as those who gave up their aspirations might find life equally intolerable. Jane Addams has described the years of backaches, depression, and purposelessness that followed her graduation from college. She even consulted Weir Mitchell, with little benefit. She diagnosed her problem as an inability to find a practical way to fulfill the ideals she had acquired in college and a disinclination to follow the course favored by her stepmother, including marriage and the dilettantish pursuit of culture. For Jane Addams and, she believed, for others like her, the decision to found a social settlement and create a new kind of community proved immensely liberating.[38] Charlotte Perkins Gilman experienced a more severe breakdown following her marriage and birth of a daughter. Her vague but exalted hopes of helping mankind seemed threatened by these events, so inescapable a part of most women's lives. In her case, Mitchell's advice compounded her difficulties and reduced her to playing with a rag doll on the floor. Her symptoms finally abated when she separated from her husband and began to pursue an independent course as a writer and lecturer.[39]

Because evidence about sexual behavior is harder to come by than information about vocational and religious conflict, it is difficult to assess its role in neurasthenia. Beard for one was acutely sensitive to the difficulties that contemporary sexual mores posed for his patients. It is possible that he had personally experienced such stress, for shortly after his engagement he asked God's blessing for his spiritual interests. He went on to declare: "The most solemn and weighty of any experience with the exception of religious experience is the love life of a man."[40]

In his posthumously published *Sexual Neurasthenia*, Beard insisted that sexual complaints had been vastly underestimated as a cause of nervousness, in men especially. He believed that sexual desire, like neurasthenia itself, plagued the sensitive men and women of the middle classes more than those of phlegmatic temperament who lived and worked outdoors. Masturbation he viewed as a nearly universal practice, for women as well as men, and did not think it invariably harmful if not begun too early in life or indulged in too often. As for other sexual difficulties, such as impotence and nocturnal emissions, Beard advised his patients not to worry about them: "Live generously. Work hard. . . . As soon as convenient, get married, but at all events keep diligently at work." Most important, he offered reassurance: "*I have known personally of very many young men who have passed through difficulties of the kind and are now well and the fathers of healthy families.*" Perhaps it was advice of this sort that prompted the comment, by a minister-friend at the memorial service for Beard, that: "Many joy children were born of his kindly words and kindly deeds, while of sad ones there were none to moan."[41]

The self-study of a neurasthenic patient, herself a specialist in mental and nervous disorders, suggests some of the conflicts that must have been central to many neurasthenic individuals, particularly those who resigned themselves to lives of partial nervous invalidism. Written in 1910 with pre-Freudian innocence, *The Autobiography of a Neurasthene* by Margaret Cleaves is a classic study of unresolved dependency needs that were at least partly met by her long-term relationship with her physician.[42]

Dr. Cleaves describes herself as hardworking to a fault, so completely devoted to her patients that "they are my family and my friends. I have none other, and science is my mistress." Overwork led first to a "sprained" brain and later to a "complete crash," accompanied by the sensation of hot blood pouring into her ears, an inability to concentrate or to "bear a touch heavier than the brush of a butterfly's wing," depression, copious weeping, fears of going insane, and other typical neurasthenic symptoms. Learning to live within the margin of her slender nervous endowment proved difficult, but essential, for she suffered "utter lassitude of body," "weariness of mind," and a "sense of physiologic sin" from the slightest indiscretion, even an excess in diet. Social events proved particularly tiring, for she could not control them. Always she fought against her illness, which she took pains to distinguish from hysteria.

Between acute attacks she carried on her work. But even as she took pride in her ability to care for her patients, it is clear that she resented her responsibilities, particularly because there "was no one to look after [her] needs." She attributed her

illness (which she considered constitutional) to feeding insufficiencies in infancy, aggravated by the death of her father when she was 14. Thus she notes that the too early arrival of a younger sister interfered with her babyhood by depriving her of milk. Upbraided throughout her life for her failure to eat, she attributed her later preference for milk products to this early deprivation. When she was acutely ill, milk was often her only source of nourishment. She thought of her father, a physician after whom she seems to have modeled herself, as her best friend and, following the death of the family's only son, tried to become her "father's boy." She must bitterly have resented his death, even as it devastated her, for she insisted that he would have protected her against the stresses and strains she encountered in later life. For years she had a recurrent dream of being a child cradled in her father's arms. The dream disappeared after her most severe breakdown, and she missed the comfort it had afforded her.

The patient was fortunate enough to find a sympathetic physician who cared for her for many years, often visiting her daily during her acute attacks. If he did not completely understand her condition—at least until he had himself suffered a neurasthenic breakdown—he was compassionate: "I told him all this tale of woe, of my past life . . . [and] laid bare my soul to my professional confessor." She depended on her physician greatly, and in times of special need on a trained nurse as well. When others responded to her needs, she reported: "It seemed worthwhile to have suffered for the sake of all this comfort." Her course of treatment—rest, limitation of activities, tonics, massage—was designed to replenish her meager supply of "neuronic energy." But given this patient's personality and her isolated life in New York City, the close relationship with her physician-confessor, by providing a substitute for other forms of intimacy, was obviously the crucial element.

The patient's struggles with her propensity toward invalidism were familiar enough to therapists, who insisted that each case required individualized treatment. Prescribing rest for one patient might be restorative, while for another with similar symptoms, it could be completely wrong. Clinicians thus recognized that the relationship between doctor and patient was often the most potent agency in effecting a cure. Given contemporary insistence that disease was an entirely objective phenomenon, they could not pursue such insights very far. Beard, for example, outraged fellow members of the American Neurological Association when he reported a series of experiments with "definite expectation"—what a later generation called suggestion—in which he cured patients of rheumatism and neuralgic sleeplessness by prescribing placebos. One colleague denied the existence of mental therapeutics entirely, a second considered it more dangerous than handling the most powerful drugs, while still another claimed that doctors had known about royal touch cures for centuries, but before practicing such deceits should "give up our medicines and enter a convent."[43]

The therapeutic guidelines of S. Weir Mitchell, member of Philadelphia's upper class and a popular novelist, proved less controversial. Mitchell first tried out the rest cure on Civil War soldiers suffering from acute exhaustion brought on by marching. He did not repeat it until 1874 when, despairing of any other treatment, he ordered an exhausted invalid to bed. He carried the principle of rest to what he later admitted was "an almost absurd extreme." The patient—a 95-pound invalid who had tried every available cure—was fed and washed by others, forbidden to read, use her hands, or talk. At first a maid even turned her when she wished to move. Mitchell subsequently systematized the treatment to include total isolation of the patient from the family, a trained nurse, a carefully regulated diet (often limited initially to milk), tonics for the nerves, rest, and massage. The treatment's success could be explained in the somatic terms so appealing to this generation, and Mitchell emphasized the benefits of building up the patient's fat and blood by this method.[44]

But Mitchell also appreciated the moral aspects of the rest cure. The separation of patients from the moral poison of their accustomed environments, especially the attentions of too solicitous relatives, was often an essential condition for recovery. Isolation also enhanced the physician's influence over the patient, which Mitchell considered of supreme importance: "The man who can insure belief in his opinions and obedience to his decrees secures very often most brilliant and sometimes easy success." Confidence in the physician produced "that calmness of trustful belief which alone will secure the rest of mind we want." At first

he found it surprising "that we ever get from any human being such childlike obedience. Yet we do get it, even from men."[45]

The similarity between the rest cure—with its bland diet, lack of external stimuli, and complete dependence on the physician—and infancy is apparent. Indeed, the enforced regression may well account for its success. The rest cure permitted individuals who ordinarily survived only by desperate effort to remove themselves from daily life and to submit for a time to the attentions of a charismatic physician like Mitchell. The physician in turn imposed reciprocal obligations. During convalescence, Mitchell lectured patients on the value of self-control and used his by then considerable influence to exact a "promise to fight every desire to cry, or twitch, or grow excited."[46] The paternalism of this therapy may help to explain why Charlotte Perkins Gilman and Jane Addams —women who temperamentally rejected the subordinate role assigned to their sex—were among Mitchell's most conspicuous failures.

Clearly there was often a therapeutic fit between physicians like Beard and Mitchell who had mastered their own nervous crises and their neurasthenic patients, many of whom—like the doctors themselves—were from the middle and upper classes. But class was not the sole determinant of a physician's response to patients. A. A. Brill, one of Freud's earliest American disciples, described the rapt attention with which as a medical student he attended the clinic on neurasthenia: "In contrast to the psychotics, the neurasthenics inspired one with a sympathetic interest; they spoke feelingly about their symptoms and apparently wanted to be helped."[47] What more could a young physician, eager to be of service, ask of a patient?

The perception of pain, the significance attached to symptoms, even the symptoms themselves vary greatly, depending not only on individual personality needs but on class and ethnic patterns. Today middle-class individuals are more willing to consult psychiatrists and to discuss emotional problems. And, despite the somatic orientation of medicine in the late 19th century, articulate individuals like William James often considered their illness in the context of their search for a meaningful personal identity.[48]

Although working-class men and women may lack a vocabulary of psychological distress, they are by no means immune from the effects of emotional stress; indeed, today they tend to be more subject to psychophysiological illnesses than members of other social groups. Recent clinical and sociological studies also indicate that visits to physicians for minor symptoms are often prompted by such needs as a desire for reassurance, for a close relationship with someone, for sanction to escape onerous duties or conflicts — needs which are often intensified during periods of severe psychological stress.[49]

It is likely that also in the late 19th century many of the conflicts of less articulate individuals manifested themselves in the myriad of physical symptoms that constitute the central clinical picture of neurasthenia. Not only were working-class patients treated for neurasthenia in outpatient clinics, but they sometimes entered Massachusetts General Hospital (then primarily an institution for charity patients) for extended periods. Nor were physicians unsympathetic to such patients. Hospital case records were not devoid of moral judgments, but the individuals described as "stupid," "lacking gumption," or "intent on deception" were more often diagnosed as hysterical than as neurasthenic. Doctors carefully recorded the complaints of individuals who were run down or "unable to keep about" after overworking or an imperfect recovery from an illness. Patients might complain of sinking feelings about the heart, an inability to bear the weight of their own hands, seeing stars, sensations of smothering, and "bearing down" pains. Their physical symptoms included palpitations and shortness of breath and a rich variety of gastric complaints (anorexia, vomiting, belching, constipation). The interpretation of these symptoms was entirely somatic. An occasional entry reported a recent death in the family, but attributed the breakdown to excessive exposure to cold or rain at the funeral rather than to the psychological effects of the loss.[50]

What is most surprising is that cigarmakers, millworkers, seamstresses, and housewives received modified versions of the rest cure for weeks and even months. Like the middle-class patients seen in private practice, they received a variety of physical therapies — including tonics, bromides, cannabis, massage, and blisters over tender spots. Special diets ranged from milk, cream toast, and eggnogs to oysters, whiskey, sherry, and beer. The

entry for a particularly frail woman read, "keep her quiet and stuff with food." The treatment seemed to work, for within three weeks the patient left the hospital much relieved, with the notation that "rest was apparently all that she needed." Many patients seemed to enjoy their hospital stays — one entry recorded a patient who "seemed disposed to remain indefinitely" — and a few kept their physicians informed of their latest symptoms after discharge. Since so many of these patients were single, it is likely that their illness and hospital sojourns provided some with psychological as well as physical care that they could obtain in no other way.[51]

During its brief reign as the national disease, neurasthenia gave physicians a rationale for diagnosing and treating many types of stress. Whatever the limitations of their construct, physicians like Beard and Mitchell pioneered in developing respectable therapies for patients with problems otherwise excluded by medicine and psychiatry. Although asylum superintendents maintained that neurasthenia might lead to insanity if not treated early enough, their isolation from general medicine and restricted conception of their role gave them no way of reaching men and women before serious trouble occurred. The rest cure and related therapies provided individuals with alternatives to inaction or incarceration.

During the first two decades of the 20th century the scope of psychiatry expanded almost beyond recognition. Physicians openly practiced psychotherapy in offices and in outpatient clinics in general and psychiatric hospitals. Some participated in prophylactic programs in schools, prisons, and industry. Most practitioners still worked in mental hospitals, but professional spokesmen insisted that psychiatry must concern itself not only with the psychoses but with "the smallest diseases and the minutest defects of the mind" and even with the efficiency of normal individuals. The new practitioner was "educator, preacher, sociologist" as well as asylum superintendent and dispenser of drugs.[52]

Specialists in the functional nervous disorders had pioneered in the expansion of the physician's social role. Even by diagnosing neurasthenia, they were interpreting behavioral symptoms that some found morally reprehensible (an inability to work for no apparent cause, compulsive or phobic behavior, bizarre thoughts) as signs of illness rather than wilfulness. They thus legitimized the right of individuals with such difficulties to be considered, and to consider themselves, victims of disease, and their own right as healers, to treat them.

Beard went further than most in asserting the physician's obligation to become a power in society. He not only insisted that neurasthenia be taken seriously, but urged that the categories kleptomania, inebriety, and pyromania—all safely medical—replace the traditional moralistic designations of stealing, drunkenness, and arson. A rebel against the evangelical faith of his childhood, Beard relished the substitution of physician for priest as arbiter of social and personal mores. Mitchell, noting the similarity between the physician's role and that of the priest, also thought members of his profession more fitted to probe human character: "The priest hears the crime or folly of the hour, but to the physician are oftener told the long, sad tales of a whole life."[53]

So much attention to a disease that could easily have been dismissed as minor also reveals a changed attitude toward health and disease. Long before the popularization of psychoanalysis, physicians interested in mental and nervous disorders proclaimed the relativity of health and illness. One superintendent declared that "perfect health of mind is probably . . . exceptional." And an influential lay philanthropist went so far as to claim: "The question to be considered is, not whether such and such a person is insane,—that is, indisposed mentally: of course he is, more or less, like the rest of us,—but, *How much* out of health is he?" Many no doubt reached such conclusions on the basis of personal experience. A fictional physician drawn by Weir Mitchell—a self-portrait—noted that even "to the most healthy nature, at times [come] inexplicable desires, moments of unreason, impulses which defy analytic research, even brief insanities." To the extent that individuals considered such conditions mental aberrations rather than sinful thoughts, they would consult physicians rather than ministers.[54]

The relationships between symptoms and diagnosis, disease and culture, doctors and patients are inevitably complex. Any attempt to understand them historically must take account of the clinical context in which doctors and patients interact; certainly this must be the case for a disease as subjective as neurasthenia. The available clinical materials suggest that neurasthenia was a complex reality for the doctors and patients charged with interpreting puzzling mental and physical difficulties they did not fully understand. If the particular insights of late 19th-century physicians into the psychological and psychophysiological aspects of illness disappoint us, it is not altogether certain that we have, even today, found satisfactory solutions to conditions of this sort.

## NOTES

Work on this article was greatly assisted by fellowships from the Radcliffe Institute and the Peter B. Livingston Fund. I am indebted to Phyllis Ackman, Martin Duberman, Nathan G. Hale, Jr., Dolores Kreisman, Charles E. Rosenberg, Barbara G. Rosenkrantz, Bennett Simon, and Martha Vicinus for their comments on earlier drafts and to Catherine Lord for research assistance. I also want to thank Dr. G. Octo Barnett and James Vaccarino for permission to use the medical records of the Massachusetts General Hospital, 1875–1900.

1   The best analysis of Beard's career is Charles E. Rosenberg, "The place of George M. Beard in nineteenth-century psychiatry," *Bull. Hist. Med.*, 1962, *36*: 245–259. See also Henry Alden Bunker, Jr., "From Beard to Freud: a brief history of the concept of neurasthenia," *Med. Rev. Rev.*, 1930, *36*: 108–114.

2   George M. Beard, *A Practical Treatise on Nervous Exhaustion (Neurasthenia): Its Symptoms, Nature, Sequences, Treatment*, 2nd ed., rev. (New York, 1880), pp. 11–85. See also George M. Beard, *American Nervousness: Its Causes and Consequences* (New York, 1881), pp. 7–8.

3   "The question of the existence of neurasthenia," *Med. Rec.*, 1886, *29*: 185–186.

4   Beard, *Nervous Exhaustion*, pp. 85, 80.

5   George M. Beard, *Sexual Neurasthenia (Nervous Exhaustion): Its Hygiene, Causes, Symptoms, and Treatment, with a Chapter on Diet for the Nervous*, ed. A. D. Rockwell (New York, 1884), p. 36; cf. pp. 61–62 and Beard, *American Nervousness*, p. 9.

6   Beard, *American Nervousness*, pp. 96–192.

7   Beard, *Nervous Exhaustion*, p. xix; Edward Cowles, "Neurasthenia and its mental symptoms," *Boston Med. & Surg. J.*, 1891, *125*: 49–52, 73–76, 97–100,

125-128, 153-157, 181-186, 209-214; Robert T. Edes, "The New England invalid," *Boston Med. & Surg. J.*, 1895, *133*: 53-57, 77-81; 101-107; Beard, *Nervous Exhaustion*, 4th ed., rev. and enl. A. D. Rockwell (New York, 1901), p. 3. Numerous references to neurasthenia may be found in the several series of the *Index-Catalogue of the Library of the Surgeon General's Office.*

8   Quoted in A. A. Brill, "Diagnostic errors in neurasthenia," *Med. Rev. Rev.*, 1930, *36*: 123.

9   I. S. Wechsler, "Is neurasthenia an organic disease?" *Med. Rev. Rev.*, 1930, *36*: 115-121; I. S. Wechsler, "The psychoneuroses and the internal secretions," *Neurol. Bull.*, 1919, *2*: 199-208; Edes, "The New England invalid," pp. 78-80.

10  On the shift in diagnostic styles, see Henri F. Ellenberger, *The Discovery of the Unconscious: The History and Evolution of Dynamic Psychiatry* (New York, 1970); and Nathan G. Hale, Jr., *Freud and the Americans: The Beginnings of Psychoanalysis in the United States, 1876-1917* (New York, 1971), esp. pp. 71-173.

11  See, for example, Charles L. Dana, "The partial passing of neurasthenia," *Boston Med. & Surg. J.*, 1904, *150*: 339-344, and G. Alder Blumer, "The coming of psychasthenia," *J. Nerv. & Ment. Dis.* 1906, *33*: 336-353. Widely used in World War I, the term *neurasthenia* largely disappeared in the United States by the 1930s and reappeared in the 1968 diagnostic manual of the American Psychiatric Association. See John C. Chatel and Roger Peele, "A centennial review of neurasthenia," *Am. J. Psychiatry*, 1970, *126*: 1404-1413.

12  Leonard Woolf, *Beginning Again: An Autobiography of the Years 1911 to 1918* (New York, 1964), pp. 75-76.

13  Rosenberg, "The place of George M. Beard." Cf. Chatel and Peele, "A centennial review," Bunker, "From Beard to Freud," and S. P. Fullinwider, "Neurasthenia: the genteel caste's journey inward," *Rocky Mount. Social Sci. J.*, 1974, *2*, 1-9.

14  John S. Haller, Jr., and Robin M. Haller, *The Physician and Sexuality in Victorian America* (Urbana and Chicago, 1974), pp. 5-43.

15  Michael Balint, *The Doctor, His Patient and the Illness*, 2nd ed. rev. (London, 1964), p. 41. This work is an excellent introduction to the psychological aspects of general medicine.

16  Richard Harrison Shryock, "The interplay of social and internal factors in modern medicine: an historical analysis," in *Medicine in America: Historical Essays* (Baltimore, 1966), pp. 307-332; Richard Harrison Shryock, *The Development of Modern Medicine: An Interpretation of the Social and Scientific Factors Involved* (New York, 1947), pp. 248-303.

17  Cf. Erwin H. Ackerknecht, *Rudolf Virchow: Doctor, Statesman, Anthropologist* (Madison, 1953). For a critical view of the laboratory approach to medicine, see Knud Faber, *Nosography: The Evolution of Clinical Medicine in Modern Times*, 2nd ed. rev. (New York, 1930), esp. pp. 68-71, 76, 87.

18  On the ambiguities of medical practice in the late 19th century, see Charles Rosenberg, "The practice of medicine in New York a century ago," *Bull. Hist. Med.*, 1967, *41*: 223-253.

19  There is no adequate history of neurology in English. But see Erwin Ackerknecht, *A Short History of Psychiatry*, trans. Sulammith Wolff (London and New York, 1959).

20  On early American neurology, see Charles L. Dana, "Early neurology in the United States," *J.A.M.A.,* 1928, *90*: 1421-1424; Louis Casamajor, "Notes for an intimate history of neurology and psychiatry in America," *J. Nerv. & Ment. Dis.*, 1943, *98*: 600-608; and Barbara Sicherman, "The quest for mental health in America, 1880-1917," (Ph.D. dissertation, Columbia Univ., 1967), pp. 35-45, 231-239.

21  Beard, *Sexual Neurasthenia*, pp. 32-33; and Beard, *Nervous Exhaustion*, pp. 86-117. For contemporary views on this type of illness, see Gerald Chrzanowski, "Neurasthenia and hypochondriasis," in Alfred M. Freedman and Harold I. Kaplan, *Comprehensive Textbook of Psychiatry* (Baltimore, 1967), pp. 1163-1168, and David Mechanic, "Social psychological factors affecting the presentation of bodily complaints," *New Eng. J. Med.*, 1972, *286*: 1132-1139.

22  S. Weir Mitchell, *Rest in Nervous Disease: Its Use and Abuse*, in *A Series of American Clinical Lectures*, ed. E. C. Seguin, I (New York, 1875), 94; Beard, *Nervous Exhaustion*, p. 103; A. S. Myrtle, "On a common form of impaired vitality," *Med. Press Circular*, 1874, *17*: 375-376. Cf. Carroll Smith-Rosenberg, "The hysterical woman: sex roles and role conflict in 19th-century America," *Social Research*, 1972, *39*: 652-678; and Ilza Veith, *Hysteria: The History of a Disease* (Chicago, 1965).

23  Esther Fischer-Homberger, "Hypochondriasis of the eighteenth century—neurosis of the present century," *Bull. Hist. Med.*, 1972, *46*: 391-401.

24  Cf. Ann Douglas Wood, "'The fashionable diseases': women's complaints and their treatment in nineteenth-century America," *J. Interdisc. Hist.*, 1973, *4*: 25-52; Carroll Smith-Rosenberg and Charles Rosenberg, "The female animal: medical and biological views of woman and her role in nineteenth-century America," *J. Am. Hist.*, 1973, *60*: 332-356; and Regina Morantz, "The lady and her physician," in *Clio's Consciousness Raised: New Perspectives on the History of Women*, ed. Mary S. Hartman and Lois Banner (New York, 1974), pp. 38-53.

25  See Joseph Collins and Carlin Phillips, "The etiol-

ogy and treatment of neurasthenia. An analysis of three hundred and thirty-three cases," *Med. Rec.*, 1899, *55*: 413–422; and Paul Schilder,"Neurasthenia and hypochondria: introduction to the study of the neurasthenic-hypochondriac character," *Med. Rev. Rev.*, 1930, *36*: 165.

26  Beard, *Nervous Exhaustion*, pp. 96–98.

27  *Ibid.*, p. 80. Mitchell too suffered from neurasthenia. See Margaret C.-L. Gildea and Edwin F. Gildea, "Personalities of American psychotherapists," *Am. J. Psychiatry*, 1945, *101*: 464–466; and Anna Robeson Burr, *Weir Mitchell: His Life and Letters* (New York, 1929).

28  George M. Beard, "The problems of insanity," *Physn. & Bull. Medico-Legal Soc.*, 1880, *13*: 244; Cowles, "Neurasthenia," p. 50.

29  *The Letters of Virginia Woolf. Volume I: 1888–1912*, ed. Nigel Nicolson and Joanne Trautmann (New York and London, 1975), pp. 141–142.

30  The classic work on the relationship between social class and the diagnosis and treatment of psychiatric illness is August B. Hollingshead and Frederick C. Redlich, *Social Class and Mental Illness: A Community Study* (New York, 1958). Gerald N. Grob discusses the ways class, race, and ethnicity influenced treatment in mental hospitals. See *Mental Institutions in America: Social Policy to 1875* (New York, 1973), esp. pp. 221–256.

31  Edward C. Mann, "A plea for lunacy reform," *Medico-Legal J.*, 1884, *1*: 159; discussion of William A. Hammond, "The non-asylum treatment of the insane," *Tr. Med. Soc. St. N.Y.* (1879), p. 297.

32  E. H. van Deusen, "Observations on a form of nervous prostration (neurasthenia), culminating in insanity," *Am. J. Insanity*, 1869, *25*: 445–461; S. Weir Mitchell, "Clinical lecture on nervousness in the male," *Med. News Libr.*, 1877, *35*: 177–184. See also Cecil MacCoy, "Some observations on the treatment of neurasthenia at the dispensary clinic," *Brooklyn Med. J.*, 1903, *17*: 399–401; and annual reports of Boston City and Massachusetts General Hospitals.

33  Collins and Phillips, "Treatment of neurasthenia," pp. 413–422. My own research in Massachusetts General Hospital records reveals a similarly high proportion of neurasthenic patients between the ages of 20 and 40 and an even higher proportion of single patients.

34  Beard, *American Nervousness*, pp. 282–284.

35  Beard's case is discussed in Barbara Sicherman, "The paradox of prudence: mental health in the gilded age," *J. Am. Hist.*, 1976, *62*: 890–912. The quotation from the minister appears in *Sermon by the Rev. J. L. Willard, of Westville, Connecticut at the Funeral Services of Elizabeth A. Beard. Together with Comments upon the Life and Career of the Late Dr. George M. Beard* (Grand Hotel, New York [1883]), p. 4, in George M. Beard Papers, Yale University Library, New Haven, Conn.

36  In addition to works discussed in n. 22 and n. 24, see Hale, *Freud and the Americans*, pp. 24–46; and Charles E. Rosenberg, "Sexuality, class and role in 19th-century America," *Am. Quart.*, 1973, *25*: 131–153.

37  Cushing Strout, "William James and the twice-born sick soul," in *Philosophers and Kings: Studies in Leadership*, ed. Dankwart A. Rustow (New York, 1970), pp. 491–511; Erik H. Erikson, *Identity: Youth and Crisis* (New York, 1968), pp. 19–22, 150–155. Compare the similar case of G. Stanley Hall, the psychologist who later formulated the modern concept of adolescence, in Dorothy Ross, *G. Stanley Hall: The Psychologist as Prophet* (Chicago, 1972), pp. 309–340.

38  Jane Addams, *Twenty Years at Hull-House. With Autobiographical Notes* (New York, 1911), pp. 64–88, 113–127. Cf. Allen F. Davis, *American Heroine: The Life and Legend of Jane Addams* (New York, 1973), pp. 24–37.

39  Charlotte Perkins Gilman, *The Living of Charlotte Perkins Gilman: An Autobiography* (New York, 1975; originally published in 1935), pp. 78–106. See also her short story about the same events, "The yellow wall-paper," reprinted in *The Oven Birds: American Women on Womanhood, 1820–1920*, ed. Gail Parker (Garden City, 1972), pp. 317–334.

40  George M. Beard, "Private Journal," p. 217, Beard Papers.

41  Beard, *Sexual Neurasthenia*, pp. 102–103, 122, 119–120; Willard, Beard Papers, p. 4.

42  Margaret A. Cleaves, *An Autobiography of a Neurasthene. As Told by One of Them and Recorded by Margaret A. Cleaves* (Boston, 1910). Although presented as an astold-to autobiography, this work is probably the story of Margaret Cleaves herself. Insofar as they are known, the facts of Margaret Cleaves's family background, early life, and professional career closely resemble those of the subject of the autobiography.

43  "American Neurological Association," *J. Nerv. & Ment. Dis.*, 1876, *3*: 429–437.

44  S. Weir Mitchell, "The evolution of the rest treatment," *J. Nerv. & Ment. Dis.*, 1904, *31*: 368–372; Mitchell, *Rest in Nervous Disease*, esp. pp. 94–96; S. Weir Mitchell, *Fat and Blood: An Essay on the Treatment of Certain Forms of Neurasthenia and Hysteria*, 5th ed. (Philadelphia, 1888); and S. Weir Mitchell, *Lectures on Diseases of the Nervous System, Especially in Women*, 2nd ed. rev. (Philadelphia, 1885), esp. pp. 265–283.

45 Mitchell, *Fat and Blood*, pp. 40–42, 47–49, 55–62; Mitchell, *Rest in Nervous Disease*, p. 84.

46 Mitchell, *Rest in Nervous Disease*, p. 94; Mitchell, *Diseases of the Nervous System*, p. 38. For a discussion of regression as a psychoanalytic technique, see Karl Menninger, *Theory of Psychoanalytic Technique* (New York, 1958), esp. pp. 43–76.

47 Brill, "Diagnostic errors in neurasthenia," p. 122.

48 Cf. Dewitt L. Crandell and Bruce P. Dohrenwend, "Some relations among psychiatric symptoms, organic illness, and social class," *Am. J. Psychiatry,* 1967, *123*: 1527–1538; and Mechanic, "Bodily complaints," pp. 1132–1139. See also William James's letters to James Jackson Putnam in the James Jackson Putnam Papers, at The Francis A. Countway Library of Medicine, Boston.

49 Cf. John D. Stoeckle, Irving K. Zola, and Gerald E. Davidson, "The quantity and significance of psychological distress in medical patients: some preliminary observations about the decision to seek medical aid," *J. Chron. Dis.*, 1964, *17*: 959–970.

50 The material in the next two paragraphs is drawn from Massachusetts General Hospital, Medical Records (East and West Wings), 1880–1900. See, for example, Vol. 381 (1885), p. 82, and Vol. 455

(1893), p. 124. For judgmental comments, see Vol. 349 (1880), p. 198; Vol. 381 (1885), p. 250. Charles Rosenberg informs me that he found similar material on working-class patients at Pennsylvania General Hospital.

51 *Ibid.*, Vol. 487 (1897), p. 42. One of these letters appears in Vol. 451 (1893), p. 56. The comment about wanting to stay refers to the same patient during a second hospitalization. Cf. Vol. 457 (1894), p. 306.

52 E. E. Southard, "Cross sections of mental hygiene, 1844, 1869, 1894," *Am. J. Insanity*, 1919, *76*: 109; Charles L. Dana, "The future of neurology," *J. Nerv. & Ment. Dis.*, 1913, *40*: 753–757.

53 George M. Beard, *Our Home Physician: A New and Popular Guide to the Arts of Preserving Health and Treating Disease* (New York, 1870), pp. xxi, 672; Mitchell, *Doctor and Patient*, 3rd ed. (Philadelphia, 1889), p. 10; cf. p. 6.

54 Peter Bryce, "The mind and how to preserve it," *Tr. Med. Assn. St. Ala.*, 1880, p. 260; Philip Garrett, "President's address," *Proc. Nat. Conf. Charities & Correction*, 1885, *12*: 20; S. Weir Mitchell, *Dr. North and His Friends* (New York, 1900), p. 389.

# Therapeutics

Therapeutics, the means of treating illness, is the core of medical practice. Until recently, however, American historians have paid little attention to this important branch of medical history. Prior to the 20th century, with its chemotherapy and antibiotics, regular physicians possessed only a handful of specific remedies, one of the most valuable of which was quinine, used to treat malaria and other fevers. In the absence of specific therapeutic agents, early 19th-century physicians focused their efforts on restoring the body to its "natural" state. To accomplish this, they often bled or blistered their patients, purged them with calomel, or induced vomiting with tartar emetic—measures that came to symbolize the regular practice of medicine. For reasons explored by John Harley Warner, medical theory and practice sometimes varied considerably from region to region.

The therapeutic revolution described by Charles E. Rosenberg occurred in the middle third of the 19th century, when regular physicians turned increasingly from depletive to supportive therapies. Among the many factors contributing to this change were the criticisms from irregular practitioners, who ridiculed the "heroic" practices of their rivals. These sectarian physicians, many of whom possessed M.D. degrees, offered the sick a range of alternatives to regular medicine, from the infinitesimal doses of the homeopaths to the water cures of the hydropaths. By the close of the century these sectarians, primarily homeopaths and eclectics (who relied on botanic remedies), constituted an estimated 16 to 24 percent of all American practitioners. By this time, however, their methods of healing differed little in practice from those of regular physicians, and in the 20th century the old sectarians faded away, leaving the field to newcomers like osteopaths and chiropractors.

Medical therapy, as James Harvey Young shows, did not always involve a physician, either orthodox or heterodox. Throughout history many people have chosen to treat themselves, while others have sought help from faith healers, quacks, and assorted personnel on the fringes of the healing arts. Self-treatment has long been practiced by persons lacking access to physicians, wanting to save money, or simply embarrassed by the prospect of discussing delicate problems. In times of need they have often turned for advice to a do-it-yourself manual, a friend, or perhaps a patent-medicine peddler. Not infrequently, they have supplemented a physician's prescription with over-the-counter drugs or concoctions of their own making.

Quacks offered still other varieties of therapy, usually secret and expensive. During the middle decades of the 19th century, when licensing laws were nonexistent and anybody could be a "doctor," these greedy pretenders to medical knowledge flourished openly. And even today, quackery remains a thriving business, annually milking hapless citizens of millions of dollars for worthless cures.

# 3

## The Therapeutic Revolution: Medicine, Meaning, and Social Change in 19th-Century America

### CHARLES E. ROSENBERG

Medical therapeutics changed remarkably little in the two millennia preceding 1800; by the end of the century, traditional therapeutics had altered fundamentally. This development is a significant event, not only in the history of medicine, but in social history as well. Yet historians have not only failed to delineate this change in detail, they have hardly begun to place it in a framework of explanation which would relate it to all those other changes which shaped the 20th-century Western world.

Medical historians have always found therapeutics an awkward piece of business. On the whole, they have responded by ignoring it.[1] Most historians who have addressed traditional therapeutics have approached it as a source of anecdote, or as a murky bog of routinism from which a comforting path led upward to an ultimately enlightened and scientifically based therapeutics. Isolated incidents such as the introduction of quinine or digitalis seemed only to emphasize the darkness of the traditional practice in which they appeared. Among 20th-century students of medical history, the generally unquestioned criterion for understanding pre-19th-century therapeutics has been physiological, not historical: did a particular practice act in a way that 20th-century understanding would regard as efficacious? Did it work?

Yet therapeutics is after all a good deal more than

a series of pharmacological or surgical experiments. It involves emotions and personal relationships, and incorporates all of those cultural factors which determine belief, identity, and status. The meaning of traditional therapeutics must be sought within a particular cultural context; and this is a task more closely akin to that of the cultural anthropologist than the physiologist. Individuals become sick, demand care and reassurance, and are treated by designated healers. Both physician and patient must necessarily share a common framework of explanation. To understand therapeutics in the opening decades of the 19th century, its would-be historian must see that it relates, on the one hand, to a cognitive system of explanation, and, on the other, to a patterned interaction between doctor and patient, one which evolved over centuries into a conventionalized social ritual.

Instead, however, past therapeutics has most frequently been studied by scholars obsessed with change as progress and concerned with defining such change as an essentially intellectual process. Historians have come to accept a view of 19th-century therapeutics which incorporates such priorities. The revolution in practice which took place during the century, the conventional argument follows, reflected the gradual triumph of a critical spirit over ancient obscurantism. The increasingly aggressive empiricism of the early 19th century pointed toward the need for evaluating every aspect of clinical practice; nothing was to be accepted on faith, and only those therapeutic modalities which proved themselves in controlled clinical trials were to remain in the physician's arsenal. Spurred by such arguments, increasing numbers of physicians grew sceptical of their ability to alter the course of particular ills, and by mid-century (this

CHARLES E. ROSENBERG is Professor in the Department of History and Sociology of Science at the University of Pennsylvania, Philadelphia, Pennsylvania.

Reprinted with permission from *The Therapeutic Revolution: Essays in the Social History of American Medicine*, edited by Morris J. Vogel and Charles E. Rosenberg (Philadelphia: University of Pennsylvania Press, 1979), pp. 3–25. A somewhat different version of this paper appeared in *Perspectives in Biology and Medicine*, 1977, *20*: 485–506.

interpretation continues), traditional medical practice had become far milder and less intrusive than it had been at the beginning of the century. Physicians had come to place ever-increasing faith in the healing power of nature and the natural tendency toward recovery which seemed to characterize most ills.

This view of change in 19th-century therapeutics constitutes accepted wisdom, though it has been modified in recent years. An increasingly influential emphasis sees therapeutics as part of a more general pattern of economically motivated behavior which helped to rationalize the regular physician's place in a crowded marketplace of would-be healers.[2] Thus the competition offered by sectarians to regular medicine in the middle third of the century was at least as significant in altering traditional therapeutics as a high-culture-based intellectual critique; the sugar pills of homeopathic physicians or baths and diets of hydropaths might possibly do little good, but could hardly be represented as harmful or dangerous in themselves. The often draconic treatments of regular physicians — the bleeding, the severe purges and emetics — constituted a real handicap in competing for a limited number of paying patients, and were accordingly modified to fit economic realities. Indeed, something approaching an interpretive consensus might be said to prevail in historical works of recent vintage, a somewhat eclectic, but not illogical position which views change in 19th-century therapeutics as proceeding both from a high-culture-based shift in ideas and the sordid realities of a precarious marketplace.

Obviously, both emphases reflect a measure of reality. But insofar as they do, they serve essentially to identify sources of instability in an ancient system of ideas and relationships; they do not explain these ideas and relationships. For neither deals with traditional therapeutics as a meaningful question in itself. As such, therapeutic practices must be seen as a central component in a particular medical system, a system characterized by remarkable tenacity over time.[3] The system must, that is, have worked, even if not in a sense immediately intelligible to a mid-20th-century pharmacologist or clinician. I hope in the following pages to suggest, first, the place of therapeutics in the configuration of ideas and relationships which constituted medicine at the beginning of the

19th century, and then the texture of the change which helped to create a very different system of therapeutics by the end of the century.

The key to understanding therapeutics at the beginning of the 19th century lies in seeing it as part of a system of belief and behavior participated in by physicians and laymen alike. Central to the logic of this social subsystem was a deeply assumed metaphor — a particular way of looking at the body and of explaining both health and disease. The body was seen, metaphorically, as a system of dynamic interactions with its environment. Health or disease resulted from a cumulative interaction between constitutional endowment and environmental circumstance. One could not well live without food and air and water; one had to live in a particular climate, subject one's body to a particular style of life and work. Each of these factors implied a necessary and continuing physiological adjustment. The body was always in a state of becoming — and thus always in jeopardy.

Two subsidiary assumptions organized the shape of this lifelong interaction. First, every part of the body was related inevitably and inextricably with every other. A distracted mind could curdle the stomach; a dyspeptic stomach could agitate the mind. Local lesions might reflect imbalances of nutrients in the blood; systemic ills might be caused by fulminating local lesions. Thus the theoretical debates which have bemused historians of medicine over local as opposed to systemic models of disease causation, solidistic versus humoral emphases, models based on tension or laxity of muscle fibres or blood vessels — all served the same explanatory function relative to therapeutics; all related local to systemic ills; they described all aspects of the body as interrelated; they tended to present health or disease as general states of the total organism. Second, the body was seen as a system of intake and outgo — a system which had, necessarily, to remain in balance if the individual were to remain healthy. Thus the conventional emphasis on diet and excretion, perspiration, and ventilation. Equilibrium was synonymous with health, disequilibrium with illness.

In addition to the exigencies of everyday life which might destablilize the equilibrium which constituted health, the body also had to pass through several developmental crises inherent in the design of the human organism. Menstruation and menopause in women, teething and puberty in both sexes — all represented points of potential danger, moments of structured instability, as the body established a new internal equilibrium.[4] Seasonal changes in climate constituted another kind of recurring cyclical change which might imply danger to health and require possible medical intervention: thus the ancient practice of administering cathartics in spring and fall to help the body adjust to the changed seasons. The body could be seen, that is — as in some ways it had been since classical antiquity — as a kind of stewpot, or chemico-vital reaction, proceeding calmly only if all its elements remained appropriately balanced. Randomness was minimized, but at a substantial cost in anxiety; the body was a city under constant threat of siege, and it is not surprising that early 19th-century Americans consumed enormous quantities of medicines as they sought to regulate assimilation and excretion.

The idea of specific disease entities played a relatively small role in such a system. Where empirical observation pointed unavoidably toward the existence of a particular disease state, physicians still sought to preserve their accustomed therapeutic role. The physician's most potent weapon was his ability to "regulate the secretions" — to extract blood, to promote the perspiration, or the urination, or defecation which attested to his having helped the body to regain its customary equilibrium. Even when a disease seemed not only to have a characteristic course, but (as in the case of smallpox) a specific causative "virus," the hypothetical pathology and indicated therapeutics were seen within the same explanatory framework.[5] The success of inoculation and later of vaccination in preventing smallpox could not challenge this deeply internalized system of explanation. When mid-18th and early 19th-century physicians inoculated or vaccinated, they always accompanied the procedure with an elaborate regimen of cathartics, diet, and rest. Though such elaborate medical accompaniments to vaccination might appear, from one perspective, as a calculated effort to increase the physician's fees, these preparations might better be seen as a means of assimilating an anomalous procedure into the physician's accustomed picture of health and disease.

The pedigree of these ideas can be traced to the rationalistic speculations of classical antiquity. They could hardly be superseded, for no information more accurate or schema more socially useful existed to call them into question. Most important, the system provided a rationalistic framework in which the physician could at once reassure the patient and legitimate his own ministrations. It is no accident that the term *empiric* was pejorative until the mid-19th century, a reference to the blind cut-and-try practices which regular physicians liked to think characterized their quackish competitors. The physician's own self-image and his social plausibility depended on the creation of a shared faith — a conspiracy to believe — in his ability to understand, and rationally manipulate the elements in this speculative system. This cognitive framework and the central body metaphor about which it was articulated provided a place for his prognostic, as well as his therapeutic, skills; prognosis, diagnosis, and therapeutics had all to find a consistent mode of explanation.

The American physician in 1800 had no diagnostic tools beyond his senses, and it is hardly surprising that he would find congenial a framework of explanation which emphasized the importance of intake and outgo, the significance of perspiration, of pulse, of urination and menstruation, of defecation, and of the surface eruptions which might accompany fevers or other internal ills. These were phenomena which he as physician, the patient, and the patient's family could see, evaluate, and scrutinize for clues to the sick man's fate. These biological and social realities had several implications for therapeutics. Drugs had to be seen as adjusting the body's internal equilibrium; in addition, the drug's action had, if possible, to alter these visible products of the body's otherwise inscrutable internal state. Logically enough, drugs were not ordinarily viewed as specifics for particular disease entities; materia medica texts were generally arranged not by drug or disease, but in categories reflecting the drug's physiological effects: diuretics, cathartics, narcotics, emetics, diaphoretics. Quinine, for example, was ordinarily categorized as a tonic and prescribed for numerous conditions other than malaria.[6] Even when it was employed in "intermittent fever," quinine was almost invariably prescribed in conjunction with a cathartic; as in the case of vaccination, a drug with a disease-specific efficacy ill-suited to the assumptions of the physician's underlying cognitive framework was assimilated to it. (Significantly, the advocacy of a specific drug in treating a specific ill was ordinarily viewed by regular physicians as a symptom of quackery.)

The effectiveness of the system hinged to a significant extent on the fact that all the weapons in the physician's normal armamentarium worked: "worked," that is, by providing visible and predictable physiological effects; purges purged, emetics vomited, opium soothed pain and moderated diarrhea. Bleeding, too, seemed obviously to alter the body's internal balance, as evidenced both by a changed pulse and the very quantity of the blood drawn.[7] Blisters and other purposefully induced local irritations certainly produced visible effects —and presumably internal consequences proportional to their pain, location, and to the nature and extent of the matter discharged.[8] Not only did a drug's activity indicate to both physician and patient the nature of its efficacy (and the physician's competence) but it provided a prognostic tool, as well; for the patient's response to a drug could indicate much about his condition, while examination of the product elicited—urine, feces, blood, perspiration—could shed light on the body's internal state. Thus, for example, a patient could report to her physician that

> the buf on my blood was of a blewish Cast and at the edge of the buf it appeared to be curded something like milk and cyder curd after standing an hour or two the water that came on the top was of a yellowish cast.[9]

The patient's condition could be monitored each day as the doctor sought to guide its course to renewed health.

The body seemed, moreover, to rid itself of disease in ways parallel to those encouraged or elicited by drug action. The profuse sweat, diarrhea, or skin lesions often accompanying fevers, for example, all seemed stages in a necessary course of natural recovery. The remedies he employed, the physician could assure his patients, only acted in imitation of nature:

> Blood-letting and blisters find their archtypes in spontaneous haemmorrhage and those sero-plastic exudations that occur in some stage of almost every acute inflammation; emetics, cathartics, diuretics, diaphoretics, etc. etc. have each and all

of them effects in every way similar to those arising spontaneously in disease.[10]

Medicine could provoke or facilitate, but not alter, the fundamental patterns of recovery inherent in the design of the human organism.

This same explanatory framework illuminates as well the extraordinary vogue of mercury in early 19th-century therapeutics. If employed for a sufficient length of time and in sufficient quantity, mercury induced a series of progressively severe and cumulative physiological effects: first, diarrhea, and ultimately, full-blown symptoms of mercury poisoning. The copious involuntary salivation characteristic of this toxic state was seen as proof that the drug was exerting an "alterative" effect—that is, altering the fundamental balance of forces and substances which constituted the body's ultimate reality. Though other drugs, most prominently arsenic, antimony, and iodine, were believed able to exert such an "alterative" effect, mercury seemed particularly useful because of the seemingly unequivocal relationship between varying dosage levels and its consequent action (and the convenient fact that it could be administered either orally or as a salve).[11] Moderate doses aided the body in its normal healing pattern, while in larger doses, giving mercury could be seen as a forceful intervention in pathological states which had a doubtful prognosis. Mercury was, in this sense, the physician's most flexible, and, at the same time, most powerful weapon for treating ailments in which active intervention might mean the difference between life and death. In such cases he needed a drug with which he might alter a course toward death—one stronger than those with which he routinely modified the secretions and excretions in less severe ailments.

Both physician and layman shared a similar view of the manner in which the body functioned, and the nature of available therapeutic modalities reinforced that view. The secretions could be regulated, a plethoric state of the blood abated, the stomach emptied of a content potentially dangerous. Recovery must, of course, often have coincided with the administration of a particular drug and thus provided an inevitable post hoc endorsement of its effectiveness. A physician could typically describe a case of pleurisy as having been "suddenly relieved by profuse perspiration" elicited by the camphor he had prescribed.[12] Fevers seemed, in fact, often to be healed by the purging effects of mercury or antimony. Drugs reassured insofar as they acted, and their efficacy was inevitably underwritten by the natural tendency toward recovery which characterized most ills. Therapeutics thus played a central role within the system of interaction between doctor and patient; on the cognitive level, therapeutics confirmed the physician's ability to understand and intervene in the ongoing physiological processes which defined health and disease; on the emotional level, the very severity of drug action assured the patient and his family that something was indeed being done.

In the medical idiom of 1800, "exhibiting" a drug was synonymous with administering it (and the administration of drugs so routine that "prescribing for" was synonymous with seeing a patient). The use of the term *exhibit* was hardly accidental. For the therapeutic interaction we have sought to describe was a fundamental cultural ritual, in a literal sense—a ritual in which the legitimating element was, in part at least, a shared commitment to a rationalistic model of pathology and therapeutic action. Therapeutics served as a pivotal link in a stylized interaction between doctor and patient, encompassing organically (the pun is unfortunate but apposite) the cognitive and the emotional within a framework of rationalistic explanation.[13] To "exhibit" a drug was to act out a sacramental role in a liturgy of healing. The analogy to religious ritual is not exact, but it is certainly more than metaphorical. A sacrament, after all, is conventionally defined as an external, visible symbol of an invisible, internal state. Insofar as a particular drug caused a perceptible physiological effect, it produced phenomena which all— the physician, the patient, and the patient's family — could witness (again the double meaning, with its theological overtones, is instructive), and in which all could participate.

This was a liturgy calculated for the sickroom, of course, not for church. And indeed, the efficacy and tenacity of this system must be understood in relation to its social setting. Most such therapeutic tableaux took place in the patient's home, and thus the healing ritual could mobilize all of those community and emotional forces which anthropologists have seen as fundamental, in their observations of medical practice in traditional, non-

Western societies. Healing, in early 19th-century America, was in the great majority of cases physically and emotionally embedded in a precise, emotionally resonant context. The cognitive aspects of this system of explanation, as well, were appropriate to the world view of such a community. The model of the body, and of health and disease, which we have described was all-inclusive, antireductionist, capable of incorporating every aspect of man's life in explaining his physical condition. Just as man's body interacted continuously with his environment, so did his mind with his body, his morals with his health. The realm of causation in medicine was not distinguishable from the realm of meaning in society generally.

There was no inconsistency between this world of rationalistic explanation and traditional spiritual values. Few Americans in the first third of the century felt any conflict between these realms of reassurance. If drugs failed, this expressed merely the ultimate power of God, and constituted no reason to question the truth of either system of belief. Let me quote the words of a pious mid-century physician who sought in his diary to come to terms with the dismaying and unexpected death of a child he had been treating; "the child seemed perfectly well," the troubled physician explained,

> till it was attacked at the tea table. Remedies, altho' slow in their action, acted well, but were powerless to avert the arm of death. The decrees of Providence . . . cannot be set aside. Man is mortal, and tho' remedies often seem to act promptly and effectually to the saving of life— they often fail in an unaccountable manner! "So teach me to number my days that I may apply my heart unto wisdom."[14]

The Lord might give and the Lord take away— but until he did, the physician dared not remain passive in the face of those dismaying signs of sickness which caused his patient anxiety and pain.

The physician's art, in the opening decades of the 19th century, centered on his ability to employ an appropriate drug, or combination of drugs and bleeding, to produce a particular physiological effect. This explains the apparent anomaly of physicians employing different drugs to treat the same condition; each drug, the argument followed, was equally legitimate, so long as it produced the desired physiological effect. The selection of a proper

drug or drugs was no mean skill, authorities explained, for each patient possessed a unique physiological identity, and the experienced physician had to evaluate a bewildering variety of factors, ranging from climatic conditions to age and sex, in the compounding of any particular prescription. A physician who knew a family's constitutional idiosyncracies was necessarily a better practitioner for that family than one who enjoyed no such insight — or even one who hailed from a different climate, for it was assumed that both the action of drugs and reaction of patients varied with season and geography.[15] The physician had to be aware, as well, that the same drug in different dosages might produce different effects. Fifteen grams of ipecac, a young southern medical student cautioned himself, acted as an emetic, five induced sweating, while smaller doses could serve as a useful tonic.[16]

The same rationalistic mechanisms which explained recovery explained failure as well. One could not predict recovery in every case; even the most competent physician could only do that which the limited resources of medicine allowed — and the natural course of some ills was toward death. The treatment indicated for tuberculosis, as an ancient adage put it, was opium and lies. Cancer, too, was normally incurable; some states of disequilibrium could not be righted.

Early 19th-century American physicians unquestionably believed in the therapeutics they practiced. Physicians routinely prescribed severe cathartics and bleeding for themselves, and for their wives and children. A New England physician settling in Camden, South Carolina, for example, depended for health in this treacherous climate upon his accustomed cathartic pills. "Took two of the pills last night," he recorded in his diary; "they have kept me busy thro' the day and I now feel like getting clear of my headache."[17] Even when physicians felt some anxiety in particular cases, they could take assurance from the knowledge that they were following a mode of practice endorsed by rational understanding and centuries of clinical experience. A young New York City physician, in 1795, for example, felt such doubts after having bled and purged a critically ill patient:

> I began to fear that I had carried the debilitating plan too far. By degrees I became reassured; and

when I reflected on his youth, constitution, his uniform temperance, on the one hand; and on the fidelity with which I had adhered to those modes of practice recommended by the most celebrated physicians, on the other, I felt a conviction that accident alone, could wrest him from me.[18]

Such conviction was a necessary element in medical practice; without belief, the system could hardly have functioned.

Individuals from almost every level in society accepted, in one fashion or another, the basic outlines of the world-view which we have described. Evidence of such belief among the less articulate is not abundant, but it does exist. Patients, for example, understood that a sudden interruption of perspiration might cause cold or even pneumonia, that such critical periods as teething, puberty, or menopause were particularly dangerous. The metabolic gyroscope which controlled the balance of forces within the body was delicate indeed, and might easily be thrown off balance. Thus it was natural for servants and laborers reporting the symptoms of their fevers to an almshouse physician to ascribe their illnesses to a sudden stoppage of the perspiration.[19] It was equally natural for young ladies complaining of amenorrhea to ascribe it to a sudden chill. The sudden interruption of any natural evacuation would presumably jeopardize the end implicit in that function; if the body did not need to perspire in certain circumstances, or discharge menstrual blood at intervals, it would not be doing so.[20] These were mechanisms through which the body maintained its health-defining equilibrium — and could thus be interrupted only at great peril.

Such considerations dictated modes of treatment, as well as views of disease causation. If, for example, the normal course of a disease to recovery involved the formation of a skin lesion, the physician must not intervene too aggressively and interrupt the process through which the body sought to rid itself of offending matter. Thus a student could record his professor's warning against the premature "exhibition" of tonics in a continued fever; such stimulants were "highly prejudicial they lock in the disease instead of liberating it from the system. After evacuations have been premised," the young man continued, "then the tonic medicine may be employed."[21] Yet physicians assumed that fevers normally accompanied by skin lesions could not "find resolution" without an appropriately bountiful crop of such blisters; and if they seemed dilatory in erupting, the physician might appropriately turn to blisters and counter-irritation in an effort to encourage them. To "drive them inward," on the other hand, was to invite far graver illness. In such ailments it was the physician's task to prescribe mild cathartics, in an effort to aid the body in its efforts to expel the morbid material. Mercury, for example, might be desirable in small doses but perilous in "alterative" ones. In any case, however, it was the physician's primary responsibility to "regulate or restore" the normal secretions whenever they were interrupted; chronic constipation, or diarrhea, or irregular menstruation simply implied active steps on the physician's part. In constipation, mild cathartics were routine; in amenorrhea, drugs to restore the flow (emmenagogues) were indicated. (The use of emmenagogues could represent an ethical dilemma to physicians who feared being imposed upon by seemingly innocent young ladies who sought abortifacients under the guise of a desire to restore the normal menstrual cycle interrupted by some cause other than pregnancy.) [22]

The widespread faith in emetics, cathartics, diuretics, and bleeding is evidenced, as well, by their prominent place in folk medicine. Domestic and irregular practice, that is, like regular medicine, was shaped about the eliciting of predictable physiological responses; home remedies mirrored the heroic therapeutics practiced by regular physicians. In the fall of 1826, for example, when a Philadelphia tallow chandler fell ill, he complained of chills, pains in the head and back, weakness in the joints, and nausea. Then, before seeing a regular physician, he

> was bled till symptoms of fainting came on. Took an emetic, which operated well. For several days after, kept his bowels moved with Sulph. Soda, Senna tea etc. He then employed a Physician who prescribed another Emetic, which operated violently and whose action was kept up by drinking bitter tea. [23]

Only after two more days did he appear at the Alms-House Hospital. Physicians sceptical of traditional therapeutics complained repeatedly of lay expectations which worked against change; medi-cal men might well be subject to criticism if they should, for example, fail to bleed in the early stages of pneumonia. Parents often demanded that physicians incise the inflamed gums of their teething infants so as to provoke a "resolution" of this developmental crisis. Laymen could, indeed, be even more importunate in their demands for an aggressive therapy than the physicians attending them thought appropriate. The indications for bleeding, for example, were carefully demarcated in formal medical thought, yet laymen often demanded it even when the state of the pulse and general condition of the patient contraindicated loss of blood. Some patients demanded, as well as expected, the administration of severe cathartics or emetics; they suspected peril in too languid a therapeutic regimen.

Botanic alternatives to regular medicine in the first third of the century were also predicated upon the routine use of severe cathartics and emetics of vegetable origin. (In the practice of Thomsonian physicians, the most prominent organized botanic sect, such drugs were supplemented by sweatbaths designed, in theory, to adjust the body's internal heat through the eliciting of copious perspiration.) [24] Botanic physicians shared many of the social problems faced by their regular competitors; they dealt with the same emotional realities implicit in the doctor-patient relationship, and in doing so appealed to a similar framework of physiological assumption.

Nevertheless, there were differences of approach among physicians, and in the minds of a good many laymen who questioned both the routinism and the frequent severity of traditional therapeutics. (The criticisms which greeted the atypically severe bleeding and purging advocated by Benjamin Rush are familiar to any student of the period.) America, in 1800, was in many ways already a modern society, diverse in religion, in class, and in ethnic background. It would be naive to contend that the unity of vision which presumably united most traditional non-Western cultures in their orientation toward particular medical systems could apply to this diverse and changing culture. Yet, as we have argued, there were surprisingly large areas of agreement. Even those Americans sceptical of therapeutic excess and inconsistency (and, in some cases, more generally of the physician's authority) did not question the fundamental structure of the body metaphor which I have described, however much they may have doubted the possible efficacy of medical intervention in sickness.[25]

In describing American medical therapeutics in the first quarter of the 19th century we have been examining a system already marked by signs of instability. Fundamental to this instability was rationalism itself. A key legitimating aspect of the traditional cognitive model was its rationalistic form (even if we regard that rationalism as egregiously speculative); yet by 1800, this structure of explanation was tied irrevocably to the institutions and findings of world science. And as this world changed and provided data and procedures increasingly relevant to the world of clinical medicine, it gradually undercut that harmony between world-view and personal interaction which had characterized therapeutics at the opening of the century.

By the 1830s, criticism of traditional therapeutics had become a cliché in sophisticated medical circles; physicians of any pretension spoke of self-limited diseases, of scepticism in regard to the physician's ability to intervene and change the course of most diseases, of respect for the healing powers of nature. This point of view emphasized the self-limiting nature of most ailments, and the physician's duty simply to aid the process of natural recovery through appropriate and minimally heroic means. "It would be better," as Oliver Wendell Holmes put it in his usual acerbic fashion, "if the patient were allowed a certain discount from his bill for every dose he took, just as children are compensated by their parents for swallowing hideous medicinal mixtures."[26] Rest, a strengthening diet, or a mild cathartic were all the aid nature required in most ills. In those ailments whose natural tendency was toward death, the physician had to acknowledge his powerlessness and simply try to minimize pain and anxiety. This noninterventionist position was accompanied by increasing acceptance of the parallel view that most diseases could be seen as distinct clinical entities, each with a characteristic cause, course, and symptomatology.

These positions are accepted by most historians as reflecting the fundamental outline for the debate over therapeutics in the middle third of the 19th century. And, as a matter of fact, it does describe a significant aspect of change — the influence of high-culture ideas and of a small opinion-forming group in gradually modifying the world-view of a much larger group of practitioners and, ultimately, of laymen. But when we try to evaluate the impact of such therapeutic admonitions on the actual practice of physicians, realities become a good deal more complex. Medical practice was conducted at a number of levels — intellectual, economic, and regional — but demonstrated in each the extraordinary tenacity of traditional views.

American physicians were tied to the everyday requirements of the doctor-patient relationship and thus, even among the teaching elite, no mid-century American practitioner rejected conventional therapeutics with a ruthless consistency. The self-confident empiricism which denied the efficacy of any therapeutic measure not proven efficacious in clinical trials seemed an ideological excess suited to a handful of European academics, not to the realities of practice. It is no accident that the radically sceptical position was christened "therapeutic nihilism" by its critics. Nihilism, with its echoes of disbelief and destructive change, of "total rejection of current religious beliefs and morals" (to borrowing a defining phrase from the *Oxford English Dictionary*) was not chosen as a term of casual abuse, but represented precisely the gravity of the challenge to a traditional world-view implied by a relentless empiricism, and by the materialism which seemed so often to accompany it.

There were enduring virtues in the old ways. "There is," as one leader in the profession explained, "a vantage ground between the two extremes, neither verging towards meddlesome interference on the one hand, nor imbecile neglect on the other."[27] The physician had to contend, moreover, with patient expectations: "the public," as another prominent clinician put it, "expect something more of physicians than the power of distinguishing diseases and of predicting their issue. They look to them for the relief of their sufferings, and the cure or removal of their complaints."[28]

The physician still had to create an emotionally, as well as intellectually, meaningful therapeutic regimen; and throughout the middle third of the 19th century, this meant the administration of drugs capable of eliciting a perceptible physiological response. No mid-century physician doubted the efficacy of placebos (as little as he doubted that the effectiveness of a drug could depend on his own manner and attitude), but in a grave illness the physician's own awareness of their inertness made it impossible for him to rely on sugar or bread pills and the healing power of nature. One medical man, for example, after conceding the uselessness of every available therapeutic means in cholera, still contended that "a noble profession whose aims and purpose are the preservation of human life, should not be content with anything short of the adoption of remedial measures for so fatal a disease, which promise positive and beneficent results in every individual case."[29] Hospital case records indicate that even elite physicians maintained a more than lingering faith in cathartic drugs throughout the middle third of the century. (And in hospital practice, economic considerations could have played no role in the doctor's willingness to prescribe.)

Physicians shaped a number of intellectual compromises in order to maintain such continuity with traditional therapeutic practice. Despite the growing plausibility of views emphasizing disease specificity, for example, most physicians still maintained an emphasis on their traditional ability to modify symptoms. The older assumption that drugs acted in a way consistent with the body's innate pattern of recovery was easily shifted toward new emphases; the physicians's responsibility now centered on recognizing the natural course of his patient's ailment and supporting the body in its progress to renewed health with an appropriate combination of drugs and regimen; even the course of a self-limited disease might be shortened, its painful symptoms mitigated. The secretions had still to be regulated, diet specified and modified, perhaps a plethora of blood lessened by cupping or leeching. Even in ills whose natural course was to death, the physician might still avail himself of therapeutic means to ease that grim journey. Finally, no one doubted, there were ailments in which the physician's intervention could make the difference between life and death; scurvy, for example, was often cited as a disease "that taints the whole system, [yet] yields to a mere change in diet."[30] The surgeon still had to set bones, remove foreign bodies, drain abscesses.

Second, even an explicit affirmation of the natural tendency to recovery, in most ills, did not obviate the place of traditional views of the body in explaining that recovery. Physicians, for example, spoke habitually of "vital power" and the need to support that vitality if the natural healing tendency were to manifest itself. The body could, that is, still be seen in traditional holistic terms, "vital power" constituting the sum of all its internal realities, and, by implication, a reflection of the body's necessary transactions with its environment. The use of the term *vital power* suggests, moreover, how deeply committed the medical profession still was to the communication of meaning through metaphor—in this case, a metaphor incorporating a shorthand version of the age-old view of the body which we have outlined, yet appearing in the necessary guise of scientific truth.

The decades between 1850 and 1870 did see an increased emphasis on diet and regimen among regular physicians, most strikingly a vogue for the use of alcoholic beverages as stimulants. It is hardly surprising that one reaction to the varied criticisms of traditional therapeutics was the acceptance of a "strengthening and stimulating" emphasis in practice; the new emphasis responded not only to criticisms by sectarian healers of "depleting" measures, such as bleeding and purging, but preserved an active role for the physician within the same framework of attitudes toward the body which had always helped order the doctor-patient relationship.

Practice changed a good deal less than the rhetoric surrounding it would suggest. "Nature," a South Carolina medical man explained to a patient troubled by a "derangement of the Abdominal organs," in 1850, "must restore their natural condition by gradually building them up anew, and time is necessary for the accomplishment of this." But, the physician continued, drug treatment was appropriate as well:

> The Medicinal treatment is to aid nature, by correcting irregularities and meeting untoward symptoms as they may occur. The Medicinal treatment consisted of an Alterative course of Tonics, chiefly Metallic, not Mercurial—so combined with Laxatives as to regulate the Secretions of the Digestive organs.[31]

Less aggressive than it might have been a generation earlier, such a course of treatment still allowed the physician an active role.

The inertia of traditional practice was powerful

indeed; older modes of therapeutics did not die, but, as we have suggested, were employed less routinely, and drugs were used in generally smaller doses. Dosage levels decreased markedly in the second third of the century, and bleeding, especially, sank into disuse. The resident physician at the Philadelphia Dispensary could, for example, report, in 1862, that of a total of 9,502 patients treated that year, "general blood-letting has been resorted to in one instance only, . . . cupping twelve times and leeching thrice."[32] Residents at Bellevue in New York and at Boston's Massachusetts General Hospital had reported the previous year that bloodletting was "almost obsolete."[33] Mercury, on the other hand, still figured in the practice of most physicians; even infants and small children endured the discomfort of mercury poisoning until well after the Civil War. Purges were still administered routinely in spring and fall to facilitate the body's adjustment to the changing seasons. The blisters and excoriated running sores so familiar to physicians and patients at the beginning of the century were gradually replaced by mustard plasters or turpentine applications, but the ancient concept of counterirritation still rationalized their use. Even bleeding still lingered, though increasingly in the practice of older men, and in less cosmopolitan areas. To divest themselves of such reliable means of regulating the body's internal equilibrium was, older physicians contended, to succumb to an intellectual fad with no compensation other than a morally irresponsible, if intellectually modish, emphasis on the healing powers of nature. It seemed to many physicians almost criminal to ignore their responsibility to regulate the secretions, even in ailments whose natural course was toward either death or recovery. Hence the continued vogue of cathartics and diuretics (though emetics, like bleeding, faded in popularity as the century progressed).

The debate over therapeutics was characterized more by moderation than by a full-fledged commitment to either the old, or to the new and radically sceptical. Few physicians occupied either of these extreme positions. In the intellectual realm as well as in that of practice, clinicians sought, in a number of ways, to insure the greatest possible degree of continuity with older ideas. When smaller doses seemed as efficacious as those heroic prescriptions they had employed in their youth, it

could be explained as a consequence of change in the prevailing pattern of disease incidence and perhaps even in the constitution of Americans.[34] More fundamentally, most physicians still found it difficult to accept the reductionist implications of the view that disease ordinarily manifests itself in the form of discrete clinical entities, with unique causes, courses, and pathologies. Physicians still spoke of epidemic influences, of diarrheas shifting into cholera, or minor fevers efflorescing into typhoid or yellow fever, if improperly managed.[35] The system was rich in confirmatory evidence; did not cases of "incipient" yellow fever and cholera recover, if treated in timely fashion? Traditionalists still found it natural to speak of general constitutional states — sthenic or asthenic — as underlying the symptomatology of particular ills or the response of the body to particular drugs. Drugs, on the other hand, were still assumed to reflect the influence of climate in their action. Man was still an organism reacting unceasingly, and at countless levels, with its environment.

Perhaps most significantly, even those who were most radical in their criticisms of traditional routinism and severity of dosage still emphasized that the physician's therapeutic effectiveness depended, to a good extent, on his familiarity with the patient's constitutional idiosyncracies. "No two patients have the same constitutional or mental proclivities," the *Boston Medical and Surgical Journal* editorialized in 1883: "No two instances of typhoid fever or of any other disease, are precisely alike. No 'rule of thumb,' no recourse to a formula-book, will avail for the treatment even of the typical diseases."[36]

Indeed, it was not until the very end of the 19th century that an outspoken and thoroughgoing therapeutic scepticism came actually to be pronounced from some of America's most prestigious medical chairs. "In some future day," as one authority put it,

> it is certain that drugs and chemicals will form no part of a scientific therapy. This is sure to be the case, for truth is finally certain to prevail. . . . The principal influence or relation of materia medica to the cure of bodily disease lies in the fact that drugs supply material upon which to rest the mind while other agencies are at work in eliminating disease from the system, and to the drug is frequently given the credit. . . . Sugar of milk

tablets of various colors and different flavors constitute a materia medica in practice that needs for temporary use only, morphin, codein, cocain, aconite and a laxative to make it complete.[37]

A dozen drugs, a Hopkins clinician argued, "suffice for the pharmaco-therapeutic armamentarium of some of the most eminent physicians on this continent."[38] Not surprisingly, the sometimes aggressive deprecation of therapeutic routinism by such leaders in the profession as William Osler or Richard Cabot still provoked aggressive counterattack. "Expectant treatment," Abraham Jacobi contended bitterly, in 1908, "is too often a combination of indolence and ignorance. . . . Expectant treatment is no treatment. It is the sin of omission, which not infrequently rises to the dignity of a crime."[39] Not all medical men were willing or able to accept the newer kind of reassurance which characterized the world of scientific medicine.

Indeed, many 19th-century American physicians were keenly aware of a potential inconsistency between the demands of science and those of clinical practice—and, by implication, of humanity. This perceived conflict had a pedigree extending backward to at least the presidency of Andrew Jackson, while it is hardly a moot question today. The debate over therapeutics naturally reflected this conflict of values. "The French have departed too much from the method of Sydenham and Hippocrates to make themselves good practitioners," an indignant New York physician complained in 1836. "They are tearing down the temple of medicine to lay its foundations anew. . . . They lose more in Therapeutics than they gain by morbid anatomy—They are explaining how men die but not how to cure them."[40] To some American medical teachers, the newly critical demands of the Paris Clinical School and its emphasis on reevaluating traditional therapeutics in the light of "numerical" standards seemed almost antisocial, a reversion to a sterile and demeaning empiricism.

> The practice of medicine according to this view, is entirely empirical, it is shorn of all rational induction, and takes a position among the lower grades of experimental observations, and fragmentary facts.[41]

The polarization of values implied by such observations grew only more intense in the second half of the century, as traditionally oriented physicians expressed their resentment of a fashionable worship of things German, and what they felt to be a disdain for clinical acumen. The appeal of the laboratory and its transcendent claims seemed to many clinicians a dangerous will-o-the-wisp. Even S. Weir Mitchell, one-time experimental physiologist, could charge that "out of the false pride of the laboratory and the scorn with which the accurate man of science looks down upon medical indefiniteness, has arisen the worse evil of therapeutic nihilism."[42] The danger, as another prominent chairholder put it, was that young men, "allured by the glitter of scientific work, will neglect the important and really more difficult attainments of true professional studies."[43] To some extent, of course, this was a conflict between the elite and the less favored; but it was, as well, a clash of temperament and world-view within America's medical elite. Willingness to accept the emotional and epistemological transcendence of science, even at the expense of traditional clinical standards, provided an emotional fault line which marked the profession throughout the last two-thirds of the century and paralleled the kind of change and conflict implied by modernization in other areas of society.

In the second half of the 20th century, the relationship between doctor and patient is much altered; its context has, in the great majority of cases, shifted from the home to some institutional setting. The healer is in many cases unknown, or known only casually, to the patient. Even the place of drug therapeutics has changed, changed not only in the sense that the efficacy of most drugs is beginning to be understood, but in the social ambience which surrounds their use. The patient still maintains a faith in the physician's prescription (often, indeed, demands such a prescription) but it is a rather different kind of faith than that which shaped the interaction of physician, patient, and therapeutics at the beginning of the 19th century.

Clearly the physician and the great majority of his patients no longer share a similar view of the body and the mechanisms which determine health and disease. Differing views of the body and the physician's ability to intervene in its mysterious opacity divide groups and individuals, rather than unifying, as the widely disseminated metaphorical view of body function had still done in 1800. Physician and patient are no longer bound together by the physiological activity of the drugs administered. In a sense, almost *all* drugs now act as placebos, for with the exception of certain classes of drugs, such as diuretics, the patient experiences no perceptible physiological effect. He does ordinarily have faith in the efficacy of a particular therapy, but it is a faith based not on a shared nexus of belief and participation in the kind of experience we have described, but rather on confidence in the physician and his imputed status, and, indirectly, in that of science itself. Obviously, one can draw facile parallels to many other areas in which an older community of world-view and personal relationship has been replaced by a more fragmented and status-oriented reality. Such observations have become commonplace, as we try to ascertain the shape of a gradually emerging modernity in the 19th-century West.

It is less easy to evaluate the moral implications of such change, and its existential meaning for the participants in the healing ritual. Our generation is tempted by an easy romanticization of the loss of community; it would be tempting, that is, to bewail the destruction of a traditional medicine, of a nexus of shared belief and assured relationship. Clearly we have lost something; or, to be more accurate, something has changed. But it would be arrogant indeed to dismiss the objective virtues of modern medicine with the charge that it is somehow less meaningful emotionally than it was in 1800. For after all, if we have created new dimensions of misery through technology, we have allayed others. To the historian familiar with 19th-century medicine and conditions of life, it would be naive indeed to dismiss the compensatory virtues of 20th-century medicine — its humane failings notwithstanding.

## NOTES

This discussion is abstracted from a larger projected history of medical care in America between 1790 and 1910. I would like to acknowledge the support of the Rockefeller Foundation during the academic year 1976–1977. I should also like to acknowledge the advice and encouragement given to me over many years by my teachers Erwin H. Ackerknecht and the late Ludwig Edelstein. My colleagues Drew Gilpin Faust, Saul Jarcho, Owsei Temkin, and Anthony F. C. Wallace read the manuscript carefully and made a number of important suggestions. A somewhat different version of this paper appeared in *Perspectives in Biology and Medicine*, 1977, *20*: 485–506.

1   For examples of work which try to place traditional therapeutics in a more general framework, see Erwin H. Ackerknecht, "Aspects of the history of therapeutics," *Bull. Hist. Med.,* 1962, *36*: 389–419 and his *Therapie von den Primitiven bis zum 20. Jahrhundert* (Stuttgart: Ferdinand Enke, 1970), and Owsei Temkin, "Therapeutic trends and the treatment of syphilis before 1900," *Bull. Hist. Med.,* 1955, *29*: 309–316.

2   For an example of this position, see William Rothstein, *American Physicians in the Nineteenth Century. From Sects to Science* (Baltimore and London: Johns Hopkins Press, 1972).

3   Within the meaning of the term *therapeutics*, I include any measures utilized by physicians or laymen in hopes of ameliorating or curing the felt symptoms of illness. In the great majority of instances this implied the administration of some drug, but might often include bleeding, and alterations in diet or other aspects of life style. This paper avoids the question of surgery and its place in the cognitive system which explained nonsurgical therapeutic practices.

4   For a more detailed discussion of one such cyclical crisis, see Carroll Smith-Rosenberg, "Puberty to menopause: The cycle of femininity in nineteenth-century America," *Feminist Stud.,* 1973, *1*: 58–72.

5   In some ways, it should be emphasized, constitutional ills fit more easily into this model than the acute infectious — and especially epidemic — ills. Cancer or tuberculosis, for example, could naturally be seen as resulting from long-term problems of assimilation. Acute and especially epidemic diseases seemed more sharply defined in time and, ordinarily, in their courses; nevertheless, the pathological mechanisms which caused the symptoms constituting the disease were still represented in terms similar to those we have described.

6   Digitalis was, similarly, categorized as a diuretic and prescribed in many cases in which the edema which indicated its employment was unrelated to a cardiac pathology.

7   The rapid fluid loss in severe bloodletting or purging might indeed lower temperature, while extremely copious bloodletting quieted agitation, as well!

8  The vogue of blisters, plasters and other purposeful excoriation or irritation of the skin was related, as well, to the prevailing physiological assumptions concerning the interdependence of all parts of the body, and the necessary balancing of forces which determined health or disease. Thus, for example, the popularity of "counterirritation," in the form of skin lesions induced by the physician through chemical or mechanical means, was based on the assumption that the excoriation of one area and consequent suppuration could "attract" the "morbid excitement" from another site to the newly excoriated one, while the exudate was significant in possibly allowing the body an opportunity to rid itself of morbid matter, and of righting the disease-producing internal imbalance. Such a path to healing could follow natural, as well as artificial, lesions. "Every physician of experience," one contended as late as 1862, "can recall cases of internal affections, which, after the use of a great variety of medicines, have been unexpectedly relieved by an eruption on the skin: or of ailments of years' continuance, which have been permanently cured by the formation of a large abscess." John P. Spooner, *The Different Modes of Treating Disease: Or The Different Action of Medicines on the System in an Abnormal State* (Boston: David Clapp, 1862), p. 17.

9  Mary Ballard to Charles Brown, May 12, 1814, Charles Brown Papers, College of William and Mary, Williamsburg, Virginia.

10  E. B. Haskins, *Therapeutic Cultivation; Its Errors and Its Reformation; An Address Delivered to the Tennessee Medical Society, April 7, 1857* (Nashville, Tenn.: Cameron and Fall, 1857), p. 22.

11  Bleeding in a single large quantity was also seen as exerting such an alterative effect (and thus might be indicated where a number of smaller bleedings would have the opposite and undesirable effect). The term *alterative* was, in addition, most frequently associated with the treatment of long-standing constitutional ills, in the words of one physician, "subverting any vitiated habit of body or morbid diathesis existing." Samuel Hobson, *An Essay on the History; Preparation and Therapeutic Uses of Iodine* (Philadelphia: the author, 1830), p. 22 n.

12  Benjamin H. Coates, Practice Book, entry for Feb. 25, 1836, Historical Society of Pennsylvania, Philadelphia.

13  For parallel discussion of medical explanation in relation to cosmology and symbolic form, see: Victor Turner, *The Forest of Symbols: Aspects of Ndembu Ritual* (Ithaca: Cornell Univ. Press, 1967); Mary Douglas, *Purity and Danger. An Analysis of Concepts of Pollution and Taboo* (London: Routledge and Kegan Paul, 1966); Douglas, *Natural Symbols, Explorations in Cosmology* (New York: Pantheon, 1970).

14  Diary of Samuel W. Butler, July 25, 1852, Historical Collections, College of Physicians of Philadelphia.

15  As Benjamin Rush could explain to an English correspondent, for example: "The extremes of heat and cold, by producing greater extremes of violence in our fevers than in yours, call for more depletion, and from more outlets, than the fevers of Great Britain." Rush to John Coakley Lettsom, May 13, 1804, L. H. Butterfield, ed., *Letters of Benjamin Rush*, 2 vols. (Princeton, N.J.: American Philosophical Society, 1951), II, 881.

16  Anonymous notebook, Materia Medica Lectures of John P. Emmett, University of Virginia, 1834–36, Perkins Library, Duke University, Durham, N.C.

17  The "busy" referred to the "operation" of the drug, not to the physician's schedule! Diary of William Blanding, July 4, 1807, South Caroliniana Library, University of South Carolina, Columbia. As usual, Benjamin Rush was particularly enthusiastic. "Ten of my family have been confined with remitting fevers," he wrote to John Redman Coxe on Oct. 5, 1795. "Twenty-four bleedings in one month have cured us all. I submitted to two of them in one day. Our infant of 6 weeks old was likewise bled twice, and thereby rescued from the grave." *Letters*, II, 763.

18  Entry for Sept. 18, 1795. *The Diary of Elihu Hubbard Smith (1771–1798)* (Philadelphia: American Philosophical Society, 1973), p. 59.

19  Such comments were made to examining physicians: for example, by laborer James McSherry, 39, and houseworker Sarah Mullin, 19, at the Philadelphia Alms-house, Hospital Casebook, 1824–1827, Records of the Board of Guardians of the Poor, Philadelphia City Archives.

20  The logic of the system is usefully illustrated by the assumption that suppressed menstruation would cause a plethora, or superabundance of blood. During pregnancy, it was believed that the blood was utilized by the developing embryo, during lactation, by the body's need to produce milk for the nursling. If the mother became ill and the infant stopped nursing, a student in David Hosack's lectures noted during the winter of 1822–1823, the lancet might be needed to "take off" the "plethora induced by the stoppage of the monthly discharge." J. Barratt, Medical Notebook, Lecture 49th, South Caroliniana Library, University of South Carolina, Columbia. "A partial suppression of the menses," a house-pupil at the Philadelphia Alms-House noted in 1825, "is sometimes the cause of Plethora. Give first an emetic of ipecac and then a laxative." Un-

paged medical notebook in the Nathan Hatfield Papers, Historical Collections, College of Physicians of Philadelphia.

21  Abraham Bitner, "Notes taken from the Philadelphia Alms-House, Nvr. 1824," p. 3. Historical Collections, College of Physicians of Philadelphia.

22  Pious physicians sometimes found it difficult to balance their professional desire to restore a normal menstrual flow against a fear of being placed in the position of inducing abortion. For an example, see Diary of R. P. Little, Nov. 28, 1842, Trent Collection, Duke University Medical Library, Durham, N.C.

23  Case of George Devert, Nov. 15, 1826, Hospital Casebook, 1824–27, Philadelphia City Archives.

24  The most detailed account of the Thomsonian movement is still that by Alex Berman, "The Impact of the nineteenth-century botanico-medical movement in American pharmacy and medicine" (Ph.D. dissertation, Univ. of Wisconsin, 1954); Berman, "The Thomsonian movement and its relation to American pharmacy and medicine," *Bull. Hist. Med.,* 1951, *25*: 405–428; 1951, *25*: 519–538.

25  The absolute rejection of traditional therapeutics enunciated by mid-century hydropaths and other evangelically oriented critics of medicine did not involve a rejection of the central body metaphor, but rather an absolute rejection of "artificial" drugs and bleeding. They did not question, but, on the contrary, emphasized the traditional view of the body; it served, indeed, as the logical basis for their dismissal of conventional therapeutics. They emphasized instead the body's capacity to heal itself when aided by appropriate regimen alone. The physician's therapeutic intrusions into that system seemed literally blasphemous.

26  Holmes, *Valedictory Address, Delivered to the Medical Graduates of Harvard University, at the Annual Commencement, . . . March 10, 1858* (Boston: David Clapp, 1858), p. 5.

27  T. Gaillard Thomas, *Introductory Address Delivered at the College of Physicians and Surgeons, New York, October 17th, 1864* (New York: 1864), p. 31.

28  Jacob Bigelow, *Brief Expositions of Rational Medicine, to Which Is Prefixed the Paradise of Doctors . . .* (Boston: Phillips, Sampson and Co., 1858), p. iv.

29  A. P. Merrill, *Med. Rec.,* 1866, *1*: 275.

30  C. W. Parsons, *An Essay on the Question, Vis Medicatrix Naturae, How Far Is It to Be Relied on in the Treatment of Diseases?* Fiske Fund Prize Dissertation No. 11 (Boston: printed for the Rhode Island Medical Society, 1849), p. 7.

31  Edmund Ravenel to unknown correspondent, draft [Nov. 1850], Ford-Ravenel Collection, South Carolina Historical Society, Charleston.

32  Report of the Resident Physician, Philadelphia Dispensary, *Rules of . . . with the Annual Report for 1862* (Philadelphia: J. Crummill, 1863), pp. 12–13.

33  O. W. Holmes, *Medical Essays* (Boston and New York: Houghton Mifflin, 1911), p. 258. Cited from an essay published originally in 1861.

34  See, for example, Samuel Henry Dickson, "Therapeutics," *Richmond Med. J.,* 1867, *3*: 12; Jared Kirtland, *An Introductory Lecture, on the Coinciding Tendencies of Medicines* (Cleveland: M. C. Younglove, 1848), p. 7.

35  A New Orleans physician could, for example, write in 1849 that "we have some cases of *Yellow Fever* — that is, they are yellow fever at the death, though but few look like it at the *beginning*. It is the mildest type of Intermittent and Remittent fever, of which 99 in the 100 cases can be cured if taken in time and properly treated, but *neglected* or *maltreated* [they shift into classic yellow fever]." E. D. Fenner to James Y. Bassett, Sept. 18, 1849, Bassett Papers, Southern Historical Collection, University of North Carolina, Chapel Hill.

36  "Routine Practice," Jan. 11, 1883, *108*: 43.

37  Elmer Lee, "How far does a scientific theory depend upon the materia medica in the cure of disease," *J.A.M.A.,* Oct. 8, 1898, *31*: 827.

38  Lewllys F. Barker, "On the present status of therapy and its future," *Johns Hopkins Hosp. Bull.,* 1900, *11*: 153. Critics of his sceptical position, the often acid William Osler put it, "did not appreciate the difference between the giving of medicines and the treatment of disease." *The Treatment of Disease. The Address in Medicine before the Ontario Medical Association, Toronto, June 3, 1909* (London: Oxford, 1909), p. 13.

39  Abraham Jacobi, "Nihilism and drugs," *N.Y. St. J. Med.,* Feb. 1908, *8*: 57–65.

40  Alexander H. Stevens to James Jackson, Apr. 14, 1836, James Jackson Papers, Francis Countway Library of Medicine, Boston.

41  L. M. Lawson, *Western Lancet,* 1849, *9*: 196.

42  Mitchell, *The Annual Oration before the Medical and Chirurgical Faculty of Maryland, 1877* (Baltimore: Inness and Co., 1877), p. 5.

43  Roberts Bartholow, *The Present State of Therapeutics: A Lecture Introductory to the Fifty-sixth Annual Course in Jefferson Medical College . . . October 1, 1879* (Philadelphia: J. B. Lippincott, 1879), p. 21.

# 4

## The Idea of Southern Medical Distinctiveness:
## Medical Knowledge and Practice in the Old South

### JOHN HARLEY WARNER

The historian seeking to assess in what ways medical knowledge and practice in the Old South differed from that in the North must inevitably come to terms with the fact that antebellum southern physicians themselves assertively proclaimed that their region was indeed medically distinctive. The argument for southern medical particularity pervades the medical literature and archival records that constitute the historian's primary texts. Yet the ubiquity of this argument does nothing to clarify how it should be read or interpreted. Was it primarily a political manifesto embodying the physician's contribution to southern nationalism, a reflection of invidious economic motives, a normative statement placed in aid of professional reform, or a prudent medical assessment of existential regional differences? I have elected herein to locate the argument for the distinctiveness of southern knowledge and practice within the context of national medical thought as the inescapable prerequisite to evaluating the extent and meaning of its peculiarly southern character.

My initial thesis is a simple one. In its underlying premises, logic, and even in the nature of its content, there was nothing inherently distinctive about the argument for southern medical distinctiveness. The sources, substance, and structure of the knowledge that purportedly guided medical practice in the North and South were remarkably similar in ways that are often taken for granted, but which are nonetheless important. At the same time,

the social production and dissemination of the argument for regional medical singularity in the South did take on characteristics that set it apart from its conceptual analogs in other regions. The South was distinctive not in possessing medical knowledge and practice avowedly molded to its peculiarly regional needs, but rather in the fervor with which physicians exploited and proselytized its medical particularity.

Southern physicians, especially from the early 1830s, pointed to a variety of factors that distinguished the South's medical character, and which dictated modifications in the medical knowledge and practice appropriate elsewhere. Historians have identified these influences upon southern practice, and analyzed their implications.[1] Geographic patterns of disease distribution, virulence, and classification; the large population of blacks and relatively small proportion of recent European immigrants in the South; and regional peculiarities in climate, topography, and diet purportedly demanded the existence of distinctively southern rules for diagnosis, prognosis, and treatment.

Physicians most often drew these diverse factors together into a coherent argument for southern medical distinctiveness when establishing the premises for institutional separatism. If southern knowledge and practice were necessarily different from those elsewhere, the reasoning of this argument went, then southern medical schools, literature, and societies became the necessary forums for generating and transmitting knowledge matched to the needs of southern medical practice.[2] But while such uses of the argument for southern medical distinctiveness to legitimize and direct institutional development resembled calls for separatism in other realms of southern life, such

JOHN HARLEY WARNER is a Research Fellow at the Wellcome Institute for the History of Medicine, London, England.

From the forthcoming book, *Science and Medicine in the Old South*, edited by Ronald L. Numbers and Todd L. Savitt.

as creative literature, liberal education, agriculture, and religion, the meaning of this argument must be discerned not only within the context of southern culture and its values, but also those of medicine.

John McCardell has noted that antebellum calls for southern cultural distinctiveness in such endeavors as liberal education rarely engendered concrete proposals regarding the form such beliefs should take in practice,[3] and this was not infrequently the case in medicine as well. However, southern physicians often were explicit about the ways their region's peculiarities should direct altered behavior at the patient's bedside. This was especially true in medical therapeutics. For example, the climate and topography of the South encouraged the production of noxious miasmata or malaria by the action of solar heat on decaying animal and vegetable matter, particularly in low, damp, swampy areas. The malarial influence in some parts of the South purportedly altered the character of all diseases occuring in these regions, demanding concomitant modifications in treatment. "Periodicity is frequently smuggled into the system," a Louisiana physician noted, and therefore in miasmatic regions if periodicity was *"even suspected, the experiment of giving quinine should be fairly tried."*[4] Not only was the southern physician to use quinine more readily than his northern counterpart, but he was also to be guided by different dosage rules adjusted to his patients' constitutions. Thus a Virginia medical professor could claim that individuals "fetched up" on malaria required larger doses of quinine to effect a cure than similarly afflicted patients who had recently arrived in a malarious district.[5]

The southern environment, physicians maintained, affected in a like fashion dosages and frequency of use of calomel, a mercurial purgative thought to stimulate the liver's activity. In the South both malaria and heat from the sun continually stimulated the liver, a student attending medical lectures in Charleston in the late 1830s typically reasoned, exhausting that organ and leaving it debilitated. To therapeutically arouse torpid southern livers, calomel was given "in the treatment of the diseases of the South generally[,] . . . because the liver is virtually the 'scape goat' for almost all the affections of the other organs . . . in Southern latitudes."[6] A Georgia student at-

tending the same school several years earlier explained in his thesis that because southerners' livers were so dulled, calomel was "required to be administered in doses nearly twice as large in the south as in the north" in order to elicit the same physiological response. "We are," he continued, "compelled to resort to what would be considered by northern practitioners, enormous doses of calomel, without which, we would be continually foiled in our attempts to cure the biliary disorders of the south." Northern judgments on calomel use, grounded upon northern experience, were irrelevant, for "a larger dose of any medicine will be required in a southern climate to produce a given effect in a disease where the liver is deeply implicated than in a northern, in consequence of the continued excitement — to which this organ is subjected in southern latitudes."[7]

The place southern physicians assigned to venesection in their practice, compared with that of the North, presented an inverted image of the patterns exhibited by quinine and calomel. "The general experience of physicians," one southern practitioner commented on pneumonia, "is, that the loss of much blood is not so well borne, nor its curative influence so favorably exerted in this as in Northern climates."[8] Both plethora and systemic overstimulation, conventional indications for therapeutic depletion by venesection, were identified with cold climates, and therefore bloodletting was regarded as more appropriate for northern constitutions and diseases. A physician in Monroe, Louisiana, typically noted in his diary in 1819 that the fevers prevailing in his region were sufficiently debilitating so "as not to admit the cure of the Lancet except in very few cases and those of persons who had lately arrived from the North and were very robust."[9] Eli Geddings, lecturing on the institutes and practice of medicine at the Medical College of South Carolina in 1861, told his students that not only venesection but antiphlogistic therapies in general were ill suited to the conditions of southern practice. But he cautioned his pupils that if they moved to another region, its environment could well demand the use of the lancet. "I wish you to understand," he told them in a lecture on pneumonia, "that the treatment, I am now to recomend is not designed for the disease, as it occurs now. But as many of you may practice in other parts of the world, it is my duty to state to you the management of the inflammatory variety. The treatment of the later is in the main antiphlogistic."[10]

Not all categories of medical knowledge were affected by such regional considerations in the same way. Physicians were very selective in the aspects of medicine they identified as regionally variable, and premised their judgments upon a fundamental division of medicine into knowledge about medical practice on the one hand and about the basic sciences on the other. Even the most strident proponents of a distinctive southern medicine held that the principles of anatomy, chemistry, and physiology, as well as the mechanical manipulations of dentistry and surgery, were not modified by local conditions, and were therefore universal in their generation and validation. But this was not true of region-specific knowledge about medical practice, encompassing diagnosis, prognosis, and medical therapeutics, which physicians claimed was distinctively southern. Edward Hall Barton, a Louisiana spokesman for southern medical distinctiveness and the case for educational separatism it supported, could state with conviction in 1835 that "southern practitioners *must* be taught in the south" and yet be innocent of duplicity when he qualified this claim in his next sentence, saying, "These remarks are not at all intended to deny that the principles of medicine are universal, and that they are, in general, the same every where; but the very nature of man is so modified by the diversities of climate, that it is often indispensible to have a personal experience of them to make successful applications."[11]

William W. Cozart, a North Carolina student attending medical lectures in Charleston, developed this theme in his thesis entitled "The Place where Southern Students Should Acquire Their Medical Knowledge" (1856). "The general principles of Medicine may be communicated by teachers that are competent without regard to locality," he asserted.

> But the case is different in respect to particular ones, and their application to practice; those differing wherever the peculiarities of localities differ. And it is well known by the medical profession that diseases are modified by these places, and other circumstances; and in order that these indications should be met successfully, the adaptation of the treatment must be varied accord-

ingly. The faculties of every institution teaches what they have observed of diseases, and the plan they pursued in the treatment of them, during their own practice. In fact, their practice is their teaching. And as the northern diseases differ materially in their characters from the southern, the advantages therefore, southern students have by attending southern Colleges are no doubt considerable.

The southern graduate of a Philadelphia or New York medical school, Cozart claimed, "returns home in high spirits and with bright anticipations, 'sticks out his shingle,' ready and very willing to go to work." But however thorough his knowledge of medical science, he was destined to fail in practice, treating his first patients, in accordance with northern teachings, with general bloodletting and sedative medicines that produced dire results. "Now his bright anticipations are clouded; disappointments discourage him; and a sad experience teaches him that the instructive lessons of a northern institution will not answer, in the treatment of southern diseases. He cannot now under the circumstances establish an extensive practice," Cozart concluded; "the confidence of the people in him is shaken, he is neglected; despised, and soon forgotten."[12]

The plain fact that the precepts informing medical practice were region-specific, as well as southern physicians' inclination to stress the dissimilarities between medicine in their region and elsewhere, tend to overemphasize the fractionalization of medical knowledge during the antebellum period. Underlying the regionally variable character of medicine as a body of knowledge was the basic assumption that the attributes of knowledge in the North and South were identical. The same fundamental rules directed the generation and validation of medical knowledge in both the North and South. This is crucial for assessing the argument for southern medical distinctiveness, for it means that those physicians who vigorously affirmed the particularity of southern medical knowledge at the same time unwaveringly maintained that a single epistemology governed knowledge regarding medical practice in all regions.

The basis for southern physicians' argument for regional medical distinctiveness, the idea that the knowledge best suited to southern practice had to be produced and tested in the South to match southern circumstances, therefore was fundamentally grounded upon an aspect of medical knowledge, its epistemology, that they shared with American physicians elsewhere and deemed to be universal. The growing allegiance to empiricism that came to dominate clinical epistemology from the 1820s implied that the knowledge most appropriate to guide practice was that gained within a context closely resembling the one in which it was to be applied in both type of patient and physical and social environments. By close observation of the effects of treatments for a patient with particular symptoms, habits, constitution, and surroundings, the physician derived therapeutic precepts that would be reliable under similar conditions; but whether or not these precepts were transferable to other conditions had to be ascertained independently. Knowledge befitting southern medicine was, accordingly, most suitably acquired through direct experience with southern practice. This was not an oddly southern perception: physicians in all parts of the United States drew similarly localistic conclusions from the same epistemological precepts. Moreover, by avowedly sharing the assumptions about the nature of medical knowledge held by other American physicians, southern practitioners were constrained to construct a distinctively southern body of knowledge and practice within the limits imposed by this epistemology. It was precisely because an epistemology that could justify the existence of distinctive local knowledge dominated regular medical thought in all regions of America, and because it plainly supplied the premises for erecting and legitimizing a singularly southern medicine, that the southern argument for regional medical distinctiveness was in itself not at all distinctive.

In fact, the notion that there must be a separate body of medical knowledge for the South was only one expression of the principle of specificity, a principle central to the belief system of American physicians of all regions. Medical treatment was not specific to disease (indeed, disease-specific treatment implied a routinism that was a stigma of quackery), but did have to be sensitively matched to the specific characteristics of individual patients and the peculiarities of the environments in which they became ill and were treated.[13] Therapeutic principles that aptly directed the treatment of immigrants might be invalid as guides to the treatment of native-born patients, and analogous discriminations were based upon age, gender, social class, and moral status. It was entirely in keeping with the doctrine of specificity that physicians were able to develop notions about the peculiarity of Negro physiology and therapeutic requirements that were sustained by prevailing medical theory.

Medical management was similarly specific to such idiosyncrasies of place as climate, population density, and topography. For example, American physicians commonly held that the physical and social environments of a city molded the constitutions of its inhabitants and their diseases in ways that required treatments unlike those for rural populations. A Boston practitioner, struck in 1843 by the more malignant character of fevers in the surrounding countryside, typically wondered "whether the stronger febrile tendency in places which have so much the advantage of the city in purity of air, &c., may not depend somewhat upon the more stimulating and gross diet made use of in the country, especially in the excess of animal food?"[14] Medical literature often depicted conventional images of the robust farmer and the debilitated city dweller, applying these caricatures to pathological conditions and to the therapeutic measures called for by them. "The peculiar mode of living in large cities," a professor of medicine in Lexington, Kentucky, told his students in 1838, changed the type of inflammation found in urban residents. "Their diseases," he proposed, "are much more of a nervous character than sanguinous. The treatment of the same disease, Erysipelas for instance, in one of those large towns and here would be entirely different[;] in one case you would stimulate[,] in the other debilitate."[15] Knowledge generated by urban practice was of dubious relevance for the country physician, for it might, as in this instance, dictate the opposite of the treatment actually required by the individual case.

Similar considerations informed American physicians' attitudes toward European therapeutic knowledge. A western practitioner visiting London in 1845 was impressed by the extent to which treatment for inflammatory affections differed from the therapeutic strategy that would have been pursued in the United States. "A course of practice which with us would prove successful," he wrote to the readers of the *Western Lancet*, which he edited, "would necessarily be fatal here from its very activity." Particularly surprised by the success achieved in London with very limited therapeutic use of calomel and bloodletting, he attributed the former to "the debilitated and broken down constitutions so commonly met with here," and said of the latter,

> That bleeding should be tolerated here to a less extent than in the United States, is not surprising; and that tonics and stimulants should find an extensive and appropriate application, is what might be anticipated from the habits and other modifying circumstances that so powerfully influence the constitutions of the inhabitants of London; and hence it is that iron, quinine, porter, wine &c, are frequently employed, when an American physician would resort to depletion.[16]

Instruction given in American medical schools reflected these perceptions. A South Carolinian attending medical lectures at Transylvania University in 1828 recorded in his class notebook that inflammation was "modified by a variety of circumstances. . . . [L]ocation or situation modified [it]. In *Paris* we would stimulate by Porter, Bark &c — In Kentucky we would bleed & purge."[17]

The sorts of factors that made urban knowledge suspect for rural patients and European knowledge suspect for American patients also led physicians in all regions of the United States to maintain that therapeutic and prognostic knowledge suitable for one part of the country might be inapplicable or even dangerous in another. A type of perception common during the first two-thirds of the 19th century was reflected by the medical student in Cincinnati who, summarizing his teacher's comments in 1834, wrote in his class notes: "Says 10 grs. of calomel is as effectual in Pennsylvania, as 50 in the Valey of the Mississippi."[18] Knowledge about practice could not be freely transferred from one region to another, but rather had to be revalidated for use in a context other than that in which it was produced. "It may be proper to state my practice has been chiefly within the city of Boston," a physician of that city stated as a prefacing caveat to reporting his own experiences using the lancet and leeches in treating scarlatina. "As the situation of the place, and of course, its climate and soil, the customs and manners of the inhabitants, may have great influence in varying the type of acute diseases, a difference in the mode of treatment [else-where] may not only be proper, but required."[19] There was no fundamental difference between the assumptions about medical knowledge underlying his remarks and those supporting the argument for southern medical distinctiveness.

One of the most persistent misconceptions about medical practice in antebellum America is that treatment was generally rote,[20] but this is belied by extant indicators of actual practice. While in principle physicians' commitment to specificity dictated treatment that varied according to circumstances, among the most striking features of records of practice from the period are the complexity and diversity that marked prescribing habits. Like their counterparts in other regions of the country, most southern practitioners were not doctrinaire in their therapeutic practices, and did not routinely bleed or give calomel, quinine, or opium. As the principles articulated by the theorists of southern medicine predicted, calomel and quinine were undeniably among the most widely prescribed drugs; however, even these medicaments were not given as a matter of course. Venesection, on the other hand, was practiced on only a small fraction of the South's sick. These usage patterns are evident in the records of practice of a dozen antebellum southern physicians selected for their geographic and temporal diversity. Venesection, for example, although declining in the South as elsewhere between the 1810s and the Civil War, was never used by these physicians on more than about 6 percent of their visits.[21] These ledgers and practice books, far from reflecting a minimalist reading of the *Pharmacopeia*, present impressive variety within each physician's armamentarium. Further evident is a striking diversity among practitioners, some with characteristic penchants reflecting in part the fact that similar therapeutic ends could sometimes be attained through a variety of means.

The widespread application of the principle of specificity to medical practice and to the assessment of medical knowledge both within and without the South plainly demonstrates that the conceptual bases of the southern argument for regional medical distinctiveness were in no way singular. It is further possible to establish the lack of southern particularity in the premises and character of the content of the argument for southern medical distinctiveness by displaying its didactic origins. Not only were the assumptions underlying this argument shared by northern physicians, but to a large extent the argument was actually acquired in the North, and through northern institutions, by southerners who brought it back to the South and exploited it.

The notion that the characteristic attributes of place modified disease and indications for treatment had been a part of medical thought for over two millennia, embodied most prominently in the Hippocratic treatise *On Airs, Waters, and Places* and Sydenham's formulation of the epidemic constitution and its influences. But in late 18th- and early 19th-century America, a dual impetus mobilized energies to establish the particularity of American nature, including its diseases. In part, Americans were driven by an ideal of cultural independence, a desire to free themselves intellectually, as politically, from their colonial status. At the same time, they were responding to European disparagements of the New World as a habitat and charges of the inherently valetudinarian character of American nature. The late 18th-century French Buffon–de Pauw thesis in particular, which postulated the physical degeneracy of animal life in the New World, elicited a concerted effort by the Jeffersonians to vindicate their continent by demonstrating that American nature was indeed distinctive, but decidedly superior.

In medicine, the case for the exceptionalism of American nature was expressed most forcefully in the endeavor to establish that the American environment, both physical and social, shaped disease and medical need in ways that demanded the existence of a distinctively American medical practice. This position was expounded particularly in Philadelphia, the geographic epicenter of the Jeffersonian circle. For example, Benjamin Rush, professor of the theory and practice of medicine at the University of Pennsylvania from 1789 to 1813 and the most prominent medical member of the cadre of men who best represented Jeffersonian philosophy, believed that political and social organization, the physical environment, and health were all linked, making disease and treatment functions of both place and culture. Rush fully embraced the implications of this posture for medical regionalism and nationalism. Benjamin Smith Barton, another member of the Jeffersonian circle, succeeded Rush in the Pennsylvania chair and held it until his death in 1815. He shared Rush's

allegiances to medical nationalism and regionalism, and sought to further a distinctively American medicine by his own investigations on the uses of American plants in the treatment of American diseases. Barton's successor, Nathaniel Chapman, who occupied the chair from 1816 to 1850, disagreed in many respects with Rush, his preceptor, but resolutely shared the elder physician's belief in the adaptation of medicine to place. Chapman's medical nationalism, which was of an aggressively chauvinistic bent, was objectified in his founding of the *Philadelphia Journal of the Medical and Physical Sciences* in 1820 as a forum for developing an American medical culture to rival that of Europe.[22]

All three men urged in their lectures that American conditions produced more energetic diseases, which demanded more forcefully sedative treatments than those of Europe. This idea that American diseases were singularly vigorous, like Jeffersonian claims that there were live mammoths roaming somewhere on the North American continent, aided the refutation of the Buffon–de Pauw thesis by demonstrating the vitality of organic life in America on a scale unmatched in Europe. A North Carolina student attending Rush's lectures in 1811 copied in his notebook, "More attention is necessary to the natural history of the United States than would strike you at first, as our diseases differ so much from those of Europe." In most diseased conditions, "the Citizens of the United States will require . . . [copious depletion] more than the Natives of Europe."[23] Barton echoed this view in his lectures four years later. The stimulant cinchona bark, a student transcribing Barton's lectures recorded,

> has not been infrequently employed in Erysipelas particularly in Europe. But in the U. States the disease differs essentially from what it is in Europe. In Europe it is in general attended [by] prostration of strength and debility, and requires the invigorating method of cure. But in the U. States this disease is in general one of the Phlegmasia of an inflammatory character and requires the antiphlogistic method of cure.

The same pattern held in other diseases; chorea, for example, assumed a debilitated form "in the enervated and enfeebled inhabitants of Europe. But in the U. States where the Blessings of Liberty are combined with the numerous other causes in developing the Physical man, this disease is usually of the tonic and sthenic character," calling for alternating bleeding and purging.[24]

The Philadelphia faculty's allegiance to medical nationalism and regionalism was of seminal importance to the argument for southern medical distinctiveness. From the start of the century through the end of the antebellum period, Philadelphia was the most influential center for the formal training of southern physicians. A large number of southern medical students attended lectures in Philadelphia before, and even after, the emergence of southern medical schools. Moreover, when medical schools were established in the South, their faculties were substantially Philadelphia trained; when the region's first medical school opened in Charleston in 1823, nearly all of its faculty had received their formal medical education in Philadelphia. A very large proportion of the most vocal advocates of southern medical distinctiveness had attended medical lectures in Philadelphia, among them Edward Hall Barton, Daniel Warren Brickell, Samuel Adolphus Cartwright, Samuel Henry Dickson, Paul Fitzsimmons Eve, and Josiah Clark Nott. The links to Philadelphia teachings among other leading proponents of southern medical distinctiveness are less direct but nonetheless clear. For example, Erasmus Darwin Fenner, the most articulate exponent of a distinctive southern medical education, received his M.D. degree in 1830 at Transylvania University, where he studied with Charles Caldwell. A pupil of Rush at the University of Pennsylvania, where he had taught for several years prior to an altercation with his former mentor, Caldwell not only urged in his lectures at Transylvania (and, later, at Louisville) the necessity of regional and national variations in medical knowledge and practice, but Fenner also credited him with being the first to extend a recognition of medical regionalism to a coherent case for the propriety of regional medical education.[25]

The fact that in the years before the Civil War literally hundreds of southern medical students annually elected to go to Philadelphia was in no sense a denial of the singularity of southern medical practice. Just as American physicians traveled to the hospitals of Europe in growing numbers during the antebellum period to gain knowledge about medical science despite their belief that European practice was doubtfully applicable to American patients, so too southern students could seek medical knowledge in Philadelphia while remaining wary of the practical precepts taught there. Thus when a South Carolina physician considering going to Philadelphia for further professional study wrote to Josiah Nott for advice in the mid-1830s, Nott counseled that advantages for professional improvement in Philadelphia were unmatched elsewhere in the United States, but cautioned him against placing too much faith in northern practice. Nott especially recommended the opportunities for gaining pathological knowledge and studying physical diagnosis with the clinician William Wood Gerhard, adding, "You will see I think much to object to in Gerhard's practice — but he is a profound pathologist."[26]

One southerner studying in Philadelphia confidently asserted that "as for learning the theoretical part of Medicine and studying those branches on which we must found our practice (as Anatomy & Physiology) Philadelphia presents as many advantages perhaps as any other place in the united states."[27] But at the same time he recognized the advantages of home education in practice itself, and applauded a fellow North Carolinian's decision to attend medical lectures in Charleston rather than outside the South, commenting that "the practice there will correspond better with that of our country."[28] Similarly, a North Carolina physician who had received his medical training at the University of Pennsylvania and proudly referred in later years to "my old master Dr. Rush" not only named his son Benjamin Rush Norcom but also sent him to the University of Pennsylvania for medical lectures after he had completed an apprenticeship with his father. Yet, despite his overt, genuine allegiance to the Philadelphia school, the father did not question the superiority of southern therapeutic knowledge for treating patients in that region. He noted in a letter to his son in Philadelphia, "We know better, here, how to manage carolina constitutions than the Physicians of Philadelphia."[29]

One message that was crystalline in the lectures delivered at the University of Pennsylvania attended by many of the southerners who led the drive for regional medical distinctiveness was that medical practice necessarily differed in the North and South. Rush told his students that such differentiae of the regions as climate, miasmatic exhalations, diet, dress, work habits, and social structure altered the symptoms of diseases and appropriate therapeutics, stating unambiguously, "Diseases of warm & cold climates require different treatment."[30] Chapman, acknowledging the same fact, at times explicitly qualified therapeutic dicta in his lectures by saying that they might be inapplicable in hot climates.[31] "Do not prescribe for the name of the disease," a southern student attending Chapman's lectures in Philadelphia copied into his notebook.

> The same disease varies at different seasons and in different parts of the Country. In no one is this more illustrated than in bilious Fever[.] In this City and section of the Country it is a disease very different in its nature and requiring different treatment from what it is farther to the South. Here it is almost uniformly inflamatory, exacting for its management the very constant and profuse use of the lancet, but in the Carolinas and Georgia this must be wholly laid aside, or sparingly & discriminately employed.[32]

In another lecture Chapman noted that "the mercurial treatment of dysentery is much more called for in warm climates, where the liver is generally affected."[33] Indeed, prevailing southern judgments on the necessary peculiarities of the use of venesection, calomel, and quinine in that region are all apparent in Philadelphian teachings.

Lectures at other northern schools where southern students matriculated conveyed a similar message. David Hosack, who had received his M.D. degree at the University of Pennsylvania in 1791, routinely drew attention to regional diversity in medical practice in his lectures at the College of Physicians and Surgeons in New York, where he taught from 1807 to 1826. "As each climate produces particular diseases," he observed, "attention should be paid to it. In warm climates, most disorders arise from debility." But, he continued,

> in cold climates there is considerable vigour in the system, together with nervous energy. The inhabitants of the North* are for the most part exempt from those bilious disorders, consequent to warm climates, but they are subject to Inflammatory affections and bear copious depletion, and are also more able to undergo the operation of medicine than those of a warmer region.[34]

Regional variations in individual therapeutic practices, such as the use of cinchona bark, were accounted for within this framework. "In hot climates," Hosack explained, "the bark is resorted to because they have to counteract the putrescent tendency[,] but in this climate it is injurious and useless."[35]

In saying that medical knowledge and practice in their region were distinctive, southern physicians were, then, not unique. Nor was there anything in its essence idiosyncratic about the premises underlying their case for regional distinctiveness or about the rules they used in its formulation. Yet, in one respect, the argument for southern medical distinctiveness was singular — not in its content, or assumptions about medical knowledge and practice, but in the emotion, the force, the stridency that informed the way it was argued.

The stridency of the argument for southern medical distinctiveness is revealed by the tenor of rhetoric in which it was voiced, rhetoric characterized by an urgency seldom so persistently expressed in regular medical literature, save for denunciations of medical sectary. Physicians frequently cast their case for the individuality of southern practice in language that evoked the crusading sense of a sociopolitical movement, as when the editors of a New Orleans journal urged that in medical education, "It is the 'manifest destiny' of the South to become each year more and more independent."[36] "Too long has the South been slumbering in inactivity," charged a Georgia medical editor urging the same point. "Hitherto she has been the passive pupil of science, content to draw her knowledge from foreign sources; but the voice that drives away her slumbers shall arouse her to emulation, and the South shall disdain to borrow what she can herself so copiously supply."[37] It was not accidental that the advocates of southern medical distinctiveness often chose agricultural metaphors to present their case in ways calculated to produce emotional resonance in their readers or listeners; as Drew Gilpin Faust has shown, the images of agriculture offered exceptionally potent symbols through which southerners could better understand and express the sources of stress within the social order.[38] "The most scientific farmer in England will not be equal to the Southern planter in growing cotton, sugar, rice, maize, [or] tobacco," asserted Bennet Dowler, a New Orleans physician and physiologist. Similarly, he claimed, "The British physician may know more of the typhus fever among the paupers of his native land, than the Southern physician; but the former might not be equal to the latter in the medical treatment of negroes and whites in the Southern States."[39] As a Tennessee practitioner argued, "Medicine, like disease, must spring from the very elements, soil, sunshine, moisture, etc., that produce disease."[40]

The fact that southern physicians saw the case for southern medical distinctiveness as an inspiration for medical activity further exhibits the peculiar strength of this idea in the South. This is best demonstrated by the express modeling of southern schools and literature in conformity with the ideal of a distinctive southern practice, but it is also illustrated by other forms of action less arguably motivated by economics. Medical societies used regional specificity as a rationale for investigating the peculiarities of climate, disease, and treatment in their locales, and the products of this enterprise offer the best counterexample to the largely correct assertion that antebellum medical societies were sociopolitical organizations void of serious scientific activity.[41] Reports on the topography, meteorology, diseases, and therapeutics of a single county or district abounded in late antebellum southern medical journals, and many medical theses were of the same genre. "It is a fact which reason would suggest, and which experience has verified, that the varied circumstances of soil, climate & local peculiarities presented by a country, do in numerous ways engender and modify disease," a student at the Medical Department of the University of Nashville began his thesis in 1851. "Hence the necessity of investigating these circumstances and peculiarities, that we may be able . . . to treat disease more successfully."[42] A student at the Medical College of the State of South Carolina who wrote his thesis on "The Topography of South Alabama and the Diseases Incident to Its Climate" (1843) similarly noted that study of the modifying influences of a particular region was an obligation of a proper physician.[43] That the argument for southern medical distinctiveness often explicitly informed such endeavors demonstrates that the force powering it was sufficient to direct action as well as engender rhetoric.

Medical theory regnant during the antebellum period and the unmistakable diversity presented by the American habitat and peoples were sufficient to make the serious discussion of regional differences by physicians inevitable. But they do not explain why southern physicians so energetically took up the case for medical specificity in their region as their own and aggressively pleaded its cardinal importance in directing southern medicine. Southern physicians recognized that the doctrine of specificity, duly applied to the environmental variation existing within the South, pointed to substantial fluctuations in medical practice in different sections of their region. Yet, while they acknowledged the importance of this diversity (hence the abundance of local studies), southern physicians placed far greater emphasis upon those modifying circumstances that characterized the South as a discrete unit. Further, they proselytized the idea of southern medical distinctiveness with a vigor unmatched in other regions of America in analogous contexts; neither northern attention to America's dissimilarities from Europe nor western emphasis upon the disparities between its environment and that of the Northeast exhibited such zeal. That emotion, that force is what must be explained to understand what was uniquely southern about the argument for southern medical distinctiveness.

Much of the force that impelled the case for southern medical particularity must be ascribed to the same engines that drove southerners from a variety of occupations in their rising defense of the southern way of life. It was patently not by happenstance that the growing preoccupation with regional distinctiveness in southern medicine chronologically paralleled the larger movement in the South toward economic, cultural, and political sectionalism and nationalism from the early 1830s. Tensions inevitably engendered by the South's colonial agrarian economy, reliance upon slavery, and diminished political power, augmented by a regional sensibility piqued by external charges of immorality, intellectual sloth, and social retrogression, imbued all questions of the region's particularity with a strong emotional vibrancy. Further, southern medical editors and educators, functioning within a medical marketplace in which competition for subscribers and students was acute, had a potent economic incentive for using the argument for southern medical distinctiveness to underscore the advantages of regional medical literature and schools. All of these considerations are cogent, and important. Nevertheless, implying that southern physicians promoted their arguments for southern medical distinctiveness simply because they were southerners, or because they were driven by invidious economic incentives, explains away as much as it explains.

The force that propelled the argument for southern medical distinctiveness was in large measure a product of anxieties experienced by southern physicians whose identities, and not just livelihoods, were bound up with both their region and profession. The pivot upon which physicians' anxieties turned was the low, marginal status of the medical profession in the South, a phenomenon expressed in several interrelated ways. To begin with, southern physicians routinely lamented the low esteem in which their profession as a whole was held by the public. The notorious difficulty of maintaining a financially successful practice, they maintained, manifested a dearth of public faith and support for regular physicians, a circumstance encouraged by sectarian competition and displayed by sectarian successes. Moreover, southern physicians were acutely aware of the disparaging judgments pronounced upon the medical endeavor in their region by prominent members of the medical profession in the North. Authoritative northern assertions of the inferiority of southern practices and theories were made more grating by the undeniable institutional and intellectual dependence upon the North by southern practitioners. Finally, thinking southern physicians plainly perceived intellectual lethargy to be a characteristic feature of the medical profession in their region, and regarded the lack of an active professional community to appreciate and reward medical enterprise as both a cause and illustration of the region's professional degradation.

Many southern physicians saw in the celebration of southern medical distinctiveness a means of alleviating the anxieties that stemmed from the low status of the medical profession in the South. The singular force that drove this argument and the ways that southern physicians believed it was linked to both the sources and solutions of the profession's distress are discerned in a reconstruction of medical history that became common in the late antebellum South. During the 1840s and 1850s, such self-proclaimed leaders of southern medicine as Cartwright, Dowler, Fenner, and Nott fashioned

a Whiggish reconstruction of professional history that took on the role and form of a distinctively southern professional myth. Constructed to explain the low status of medicine in the South and the means of its elevation, this mythologized history was driven by the same animus that imparted such force to the argument for the distinctiveness of southern medical practice.

The "true regular science of medicine," this history held, originated in a southern climate, the Greece of Hippocrates, and in this southern cradle it approached perfection. Erected from observations of southern climates, constitutions, and diseases, the principles of this medicine were matched to southern needs, and were still suited to many of the medical needs of the American South. But southern medicine, boasting an unrivaled intellectual vitality at a time when, according to Fenner, "London and Paris, Edinburgh, Dublin and Vienna, were in a state of barbarism,"[44] did not retain its dominance. Medicine flourished in the southern latitude of Rome "until," as one Atlanta professor told an entering class of medical students, "the floods of vandal barbarism poured down upon the doomed city, from the plains of the North, and bore off upon their dark and turbid bosom, almost every trace of learning and refinement."[45] The looted remnants of superior southern medicine were taken to cold latitudes, and there were distorted to meet northern needs.

The objective of this historical account was to show that the medicine practiced by some regular southern physicians in mid-19th-century America, and learned by them through northern institutions, was not true regular medicine, but rather a "reformed" system suited to the climate of the northern parts of America and Europe. According to the historical narrative, which was cast in a loose temporal framework typical of myth, medical sovereignty passed almost directly from Rome to Edinburgh, a city characterized as a cold, desolate outpost on the northernmost boundary of civilization. There, medicine was reformed to suit the peculiar requirements of the Edinburgh environment; according to Cartwright, "a new nomenclature was there made to embrace the new order of diseases observed, new theories invented, and a new practice adopted to suit the diseases in that little hyperborean corner of the globe."[46] This reformed system of medicine was transplanted to

America when pupils of the Edinburgh school established what Cartwright called a branch school in Philadelphia, at the University of Pennsylvania, and taught Edinburgh medicine until it attained national dominance.[47]

However, this reformed system was fundamentally inappropriate for southern medical practice. Treatment as it was transformed to suit a northern climate "under the auspices of Cullen and his followers," an Alabama physician told the delegates to the state medical association's annual meeting in 1855, "became quite too frigid for the ardent temperament and more relaxed system of our 'Sunny South.'"[48] Northern lecturers and writings therefore taught a reformed system of medical knowledge and practice fitting for their regions, but deceptive and dangerous for the southern practitioner. Much of the uncertainty and want of confidence that did exist in southern practice was due to the reliance of some southern physicians upon improper northern authority, a continual source of corruption, rather than upon their own experience at the southern bedside or the observations of other physicians practicing in the South. The underlying message this version of medical history bore was that physicians of the South could elevate their professional standing and regain for the South its position of leadership in medicine by throwing off the hegemony of a reformed system of medicine never designed for use in the South, by observing southern diseases and treatments for themselves, and by restoring true regular medicine.

The same historical framework was also used to account for the flourishing state of medical sectarianism in the South. The Edinburgh reform, in Cartwright's assessment, "was all well enough for that little place on the globe, but it went farther and imposed the same reformed physic on the rest of the world."[49] To meet Edinburgh's sthenic, inflammatory fevers, the diseases of "a climate that almost forces the red blood through the skin," northern reformers had properly relied principally on the lancet and antiphlogistic drugs. However, adherence to this treatment was harmful in dealing with southern fevers, which were often of a more debilitated or asthenic character, leading to unsuccessful therapeutic management that encouraged public disillusionment with the regular profession and fostered the rise of quackery. Moreover, Cartwright argued, stimulants and hot fiery drugs

such as peppers, which were called for by diseases in the South, had been cast out from the reformed armamentarium because they were not useful in treating the diseases of Edinburgh. Cayenne pepper, a mainstay of Thomsonian practice, was therefore more appropriate to the needs of southern patients than were many of the remedies of the reformed system of medicine practiced by regular physicians, a situation that accounted for Thomsonian successes.[50] The regrettable allegiance of some physicians to medical knowledge of European and northern provenance blinded them to the value of drugs such as red pepper and lobelia in treating southern diseases, Cartwright confided in a letter to a nonphysician friend, driving many patients to embrace Thomsonianism and reject the regular profession.[51]

The use of history as a tool for explanation, legitimation, and affirmation of links with tradition was commonplace in 19th-century American medicine. For some southern physicians, the retelling of this particular account of the historical course of southern medicine assumed the cadence of a ritual. A stylized narrative recounted as a preface to calls for professional vigor and improvement in southern medicine, the story served functions conventionally attributed to myth. It explained why medicine in the South occupied its present degraded status, and how this had come to be. Further, it exemplified proper values for the professional culture, clarifying what was important, and set role models. For example, Hippocrates was the archetypal southern physician, for rather than relying on established wisdom he observed for himself southern diseases, peoples, and environments, thereby developing morbid natural histories and therapeutic strategies appropriate to southern patients.[52] Moreover, this story aided the legitimation of a self-conscious effort to develop, or redevelop, a distinctive southern medicine by demonstrating its ancient roots and modern corruption. The repetition of this narrative was also a source of creative power and control. It projected a model of professional redemption bearing the message that in order to elevate in their region what Eve called "this much abused, but little comprehended, this neglected and now degraded, this noble, this God-like Profession,"[53] southern physicians needed to follow the Hippocratic example, recognize the distinctive character of southern medicine, and liberate themselves from northern and European authority.

Regarded within the context of this reconstruction of professional history and the functions it was designed to serve, the argument for southern medical distinctiveness clearly had taken on attributes that Clifford Geertz has ascribed to ideologies. "The attempt of ideologies to render otherwise incomprehensible social situations meaningful, to so construe them as to make it possible to act purposefully within them," he suggests, accounts for "the intensity with which, once accepted, they are held."[54] Geertz's model of an ideology as a response to social, cultural, and psychological strains helps to clarify the strident advocacy by physicians of the idea of southern medical distinctiveness, which made understandable the degraded status of the medical profession in the South. The specific contours of these strains as southern physicians experienced them are plainly identified by the problems this reconstructed professional history sought to explain and begin to resolve. Southern physicians had developed a minority consciousness like that of their region. Aware of their collective loss of status, southern physicians saw themselves located on the periphery of creative activity and institutional power in medicine, and their rhetoric lucidly reveals their experience of marginality, isolation, and alienation.[55] Assessing their position vis-à-vis the North, thinking physicians in the South perceived a disturbing dependency, inferiority, and consequent humiliation.

A fervently argued case for southern medical distinctiveness represented one means of alleviating these burdens. As I have suggested elsewhere, the preoccupation of some southern physicians with their region's peculiar medical problems, and with the need for a singularly southern body of medical knowledge and practice this implied, was driven by a reform animus.[56] Medical men in the South saw in the argument for southern medical distinctiveness a platform for energizing and thereby elevating the medical profession in their region. A distinctive southern medicine promised to remedy the low standing of the profession in the South by raising the public's regard for regular physicians' abilities to heal, thereby scotching sectarian competition; by releasing southern practitioners from their dependence upon the North and Europe, opening up the possibilities of scientific and institutional parity; and by activating the medical community, augmenting both its cognitive and social power. This argument was of special importance to the southern physician with intellectual aspirations, for it offered an avenue to the justification and vitalization of the intellectual life of medicine in the South.

Thus while the basic assumptions about the nature of medical knowledge that underlay the argument for southern medical distinctiveness were shared by physicians outside the South as well as within it, its energetic promulgation was at once a response to the epidemiological, ethnic, and climatic realities of the southern environment; a tool in southern competition for economic advantage and social influence with the traditional loci of professional power, northern medical institutions; and a contribution to the growing impulse toward southern nationalism. But at the most fundamental level, the case for the particularity of southern medical practice was driven by anxieties and needs that pertained especially to the situation of the thinking physician who practiced his profession in the South. It was the promise that such physicians saw in the idea of a distinctively southern medicine to motivate action, to catalyze the realization of their aspirations for the medical profession in the South, that accounts in large measure for the intensity with which they asserted their region's medical singularity. In this respect, the argument for southern medical distinctiveness was distinctively southern.

Yet, at the core of this judgment of distinctiveness is an inescapable irony. There can be no doubt that the collective experience of physicians in the antebellum South is properly characterized by their self-perceived marginality, isolation, low professional status and lack of community appreciation, economic uncertainty, dependence upon external sources for innovation and external institutions for the dissemination of knowledge, as well as by defensiveness rooted in a consciousness of inferiority. But in varying degrees, and with due regard to the cultural diversity existing within the profession, these same attributes precisely characterize the experience of the American physician during the same period. Isolated from the medical centers of Europe yet dependent upon them for both new knowledge and synthetic instruction; working in a profession accorded a dubiously high standing in American society; competing for uncertain financial security with irregulars whom society granted equal legal, and often social, status; alienated from European physicians researching on the cutting edge of medical science, and within an American culture known for its valuation of practice over learning; and conscious of their inferiority to Europe in medical institutions and the pursuit of medical science, American physicians, taken as a whole, mirrored an image of the problems of southern physicians that was dimmer but nonetheless whole. The experience of the physician in the Old South, embodying in exaggerated form anxieties of their professional counterparts in other regions, may best epitomize the experience of the antebellum American physician. Regarded in this way, the argument for southern medical distinctiveness was in its essence a southern response to problems felt in varying degrees by medical practitioners in all regions of America.

## NOTES

This paper was supported in part by NIH Grant 03910-01, -02 from the National Library of Medicine; an award from an Arthur Vining Davis Foundation grant to the Department of Social Medicine and Health Policy, Harvard Medical School; a Charlotte W. Newcombe Dissertation Fellowship; and NSF Grant SES-8107609. I am most grateful for this support.

1 Among the most useful studies are James O. Breeden "States-rights medicine in the Old South," *Bull. N.Y. Acad. Med.*, 1968-1969, *52*: 29–45; John Duffy, "Medical practice in the ante bellum South," *J. Southern Hist.*, 1959, *25*: 53–72; *idem*, "A note on antebellum southern nationalism and medical practice," *J. Southern Hist.*, 1968, *34*: 266–276; James Denny Guillory, "Southern nationalism and the Louisiana medical profession, 1840–1860" (M.A. thesis, Louisiana State Univ., 1965); Mary Louise Marshall, "Samuel A. Cartwright and states' rights medicine," *New Orleans Med. & Surg. J.*, 1940, *93*: 74–78; and Richard Harrison Shryock, "Medical practice in the Old South," *South Atlantic Quart.*, 1930, *29*: 160–178.

2 On the use of this argument to support medical schools, see John Duffy, "Sectional conflict and medical education in Louisiana," *J. Southern Hist.*, 1957, *23*: 289–306, and John Harley Warner, "A southern medical reform: the meaning of the antebellum argument for southern medical education," *Bull. Hist. Med.*, 1983, *57*: 364–381.

3 John McCardell, *The Idea of a Southern Nation: Southern Nationalists and Southern Nationalism, 1830–1860* (New York and London: W. W. Norton and Co., 1979), pp. 204–205. Of an extensive historical literature analyzing antebellum southern calls for cultural distinctiveness and self-sufficiency, McCardell gives the most synthetic account.

4 W[illia]m A. Booth, "Observations and remarks upon the action of the sulphate of quinine," *New Orleans Med. & Surg. J.*, 1848–1849, *5*: 15–16, quotation on p. 16.

5 William Octavius Eversfield, Notes from Lectures on Therapeutics and Materia Medica by Dr. [John Staige] Davis, University of Virginia, 1859–1860, lecture of May 12, 1860, William Octavius Eversfield Notebooks, Manuscripts Department, Alderman Library, University of Virginia, Charlottesville.

6 John P. Caffry, "A thesis on calomel in southern fevers" (M.D. thesis, Medical College of the State of South Carolina, 1839), South Carolina Room, Main Library, Medical University of South Carolina, Charleston. My intention here is to stress the perceived links during the antebellum period between environment and therapeutic knowledge and practice; accordingly, I have chosen not to explicate the substantial diversity of opinion that existed on most therapeutic questions or the change in belief over time.

7 Jeremiah Butt, Jr., "A dissertation on the influence of climate" (M.D. thesis, Medical College of the State of South Carolina, 1835), South Carolina Room, Main Library, Medical University of South Carolina. The original orthography is preserved in all quotations.

8 "Dr. Ames on the treatment of pneumonia," *New Orleans Med. & Surg. J.*, 1853, *10*: 417–441, quotation on p. 423.

9 R. F. McGuire, Diary, 1818–1852, Ouachita Parish, Monroe, Louisiana, entry for Dec. 18, 1819, Department of Archives, Library, Louisiana State University, Baton Rouge.

10 Simon Baruch, Notes on Lectures of E[li] Geddings, Institutes and Practice of Medicine, Delivered at the Medical College of South Carolina, 1860–1861, lecture of Feb. 18, 1861, Special Collections, Robert W. Woodruff Library, Emory University, Atlanta, Georgia.

11 Edward H. Barton, *Introductory Lecture on the Climate and Salubrity of New-Orleans, and Its Suitability for a Medical School* (New Orleans: E. Johns & Co., 1835),

p. 21; and see *idem*, *The Application of Physiological Medicine to the Diseases of Louisiana* (Philadelphia: Jos. R. A. Skerrett, 1832). Dale C. Smith, in his comments on the version of my essay discussed at the Second Barnard-Millington Symposium on Southern Science and Medicine, Jackson, Mississippi, Mar. 18, 1983, made an intriguing suggestion about what he aptly terms "the gray area of . . . pathology," in which the extremes of universality and regional specificity represented by, say, chemistry and medical therapeutics became shaded. He suggested that from the 1830s southern physicians may have been less likely than their counterparts elsewhere to accept "the new pathology," that is, an increasingly disease-specific pathology and the universalizing notion of discrete disease entities it implied. Both Smith's suggestion and the explanation for this phenomenon deserve further study.

12  William W. Cozart, "An inaugural dissertation on the place where southern students should acquire their medical knowledge" (M.D. thesis, Medical College of the State of South Carolina, 1856), South Carolina Room, Main Library, Medical University of South Carolina.

13  Typically, a student attending medical lectures at the University of Michigan recorded in his class notes on therapeutics the "circumstances which modify indications" for treatment: "Age of patient. The Sex. . . . A good Constitution. . . . The Temperament. The disease going on in the organ. Idiosyncrasies, or personal peculiarities. Variation of the pulse. Habits of the patient. Tolerance of medicines. Climate. The prevailing epidemic influence. Race. Profession. Severity of disease." John B. Rice, Fremont, Ohio, Notes on Lectures of Prof. Alonzo B. Palmer, Materia Medica and Therapeutics, University of Michigan College of Medicine and Surgery, Ann Arbor, Mich., Dec. 4, 1855, John B. Rice Papers, Rutherford B. Hayes Library, Fremont, Ohio.

14  L. C., "Prevailing fevers in country towns," letter to the editor, Boston, Nov. 29, 1843, *Boston Med. & Surg. J.*, 1843, *29:* 359.

15  R. T. Dismukes, Notes on Lectures of B[enjamin] W[inslow] Dudley, Professor of Anatomy and Surgery in the Medical Department of Transylvania University, Lexington, Kentucky, 1838–1839, Manuscript Department, Perkins Library, Duke University, Durham. Statements of such perceptions, although fully sustained by medical theory, were at times clearly propelled by proprietary interests as well. For example, a medical professor at a rural school in upstate New York proposed to his students in 1846, "Let a student from the country take a course of instruction in the hospitals of one of our large cities and then let him go home and commence practice among the yeomanry of his native town, and he will soon find that he has a set of very different patients[,] a different class of diseases[,] and that [these] require a very different course of treatment from those he found in the hospitals." Daniel D. Slanson, Medical Daybook, 1846–1877, introductory lecture by Prof. [James] Webster, Geneva College, 1846, Daniel D. Slanson Papers, Department of Archives, Library, Louisiana State University.

16  L[eonidas] M[oreau] Lawson, "Foreign correspondence," *Western Lancet*, 1845–1846, *4:* 145–153, quotation on pp. 150–151. On the notion that American medical knowledge and practice must be distinct from that of Europe, and the changing course of this idea, see Ronald L. Numbers and John Harley Warner, "The maturation of American medical science," Ch. 8, this volume; also in *Scientific Colonialism, A Cross-Cultural Comparison*, ed. Nathan Reingold and Marc Rothenberg (Washington, D.C.: Smithsonian Institution Press, forthcoming).

17  [Lawrence] Jefferson Trotti, Notebook, MS bound with catalogue from Transylvania University, 1828, Special Collections and Archives, Frances Carrick Thomas Library, Transylvania University, Lexington.

18  John Leonard Riddell, Manuscript Volumes, Vol. XXVI, Minutes of lectures delivered at the Medical College of Ohio, in the winter of 1834–35, lecture of Dr. [Jesse] Smith, Nov. 5, 1834, Special Collections Division, Howard-Tilton Memorial Library, Tulane University, New Orleans.

19  "Extract from Dr. Ingalls's letter on scarlatina," *Boston Med. & Surg. J.*, 1837, *17:* 239–240, p. 239.

20  Exceptions are Charles E. Rosenberg's excellent explication of the structure of therapeutic thought and practice, "The therapeutic revolution: medicine, meaning, and social change in nineteenth-century America," in *The Therapeutic Revolution: Essays in the Social History of American Medicine*, ed. Morris J. Vogel and Charles E. Rosenberg (Philadelphia: Univ. of Pennsylvania Press, 1979), pp. 3–25, also ch. 3 of this volume; and two numerical exhibitions of the complexity of therapeutic practice based upon physicians' practice books and prescription records: David L. Cowen, Louis D. King, and Nicholas D. Lordi, "Nineteenth century drug therapy: computer analysis of the 1854 prescription file of a Burlington pharmacy," *J. Med. Soc. N.J.*, 1981, *78:* 758–761, and J. Worth Estes, "Therapeutic practice in colonial New England," in *Medicine in Colonial Massachusetts, 1620–1820*, ed. Philip Cash, Eric H. Christianson, and J. Worth Estes (Boston: The

Colonial Society of Massachusetts, 1980), pp. 289–383.

21 The records upon which this figure is based, which usually were kept primarily for financial purposes, are restricted to those of physicians whose practices were for the most part made up of individual patients, slave and free. Excluded therefore are hospital records and the records of physicians who practiced substantially on large plantations, in which entries often described the services rendered to a group of slaves in the aggregate rather than the itemized care of individuals. The percentages calculated for each set of records represent the proportion of debt entries (that is, a physician's entries into his record book of the services provided and drugs prescribed to a patient) in which venesection appeared. While individual drug treatments were often entered only as "medicine" or "prescription," venesection, as a surgical procedure, was conventionally identified by name, permitting meaningful comparison among various physicians' records. Ordinarily, a practitioner made a separate entry into his ledger each time he visited a patient, though it is not always possible to determine this with certainty. The samples taken from each set of records represent varying proportions of the total number of entries, never under 10 percent and in some instances encompassing the entire source. Care was taken, however, to draw a representative seasonal cross section of each physician's practice, to avoid skewing the sample by an undue stress on hot or cold months.

The following records were used: Anonymous, Doctor[']s Journal, 3 vols. [labeled University of Alabama Medical Department], 1850–1852, 1853–1856, 1856–1858, University Archives, William Stanley Hoole Special Collections Library, Amelia Gayle Gorgas Library, University of Alabama, University, Alabama; O. L. Collins, Account Book, Chipola, St. Helena Parish, Louisiana, 1857–1871, Department of Archives, Library, Louisiana State University; John Hainey Davis, Account Book, 1827–1843, South Caroliniana Library, University of South Carolina, Columbia, South Carolina; William Dawson Dorris, Ledgers, 3 vols. [internally identified as near Nashville, Tennessee], 1836–1843, 1841–1844, and 1849–1856, History Room, Library, University of South Florida Medical Center, Tampa; C. A. Hentz, Medical Diary, Quincy, Florida, 1858–1862, Vol. XIV, Hentz Family Papers, Southern Historical Collection, University of North Carolina at Chapel Hill, Chapel Hill; Samuel Holt, Ledger, Montgomery, Alabama, 1847–1848; Samuel Holt Papers, Maps and Manuscripts Division, State of Alabama Department of Archives and

History, Montgomery; Bartlett Jones, Record Book [South Carolina], 1817–1828, Southern Historical Collection; Lueco Mitchell, Account Book, Salisbury, North Carolina, 1823–1830, Harnett County Papers, Southern Historical Collection; Benjamin and Benjamin West Robinson, Account Books, Fayetteville, North Carolina, 1805–1863, Southern Historical Collection; Robert H. Ryland, Record Book, 1849–1856, Robert H. Ryland Papers, Department of Archives, Library, Louisiana State University; Henry Frederick Shugart, Account Book [Middleton?], Mississippi, 1835–1837, microfilm copy in Manuscripts and Archives, Mississippi Department of Archives and History, Jackson; M. L. Traviss, Daybook, Benton County, Tennessee, 1843–1861, Archives and Manuscripts Section, Tennessee State Archives and Library, Nashville.

22 Daniel J. Boorstin, *The Lost World of Thomas Jefferson* (New York: Henry Holt and Co., 1948); [Nathaniel Chapman], "Prospectus," *Philadelphia J. Med. & Phys. Sci.*, 1820, *1:* vii–xii; Gilbert Chinard, "Eighteenth century theories on America as a human habitat," *Proc. Am. Phil. Soc.*, 1947, *91:* 27–57; Antonello Gerbi, *The Dispute of the New World: The History of a Polemic, 1750–1900* (Milano-Napoli: Ricardo Riccardi Editore, 1955; trans. Jeremy Moyle, Pittsburgh Univ. Press, 1973); George Rosen, "Political order and human health in Jeffersonian thought," *Bull. Hist. Med.*, 1952, *26:* 32–44. The division of medical knowledge into universal medical principles and region-specific tenets of practice is apparent in Jeffersonian medical nationalism. While medicine as a practice was to be distinctively American, as Perry Miller noted, "In Barton's thought, as in Benjamin Franklin's, there could be no question of producing some uniquely American scientific doctrine" (*The Life of the Mind in America: From the Revolution to the Civil War* [New York: Harcourt, Brace & World, 1965], p. 270).

23 James P. Miller, Notes on Doctor Rush's Lectures Delivered 1811–12 in the University of Pennsylvania, lecture of Nov. 24, 1811, Manuscripts Department, William R. Perkins Library, Duke University, Durham, North Carolina.

24 James Rackliffe, Notes on the Lectures of Benjamin S. Barton, Philadelphia, lecture of Nov. 1, 1815, Trent Collection, Duke University Medical Center Library, Durham, North Carolina.

25 E. D. Fenner, "Introductory lecture delivered at the opening of the New Orleans School of Medicine, on the 17th Nov., '56," *New Orleans Med. News & Hosp. Gaz.*, 1856–1857, *3:* 577–600, quotation on p. 597; *Autobiography of Charles Caldwell, M.D.* (Philadelphia, 1855; reprinted New York: Da Capo Press, 1968), pp. 358–359.

26  [Josiah Clark Nott] to James M. Gage, New Or-
    leans, Mar. [1837], James M. Gage Papers, South-
    ern Historical Collection.
27  James K. Nisbet to N[athaniel] E. McCleeland,
    Philadelphia, Feb. 26, 1830, McCleeland Family
    Papers, Southern Historical Collection.
28  *Ibid.*, Sept. 18, 1830.
29  Ja[me]s Norcom to Benjamin Rush Norcom, Eden-
    ton, North Carolina, Feb. 21, 1832, Dr. James Nor-
    com and Family Papers, North Carolina State Ar-
    chives, Raleigh. His mention of Rush is in Ja[me]s
    Norcom to John Norcom [son in Washington,
    North Carolina], Edenton, North Carolina, Feb. 18,
    1846, Dr. James Norcom and Family Papers.
30  John Austin, Notes on the Lectures of Benjamin
    Rush, 1809, Historical Collection, Rudolph Matas
    Medical Library, Tulane University Medical Cen-
    ter, New Orleans; and P. Washington Little, Note-
    book of Lectures by Rush 1805–06, Notes on physi-
    ology, pathology, &c &c &c delivered at the Univ.
    of Pennsylvania, Trent Collection, Duke Univer-
    sity Medical Center Library.
31  Samuel Murphy, Notes from Doctor [Nathaniel]
    Chapman's Lectures, 1830, 2 vols., Vol. I, Univer-
    sity of Pennsylvania Archives, Philadelphia.
32  Benjamin Huger, Notes on Materia Medica from
    Lectures Delivered by Nathaniel Chapman, 1816,
    2 vols., Vol. I, Waring Historical Library, Medical
    University of South Carolina, Charleston.
33  Samuel Barrington, Notes on the Practice of
    Medicine Taken from the Lectures of N. Chap-
    man, M.D. Professor of the Institutes & Practice
    of Physic &c., in the University of Pennsylvania,
    1818–19, 1820–21, 1821–22, History of Medicine
    Division, National Library of Medicine, Bethesda,
    Maryland.
34  Buckner Hill, [Notes on Hosack's Lectures, Vol.
    I], commenced Nov. 1, 1824, Buckner Hill Note-
    books, North Carolina State Archives. The aster-
    isk in the quoted comments led to the following ad-
    dition at the bottom of the page: "* Inhabitants of
    the North, do not require the same treatments (of
    tonics) as those in southern climates." And see
    Thomas A. Brayton, Notes on Lectures on [the]
    Theory & Practice of Physic by David Hosack,
    M.D., 1823, lectures for Nov. 11 and 14, 1823,
    Thomas A. Brayton Papers, Rare Books and Manu-
    scripts Division, The New York Public Library,
    (Astor, Lenox, and Tilden Foundations), New York.
35  John Barratt, Lecture Notes [on Lectures of Dr.
    Hosack], New York, 1822, South Caroliniana Li-
    brary, University of South Carolina; and see David
    Hosack, Notes on the Lectures on the Theory and
    Practice of Physic and Clinical Medicine Taken by
    George B. McKnight, 1814–1816, Joseph M. Toner

    Papers, Manuscript Division, Library of Congress,
    Washington, D.C.
36  "Medical sectionalism," *New Orleans Med. News &
    Hosp. Gaz.* 1857–1858, *4:* 156–158, quotation on
    p. 158.
37  "Atlanta medical colleges," *Georgia Med. & Surg. En-
    cyc.,* 1860, *1:* 44. When the Philadelphia medical
    author and editor John Bell assailed pleas for pecu-
    liarly southern medical literature and education as
    "states-rights medicine," it was the stridency of this
    use of the argument for southern medical distinc-
    tiveness and not the assumed need for regional
    specificity to which he objected. He defended the
    pertinence of northern teachings (and especially his
    own recent treatise on practice) to southern prac-
    tice by affirming that northern authors and pro-
    fessors recognized the individuating factors that
    characterized various regions and took them into
    account. "It should be remembered, that our north-
    ern lecturers and writers on systematic medicine
    still continue the old fashion of pointing out the
    modifications in fevers and other diseases arising
    from the difference of locality and climate in gen-
    eral, as well as from manner of living, age, and sex,"
    he asserted. "They are not quite like moles, whose
    purblind vision prevents their seeing beyond their
    own habitations; but, on the contrary, they extend
    their investigations over the whole habitable world,
    making collections from all quarters, which they
    afterwards arrange and place on the altar of sci-
    ence; as an offering to their countrymen through-
    out the whole United States" ("Dr. Cartwright's
    Address—States-Rights Medicine," *Bull. Med. Sci.,*
    1846, *4:* 207–213, quotation on p. 212). The term
    Bell coined, *states-rights medicine,* was a damning epi-
    thet created by a self-interested critic of the move-
    ment for southern medical distinctiveness, not an
    objective appraisal of the movement's animus.
38  Drew Gilpin Faust, "The rhetoric and ritual of ag-
    riculture in antebellum South Carolina," *J. South-
    ern Hist.,* 1979, *45:* 541–568; and Dorse Harland
    Hagler, "The agrarian theme in southern history
    to 1860" (Ph.D. dissertation, Univ. of Missouri,
    1968).
39  B. Dowler, "A review of medical literature, includ-
    ing critical remarks on Professor Palmer's report
    on that subject, as published in the Transactions
    of the American Medical Assocation, Vol. XI," *New
    Orleans Med. & Surg. J.,* 1859, *16:* 441–451, quota-
    tion on p. 446.
40  S. P. Crawford, "Southern medical literature," *Nash-
    ville Med. & Surg. J.,* 1860, *18:* 195–198, p. 198; and
    see Samuel A. Cartwright, "Report on the locality
    of plants, or the law of the vegetable kingdom, giv-
    ing to some plants peculiar or superior properties,

in certain localities, not possessed by the same plants elsewhere, and the application of this law to the cane and cotton plants," *New Orleans Med. & Surg. J.*, 1853, *10*: 1–12; J[uriah] H[arriss], "Our journal," *Savannah J. Med.*, 1858, *1*: 126–128, pp. 127–128; and "Salutatory," *Charleston Med. J. & Rev.*, 1860, *15*: 131–133, p. 131.

41 For example, see J. P. Barratt, "Transactions of the South Carolina Medical Association," *Charleston Med. & Surg. Rev.*, 1856, *11*: 178–198, pp. 180, 183; A. H. Buchanan, "Address delivered at the first annual meeting of the Nashville Medical Society," *Nashville Med. & Surg. J.*, 1859 *17*: 193–199, p. 199; and P. H. Lewis, "A medical history of Alabama," *New Orleans Med. & Surg. J.*, 1846–1847, *3*: 691–706, and 1847–1848, *4*: 3–34, 151–177.

42 James A. Briggs, "An inaugural dissertation on the medical topography and diseases of Warren County, Ky." (M.D. thesis, Medical Department of the Univ. of Nashville, 1851), Special Collections, Medical Center Library, Vanderbilt University, Nashville. Physicians further claimed that they must study disease in its local milieu in order to determine its etiology and behavior. Such local knowledge would direct prudent activity in the face of epidemics, and thereby protect the health and commerce of their region. See Margaret Ellen Warner, "Public health in the New South: government, medicine and society in the control of yellow fever" (Ph.D. dissertation, Harvard Univ., 1983), Ch. 1.

43 Thomas Hunter, "A dissertation on the topography of south Alabama and the diseases incident to its climate" (M.D. thesis, Medical College of the State of South Carolina, Charleston, 1843), South Carolina Room, Main Library, Medical University of South Carolina. To be sure, such local studies were common in the North and especially the West as well; but their pursuit in these regions did not display the extent of explicitly sectional ardor that animated investigations in the South.

44 Fenner, "Introductory lecture," p. 587.

45 Alexander Means, "An address to the second course of lectures in the Atlanta Medical College," *Atlanta Med. & Surg. J.*, 1855–1856, *1*: 707–723, p. 708; and see Bennet Dowler, "Progress of medicine," *New Orleans Med. & Surg. J.*, 1856, *12*: 220–221, and J. C. Nott, "Medical schools," *New Orleans Med. & Surg. J.*, 1857, *14*: 353–357, p. 353. A variation of the same theme illustrated the deterioration of southern medicine by contrasting not ancient Greece and Rome with Edinburgh and Philadelphia, but instead the colonial South with the mid-19th-century South; see Fenner, "Introductory lecture," pp. 587, 597, and E. D. Fenner, "Introductory address," *Southern Med. Rep.*, 1850, *1*: 7–13, on pp. 8–9.

46 Samuel A. Cartwright, "Malum Egyptiäcum, cold plague, diphtheria, or black tongue," *New Orleans Med. & Surg. J.*, 1859, *16*: 378–388, 797–821, quotation on p. 380.

47 *Ibid.*, p. 815.

48 W. Taylor, "Annual oration," in *Transactions of the Medical Association of the State of Alabama at Its Eighth Annual Session, Begun and Held in the City of Mobile, February 5,-6,-7, 1855. Together with the Code of Medical Ethics and a History of Members* (Mobile: Middleton, Harris & Co., 1855), pp. 117–129, on p. 120.

49 Sam[ue]l A. Cartwright to Rezin Thomson, New Orleans, June 15, 1856, *Nashville Med. & Surg. J.*, 1856, *11*: 212–216, quotation on p. 214.

50 *Ibid.*; Cartwright, "Malum Egyptiäcum," pp. 380–388, 800–817; *idem, The Pathology and Treatment of Cholera: With an Appendix, Containing His Latest Instructions to Planters and Heads of Families (Remote from Medical Advice) in Regards to Its Prevention and Cure* (New Orleans: Spencer and Middleton's "Magic Press" Office, 1849). Attributing southern problems to northern sources became a convention in southern medical literature. When the editors of the *New Orleans Medical and Surgical Journal* referred to sectarians as "the Goths and Vandals of empiricism," the point that these were tribes of barbarian northerners who swept down to loot and destroy a superior southern civilization was unambiguous. (See editors' introduction to Samuel A. Cartwright, "Address delivered before the medical convention, in the city of Jackson, January 13, 1846," *New Orleans Med. & Surg. J.*, 1845–1846, *2*: 724–733, p. 729.) Similarly, southerners pointed again and again to the facts that Samuel Thomson was a New Englander and Samuel Hahnemann a European.

51 Samuel A. Cartwright to John Francis Hamtramck Claiborne, [New Orleans?], Apr. 26, 1856, John Francis Hamtramck Claiborne Papers, Southern Historical Collection.

52 Another model physician was James Johnson, the British physician who, according to Fenner, discovered the fallacy of relying on northern authority in southern diseases and observed for himself the influence of hot climates upon European constitutions; see E. D. F[enner], "[Review of] *The Influence of Tropical Climates on European Constitutions*, by James Johnson . . . and Ranald Martin," *New Orleans Med. & Surg. J.*, 1846–1847, *3*: 381–385.

53 Paul F. Eve, "Address to the class, on opening the course of lectures in the Medical College of Georgia, the 17th of October, 1837," *Southern Med. & Surg. J.*, 1838, *2*: 1–12, quotation on p. 11.

54 Clifford Geertz, "Ideology as a cultural system," in *Ideology and Discontent*, ed. David Apter (New York: Free Press of Glencoe, Macmillan Company, 1964),

pp. 47–77, quotation on p. 64. Aptly for the historian's purposes, Geertz quotes Talcott Parsons's observation: "The concept of strain is not in itself an explanation of ideological patterns but a generalized label for the kinds of factors to look for in working out an explanation" (p. 54).

55 Everett Mendelsohn, speaking of groups holding an alternative conception of nature and socially and cognitively alienated from the centers of scientific power, has noted: "One of the characteristics that has impressed me about these activities at the margin of orthodox and established science and medicine is the social movement nature of their organization and the intense commitment evidenced by both practitioners and lay participants. Political overtones are also often present." ("The social construction of scientific knowledge," in *The Social Production of Scientific Knowledge*, ed. Everett Mendelsohn, Peter Weingart, and Richard Whitley [Dordrecht, Holland, and Boston: D. Reidel, 1977], pp. 3–26, quotation on p. 21, n. 6.) The case of physicians in the antebellum South and their intense advocacy of the idea of southern medical distinctiveness suggests that a group of practitioners located socially and geographically on the margins, but cognitively within the mainstream, might behave in a strikingly similar fashion. An intriguing analysis of physicians' efforts to alleviate their marginality within a quite different context is Ian Inkster, "Marginal men: aspects of the social role of the medical community in Sheffield 1790–1850," in *Health Care and Popular Medicine in Nineteenth Century England*, ed. John Woodward and David Richards (London: Croom Helm, 1977), pp. 128–163.

56 Warner, "A southern medical reform." My understanding of the position occupied by the physician with intellectual aspirations in the antebellum South owes much to my reading of Drew Gilpin Faust's *The Sacred Circle: The Dilemma of the Intellectual in the Old South, 1840–1860* (Baltimore and London: Johns Hopkins Univ. Press, 1977), and "A southern stewardship: the intellectual and the proslavery argument," *Am. Quart.*, 1979, *31*: 63–80.

# 5

## Patent Medicines and the Self-Help Syndrome

### JAMES HARVEY YOUNG

"Somebody buys all the quack medicines," Oliver Wendell Holmes once wrote, "that build palaces for the mushroom, say rather, the toadstool millionaires."[1] To comprehend the kind of medical self-help that involves the use of patent medicines, therefore, we need to try to understand both parties to the transaction, the seller of the nostrums and that "somebody" who buys them.

Both seller and buyer possess complex and subtle motives; hence the task of comprehension is not easy. In his public face, advertising, the seller most often disguises or distorts his most obvious aim. And patent medicine promoters have on the whole protected their privacy with great diligence. They have in the main eschewed the art of autobiography. When biographical information has appeared, in book or magazine, it too often sounds like a mere extension of advertising. Few documented histories of proprietary medicine companies exist.[2]

Nor, on the buyer side, do we have an abundance of conscious, candid self-revelation. Proprietary users do not keep diaries of their medicine-taking habits in which they detail their symptoms and analyze their motives for purchasing a given pill or potion. So we must try to recapture the experience from piecing together evidence from the kinds of records that do exist.

Voltaire said that quackery began when the first knave met the first fool. Throughout most of history quackery has principally involved face-to-face encounter, so that the quack's presence—his per-

sonality, costume, oratory, showmanship—have overwhelmed the customer-victim. He might be selling a potion, an amulet, or a laying on of his powerful hands. Responding to the overawed reaction of those to whom he ministered, the quack often became as persuaded as did they, however unscrupulous his initial motives, that his drug, device, or manipulation possessed healing power. For, as Grete de Francesco has written, "The charlatan resembled his dupes; his, too, was a weak and disappointed nature that sought compensation in the realm of illusion, on a plane that was no longer that of the sober earth."[3] Thus both parties to the transaction could be enveloped in delusion.

Face-to-face quackery still flourishes, the quack dispensing drugs with polysyllabic chemical names, vitamins lettered far down into the alphabet, treatments with complex and impressive machines, and the laying on of hands, all done with glowing therapeutic promises. To the patient-victim it makes no difference whether his self-asserted savior lies brazenly or speaks what he himself ignorantly believes to be the truth.

Patent medicines—and devices similarly promoted—separate the proprietor from the user by one or more removes and owe their origin to the more complex and sophisticated modes of life ushered in by the commercial and the printing revolutions. Printing created the newspaper, and 17th-century English journals quickly blossomed forth with nostrum ads. *Mercurius Politicus* during 1660, for example, touted a dentifrice which would make the teeth "white as Ivory," fasten them firmly, prevent toothache, sweeten the breath, and banish cankers.[4] The ad gave a location at which customers could buy this wonder, the shop of a stationer beside St. Paul's Church. Presumably the stationer was middleman, not the dentifrice maker himself. If such a proprietor could place his prod-

JAMES HARVEY YOUNG is Charles Howard Candler Professor Emeritus of American Social History at Emory University, Atlanta, Georgia.

Reprinted with permission from *Medicine Without Doctors: Home Health Care in American History*, edited by Guenter B. Risse, Ronald L. Numbers, and Judith Walzer Leavitt (New York: Science History Publications, 1977), pp. 95–116.

uct in various London shops, as well as in shops throughout the countryside, a feat which better transportation had made easier, and could lure customers into those shops by means of printed advertising, he had expanded his potential market tremendously over that possible through face-to-face appeals. Competition developed so rapidly in this new favorable environment that, to distinguish his product from its many rivals, a promoter endowed it with badges of proprietorship, especially a container of unique design, often pictured in newspaper advertising.[5]

The evolving patent system began, during the early 18th century, to cover compound medicines. Proprietors who chose to patent their formulas boasted that this step signified governmental endorsement of therapeutic efficacy. In exchange for the dubious right to make this false claim, those securing patents had to reveal each medicine's composition. Most proprietors preferred to vend secret formulas without a patent. The term "patent medicine" came in common parlance to apply to both categories indistinguishably.

English patent medicines appeared on the American market early in the 18th century, advertised soon after the origin of the colonial press. By mid-century such advertising had become abundant, continuing to expand until tensions between colony and mother country put restrictions on trade. An odd circumstance differentiates the advertising of the same brands of patent medicines in the British and in the American press. In England the nostrum proprietor sought to transfer into print something of the high-flown harangue used by quacks in face-to-face promotion, often using for the purpose several column inches of type. In colonial America this hardly ever happened. Only a few hyperbolic pamphlets extolling the virtues of patent remedies have come down to us, and only with great rarity in the late colonial years did a nostrum ad appear smacking of the customary British vim and vigor. For the most part, colonial advertisements of the British patent medicines consist of mere names in lists. The latest ship from London had come to port, so Anderson's Scots Pills, Bateman's Pectoral Drops, Hooper's Female Pills and other familiar name-brands were now available. Customers in colonial towns bought patent medicines from many outlets; apothecaries, booksellers, goldsmiths, grocers, hairdressers,

tailors, and printers — among other tradesmen — vended them.

Why the terse, drab American advertising? For one thing, remoteness of the proprietors. Busy competing with each other at home, they had not extended their technique of grandiose promotion across the ocean. As a consequence, the American weeklies, modest in size, had not been pushed to expand advertising space so as to rival that in the more frequent and numerous English newspapers. On the American side, perhaps the medicines sold well enough without the British harangues in print. Supply may never have exceeded demand so markedly in the colonies as in the mother country. Certainly Americans lacked initiative in creating nostrums to compete with the traditional British brands, for only rarely, to judge from the press, did some colonist move an eye-water or a salve from the realm of folk medicine into commerce.[6] Americans became accustomed to dosing themselves with the British brands — many physicians prescribed them — and out of a sense of tradition and loyalty continued to use them. Indeed, when political loyalty began to wear thin, medicinal loyalty persisted, for customers so desired the brand-name British nostrums now cut off by economic warfare, that American apothecaries refilled empty bottles by the gross.

Patent medicines shared in the burst of creativity let loose by the cultural nationalism of the revolutionary generation. Made-in-America nostrums proliferated, a few of them patented when the Constitution authorized this protection to inventors, but most of them shrouded in secrecy. Competition increased and proprietors bought ever more space in the burgeoning newspapers to acclaim their own respective brands. In time, joining nationalism as a stimulating force, came the thrust for an expansion of democracy. Physicians came under suspicion because of their "heroic" bleeding and purging, a battle in which Thomsonians[7] and homeopaths were joined by patent medicine makers who boasted to an increasingly worried public about how painless, nice-tasting, and nonmineral their proprietary products were as compared with the regular doctors' lancet and mercury.[8]

Learned physicians also lost caste, along with members of other educated professions, during the cultural climate associated with Jacksonian democracy. As leaders of opinion lost this traditional role, each common man had to make up his own mind for himself. The right to do so stimulates pride, fires ambition, but also provokes anxiety. Which of the many new voices appealing for favor can be believed? Hard, sharp, unscrupulous bargaining reigns in the realms of both thought and trade. Life becomes intensely competitive. A horde of tricksters appears. Victimization runs rampant. Everybody expects roguery, anticipates being cheated, himself cheats in turn. Nor, within limits, do people mind being hoodwinked. They have made their own decisions, taken their chances in a free environment. Sometimes they are bound to lose. Indeed, clever imposture amuses them. Such a picture of the popular mind emerges from Neil Harris' brilliant book on "the art of P. T. Barnum," entitled *Humbug*.[9]

In this pervasive atmosphere of caveat emptor, American patent medicines soared. Becoming more literate through the expansion of elementary schooling, citizens read newspaper advertising and determined on their own which nostrums to buy in order to treat their ailments. Much advertising explicitly attacked the high-and-mighty arrogance of regular physicians. Whatever affliction bothered the common man, patent medicines promised a cure for it. Cholera remedies proliferated during epidemics, and year-in-year-out concern for tuberculosis received constant prodding in advertising columns. That so many nostrums contained laxative ingredients gives insight into the poor dietary habits of the mid-19th century. Constipation, indeed, appeared in much patent medicine advertising as a grim harbinger of worse ills to come. To judge from advertising also, Americans led dreary, boring, work-filled, depressing lives, and many nostrums, some containing alcohol, fell into a sort of "mood drug" category.

One such mood drug may be used for more extended illustration, not because it completely typifies 19th-century patent medicine promotion — each case history has its unique particulars — but because it reveals several significant features of the way proprietary medicines intertwined with broader facets of life.

When the panic of 1873 struck the nation, Mrs. Lydia Estes Pinkham had attained the age of 54. For 30 years she had struggled to maintain her family of three sons and a daughter — another son

had died in infancy — on the hope that one of her husband Isaac's many speculations, mainly in real estate, might handsomely pay off. None had done so, and the Depression ended all such hope and snuffed out Isaac's will to strive. In family council, Lydia and her sons took things into their own hands.[10]

Like many enterprising housewives, Lydia for years had nursed members of her family when they were ill, using remedies remembered from family tradition and gathered from medical guides which she liked to read. A particular favorite of hers, John King's *American Dispensatory*, fell into that class of popular botanical handbooks stemming from the revived interest in the vegetable kingdom stimulated by Thomsonianism. Lydia Pinkham, a good neighbor, dosed others outside her family when they were ailing. Strangers sometimes showed up at her door asking for her concoctions which they had heard about in conversation. For centuries, folklore remedies, administered gratis by grandmothers and maiden aunts, had occasionally become articles for sale under the press of financial exigency. Now in the Pinkham household the need indeed was great, and one of Lydia's favorite vegetable brews became a proprietary medicine.

The bottles filled in the Pinkham cellar kitchen in Lynn, Massachusetts, contained not only a mixture of several botanicals but a fillip of reform. For Lydia had grown up amidst freedom's ferment and had shown strong interest in many causes. Her parents had left their Friends meeting over the issue of slavery, and Lydia herself embraced strong abolitionist sentiments, belonging to the Female Anti-Slavery Society and developing an acquaintance with Garrison, Whittier, Frederick Douglass, Abby Kelley, the Grimké sisters, and other abolitionist worthies. Lydia espoused temperance, even though her Vegetable Compound was to contain 18 percent alcohol. She looked with favor on the food reform doctrines of Sylvester Graham, supported inflation through the issuance of greenbacks, welcomed phrenology, and believed with increasing intensity in spiritualism. Lydia helped establish and served as secretary for the Freeman's Institute, a group formed for the uninhibited discussion of all social ideas.

So, of course, living in this climate, Lydia believed in a larger role for women in society. As Samuel Thomson's system had sought to strike a blow for medical democracy, so Lydia E. Pinkham's Vegetable Compound sought to strike a blow for women's rights. Lydia had developed the belief that male physicians were insensitive to women's ills.[11] When testimonials began arriving in the mail praising her new proprietary, they confirmed her own conviction. "I had doctored with the physicians of this town for three years," read one such letter, "and grew worse instead of better." Lydia hoped for a more tolerant attitude than that which then prevailed toward women seeking to become doctors, and she clipped newspaper stories relating to women and medical education. Her own role with respect to women's health would be different but, as she saw it, no less important. She would bottle and sell the vegetable compound she had adapted from King's *Dispensatory* and had prescribed for women of her acquaintance who had seemed pleased with the results.

"Only a woman understands a woman's ills," Lydia believed, and this maxim became an advertising slogan, as her own dignified gray-haired countenance became her remedy's trademark. Soon her advertising urged women to write her for advice about their most intimate health problems, promising that no male eye would see the letters. For a while she penned the answers herself, but soon the pressure of work caused her to introduce other female relatives to this task, the advice now dictated to women stenographers skilled at using that new invention, the typewriter. Lydia's letters urged the use of her Compound, but also gave counsel on diet, dress, and bathing. "Keep clean inside and out" was a favorite injunction. Most letters evidently employed the imperative mode.

In the 19th century any lay person could do just what Lydia Pinkham did, devise a formula inspired or informed by whatever sources of information came to hand, and market the medicine with whatever therapeutic claims seemed likely to persuade. The marketplace groaned with packages of inert ingredients ballyhooed as cures for cancer and with opium-laden syrups vended to soothe fretful babies. Lydia Pinkham exercised more restraint than most of her fellow competitors in proprietary marketing. She had the support of eclectic medicine for most of the ingredients in her Vegetable Compound and for many of her claims. King's *American Dispensatory* praised the true uni-

corn root—her mixture also contained the false unicorn root—for "the tonic influence it exerts upon the female generative organs, giving a normal energy to the uterus, and thus proving helpful in cases where there is an habitual tendency to miscarriage."[12] King also asserted that pleurisy root had helped cure cases of prolapsus uteri. These botanicals, along with life-root, black cohosh, fenugreek seed, and that 18 percent alcohol went into Lydia's Compound. And onto the label went claims for relieving the entire gamut of women's peculiar physiological ailments.

Among those seeking to make money from offering customers self-help, temptations arise. Lydia and her sons were not immune. They had worked desperately hard to acquaint women with their product by distributing pamphlets, first in Lynn, then in other New England towns. The first sales significant enough to inscribe in a ledger were made in April 1875. Soon Daniel Pinkham journeyed to introduce the Vegetable Compound to New York City. He wrote home to brother Will: "I think there is one thing we are missing it on; and that is, not having something on the pamphlets in regard to Kidney Complaints as about half of the people out here are either troubled with Kidney complaints or else think they are. I think you better put something about Kidney complaints of both sexes in very conspicuous type on the first page. . . ."[13]

And so the Pinkham pamphlets began to promote the Compound for kidney complaints of both sexes and for ailments of men's generative organs as well. It was the appeal to women, however, that made the Compound profitable and famous, Lydia's benign face becoming no doubt the best-known feminine visage in America. Since the cut of the trademark was the only illustration of a female that many village newspapers possessed, Lydia now and then appeared as Queen Victoria.[14] The two women had been born in the same year. Indeed, a female pill which competed with the Vegetable Compound was named for Victoria's physician—a brazen act of robbery by a male American nostrum-maker, who further falsely asserted on the pill's wrapper, "Patronized by the Queen."[15]

Daniel Pinkham's attempt to open up a male market is nonetheless instructive. The maker of bottled self-help seldom strays from a prime goal, whatever his other purposes may be: to maximize sales. He has constantly done as Daniel did, observed what potential customers are suffering from in order to frame claims for what his patent medicine can do. The mercenary motive, of course, must never show. Instead, promoters presented themselves as the people's friend, the good samaritan, the ministering angel. But the basic drive for profit was always there. This still holds true in a proprietary medicine climate vastly different from that of a century ago.

In *American Self-Dosage Medicines*, I sought to focus on "the emergence from quackery of American proprietary medicines and their ascent under pressure to successive levels of greater respectability. . . ."[16] While outright quackery has not been subdued, laws regulating drugs and advertising, and developments in science and in the ethical standards of business behavior, have created the modern proprietary industry. Massive in size, it is distinctly restricted in therapeutic scope, its wares confined to treating the symptoms of minor self-limiting ailments and conditions. Yet the time-honored imperative for selling self-help still reigns, to maximize sales. A new confrontation between the proprietary industry and regulatory agencies is now in progress. Central issues relate to the effectiveness of ingredients and the legitimacy of promotional claims. Do modern proprietaries consist of an ounce of physiological efficacy and a pound of placebo? If their claims are not so outrageous as in the 19th century, do the explicit and especially the implied promises in their advertising still exceed warrant?

"Just watch television for one evening and judge for yourself," a pharmacist wrote not long ago. "See how many of life's problems are caused by commonly known diseases like 'the blahs,' or see how 'a little blue pill' can save your marriage, or witness how aspirin suddenly has become a sleeping potion, or be amazed at the myriad of psychological and sociological problems that are allegedly the result of 'irregularity.'"[17]

Another disturbing question has recently been raised—and hotly debated—respecting proprietaries. Has the enormous and unrelenting pressure of their promotion helped persuade the younger generation that drug-taking is a legitimate way of confronting troublesome problems? "Let no one delude himself into thinking," a professor of public health testified before a Senate subcommittee, "there is no nexus between excessive self-medication and use of illegal drugs. Good epidemiologic studies show that parents who use inordinate amounts of medicaments breed children who have a far greater likelihood of using illicit drugs."[18]

From what has been said so far about the sellers of patent medicines, a glimpse of the buyers already has been provided. If they do not keep self-medication diaries, they reveal themselves in other ways. Studying the advertising of successful nostrums affords clues to the motivations of those purchasing patent medicines. Private papers also offer hints. In scanning recently the accumulated papers of a farm family from rural Georgia, I found the collection filled with direct mail nostrum advertising, saved as carefully as letters from cousins in Arkansas. A student of mine has apprised me that a Georgia bishop communicated with the makers of patent medicines he took.[19] Lydia Pinkham was not unique in receiving a vast flood of incoming mail, asking advice and volunteering testimony. Other proprietors also answered their mail, prescribing their remedies over slogans like Lydia's, "Yours for Health." Most promoters were less honorable than she with respect to confidentiality, bundling up letters in huge batches, organized by symptom categories, and selling or renting them to other proprietors.[20]

The Pinkham sense of restraint passed on to Lydia's heirs. At some time before the transfer by the family of the company records to the Schlesinger Library of Radcliffe College, the thousands of candid letters written in by inquiring women were removed from the collection.[21] Thus no male eye shall ever see them. One may note a pang of regret that female researchers may not study this rich, lost source of insight into the minds and bodies of women at the end of the 19th and beginning of the 20th century.

What emerges from all these sources, of course, is that life is tough, fraught with tensions and disappointments, with boredom and worries, with minor ailments and major diseases, both of which acquire emotional overlays, while emotional concerns alone can produce distinct physiological symptoms.[22]

Self-help, of course, has a high enough percentage of success to build confidence in the means employed. If the ailment be minor and emotional, the mere act of doing something—anything—may bring relief. Even in more serious conditions, a significant placebo effect comes into play. Almost anything new that is tried helps most arthritic sufferers for a time. If the ailment be minor and self-limited and of short duration, nature achieves the cure for which a nostrum gets the credit. Modern authorities recognize that a large measure of the consumer satisfaction derived from using present-day proprietaries derives from the placebo effect.[23] Even in the gravest diseases, like cancer, some dying patients swear by quacks, parroting the charlatan's assertion that the treatment had done much good and would have cured if begun soon enough.

In the old days, many patent medicines contained much opium, truly deadening pain. Alcoholic nostrums—some as high as 80 proof—relaxed many users—some with strong temperance convictions—and temporarily gave a more cheerful prospect to gloomy circumstances. From the first, orthodox medical opinion acknowledged the effect of the 18 percent alcohol in Lydia E. Pinkham's Vegetable Compound upon a woman's mood, while not sharing Lydia's confidence in the therapeutic action of her botanicals.[24] Her proclaimed interest in the suffering of women, the promises in her advertising, the cheerful tone of her letters, no doubt her very femaleness, also helped those who dosed themselves with her proprietary. Sales held up even after the pressure of food and drug laws forced a steady retreat from the initial bold and explicit claims upon the label to such simple but subtle recommendations of the Compound "as a vegetable tonic in conditions for which this preparation is adapted."[25]

Many nostrums have recruited legions of faithful users when the ingredients could have had no helpful physiological effects at all. Ardent testimonials, and even testimony in court, supported a diabetes "cure" consisting of the abandonment of insulin in favor of saltpeter dissolved in vinegar. Such praise came from victims whose new mode of treatment already was moving them swiftly toward their graves.[26] Even in the most disastrous circumstances, self-help manages to get a good name.

Americans have been especially impatient about illness. They have wanted something done—and soon—and have been prone to take things into their own hands, *not* consulting physicians, *before* consulting physicians, *while* consulting physicians. This was true in Lydia Pinkham's day, and the attitude continues. A recent behavioral survey, financed by seven federal agencies, spoke of this widespread American trait as "rampant empiricism."[27] Basing decisions on no coherent body of health knowledge, millions of Americans think "anything is worth a try." If orthodox medicine opposes, that does not matter much. Forty-two percent of American adults, the survey revealed, would not be persuaded by almost unanimous expert opinion that a purported "cancer cure" held out false hope. One out of every 50 adults does something virtually every day, acting alone and without a physician's advice, to move his bowels. One out of eight asserted that he or she would self-medicate, without seeing a doctor, for more than two weeks while treating such symptoms as sore throat, cough, upset stomach, and insomnia.

Three out of four Americans cherish the magical belief that, no matter how sufficient their diets, taking vitamins automatically provides more energy and pep. From the ranks of this large segment of the population, stirred by promoters of the more extravagant dietary supplements and operators of health food stores, came a barrage of mail in the early 1970s descending upon Congress—a barrage said to have been of greater intensity than that provoked by Watergate—in support of a bill that would have gutted the Food and Drug Administration's controls over special dietary wares.[28] The bill swept through the Senate by a ratio of eight to one but remained bottled up in conference committee at the end of the session. The Senate bill, as the Food and Drug Commissioner saw it, was "a charlatan's dream."[29]

During the course of history, patent medicines have provided a little help to some of their users by easing minor symptoms of self-limiting ailments, by furnishing a sense of relief through the sheer act of doing something, by encouraging mood. There has been a darker side: the creation of narcotic addicts and alcoholics, the conversion of remediable into incurable ailments because of delay at the futile way-station of self-help. Self-help may not even be a proper term to apply to self-dosage with proprietary medicines. The self has hardly been a free and independent agent under the tremendous, clever pressure of advertising, the main unvarying goal of which has been rather the self-help of the advertiser than the self-help of the suffering citizen belabored to believe that whatever his trouble — from the consumption of yore to the "blahs" of recent date — some commercial pill or potion can produce a cure.

"Advertisers and flourishers know perfectly well," wrote an editorialist back in 1871, "that even the gravest and most cautious are to a certain extent touched by their appeals, and that even in the act of denunciation, the most careful often find themselves seduced."[30]

## NOTES

1  Oliver Wendell Holmes, *Medical Essays, 1842–1882* (Boston: Houghton Mifflin Co., 1892), p. 186.

2  For an example, see Robert B. Shaw, *History of the Comstock Patent Medicine Business and Dr. Morse's Indian Root Pills,* Smithsonian Studies in History and Technology, No. 22 (Washington, D.C.: Smithsonian Institution Press, 1972).

3  Grete de Francesco, *The Power of the Charlatan* (New Haven: Yale Univ. Press, 1939), pp. 27–28.

4  Cited in E. S. Turner, *The Shocking History of Advertising!* (New York: Dutton, 1953), p. 25.

5  George B. Griffenhagen and James Harvey Young, *Old English Patent Medicines in America,* Contributions from the Museum of History and Technology, Paper 10. U.S. National Museum Bulletin 218 (Washington, D.C.: Smithsonian Institution Press, 1959), pp. 155–183.

6  An example is the ointment for the itch advertised in the *Pennsylvania Gazette,* Aug. 19, 1731, by Sarah Read, publisher Benjamin Franklin's mother-in-law.

7  See Ronald L. Numbers, "Do-it-yourself the sectarian way," in *Medicine Without Doctors: Home Health Care in American History,* ed. G. B. Risse, R. L. Numbers, and J. W. Leavitt (New York: Science History Publications, 1977).

8  The discussion of American patent medicines during their formative period is based on my *The Toadstool Millionaires* (Princeton, N.J.: Princeton Univ. Press, 1961).

9  Neil Harris, *Humbug, The Art of P.T. Barnum* (Boston: Little, Brown, 1973). Harris does not explicitly point his more general analysis toward patent medicine promotion, as I have done here.

10  The discussion of Lydia E. Pinkham is based mainly on Robert Collyer Washburn, *The Life and Times of Lydia E. Pinkham* (New York: G. P. Putnam's Sons, 1931); Jean Burton, *Lydia Pinkham Is Her Name* (New York: Farrar, Straus, 1949); and J. H. Young, "Lydia Estes Pinkham," in *Notable American Women 1607–1950,* ed. Edward T. James (Cambridge, Mass.: Bellknap Press of Harvard Univ. Press, 1971), III, pp. 71–72. Martha Verbrugge of Cambridge presented a paper on Lydia Pinkham at the 1975 convention of the American Association for the History of Medicine. Since the original publication of this chapter, an excellent biography of Mrs. Pinkham has been published: Sarah Stage, *Female Complaints: Lydia Pinkham and the Business of Women's Medicine* (New York: Norton, 1979).

11  A retrospective look at this theme may be found in John S. and Robin M. Haller, *The Physician and Sexuality in Victorian America* (Urbana: Univ. of Illinois Press, 1974).

12  John King, *The American Dispensatory,* 8th ed. (Cincinnati: Wilstach, Baldwin & Co., 1870), pp. 78–79, 142–144.

13  Burton, *Lydia Pinkham Is Her Name,* p. 89.

14  *Printer's Ink,* Oct. 5, 1922, *121*: 44.

15  Richard F. Riley, "Caveat emptor — 19th century American style," *Am. Philatelist,* Jan. 1975, *89*: 31–34.

16  James Harvey Young, *American Self-Dosage Medicines, An Historical Perspective* (Lawrence, Kans.: Coronado Press, 1974), quotation on p. xiii.

17  W. James Bicket, "Autotherapy—'The Future Is Now,'" *J. Am. Pharm. Assn.,* n.s., 1972, *12*: 562.

18  Testimony of Donald B. Louria, Department of Public Health and Preventive Medicine, New Jersey College of Medicine, July 22, 1971, *Advertising of Proprietary Medicines,* Hearings before the Subcommittee on Monopoly of the Select Committee on Small Business, U.S. Senate, 92nd Congress, 1st session (Washington, D.C.: Government Printing Office, 1971), p. 509.

19  Hunnicutt Family Papers and Warren A. Candler Papers, Special Collections Department, Robert A. Woodruff Library for Advanced Studies, Emory University, Atlanta, Ga. Mark Bauman called my attention to the letters in Bishop Candler's Papers.

20  "Strictly confidential," in Samuel Hopkins Adams, *The Great American Fraud* (Chicago: P. F. Collier, 1906), pp. 142–146.

21  Conversation with Diane M. Dorsey, Archivist, The Arthur and Elizabeth Schlesinger Library on the History of Women in America, Radcliffe College, Cambridge, Mass., Oct. 8, 1971; Eva Moseley, Curator of Manuscripts, Schlesinger Library, to author, Feb. 18, 1975.

22  James Harvey Young, "The persistence of medical quackery in America," *Am. Scientist,* 1972, *60*: 318–326.

23  Joseph D. Cooper, ed., *The Efficacy of Self-Medication*, Vol. IV, Philosophy and Technology of Drug Assessment, (Washington, D.C.: Smithsonian Institution Press, 1973).

24  *J.A.M.A.,* 1939, *112*: 2082–2083; E. Lee Strohl, "Ladies of Lynn—emphasis on one," *Surg., Gynec. & Obst.*, 1957, *105*: 769–775; Oliver Field, Department of Investigation, American Medical Association, to author, July 5, 1960.

25  From label as of 1933.

26  James Harvey Young, *The Medical Messiahs* (Princeton, N.J.: Princeton Univ. Press, 1967), pp. 217–238.

27  *A Study of Health Practices and Opinions* was conducted by National Analysts, Inc., under contract and was published in 1972 by the National Technical Information Service of Springfield, Va.

28  J. H. Young, "A threat to self-dosing consumers," *Atlanta Med.,* Dec. 1974, *48*: 19, 30; *Atlanta Constitution*, June 25, 1973; *FDC Rep.,* Aug. 6, 1973, *35*: 12; Aug. 13, 1973: T&G 9; Sept. 30, 1974, *36*: T&G 9.

29  Statement by Alexander M. Schmidt, M.D., Commissioner, Food and Drug Administration, before the Subcommittee on Health, Committee on Labor and Public Welfare, U.S. Senate, Aug. 14, 1974.

30  "Thoughts on puffing," *All the Year Round*, 1871, *25*: 330.

# The Art and Science of Medicine

Colonial American physicians practiced medicine, performed surgery, and prescribed drugs. Some historians have argued that this type of general practice resulted from the democratizing effect of the New World environment on Old World distinctions that rigidly separated the duties of physician, surgeon, and apothecary. Other historians have pointed out that even in England such strict divisions of labor seldom held outside London; in the provinces medical practitioners performed all the healing arts. Besides, few members of the upper classes, to which university-educated physicians belonged, emigrated to the colonies. Thus medicine in America from the beginning fell largely into the hands of surgeon-apothecaries and others already accustomed to a mixed practice.

Most American doctors of the 18th and early 19th centuries lived in small towns or villages, where they ministered to perhaps three or four hundred families. Although they frequently kept medicines, instruments, and a few books in an office at home, they conducted most of their practice in the homes of patients, visiting them on horseback with the supplies in saddlebags. Many physicians combined the practice of medicine with some other trade, such as farming, because professional fees seldom sufficed to support a family.

Such a life left little time for the cultivation of science. As Ronald L. Numbers and John Harley Warner point out, 19th-century American physicians tended to value wealth above knowledge and to pride themselves more on their skill as practitioners of the art of medicine than on their contributions to the science of medicine. Not surprisingly, their most original advances came in the practical fields of surgery and dentistry. In 1846, William T. G. Morton, a Boston dentist, won medical immortality for demonstrating the pain-killing effects of ether in surgery. But even this widely heralded panacea, Martin S. Pernick shows, presented American physicians with an ethical dilemma: did the relief of suffering justify risking a patient's life?

The discovery of surgical anesthesia also gave physicians a decided advantage over midwives in the competition for clients, and, as Judith Walzer Leavitt demonstrates, had far-reaching consequences for the practice of obstetrics. The availability of anesthetics, in addition to the use of instruments such as forceps, hastened the medicalization of childbirth and radically altered the relationship between parturient women and their attending physicians.

By the late 20th century the old-time practice of medicine had largely disappeared. Most American physicians specialized in a particular area of medicine and practiced in groups. House calls were a nostalgic symbol of times past. Physicians no longer visited the sick; the sick visited physicians, who efficiently examined them in assembly-line fashion. As assistants multiplied and forms proliferated, many physicians began to feel more like managers than healers. In three hundred years the practice of medicine had evolved from a cottage industry into big business.

# 6

## "Science" Enters the Birthing Room: Obstetrics in America since the 18th Century

### JUDITH WALZER LEAVITT

At the end of the 18th century, Dr. William Shippen, Jr., of Philadelphia attended all the childbearing women in the well-established Drinker family. The family members chose Shippen instead of a woman midwife, in spite of their ambivalence about having a man in the traditionally all-female birthing room, because they believed the physician offered the best hope for a successful outcome. The Drinkers, and many others like them, considered themselves fortunate to be living at a time when male physicians began replacing female midwives in the birthing rooms of the American urban elite. The families expected—and believed that they received—better care at the hands of physicians than they thought possible with traditional female attendants. This article examines the promises of the new physician-directed obstetrics—beginning in the 1760s, when physicians entered obstetrics, and ending in the 1940s, after they dominated the field—and evaluates the extent to which those promises were kept.[1]

Before 1760 birth was a women's affair in the British colonies of North America. When a woman went into labor, she "called her women together" and left her husband and other male family members outside. "I went to bed about 10 o'clock," wrote William Byrd of Virginia, "and left the women full of expectation with my wife." Only in cases where women were not available did men participate in labor and delivery, and only in cases where labor did not progress normally did physicians intervene

JUDITH WALZER LEAVITT is Associate Professor of the History of Medicine, History of Science and Women's Studies at the University of Wisconsin, Madison, Wisconsin.

Reprinted with permission from the *Journal of American History*, 1983, *70*: 281–304.

and perhaps extricate a dead fetus. The midwife orchestrated the events of labor and delivery, and the women neighbors and relatives comforted and shared advice with the parturient.[2] Women suffered through the agonies and dangers of birth together, sought each other's support, and shared the relief of successful deliveries and the grief of unsuccessful ones. This "social childbirth" experience united women and provided, as Carroll Smith-Rosenberg has argued, one of the functional bonds that formed the basis of women's domestic culture.[3]

Within their own homes, birthing women controlled much of the experience of childbirth. They determined the physical setting for their births, the people to attend them during labor and delivery, and the aids or comforts employed. Midwives traditionally played a noninterventionist, supportive role in the home birthing rooms. As much as possible they let nature take its course: they examined the cervix or encouraged women to walk around; they caught the child, tied the umbilical cord, and if necessary fetched the placenta. In complicated cases, midwives might have turned the fetus—podalic version—or fortified women with hard liquor or mulled wine. They may have manually stretched the cervix or, rarely, administered ergot. Midwives spent most of their time, as the written record reveals, comforting the parturient and waiting. The other women attendants supported the midwife and the birthing woman, and the atmosphere in the birthing rooms—if everything proceeded normally—was congenial and cooperative. Parturient women, who felt vulnerable at the time of their confinements, armed themselves with the strength of other women who had passed through the event successfully.[4]

Despite the very positive aspects of social childbirth, a romantic image of childbirth in this period would be misleading. Women garnered support from their networks of companions, but they continued to fear their births because of the possibilities of death or debility that could and frequently did result from childbirth. Although statistics do not exist to measure these dangers precisely, women's fears were not unfounded. By all accounts maternal and infant mortality rates were high. Furthermore, postpartum gynecological problems resulting from unsutured perineal tears, prolapsed uteri, or vesico-vaginal and recto-vaginal fistulas caused some women extreme discomfort and disability throughout the rest of their lives. Women's fears of death and physical debility led them away from traditional birthing patterns to a long search for safer and less painful childbirths. Thus some women, especially those who were economically advantaged, tried to modify traditional births by incorporating new possibilities as they became available. Like the Drinkers, these 18th-century women readily invited physicians to attend them, despite their worries about the propriety of having men participate in intimate female events, in hopes that the "man-midwives" could provide easier and safer births.[5]

The entrance of physician-accoucheurs into the practice of obstetrics in America during the second half of the 18th century marked the first significant break with tradition. The story of this new midwifery, familiar to historians of American medicine, centers on Shippen, who in 1762 returned from his studies in London and Edinburgh and established the first systematic series of lectures on midwifery in America. Shippen initially trained both female midwives and male physicians in anatomy (including the gravid uterus), but he soon limited his lectures to male students. He established a private practice of midwifery and became a favorite of Philadelphia's established families. The Drinkers found him "very kind and attentive" during labor and delivery and noted that he remained with his patients even during protracted labors and "sleep't very little."[6]

Shippen was the most famous of late-18th-century physicians who practiced midwifery, but he was not alone. Numerous doctors expanded their practice of medicine and began to attend laboring women. The transition to male attendants occurred so easily among advantaged urban women that it can only be explained by understanding the women's impression that physicians knew more than midwives about the birth process and about what to do if things went wrong. Women overturned millennia of all-female tradition and invited men into their birthing rooms because they believed that men offered additional security against the potential dangers of childbirth. By their acknowledgement of physician superiority, women changed the fashions of childbearing and made it desirable to be attended by physicians.[7]

Women had good reason to believe that physicians could provide services that midwives could not. Many of the physicians who practiced obstetrics at the turn of the 19th century had trained in Great Britain, where a tradition of male accoucheurs had already developed. The men had access to education then denied to women, which provided theoretical understanding of female anatomy and the process of parturition. Whereas women midwives relied on practical experience and an appeal to female traditions—attributes to some extent taken for granted and unappreciated—men physicians had the extra advantage and prestige associated with formal learning. Even though most American practitioners had not attended medical school and were themselves apprentice trained, physicians carried with them the status advantages of their gender and of the popular image of superior education. Furthermore, birthing women perceived that the male presence had already contributed opium and forceps to obstetrics and promised even greater benefits in the future. The appeal to overturn tradition was strong.[8]

When Shippen attended Sally Drinker Downing's 1795 birth, which was complicated by a footling presentation, he administered opium to relieve her suffering. Two years later, faced with another of Downing's difficult labors, Shippen "was oblig'd to force her mouth open to give some thing with a view of reviving her." In 1799 Downing again suffered a protracted labor, and Shippen took 14 ounces of blood and then gave her 80 to 90 drops of liquid laudanum. According to Downing's mother, when labor still did not progress, Shippen gave "an Opium pill three grains he said, in order to ease her pain, or to bring it on more violently." When this still did not produce the desired result, Shippen threatened to use his instruments, but finally Downing delivered without them.[9]

Shippen's practice of allaying painful and lengthy labors by bleeding, giving opium, and occasionally using forceps illustrates why women wanted physicians to attend them. The prospect of a difficult birth, which all women fearfully anticipated, and the knowledge that physicians' remedies could provide relief and successful outcomes led women to seek out practitioners whose obstetric armamentarium included drugs and instruments.[10]

The promise of the new obstetrics developed in part through formal physician education in midwifery. Shippen's first lectures covered pelvic anatomy, the gravid uterus, the placenta, fetal circulation and nutrition, natural and unnatural labor, and the use of obstetrical instruments. He demonstrated on manikins and on patients—poor women for whom he provided accommodation—and used drawings and textbooks. Other physicians followed his example, and courses in midwifery became available in Boston and New York as well as in Philadelphia.

During the first half of the 19th century medical education in obstetrics expanded. To many professors and students, the subject was embarrassing, and students generally did not observe women in labor but received only a theoretical education. Samuel D. Gross, a student who observed Thomas Chalkley James teaching obstetrics at the University of Pennsylvania early in the 19th century, noticed that "it was seldom that he . . . looked squarely at his audience. His cheeks would be mantled with blushes while engaging in demonstrating some pelvic viscus, or discussing topics not mentionable in ordinary conversation. It was often painful to witness his embarrassment."[12]

Although the embarrassment of physicians about their role in obstetrics soon disappeared, the question of a man's proper behavior in a woman's birthing room continued to influence the teaching and the practice of obstetrics. Of William Potts Dewees, who succeeded James at the University of Pennsylvania, Gross observed, "he did not hesitate to call things by their proper names. No blush suffused his cheek in the lecture-room." But Dewees, whose *A Compendious System of Midwifery* went through an influential 12 editions, remained as horrified by the idea of ocular inspection as his most modest patients. Using manikins, he taught his students how to perform unsighted digital ex-

plorations of parturient women. Even when applying forceps, Dewees taught, "every attention should be paid to delicacy . . . the patient should not be exposed . . . even for the drawing off of the urine. . . . The operator must become familiar with the introduction of the instruments without the aid of sight."[13]

Students graduating from such didactic obstetrics courses were forced to enter the birthing rooms of their first patients in relative ignorance. Never having witnessed actual births, and armed with only theoretical knowledge, they must have been somewhat apprehensive. Yet doctors knew that they had to be confident to gain confidence, and they forged ahead and delivered babies. One medical graduate wrote that when he delivered his first baby he examined the laboring woman, "but whether it was head or breech, hand or foot, man or monkey, that was defended from my uninstructed finger by the distended membranes, I was as uncomfortably ignorant, with all my learning, as the foetus itself that was making all this fuss."[14] Rejecting the practical experience of the midwives' training, those physicians who had formal medical education tried to raise the practice of obstetrics to a higher level by emphasizing anatomy and physiology.

Through their theoretical training, this physician elite had the potential to expand the practice of obstetrics beyond individual experience. Apprentice-trained midwives and physicians could develop expertise only insofar as their mentors' or their own experiences took them, and wider perspectives remained elusive. But when some doctors took it upon themselves to study anatomy of the female pelvis and activity of the gravid uterus, they removed knowledge from its anchor in individual human experience and brought it to a more abstract level. Learning what was possible and probable in labor and delivery, what was normal and abnormal, provided these birth attendants with knowledge to make judgments on the individual cases they examined.

While the potential for this increased enlightenment may have existed, the question remains whether or not individual medical graduates related their theoretical knowledge to the actual cases they faced in their practices. Did male physicians enhance or improve childbirth, as women believed they would? Did "science," the symbol of the promises of physician-directed obstetrics, come to the aid of birthing women?

Either because of their training or because of families' expectations, male physicians, the apprentice-trained and medical school graduates alike, intervened in the birth process more than midwives. Walter Channing, professor of obstetrics at Harvard, advised that a doctor, when called to attend laboring women, "must do something. He cannot remain a spectator merely, where there are many witnesses, and where interest in what is going on is too deep to allow of his inaction. Let him be collected and calm, and he will probably do little he will afterwards look upon with regret."[15]

Physicians' favorite interventions during the first half of the 19th century were bloodletting, drugs, and forceps, frequently all used together. Dewees advocated substantial bloodletting. In one of his difficult cases, for example, with the woman standing on her feet, he took "upwards of two quarts" until she fainted. Dewees remarked that "every thing appeared better . . . I introduced the forceps, and delivered a living and healthy child." Physicians believed that venesection could relieve pain, accelerate labor, soften a rigid cervix, ease podalic version, and reduce inflammation. They even bled patients who were hemorrhaging, using the logic that further reducing circulation would produce blood clotting and stop the hemorrhage. They also relieved puerperal convulsions by bloodletting. In fact, as one historian has concluded, "bloodletting . . . was uncritically accepted as the fashion in early American obstetric practice."[16]

The use of opium or laudanum (tincture of opium) seems to have been equally popular among physician-accoucheurs in the 19th century. In cases of protracted labor, as in the Shippen-Downing cases cited above, physicians tried opium to accelerate cervical dilation and ease suffering. They also employed cathartics to open the bowels, ergot to stimulate contractions, tobacco infusions to encourage the cervix to dilate, and manually breaking the waters to accelerate labor. In cases of extreme need physicians could surgically separate the pubic bones to facilitate passage of the fetus's head or they could introduce the crochet, the instrument used for fetal dismemberment and extraction.[17]

The forceps constituted the favorite instrument of physician intervention, and women both feared and respected the "hands of iron." When Shippen referred obliquely to forceps in front of Sally Downing's mother, she "was afraid to ask him, least he should answer in the affermative" that he needed to use it. Her confidence in its benefits, however, remained intact. Women were grateful for the tool that could extricate a fetus in compacted labors.[18]

In 1812 a medical graduate of the University of Pennsylvania entered practice in a town where two aging physicians already practiced. These physicians "had never used forceps, and were in the habit of resorting to Smellie's scissors and the crotchet in all cases where the foetal head became obstructed in the pelvis." The young doctor soon established himself among the women in the community by successfully using forceps to deliver healthy babies who might have otherwise been destroyed. This sort of success story achieved a legendary quality in the 19th century as physicians expanded the use of forceps at the same time as they developed their practices.[19]

When well used, forceps could save lives; when misused, they could increase women's perineal lacerations and cause head injuries to the fetus. Dewees called attention to the "mischief" that forceps could cause and believed that their dangers were enhanced because physicians used them too often and unnecessarily. He cautioned: "The greatest care must be taken, before we begin our traction, that no portion of the mother is included in the locking of the blades — this must be done by passing a finger entirely round the place of union. . . . I was once called to a poor woman who had had a considerable portion of the internal face of the right labium removed, by having been included in the joint of the short forceps."[20] Physicians who had been trained to use forceps only on manikins and who were required by custom to perform the forceps operation without the benefit of sight ran considerable risk of creating new problems for the women whose obstructed labors they tried to ameliorate.

Countless stories testify to the severe lacerations 19th-century women suffered in childbirth, and they suggest an increase in the problem over what women had previously experienced. The accusation of "meddlesome midwifery" followed physician-accoucheurs, and textbooks cautioned against forceps misuse often enough to suggest that a significant problem existed. The midwifery professors repeatedly warned against unnecessary use of forceps. But their students or apprentice-trained physicians in practice in America's communities found forceps a very valuable tool, and because of their eagerness or their limited practical experience, they may have overused and misused them. Dewees observed so many cases of misused forceps that he concluded, "The forceps . . . are nearly as fatal as the crochet itself."[21]

If forceps were at fault in the "meddlesome midwifery" of the early 19th century, they were not the only problem. Almost any intervention by the physician created a potential for harm. If a birth could not proceed without help, the physician provided a service not available elsewhere and necessary to saving lives. If, however, as was statistically more probable, labor was proceeding normally and physicians intervened anyway, their actions introduced dangers not otherwise present. Dewees's caution about careful use of forceps inadvertently informs us about the concurrent dangers of infection. He taught his students to check that no part of the mother was caught in the blades of the forceps by "passing a finger entirely round the place of union." An unwashed and ungloved finger could have carried a higher risk to women's lives than a perineal laceration.

H. B. Willard, a medical graduate who practiced obstetrics in Wisconsin beginning in 1849, rarely used forceps because "the idea of instruments is *horrible* to *friends & patient* beside there is much liability to injure the parts." But Willard had no reservations about using opium and ergot, internally manipulating the fetus to change its presenting part, and routinely rupturing the waters with his fingernails. Willard chose his therapeutic activities by weighing the effects they would have on his reputation in the community. He tried not to use emetics, for example, because he knew "the idea of being vomited at such a time is exceedingly repugnant to the patient & to friends." By the same reasoning, Willard, when called to attend a laboring woman, followed Channing's dictum to do something. He knew his patients expected action. The only cases in which Willard did not interfere were those in which the baby had been born before his arrival. In those cases he might still have had opportunity to extract the placenta manually.[22]

Physicians' obstetrics courses taught them the theoretical basis of their craft, their apprenticeships gave them tools with which to effect a successful birth, but nowhere did they receive clear guidelines for the practical application of their knowledge. Doctors had numerous techniques at their command and complete leeway in their use. If physicians used forceps too often, or if they intervened in the birth process too eagerly, it was because they were more persuaded by the faces of women in agony than by the cautions of their elders. Their decisions about intervention were made on the spot and in relative isolation. Even the professors at the medical schools and the leading textbooks taught by anecdotal example, making generalizations hard if not impossible to construct. Physicians could convince themselves easily and in good conscience that their judgment to intervene in labor was in the best interests of the patient. The majority of successful outcomes in each individual's practice underlined the truthfulness of these conclusions. Early obstetric "science" provided knowledge and wherewithal, but the principles of the practical application remained at the bedside in the hands of individual, isolated doctors such as Willard.[23]

The decision of whether or not to employ the skills of the physician remained with women, where it had traditionally been. The parturient, her midwife, and her assistants frequently decided to call a doctor after labor had begun and then gave or withheld permission for each procedure suggested. Dewees, for example, after one successful forceps operation, was called to other cases because "the influence of this case upon many of the midwives of this city, procured me many opportunities of applying the forceps." Similarly the young Pennsylvania doctor's success in delivering babies using forceps led women to refuse to let other doctors use the crochet. Although physicians had broken the gender barrier and birth was no longer exclusively a women's event, women continued to hold the power to shape events in the birthing room.[24]

Despite the strength of tradition, however, birth had changed for the women who invited physicians to attend them in their homes. These women formed a minority of all birthing women, and they probably were limited geographically to the major cities and economically to the advantaged classes. Most Americans still could not afford doctors and employed midwives and delivered their babies in the same ways as their mothers and grandmothers had. But for those women who chose physicians instead of or in addition to midwives, birth became less a natural process and more an event that could be altered and influenced by a wide selection of interventions. Women and physicians realized that fate no longer held women in such a tight grip and that decisions could be made and actions could be taken that would determine what kind of a birth a woman would have and perhaps whether she and her baby lived or died. This mental perception of the ability to shape the birth experience became even more important in the second half of the 19th century when anesthesia emerged as the paramount birthing panacea.

Fanny Longfellow's exuberant description of her childbirth under ether in 1847 (the first in the United States) indicates just how ready women were to change their childbirth experiences. "I never was better or got through a confinement so comfortably," she wrote her sister-in-law. "I feel proud to be the pioneer to less suffering for poor, weak womankind. This is certainly the greatest blessing of this age, and I am glad to have lived at the time of its coming and in the country which gives it to the world."[25] By the middle of the century middle-class women had become accustomed to male birth attendants, although a large segment of the population — probably growing as immigration soared in the latter part of the century — remained faithful to female midwives and traditional birth procedures. Advantaged urban women sought every obstetric improvement that male physicians could offer because they continued to fear childbirth and its attendant discomforts. As one woman wrote about her fourth birth in 1885, "Between the oceans of pain, there stretched continents of fear; fear of death and dread of suffering beyond bearing."[26]

Women who experienced their childbirths as the hour in which they "touched the hand of death" eagerly sought relief from the frightful event. Ether and chloroform promised such relief, and women like Longfellow embraced anesthesia enthusiastically. One of Channing's patients told him after her etherized birth "how wonderful it was that she should have got through without the least suffering, and how grateful she was."[27]

Women, in fact, were initially more eager than physicians to use anesthesia. Among physicians,

there was some uncertainty about the safety of the new drugs for midwifery practice. Charles D. Meigs of Philadelphia rejected chloroform and ether and carried on a well-publicized campaign against their use, claiming that he had "not yielded to several solicitations as to its exhibition addressed to me by my patients in labour." Meigs relied upon women's painful contractions to help him determine labor's progress and believed that their inhibition would make him a less effective birth attendant.[28]

Walter Channing, one of ether's most ardent supporters, in 1848 surveyed 46 Boston-area physicians' use of anesthesia in labor and found that they held back on using the drugs except in cases when "patients have demanded it with an emphasis which could not be resisted . . . in many cases, and in the practice of some physicians, it has only been used when such demand has been made."[29] A. R. Thompson of Charlestown, Massachusetts, wrote Channing the following account, which was not unusual. "This lady had informed herself fully as to the use of ether, and had made up her mind to take it. . . . When called to her, I frankly told her that I had never used the ether, nor had I ever seen it used in any case, but that I had no prejudice against it, and would consent to its administration in her case. . . . she was resolute, and demanded the ether. . . . I poured an ounce of ether into the sponge, and the lady held it to her mouth and nose." A successful outcome and a happy patient convinced this doctor to use the drug in subsequent cases. After his second trial of ether Thompson concluded confidently, "My conviction at the time was strong, that the ether had greatly diminished the sufferings of the mother, and shortened the term of her travail for many hours."[30]

Perceptions of safety and patterns of anesthesia use varied enormously among physicians in the second half of the 19th century. The medical journals reported both safe and hazardous results of ether and chloroform in midwifery. A Massachusetts physician, for example, wrote in the *Boston Medical and Surgical Journal* that chloroform was "a dangerous and often deadly agent," and a Detroit physician concluded in the *Journal of the American Medical Association*, "I have yet to see my first case of the least evil result to mother or child." With such variation in the literature, individual physicians relied heavily on their own experiences and on the desires of their patients. A rural Iowa doctor wrote about his 500 obstetric cases: "I do not use an anaesthetic of any kind, especially in forceps cases. I want the patient to know what is going on." Another physician came to the opposite conclusion and recommended anesthesia "not only in troublesome instrumental labor, but in all cases where the pains of travail fall upon women."[31]

Many physicians felt pressed, if their time was limited and other patients were waiting, to use forceps, anesthesia, or both to direct labor into patterns under their control. This inclination was reinforced by women eagerly seeking relief from their suffering. A Colorado physician related that after several hours of hard labor one of his patients "implored me to do something, and, with many misgivings, at last I decided to use instruments [and] chloroform."[32]

Physicians came to adopt anesthesia so generally that one physician in 1895 observed that "the profession has come to regard the use of chloroform in parturition as almost utterly devoid of danger," so that "chloroform is given in labor often recklessly, carelessly, and copiously." As physicians delivered the babies, other attendants—"ignorant nurses, husbands, bystanders, and even . . . the patients themselves"—dripped chloroform or ether onto a sponge or cloth and held it to the woman's nose. No standard procedures guarded physicians' drug dosages.[33]

Physicians' reports of their obstetric practices in the second half of the 19th century indicate that use of anesthesia did not necessarily lead to increased forceps use. While doctors did come to use anesthesia routinely in forceps deliveries, the reverse was not true. Physicians did not use forceps routinely on patients to whom they gave ether and chloroform. Physicians employed forceps in approximately 8 percent of their births, whereas some used anesthesia at almost every birth they attended, and on the average about 50 percent of all physician-attended births utilized chloroform or ether.[34] Thus, despite the haphazard use of open-drop ether or chloroform and the consequent potential for overdosing, actual anesthesia use must have remained light. Profound anesthesia would have caused labor to decelerate and would have made forceps necessary to lift the baby that the woman was unable to push out. But with light analgesia physicians did not require forceps, and

in the 19th century forceps abuse did not increase as a result of increased use of anesthetics. Physicians aimed at pain relief, not total unconsciousness. If a woman administered her own drugs on a handkerchief she held up to her nose, her arm would periodically drop away, decreasing the drug dose. One physician advised maintaining what he called a "dreamy sleep, in which the patient follows in her imagination the direction of the physician." While labor progressed, he conversed with his patients about scenes from their childhood or the Sunday school picnic. One of his patients "almost immediately after the first inhalation burst out in a beautiful song, and continued singing one after another until her babe, a large boy, first child, was born."[35]

Most physicians continued to intervene in the birth process in the second half of the 19th century as they had earlier. Their safety record when measured by mortality matched the record of midwives, who continued to follow a basically noninterventionist birth policy. Dorothy Reed Mendenhall studied births in Wisconsin at the beginning of the 20th century and concluded that for both physicians and midwives maternal mortality was higher than it needed to be but that "we must admit that the midwife is, on the whole, probably less culpable in regard to the deaths of parturient women than physicians in the state."[36] Similar maternal mortality rates for midwife- and physician-attended births indicate that physicians, with all their expertise and intervention techniques, did not, as they had promised, enhance the safety of the birth experience for women. Medicine may have improved comfort levels and may have rescued some women from complicated labors, but it did not, on the whole, increase women's chances of survival.

There are other indications that physicians' techniques created new problems for birthing women and actually increased the dangers of childbirth. Inappropriate forceps use and the careless administration of ether and chloroform introduced serious lacerations and breathing disorders that otherwise might not have developed. Most significant, physicians carried puerperal fever, which was potentially disastrous, to birthing women. Because their medical practices included attending patients with communicable diseases, doctors were more likely than midwives to bring with them on their hands and on their clothing the agents of infection. Epidemics of puerperal fever developed even in the practices of physicians like H. H. Whitcomb of Norristown, Pennsylvania, who did "as little meddling as possible" in normal labor and delivery. In 1886 one of Whitcomb's parturient patients developed fever because Whitcomb brought the infection from a previous patient who had scarlet fever. That winter and spring Whitcomb transmitted the fever to 32 more birthing women.[37]

Physicians offered some women relief from suffering and aided others through compacted labors, but because of the variations in ability and practices of their birth attendants, most women continued to experience discomfort and to fear childbirth. One woman described her physician-attended delivery as "hell. . . . It bursts your brain, and tears out your heart, and crushes your nerves to bits. It's just hell."[38] Despite their continued suffering, those middle-class women who had chosen physicians to attend them did not want to return to midwives. They believed that if birth were to be eased, improvements would come from progress in medicine. Instead of turning to tradition, these women demanded more of their physicians and continued to hope that safe and comfortable deliveries would come to them from the medical world.

As the symbol of what science had to offer, anesthesia enhanced the place and role of physicians in birthing rooms across America. Women who could afford physicians and their new panacea demanded the advantages of painlessness. Despite the presence of men and modern technology in the birthing rooms, however, the birth experience of 19th-century middle- and upper-class women retained many important elements from traditional births. Anita McCormick Blaine's first childbirth in 1890 illustrates this. During her pregnancy Blaine corresponded with her mother, who was in Europe seeking a cure for a hearing loss, and sought the traditional female support network to help her through the impending crisis. "If you could but be with me now, what wouldn't I give," wrote Blaine to her mother, Nettie Fowler McCormick. Despite all of Blaine's preparations and the doctor and nurse who would attend her, McCormick yearned to be with her daughter. She wrote detailed instructions about her care, advising, for example, rubbing olive oil over the abdomen and perineal area to ease delivery. She worried that only a mother could rightfully do such an intimate job. "I don't know if you have a person you could let do it," she wrote, "but I wish I were there to do it." Blaine sequestered herself in her childhood Chicago home, where "every chair and table speaks to me of dear familiar times . . . nothing is so sweet as to feel the presence of all it reminds me of." She surrounded herself with helpers, including her old friend Harriot ("Missy") Hammond, who traveled from Virginia to be with her. Strengthened by these traditional comforts, Anita delivered her baby while under the influence of chloroform, supported by her nurse and by Hammond and attended by a male physician. Her husband waited outside. She united the old and the new in obstetric experiences and planned the whole event to meet her expectations. The doctor managed the birth in the context that the woman created.[39]

The decision-making process in the turn-of-the century birthing rooms reveals how the old and the new intermingled. Doctors, who may have had only minimal practical experience, were invited to attend women in their own homes in the presence of other women, many of whom had had considerable birth experience and had developed strong opinions about birth procedures. Within the birthing rooms, these attendants negotiated. There were desires and expectations on both sides. Women retained a lot of power in their own homes, and physicians bowed to it or risked damaging their reputations among a whole community of women and losing patients. As the new obstetrical techniques — from forceps to anesthetics — became available, they worked to the advantage of physicians, who held the monopoly over their use, while centuries of female traditions and the domestic environment in which they operated worked to the advantage of women.

Inexperienced physicians sometimes welcomed the knowledge of other attendants. Morris Fishbein admitted that he learned more from a laboring woman whose eighth birth he attended than from all his classroom experience. Other physicians found attending a birth in the presence of well-informed women intimidating. One physician recalled, "A young doctor, fresh from medical college, can pass many embarrassing moments in the presence of the neighborhood midwife." Another recalled that a mother's instructions to him "rattled me so that I hardly knew what I was doing."[40]

Women invited physicians to attend them in order to benefit from their expertise and technology, yet doctors could not obtain patients' compliance with all procedures. An Oklahoma physician explained why he could never try to shave a patient's pubic hair even though he thought it would help prevent infection. "In about three seconds after the doctor has made the first rake with his safety [razor], he will find himself on his back out in the yard with the imprint of a woman's bare foot emblazoned on his manly chest, the window sash round his neck and a revolving vision of all the stars in the firmament presented to him. Tell him not to try to shave 'em."[41] Another practitioner realized that a doctor "has his living to make and cannot be too insistent with his patient over whom, usually, he has no control." Yet physicians could not come into the birthing room and do nothing. One Kansas doctor admitted, "Perhaps the best way to manage normal labor is to let it alone, but you cannot hold down a job and do that." Women and physicians negotiated the procedures that would be used, and the result represented a compromise between the two worlds of women's tradition and men's medicine. The compromises held until the 20th century, when physician-directed obstetrics finally became master of the birthing room.[42]

At the turn of the 20th century physicians delivered approximately half of the nation's babies. Most of these births took place in the woman's home and combined aspects of traditional and modern techniques. Although most of the medical profession accepted the need for aseptic conditions—sterile gloves, shaved perineum, antiseptic infusions, sterile instruments—they could not always achieve them. Whether because of their own abilities or their patients' demands, physicians intermingled modern surgical techniques with wide individual variations and traditional practices. One physician writing in 1912 about the management of normal labor observed that only when the fetal head was resting on the perineum was it necessary "to expose the perineum so that its condition may be constantly watched." The inference, harking back to William Dewees, was that before this stage ocular examination should remain limited. Another doctor refused to shave his patients because the attempt "would cause such a violent attack of hysteria that the physician would cease to be of any

further use to that family."[43] Physician practice—susceptible to the physical environment, to the opinions of other attendants, and to the physician's own training and inclination—varied from individual to individual. Physicians acted when they were called to women in labor, but the nature of their interventions followed particular circumstances more than any predetermined science of obstetrics.

The lack of a systematic approach to the practice of obstetrics in the early 20th century can be directly traced to the quality and emphasis of obstetric education, which had not changed substantially during the 19th century. After the middle of the 19th century, "demonstrative midwifery," or teaching students by having them observe actual laboring women, became available, but many medical schools ignored this innovation and continued their didactic teaching from textbooks and manikins. In 1910, although most practitioners now received a formal medical education, many still graduated having witnessed few or no live deliveries. Such training at best prepared students to understand birth pathology and perhaps how to intervene to rescue a woman in trouble, but it did not prepare physicians to attend women in normal labor.[44]

J. Whitridge Williams, professor of obstetrics at the Johns Hopkins Medical School, surveyed obstetrics education in 1912 and concluded that the "average practitioner, through his lack of preparation for the practice of obstetrics, may do his patients as much harm as the much-maligned midwife." Williams found that most medical students had the opportunity during their training to watch only one woman deliver, and one-quarter of the medical schools admitted that their graduates were not competent to practice obstetrics. Yet most physicians did deliver babies as part of their medical practices, spending on the average approximately 30 percent of their time attending childbirth.[45] In the era when scientific investigations began to permeate the medical world, when medical schools increasingly built laboratories and trained their students in research methods and findings, and when specialization and hospital expansion transformed medical practice, physicians' obstetrical practices were characterized by individual variation and unsystematic application of general principles.

Williams believed that only the developing specialty of obstetrics practiced in the hospital setting could improve the marginal situation. Even as a significant portion of American women continued to be attended by midwives in their own homes, and most others continued to invite general practitioners to attend them at home, increasing numbers of women from the middle and upper classes became convinced that childbirth in the hospital offered them the safest experience. Many factors converged to encourage women to move to the hospital in the early years of the 20th century, including the new anesthetic agent scopolamine (best monitored in the hospital), the preference of the specialists, the growth of the hospitals themselves, and the increasing technology and ease of management in the well-equipped and well-staffed hospital setting.[46] Still seeking more comfortable births and safer deliveries with minimal negative aftereffects, many women decided to try the newest that obstetrics had to offer and go to the hospital to be attended by specialists. "I have placed myself in the hands of . . . a specialist in obstetrics," wrote Lella Secor to her mother in 1918. "I have every confidence in him, and it is a great relief."[47]

In hospital deliveries women left their family and friends at the door of the labor room and faced their birthings alone, as one account of birth in the 1930s indicated:

> Arriving [at the hospital], she is immediately given the benefit of one of the modern analgesics or painkillers. Soon she is in a dreamy, half-conscious state. . . .
>
> She knows nothing about being taken to a spotlessly clean delivery room, placed on a sterile table, draped with sterile sheets; neither does she see her attendants, the doctor and nurses, garbed for her protection in sterile white gowns and gloves; nor the shiny boiled instruments and antiseptic solutions. She does not hear the cry of her baby when first he feels the chill of this cold world, or see the care with which the doctor repairs such lacerations as may have occurred. . . . Finally she awakes in smiles, a mother with no recollection of having become one.[48]

This woman was separated from the people she loved, she was in an unfamiliar environment controlled by others, and she was unconscious during her childbirth. Women did not view the stay in the hospital as a time when they lost important parts of the traditional birth experiences, but rather as a time when they gained protection for life and health, aspects of birth that had been elusive and uncertain in the past. Women gave up some kinds of control for others because on balance the new benefits seemed more important. In seeking life and health, women relinquished consciousness and self-determination.

The hospital appealed to women because it was modern, well equipped, and staffed by experts: it represented the newest medical advance. Also, it physically separated women from their domestic chores and allowed them to relax. One wrote, "My stay in that hospital was like a lovely vacation." "I can't tell you the relief I feel as I walk out my door headed for the hospital to have a baby," wrote another. "I have nothing to worry about . . . and have only to concentrate on giving birth. All this peace of mind, plus expert medical attention, makes me wonder why anybody would consider it a 'privilege' to have her baby at home." Home did not hold for mid-20-century women the same comforts and sustenance that Blaine had found so reassuring. The "hospital is equipped with every modern device for the safe delivery of babies," wrote one mother. "Nursing and medical attention is available at any hour of the day or night. How much simpler — and more restful — to be in a hospital where babies are an accepted business."[49]

The move to the hospital was hastened by specialists' attempts to wrest birth away from general practitioners and to systematize birth procedures within the hospital setting. One very influential move in this direction was made in 1920 by Joseph B. DeLee of Chicago in the first volume of the new journal for specialists, the *American Journal of Obstetrics and Gynecology*. DeLee argued that birth was a "pathologic process" and that "only a small minority of women escape damage during labor." He continued, "So frequent are these bad effects, that I have often wondered whether Nature did not deliberately intend women should be used up in the process of reproduction, in a manner analogous to that of salmon, which dies after spawning?" Because of its dangers, DeLee believed birth needed careful monitoring in skilled hands. He recommended reducing birth to predictable patterns by using outlet forceps and episiotomy routinely and prophylactically in normal deliveries. DeLee sedated the parturient with scopolamine, allowed the cervix to dilate, gave ether during the second stage, performed an episiotomy, and lifted the fetus with forceps. He then extracted the placenta, gave ergot to help the uterus contract, and stitched the perineal cut.[50]

DeLee's operation achieved wide acceptance. It represented the new move in the 1920s and 1930s to make obstetrics scientific, systematic, and predictable by putting it under the control of the specialist. Not all specialists wanted to use prophylactic forceps, but hospital-based obstetricians did develop routines for managing childbirth that incorporated systematic use of pain-relieving drugs, labor inducers, and technological intervention. Mothers-to-be learned they could plan when and how they would have a baby, and doctors could predict the course of labor because they controlled it. "The old way [of having a baby] was no fun," wrote one father about the 1916 birth of his first daughter. In 1938 his second daughter, "was born the new way—the easy, painless, streamlined way." His wife, in consultation with her doctor, decided which day to deliver, and after a matinee and dinner went into the hospital. Pituitrin induced her labor, Nembutal and scopolamine deadened her perceptions of it, and the doctor delivered her baby. "Why, I wouldn't mind having another baby next week," she said, "if that's all there is to it."[51] Increasing numbers of middle-class women turned to the hospital and the specialist for their childbirths, believing, as one of them put it, "the vexation of hospital routine shrinks to infinitesimal importance beside the safety of the delivery room."[52]

But was streamlined childbirth safe? Had medicine at last provided safer and more comfortable childbirth for women, as it had promised since the 1760s? Observers in the 1930s realized that while the practice of obstetrics now could relieve women of much of their discomfort, childbirth remained unsafe. Maternal mortality in the 1930s remained "unnecessarily high," according to a group of concerned physicians in New York. The physicians claimed hospital deliveries contributed to the high mortality with a "high incidence of operative interference during labor . . . undertaken when there was no indication or a plain contra-indication." Birth in the hospital encouraged interference because the equipment and staff were readily accessible, and this interference increased the number of maternal deaths. Rather than making child-

birth safer, physicians in the 1920s and 1930s, according to their own evaluation, were responsible for maintaining high rates of maternal mortality.[53]

In home deliveries of the 19th century, increased anesthetic use had not caused an increase in forceps deliveries, but in hospital deliveries of the early 20th century, a direct relationship existed between anesthesia and forceps. The New York doctors noted, "The frequent use of instrumentation is based upon the easy accessibility of anaesthesia. . . . the increase in the use of anaesthesia is a factor in keeping the maternal mortality rate stationary." According to the New York study, use of anesthetic agents led directly to increased instrumentation because drugged women were less effective in pushing the baby out. Approximately 25 percent of hospital deliveries were operative. "The increase in the use of instrumentation brings with it an increased hazard," the doctors found. "Clearly a reduction of the mortality rate can be achieved through a reduction in operative interference."[54]

During the early 1930s the medical profession publicly confessed the shortcomings of its obstetric practices. Rudolph Wieser Holmes declared at a crowded American Medical Association meeting, "I have seen hundreds of women die on the delivery table because of the wrongful use of drugs." Holmes blamed his own role in accelerating scopolamine use for many of these deaths. The public health commissioner for the state of New York calculated that maternal deaths were actually increasing in the 20th century and concluded that "they represent the results of meddlesome and unskillful obstetrical practice."[55] Philadelphia doctors agreed that 56 percent of preventable maternal deaths could be blamed on physician errors of judgment and technique.[56] A national study concluded similarly that "artificial delivery is becoming increasingly frequent, especially in hospital practice," and "that interference with normal labor is accompanied by some added risk to both mother and child." Although the indictment was not universally accepted by physicians in the 1930s, the statistics indicated that going to a hospital to have a baby managed by a physician and under the influence of 20th-century drugs and instruments did not necessarily give a mother an advantage and may have put her in greater jeopardy than her neighbor who stayed home.[57]

Obstetrics by the 1930s had not achieved a record of safety commensurate with its abilities. Aided by the New York Academy of Medicine's 1933 revelations about preventable maternal and infant deaths, however, physicians moved toward regulation and standardization of hospital obstetrics practice in their attempts to decrease the overuse and misuse of drugs and operative procedures. Their success in establishing minimum standards for delivery procedures is evident in the fact that hospital births increased from 35 percent of all births in 1933 to 72 percent ten years later and "for the first time was not associated with higher rates of puerperal death." Other factors converged with hospital regulations to cause the decrease in maternal mortality after 1935. The prenatal-care movement spearheaded by middle-class women succeeded in gaining adherents and in educating the public about the importance of care during pregnancy. Probably most important in

the decelerating death rates was the wide adoption of sulfonamides, blood transfusions, and, after World War II, antibiotics, which were successful in combating infection and hemorrhaging, two of the major causes of maternal deaths. After 1935 maternal mortality fell dramatically.[58] (See Fig. 1.)

Even though birth became safer in the 1940s and 1950s, women who went to the hospital to deliver their babies — 95 percent of American women by 1955 — missed some of the features of traditional social childbirth and found hospital births sterile both in the antiseptic sense and in the human dimension. Continuing to appreciate the safety factors they acknowledged to exist for hospital births, women as early as the 1950s attacked the "cruelty in maternity wards." One woman from Elkhart, Indiana, wrote to the *Ladies' Home Journal*, which exposed these conditions: "So many women, especially first mothers, who are frightened to start out

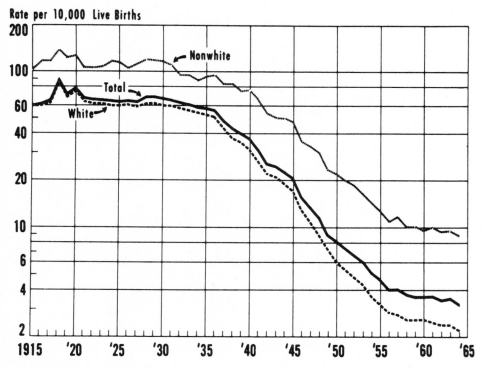

Fig. 1: Maternal mortality rates. Birth registration states or United States, 1915–1964. Source: Sam Shapiro, Edward R. Schlesinger, Robert E. L. Nesbitt, Jr., *Infant,* *Perinatal, Maternal, and Childhood Mortality in the United States* (Cambridge, Mass.: Harvard University Press, 1968), p. 145. Reprinted by permission.

with, receive such brutal inconsiderate treatment that the whole thing is a horrible nightmare. They give you drugs, whether you want them or not, strap you down like an animal." A woman from Columbus, Ohio, concurred that a new mother was "foiled in every attempt to follow her own wishes."[59] These women noticed that the physical removal of childbirth from the woman's home to the physician's institution shifted the balance of power. Birth was no longer part of the woman's domain, as it had been during all the years it remained in the home. It had become instead a medical affair run by medical professionals. Women were no longer the main actors, but instead physicians acted upon women's bodies. Women who were attended by physicians in their own homes could still determine what would happen — could refuse to be shaved or could demand ether. They still controlled much of their own births. But women who entered the birthing rooms of medicine were captured by the routine and by the expertise surrounding them. They could not decide what kind of births they would have.

Some hospitals and some doctors did not depersonalize birth with institutional routine and were able to provide satisfying birth experiences. But many women agreed with the Bozeman, Montana, mother who wrote, "The cruelest part of [hospital] childbirth is being alone among strangers." She found nothing familiar to comfort her through the difficult hours, only the routine of hospital life that she and others described as an assembly line.[60] Physician-directed hospital obstetrics had not met the expectations of American women by protecting a woman's dignity and integrity at the same time as it insured safety. Women wanted the psychologically comforting practices of their traditional birthing rooms to be incorporated into the modern practices of the birthing rooms of science.

The two images of birthing women in America — one "brought to bed" in her own home by the women she had called together and the other drugged and "alone among strangers" in an impersonal hospital — frame the American obstetric experience. The 18th-century woman felt vulnerable to death and debility despite the strength she derived from her friends; the 20th-century woman felt vulnerable to the institutional routine despite the strength she derived from encouraging

maternal-mortality statistics. Neither woman had what she knew she needed at the time of her birth: the certainty of a healthy outcome with the freedom to make choices about how to conduct the important event.

For most of American history women controlled the events in their own birthing rooms. They negotiated with their birth attendants and decided, as much as their bodies and available technology allowed, how the birth would proceed. But the physical forces of birth did not always cooperate, and women felt at the mercy of fate. When physicians entered the women's birthing rooms with the promises of increased safety, women shared their traditional jurisdiction. Forceps, therapeutic aids, and especially anesthesia seemed to offer some insurance against the uncontrollable terrors of birth. Women found that they could, if they wanted to, give their bodies up to labor and to the physician and return to consciousness after the event. Birthing women and their physicians, in the company of other women or family members, negotiated the particulars of birth procedures behind the closed doors of the birthing room and achieved a compromise that recognized the needs, wishes, and abilities of all participants.

But physicians could not achieve the safety that they had promised. While some women were relieved or saved by medical intervention, on balance women's experiences of birth were not significantly enhanced by the entrance of medicine. Physicians remained unable to control their own use of obstetric technology for the first 170 years they were engaged in delivering America's babies, and they frequently added to women's problems by increasing the danger of infection, overdosing with anesthesia, and mutilating with forceps.

In the 20th century the hospital offered an alternative that appealed to women and to doctors because it promised at last the safety that both had sought. Removing birth from women's homes seemed just another step in the progression of changing practices. But women soon discovered that the birthing rooms of medicine differed fundamentally from their own birthing rooms. In hospitals women lost the ability to make choices for themselves and surrendered to the medical community the power to determine what would be done to their bodies. The early years of hospital-based obstetrics did not even provide additional safety for women. As the doctors themselves eventually realized, the hospital made interventions so easy that doctors resorted to operations and drugs in excess of what was indicated and by their own action kept the rates of maternal mortality high. Only after 1940 did medicine begin to achieve a record of safety commensurate with the promises it had held out to women centuries earlier.

Each major transition in American childbirth history—from midwives to physicians, from home to hospital, from "hands of flesh" intervention to "hands of iron" interference—represents in a different form the lure of science and its promise to improve the childbirth experience.[61] As women and their attendants came to perceive birth as an event that could be shaped and manipulated, their *mentalité* of pathology and impending emergencies led each generation to seek its own kind of ideal childbirth. Ultimately it was the promise of continual advances that pushed birth into new patterns throughout American history. Women and their birth attendants believed that medicine could solve their birthing problems and make procreation safe, and they put their faith in scientific advances years before science had significant impact on obstetric practices. Systematic application of tested principles did not characterize obstetrics until the 20th century, yet medical activities in the birth room were valued much earlier because physicians carried an image of expertise and knowledge along with the instruments and drugs in their medical bags.

Despite the lack of a systematic practice of obstetrics, women did not want to turn back to traditional practices. Only in very recent years has any sizable group of American women tried to change direction. Today some women are trying to alter the patterns of childbirth by seeking practices that were common in the past. These women, still a minority and predominantly middle-class, search out midwives or demand that doctors turn back the clock to a time when decision making involved all the birth participants. Women in America today who are seeking to control their own births are fighting the legacy of childbirth as structured by the medical profession and are demanding that choice be reintroduced to the childbirth agenda. They are not trying to overturn science but rather to control it within the traditional female context.[62]

The two themes of social childbirth and scientific childbirth have persisted throughout American history. In the 17th and 18th centuries, social childbirth practices prevailed. The two vied for supremacy during the 19th century, and not until the middle of the 20th century did the medical model succeed in dominating American childbirth. Yet physician-directed childbirth has not met all the needs of birthing women. The pendulum swing between the two traditions has not yet found its resting place.

## NOTES

This paper was written for and first delivered at the Seventh International Symposium on the Comparative History of Medicine—East and West, Susono-Shi, Japan, Sept. 19–26, 1982. This symposium is held by the Division of Medical History, the Taniguchi Foundation.

1 Cecil K. Drinker, *Not So Long Ago: A Chronicle of Medicine and Doctors in Colonial Philadelphia* (New York, 1937), pp. 50–62; Jane B. Donegan, *Women and Men Midwives: Medicine, Morality, and Misogyny in Early America* (Westport, Conn., 1978); and Catherine M. Scholten, "'On the Importance of the Obstetrick Art': changing customs of childbirth in America, 1760 to 1825," *William & Mary Quart.*, July 1977, *34:* 426–445. The scope of the subject of changing obstetric practices necessitates a synthetic analysis and does not permit full documentation here of all the points raised.

2 Louis B. Wright and Marion Tinling, eds., *The Se-cret Diary of William Byrd of Westover, 1709–1792* (Richmond, 1941), p. 79. The phrase "called her women together" is common in early childbirth accounts. See, for example, the diary of midwife Martha Moore Ballard of Augusta, Maine, November 21, 1785—"Mrs. Cowen called her women together this evening; was safely delivered of a daughter about the middle of the night and is comfortable"—and February 18, 1786—"Mrs. Fletcher called her women again this morn, and was safely delivered of a daughter." Charles Elventon Nash, *The History of Augusta: First Settlements and Early Days as a Town, including the Diary of Mrs. Martha Moore Ballard* (1785 to 1812) (Augusta, Maine, 1904), pp. 243, 246.

3 Carroll Smith-Rosenberg, "The female world of love and ritual: relations between women in nineteenth-century America," *Signs,* Autumn 1975, *1:* 1–29. For a discussion of social childbirth, see Richard W. Wertz and Dorothy C. Wertz, *Lying-In: A*

*History of Childbirth in America* (New York, 1977), pp. 1–26.

4 On midwives' practices, see Donegan, *Women and Men Midwives*, pp. 9–11, 25, 127; Scholten, "'On the Importance of the Obstetrick Art,'" pp. 429–431, 432–434; Claire E. Fox, "Pregnancy, childbirth and early infancy in Anglo-American culture: 1675–1830" (Ph.D. dissertation, Univ. of Pennsylvania, 1966), pp. 122–127; and Janet Bogdan, "Care or cure? Childbirth practices in nineteenth century America," *Feminist Stud.*, June 1978, *4*: 94.

5 For more on women's perceptions of childbirth as a time of danger, see Judith Walzer Leavitt and Whitney Walton, "Down to death's door: women's perceptions of childbirth in America," in *Proceedings of the Second Motherhood Symposium: Childbirth: The Beginning of Motherhood,* ed. Sophie Colleau (Madison, 1982), pp. 113–36. On efforts to compute maternal mortality, see B. M. Willmott Dobbie, "An attempt to estimate the true rate of maternal mortality, sixteenth to eighteenth Centuries," *Med. Hist.*, Jan. 1982, *26*: 79–90; and Louis I. Dublin, "Mortality among women from causes incidental to childbearing," *Am. J. Obst. & Dis. Women & Children,* July 1918, *78*: 20–37.

6 Drinker, *Not So Long Ago*, pp. 60–61; Lewis C. Scheffey, "The earlier history and the transition period of obstetrics and gynecology in Philadelphia," *Ann. Med. Hist.*, May 1940, *2*: 215–216.

7 Scholten, "'On the Importance of the Obstetrick Art,'" pp. 434–436.

8 Bogdan, "Care or cure?" pp. 96–97; Donegan, *Women and Men Midwives,* pp. 141–157.

9 Drinker, *Not So Long Ago*, pp. 51–53, 58–61.

10 Jane B. Donegan argues that William Shippen practiced conservative obstetrics when compared with the "meddlesome midwifery" of others. Donegan, *Women and Men Midwives*, pp. 118–119. For more on Shippen, see Betsy Copping Corner, *William Shippen, Jr.: Pioneer in American Medical Education: A Biographical Essay* (Philadelphia, 1951).

11 Lawrence D. Longo, "Obstetrics and gynecology," in *The Education of American Physicians: Historical Essays,* ed. Ronald L. Numbers (Berkeley, 1980), pp. 205–208.

12 *Autobiography of Samuel D. Gross, M.D., with Sketches of His Contemporaries,* ed. [Samuel Weissel Gross and Albert Haller Gross], 2 vols. (Philadelphia, 1887), II, p. 240.

13 *Ibid.*, p. 247; William P. Dewees, *A Compendious System of Midwifery, Chiefly Designed to Facilitate the Inquiries of Those Who May Be Pursuing This Branch of Study* (Philadelphia, 1843), p. 289. See also Irving S. Cutter and Henry R. Viets, *A Short History of Midwifery* (Philadelphia, 1964), pp. 156–157.

14 Wertz and Wertz, *Lying-In,* p. 50.

15 Walter Channing, *A Treatise on Etherization in Childbirth. Illustrated by Five Hundred and Eighty-One Cases* (Boston, 1848), p. 229.

16 Dewees, *Compendious System,* pp. 354, 356–357; A. Clair Siddall, "Bloodletting in American obstetric practice, 1800–1945," *Bull. Hist. Med.,* Spring 1980, *54*: 101–110.

17 Bogdan, "Care or cure?" pp. 96–98; Scholten, "'On the Importance of the Obstetrick Art,'" pp. 437–439. The crochet was the classic instrument to destroy the fetus in utero and permit extraction.

18 Drinker, *Not So Long Ago*, pp. 60–61.

19 Robert P. Harris, "History of a pair of obstetrical forceps sixty years old," *Am. J. Obst. & Dis. Women & Children*, May 1871, *4*: 55–59.

20 Dewees, *Compendious System*, p. 290.

21 *Ibid.*, p. 286.

22 H. B. Willard Obstetrical Journal, June 29, 1854, p. 23, H. B. Willard Papers (State Historical Society of Wisconsin, Madison); *ibid.*, Feb. 4, 1856, p. 29. For a woman's perceptions of physicians' interventions, see Harriet Connor Brown, *Grandmother Brown's Hundred Years, 1827–1927* (Boston, 1929), p. 93.

23 See, for example, Willard Obstetrical Journal, Oct. 27, 1849, p. 3; *ibid.*, Dec. 25, 1849, p. 2; *ibid.*, May 7, 1850, p. 4.

24 Dewees, *Compendious System*, p. 281; Harris, "History of a pair of obstetrical forceps," p. 57.

25 Edward Wagenknecht, ed., *Mrs. Longfellow: Selected Letters and Journals of Fanny Appleton Longfellow (1817–1861)* (New York, 1956), pp. 129–30.

26 Elizabeth H. Emerson, *Glimpses of a Life* (Burlington, N.C., 1960), pp. 4–5.

27 Mrs. Hal Russell, "Memoirs of Marian Russell," *Colorado Magazine*, Jan. 1944, *21*: 35–36; Channing, *Treatise on Etherization*, p. 165. For more on women's fears of death and debility, see Leavitt and Walton, "Down to death's door."

28 "Dr. Meigs' reply to Professor Simpson's letter," *Med. Exam. & Rec. Med. Sci.*, Mar. 1848, *11*: 148–51. See also John Duffy, "Anglo-American reaction to obstetrical anesthesia," *Bull. Hist. Med.*, Jan.–Feb. 1964, *38*: 32–44.

29 Channing, *Treatise on Etherization*, p. 300. Walter Channing did not report what proportion of these physician-attended births used anesthesia.

30 *Ibid.*, pp. 334–335. The woman who insisted on using ether was 43 years old and had had five children.

31 B. E. Cotting, "Anesthetics in midwifery," *Boston Med. & Surg. J.*, Dec. 9, 1858, *59*: 369; Bedford Brown, "The therapeutic action of chloroform in parturition," *J.A.M.A.*, Aug. 31, 1895, *25*: 355; A. D.

Bundy, "Obstetrics in the country," *Med. & Surg. Rep.* Feb. 12, 1887, *56:* 201; D. M. Barr, "Anaesthesia in labor," *ibid.*, Mar. 13, 1880, *42:* 221.

32	Charles Fox Gardiner, *Doctor at Timberline* (Caldwell, Idaho, 1938), p. 211. See also Barr, "Anaesthesia in labor," p. 227.

33	Brown, "Therapeutic action," p. 354; Duffy, "Anglo-American reaction," p. 38. See also J. F. Ford, "Use of drugs in labor," *Wisconsin Med. J.*, Oct. 1904, *3:* 257–265.

34	Ford, "Use of drugs," pp. 257–258; Bundy, "Obstetrics in the country," pp. 200–201. In 91,000 births in Iowa physicians used forceps in 7 percent of cases. E. D. Plass and H. J. Alvis, "A statistical study of 129,539 births in Iowa, with special reference to the method of delivery and the stillbirth rate," *Am. J. Obst. & Gynec.*, Aug. 1934, *28:* 297.

35	Barr, "Anaesthesia in labor," pp. 226–227. In the 20th century, obstetricians appear to have used anesthesia with the intent to produce unconsciousness, and forceps use consequently increased.

36	Dorothy Reed Mendenhall, "Prenatal and natal conditions in Wisconsin," *Wisconsin Med. J.*, Mar. 1917, *15:* 353. See also the comments of Dorothy Reed Mendenhall and Florence Sherbon, in American Association for Study and Prevention of Infant Mortality, *Transactions of the Seventh Annual Meeting, Milwaukee, October 19–21, 1916* (Baltimore, 1917), pp. 67–68, 63–64.

37	H. H. Whitcomb, "A report of 616 cases of labor in private practice," *Med. & Surg. Reptr.*, Feb. 12, 1887, *56:* 201. Puerperal sepsis caused the largest proportion of maternal deaths at the beginning of the 20th century. See American Association for Study and Prevention of Infant Mortality, *Transactions of the Seventh Annual Meeting*, p. 67.

38	Russell Kelso Carter, *The Sleeping Car "Twilight"; or, Motherhood without Pain* (Boston, 1915), pp. 10–11.

39	Anita McCormick Blaine to Nettie Fowler McCormick, Aug. 24, 1890, folder 2B, box 46, Nancy Fowler McCormick Papers (State Historical Society of Wisconsin); McCormick to Blaine, Aug. 1890, folder 1E, box 459, *ibid.*

40	Morris Fishbein, *An Autobiography* (Garden City, N.Y., 1969), p. 25; Helen MacKnight Doyle, *A Child Went Forth: The Autobiography of Dr. Helen MacKnight Doyle* (New York, 1934), p. 322; Gardiner, *Doctor at Timberline*, pp. 211–212. See also Leon Herman, *A Surgeon Thinks It Over* (Philadelphia, 1962), p. 60.

41	S. H. Landrum to editor, *J.A.M.A.*, Feb. 24, 1912, *58:* 576. See also George S. King, *Doctor on a Bicycle* (New York, 1958), pp. 61–63; Marcus Bossard, *Eighty-One Years of Living* (Minneapolis, 1946), pp. 39–40; and Mary Bennett Ritter, *More than Gold in California, 1849–1933* (Berkeley, 1933), p. 219.

42	J. H. Mackay to editor, *J.A.M.A.*, Mar. 9, 1912, *58:* 720; J. H. Guinn to editor, *ibid*, Mar. 23, 1912; 880. Women physicians, although small in number, provided a bridge between the two worlds of domesticity and medicine, and many women who wanted the benefits of medicine within the comforting female sphere chose women doctors as birth attendants. More research is needed in this area, beginning with women's hospitals such as the New England Hospital for Women and Children, which, one could argue, tried to provide a milieu in which traditional women's supports could be maintained. See, for example, Virginia G. Drachman, "Female solidarity and professional success: the dilemma of women doctors in late nineteenth-century America," *J. Soc. Hist.*, Summer 1982, *15:* 607–619; and Regina Markell Morantz and Sue Zschoche, "Professionalism, feminism, and gender roles: a comparative study of nineteenth-century medical therapeutics," *J. Am. Hist.*, Dec. 1980, *67:* 568–588.

43	"Management of normal labor," *J.A.M.A.*, Jan. 27, 1912, *58:* 274; William M. Gregory to editor, *ibid.*, Feb. 24, 1912, 577. See also F. W. MacManus to editor, *ibid.*, Mar. 9, 1912, 720; and Landrum to editor, *ibid.*, Feb. 24, 1912, 576.

44	Longo, "Obstetrics and gynecology," pp. 211–214; Virginia G. Drachman, "The Loomis trial: social mores and obstetrics in the mid-nineteenth century," in *Health Care in America: Essays in Social History*, ed. Susan Reverby and David Rosner (Philadelphia, 1979), pp. 67–83; American Association for Study and Prevention of Infant Mortality, *Transactions of the Seventh Annual Meeting*, pp. 63–64; Francis A. Long, *A Prairie Doctor of the Eighties: Some Personal Recollections and Some Early Medical and Social History of a Prairie State* (Norfolk, Nebr., 1937), p. 29.

45	J. Whitridge Williams, "Medical education and the midwife problem in the United States," *J.A.M.A.*, Jan. 6, 1912, *58:* 1, 2, 5; R. H. Riley, "The public health aspect of the teaching of obstetrics in undergraduate medical schools," *ibid.*, Apr. 25, 1936, *106:* 1438. See also Lawrence D. Longo, "John Whitridge Williams and academic obstetrics in America," *Tr. Coll. Physicians Phila.*, Dec. 1981, *3:* 221–254.

46	I have explored some of these points elsewhere; see Judith Walzer Leavitt, "Birthing and anesthesia: the debate over twilight sleep," *Signs*, Autumn 1980, *6:* 147–164. See also Morris J. Vogel, *The Invention of the Modern Hospital: Boston, 1870–1930* (Chicago, 1980); and Judy Barrett Litoff, *American Midwives: 1860 to the Present* (Westport, Conn., 1978). The declining number of midwives in this period contributed to the trend toward hospital deliveries and was affected by many of the same factors. See Frances E. Kobrin, "The American midwife controversy:

a crisis of professionalization," *Bull. Hist. Med.*, July–Aug. 1966, *40*: 350–63; Neal Devitt, "The statistical case for elimination of the midwife: fact versus prejudice, 1890–1935," *Women & Hlth.*, Spring 1979, *4*: 81–96; *ibid.*, Summer 1979: 169–186. The midwife was the major victim of advancing obstetrics. Physicians took almost two centuries to replace midwives in America's birthing rooms, but by the 1940s medicine successfully superseded female midwifery. Since few women were obstetricians, when midwives "disappeared," women lost the occupation for their sex; they also lost with midwifery centuries of female tradition, ritual, and unity, which today they are seeking to reclaim.

47 Barbara Moench Florence, ed., *Lella Secor: A Diary in Letters, 1915–1922* (New York, 1978), p. 170.

48 Roy P. Finney, *The Story of Motherhood* (New York, 1937), pp. 6–7. See also Alan Frank Guttmacher, *Into This Universe: The Story of Human Birth* (New York, 1937), pp. 192–267.

49 Gladys Denny Schultz, "Journal mothers report on cruelty in maternity wards," *Ladies' Home Journal*, May 1958, *75*: 44; M. F. Ashley Montagu, "Babies should be born at home!" *ibid.*, Aug. 1955, *72*: 52. See also Betty MacDonald, *The Egg and I* (Philadelphia, 1945), pp. 108, 163. Betty MacDonald found the hospital a place of luxury, wonderful food, and good care — almost, she said, enough to keep her pregnant the rest of her life. Hospital stays may have looked attractive because women's own networks of home helpers were diminishing in this period. This hypothesis needs further research.

50 Joseph B. DeLee, "The prophylactic forceps operation," *Am. J. Obst. & Gynec.*, Oct. 1920, *1*: 40–41, 34–35.

51 J. P. McEvoy, "Our streamlined baby," *Reader's Digest*, May 1938, *32*: 15–16. For reaction to prophylactic forceps, see J. Whitridge Williams, "A criticism of certain tendencies in American obstetrics," *N.Y. St. J. Med.*, Nov. 1922, *22*: 493–499.

52 "I had a baby, too: a symposium," *Atlantic Monthly*, June 1939, *163*: 768. See also Lenore Pelham Friedrich, "I had a baby," *ibid.*, Apr. 1939: 461–465. Clara Rust delivered five babies at home before going to the hospital to have her sixth in 1926. She was apprehensive about leaving home but went to the hospital on the doctor's advice. Jo Anne Wold, *This Old House: The Story of Clara Rust* (Anchorage, 1976), pp. 207–208.

53 New York Academy of Medicine Committee on Public Health Relations, *Maternal Mortality in New York City: A Study of All Puerperal Deaths, 1930–1932* (New York, 1933), pp. 213–215, 125–127.

54 *Ibid.*, pp. 113–117, 126–127. An Iowa study found that 11.8 percent of all births and 23 percent of

hospital births were operative statewide. Plass and Alvis, "Statistical study," pp. 293–305.

55 "Childbirth: nature v. drugs," *Time*, May 25, 1936: 36; Matthias Nicoll, Jr., "Maternity as a public health problem," *Am. J. Public Hlth.*, Sept. 1929, *19*: 967. See also R. W. Holmes, R. D. Mussey, and F. L. Adair, "Factors and causes of maternal mortality," *J.A.M.A.*, Nov. 9, 1929, *93*: 1440–1447.

56 Philadelphia County Medical Society, Committee on Maternal Welfare, *Maternal Mortality in Philadelphia, 1931–1933* (Philadelphia, 1934), p. 130. See also New York Academy of Medicine, *Maternal Mortality*, pp. 32–38.

57 White House Conference on Child Health and Protection, *Fetal, Newborn, and Maternal Morbidity and Mortality: Report of the Subcommittee on Factors and Causes of Fetal, Newborn, and Maternal Morbidity and Mortality* (New York, 1933), pp. 14, 220. For information about the effects of instrumental deliveries on the children, see Charles Edwin Galloway, "Prevention of birth injury and its resulting mortality from the standpoint of the obstetrician," *J.A.M.A.*, Feb. 15, 1936, *106*: 505–507.

58 Joyce Antler and Daniel M. Fox, "The movement toward a safe maternity: physician accountability in New York City, 1915–1940," in *Sickness and Health in America: Readings in the History of Medicine and Public Health,* ed. Judith Walzer Leavitt and Ronald L. Numbers [Madison, 1978], p. 386; Lawrence D. Longo and Christina M. Thomsen, "The evolution of prenatal care in America," in *Proceedings of the Second Motherhood Symposium*, ed. Colleau, pp. 29–70. During the 1920s and 1930s, when increasing numbers of women moved to the hospital to have their babies, maternal mortality rates remained as high as they had been earlier in the century, approximately 60 deaths per 10,000 live births (over 100 per 10,000 for nonwhite women). See Sam Shapiro, Edward R. Schlesinger, and Robert E. L. Nesbitt, Jr., *Infant, Perinatal, Maternal, and Childhood Mortality in the United States* (Cambridge, Mass., 1968), pp. 144–145. When maternal mortality rates started falling after 1935, the decrease was not due to the hospital *per se* but to measures such as antibiotics that could have been used at home.

59 Schultz, "Journal mothers report on cruelty," pp. 44–45.

60 *Ibid.*, p. 44.

61 The dichotomy between hands of flesh and hands of iron is used particularly effectively by Adrienne Rich, *Of Woman Born: Motherhood as Experience and Institution* (New York, 1976), pp. 128–155.

62 As an example of contemporary interests, see Barbara Katz Rothman, *In Labor: Women and Power in the Birthplace* (New York, 1982).

# 7

## The Calculus of Suffering in 19th-Century Surgery

### MARTIN S. PERNICK

"I most conscientiously believe that the proud mission of the physician is distinctly twofold—namely, to alleviate human suffering, as well as preserve human life," wrote Dr. James Y. Simpson, the Edinburgh pioneer of chloroform anesthesia.[1] Doctors in Western cultures are expected to restore health and preserve life; they are also expected to combat suffering. But what is the proper professional behavior when these obligations conflict? What should a physician do when pain relief requires giving a dangerous drug—or conversely, when curing a dangerous disease requires the use of painful remedies? Should life be preserved absolutely, no matter what the cost in anguish? Should all suffering be relieved regardless of the risk to life? No sane person would want to inflict more suffering or more risk than necessary; but what constitutes "necessity," and for what ends? Should an agonized cancer patient be given a potentially deadly dose of painkillers? Should painful therapies be used to gain a brief prolongation of life in a terminal illness?

Most physicians today would agree there is *some* point at which the duty to relieve suffering overrides the duty to prolong life. But what is that point? Clearly, no one standard can provide a universal response to such conflicts. Some people risk death itself to avoid even minor pain; others suffer intense agonies to avert slight dangers. This problem of choosing between relieving suffering and preserving life is as old as medicine itself. The prehistoric healer who first discovered the blessing and the curse of the opium poppy faced an identical dilemma.

One way physicians have sought to resolve such

Martin S. Pernick is Associate Professor of History at the University of Michigan, Ann Arbor, Michigan.

Reprinted with permission from *The Hastings Center Report* April 1983, 13: 26–36.

conflicts has been to develop a common set of professional values, formal or informal ideals, which serve to guide practitioners when weighing a choice between such basic duties. But the values, which taken together constitute professionalism, are constantly subject to change, both as a result of new medical techniques and new social conditions. In conflicts between relieving and curing, for example, the medical profession has decided very differently at different times.[2]

The mid-19th century was one period of great change and conflict over such basic questions of professional values. A new social awareness of and sensitivity to suffering helped shape such disparate movements as antislavery and antivivisection. Looking back on this era, philosopher Charles Peirce proposed that the 19th century be remembered as the "Age of Pain."[3] Accompanying this change in social values was a technical revolution in the treatment of pain: the isolation of morphine, cocaine, and heroin; the invention of the hypodermic syringe; and, most dramatically, the discovery of inhalation anesthesia. These changes combined to alter profoundly the professional values of 19th-century doctors.

At the start of the 19th century, the majority tradition in Western medical ethics was hostile to any efforts at relieving suffering if they involved a risk to life. But, in the mid-1800s, a growing number of practitioners turned toward a more utilitarian professionalism, which allowed—even required—a degree of risk taking proportional to the degree of pain relieved. This revolution in professional attitudes drew upon the sentimental romanticism of literature and the arts, the benevolent humanitarianism of social reformers, the calculating mentality of the new medical statisticians, and the perfectionist naturalism of rival medical sects.

But, most fundamentally, the new medical approach to suffering was rooted in American physicians' search for a unifying, moderate consensus ideology, to reunite a seriously divided profession.

## THE SURGEON'S OUTLOOK

It is hard for us today to recreate the surgeon's feelings before anesthesia became available. The emotional ability to inflict vast suffering was perhaps the most basic of all professional prerequisites. A 19th-century anesthesia promoter recalled the procedure to repair a dislocated hip.

> Big drops of perspiration, started by the excess of agony, bestrew the patient's forehead, sharp screams burst from him in peal after peal—all his struggles to free himself and escape the horrid torture, are valueless, for he is in the powerful hands of men then as inexorable as death. . . . At last the agony becomes too great for human endurance, and with a wild, despairing yell, the sufferer relapses into unconsciousness. . . .[4]

Under such conditions, the professional values adopted by surgeons for most of Western history emphasized that saving life held absolute priority over avoiding suffering. The Hippocratic tradition even forbade physicians from providing pain relievers to patients judged incurable. The intent of such prohibitions may have been to prevent euthanasia, to protect the physician's reputation, and/or to save the patient's money. But the implication was clearly that cure, not pain relief, was the overriding medical duty.[5]

Surgical practice was not a license to torture. "On no account should one cause needless pain," Hippocrates cautioned surgeons. But no suffering that might save lives was defined to be "needless."[6] "Now a surgeon should be . . . filled with pity, so that he wishes to cure his patient, yet is not moved by his cries, to go too fast, or cut less than is necessary; but he does everything just as if the cries of pain cause him no emotion," insisted the 1st-century A.D. physician Celsus. His injunction helped define surgical professional duty for centuries thereafter.[7] Like Hippocrates, Celsus sanctioned neither callousness nor indifference. He required the surgeon to feel "pity" for the patient. But feelings of pity ought neither to affect the surgeon's actions nor to interfere with the infliction

of the vast suffering necessary to fight death. Surgeons were required to inflict tremendous suffering whenever "necessary" to save life, yet without losing their humanity in the process.

For many early-19th-century surgical students, learning to inflict pain according to these dicta of Celsus constituted the single hardest part of their professional training. Benjamin Rush's student Philip Syng Physick, the first American to gain prominence as a full-time surgeon, became so sick at his initial amputation that he had to be carried from the room in mid-operation.[8] Those who could not learn to accept the value of the suffering had to leave the profession. Samuel Cooper's early-19th-century textbook cautioned prospective young surgeons to heed the example of the Swiss physiologist Haller, who had studied diligently to become a surgeon but had failed in practice, due to his "fear of giving too much pain." Cooper told aspiring young surgeons to learn well the "excellent" precept of Celsus: "This undisturbed coolness, which is still more rare than skill, is the most valuable quality in the practice of surgery."[9]

The emotional outlook required to practice such painful cures was an acquired skill. Asa Fitch of New York, a student at Rutgers in the winter of 1828, kept a journal of the process by which the emotions of a young man were transformed into those of a professional surgeon. At the beginning, the sight of a leg amputation left him devastated.

> But, oh, how my feelings recoiled at the sight! To behold the keen shining knife drawn around the leg severing the integuments, while the unhappy subject of the operation uttered the most heart rending screams in his agony and torment, . . . to hear the saw working its way through the bone, produced an impression I can never forget.

But after only a few weeks of witnessing such pain and copying the impassivity of his professional mentors, Fitch could boast about "a most tedious and painful operation" on a young child, "I had none of the tenderness which I have always before felt on such occasions."[10]

Not surprisingly, those who managed to overcome their revulsion and master the professional ability to inflict suffering took a certain pride in their accomplishment. British surgeon John Hunter claimed that there was a certain "*éclat* generally attending painful operations, often only because they are so." And, also not surprisingly, the practice of surgery did sometimes produce callousness, despite Celsus's careful injunction.[11] One medieval authority, Henri de Mondeville, declared that the two professional prerequisites for a surgeon were a strong stomach and the ability to "cut like an executioner. . . ."[12]

While their traditions and training thus sanctioned the infliction of agonizing remedies whenever "necessary" to save life, practitioners varied widely in their concept of necessity. For most surgeons operations generally remained the last resort. Such surgical reticence derived mainly from the appalling mortality rates, the product of uncontrollable infections, hemorrhage, and shock. In major limb amputations, death rates of 30 to 50 percent were not uncommon.[13] As a result, both surgeons and patients avoided operations as long as possible (thus perhaps further inflating the surgical mortality rates). But, at least some surgeons cited suffering, not simply mortality, as their reason for avoiding the knife. An 18th-century British surgical text declared: "Painful methods are always the last remedies in the hands of a man that is truly able in his profession; and they are the first, or rather they are the only resource of him whose knowledge is confined to the art of operating."[14]

Within this general tradition, early-19th-century American physicians and surgeons gained a reputation for the particularly unrestrained infliction of excruciating remedies. Central to the notoriety of American practice as uniquely harsh and cruel was the medical system of Dr. Benjamin Rush. Rush's remedies, such as bloodletting and emetics, were based on treatments for fever that had been common to many medical systems for centuries. But he employed these procedures in an extremely heroic, unrestrained fashion. For Rush, the more dangerous the disease, the more painful the remedy must be. Rush favored "that bold humanity which dictates the use of powerful but painful remedies in violent diseases."[15]

A skilled propagandist, Rush promoted his therapies in part by convincing practitioners and patients alike that they were heroic, bold, courageous, manly, and patriotic. Americans were tougher than Europeans; American diseases were correspondingly tougher than mild European diseases; to cure Americans would require uniquely powerful doses administered by heroic American physicians.

Whether or not American physicians really inflicted more pain than Europeans, Rush's rhetoric led observers on both sides of the Atlantic to assume they did.[16] In the West especially, "mildness of medical treatment is real cruelty," wrote a popular medical author from Cincinnati. What was needed, he declared, was a "vigorous mode of practice; the diseases of our own country especially require it."[17]

The heroic reliance on massive doses and extreme measures, regardless of pain, was by no means limited to orthodox physicians. Many rival healing sects flourished in 19th-century America; some were as painful and heroic in their practices as their professional rivals. The "botanical physicians," followers of self-cure promoter Samuel Thomson, advocated many of the same therapeutic procedures as did Rush. Thomson purged, puked, and blistered excruciatingly; he differed mainly in using only natural herbal substances to produce his pharmaceuticals.

In surgery as in medicine, Americans portrayed their practice as uniquely painful. "Frontier" surgeons like Ephraim McDowell, Nathan Smith, and J. Marion Sims developed new operations which, they bragged, Europeans had been too sensitive and timid to perform. Smith's biographer boasted that "the surgeon . . . often feels it to be his duty . . . to perform a painful and hazardous operation. . . . The timid man shrinks from such high responsibility, and suffers his patient to be destroyed by disease. Such was not Dr. Smith."[18] Nationalistic Americans pointed with vast pride to the agonizing accomplishments of their surgeons as examples of the virile new culture of the young Republic. American surgeons attributed their successes in part to a frontier stoicism lacking in effete Old World practitioners; European critics denounced the American practice as an example of frontier barbarism and cruelty.[19] William Gibson's popular textbook summed up the spirit of American surgical practice in the first decades of the 19th century. Gibson advised that even the most "severe pain should never be an obstacle" to the performance of life-preserving operations.[20]

Thus, in the half century prior to the discovery of anesthesia, American physicians and surgeons generally defined professional duty as demanding the unhesitating infliction of extreme suffering in order to save lives. They were not cruel or indifferent; rather, they were totally dedicated to doing whatever seemed necessary to prevent death. Reared in this tradition, many midcentury practitioners found it understandably difficult to turn around and sanction the use of drugs that had the power to relieve suffering at the risk of life. This response can be seen most starkly in the reaction of some leading American practitioners to the discovery of anesthesia.

## THE AGE OF ANESTHESIA

On October 16, 1846, a Boston dentist named William T. G. Morton first demonstrated that the vapor of diethyl ether could prevent the pain of surgery. Within three months of this initial public experiment, the leading hospitals of New York, London, and Paris began employing ether anesthesia. By 1848, nitrous oxide (laughing gas), chloroform, and other compounds had been added to the list of known anesthetics. The use of anesthesia spread far more rapidly than such earlier innovations as smallpox vaccination, or such later discoveries as antisepsis. Vaccination remained bitterly controversial over a century after Jenner's initial experiments; antisepsis aroused strong opposition for decades after Lister's early work. Anesthetics won acceptance at most major world medical institutions within a few years of Morton's first demonstrations.[21]

But despite the unprecedented speed with which anesthesia entered practice, few surgeons then or since have regarded anesthetics as completely safe. In today's aseptic and technically sophisticated operating rooms, general anesthesia is often regarded as more risky than the surgery itself.[22] In the mid-19th century, when anesthesia was an untested, poorly understood novelty, concerns about its safety filled the medical journals. (Safety was far from the only issue. A large number of physicians felt that pain had some important — though not necessarily overriding — benefits to the patient. Other concerns involved professional power and professional etiquette.)

Mid-century surgeons thus had to decide whether the benefits of painless operations were worth the risks. Not surprisingly, more than a few insisted that the duty to preserve life absolutely outweighed the duty to relieve what one doctor revealingly termed "mere anguish."[23] Writing in the prestigious *American Journal of the Medical Sciences* in 1852, David F. Condie declared flatly, "It may be our duty to inflict pain to *save life*, but [we] can scarcely be warranted in *risking life* merely to avoid pain."[24] An opponent of chloroform based his position on "the absolute and supreme respect for human life which gives grandeur and dignity to our art." The *New York Journal of Medicine* ruled that "immunity of pain merely, should never be purchased at the risk to life."[25]

For these practitioners, the duty to preserve life was absolute; the duty to prevent suffering was recognized, but only when there was virtually no degree of physical danger involved. Thus, one young doctor admitted, "The mission of the physician is undoubtedly two-fold — to relieve human pain as well as to preserve human life. . . ." Yet one had clear priority over the other. "Endangering the life of our patient, merely for the purpose of relieving . . . from pain," he found totally "unjustifiable."[26]

These physicians, it must be emphasized, did not claim that suffering was necessarily good, nor that doctors should not try to prevent it; only that no risk to life should be taken for that purpose. Their position did not rule out the use of anesthetics, if they could be shown to have other advantages, such as saving life or preventing disease, or if the dangers could be totally eliminated. The question here was not whether anesthesia had any legitimate uses, but whether the relief of suffering ever justified the risk to life anesthetics were believed to pose. On that narrower issue, many midcentury practitioners answered "never."

## CONSERVATIVE MEDICINE

However, a growing number of other physicians angrily disagreed. They urged the use of anesthesia, based on what they claimed was a professional duty to prevent suffering, even when that meant taking some risks with life. "Pain is only evil. . . . We are not required to possess an innocuous agent" to fight it, declared New York surgeon Valentine Mott. John Erichsen's influential textbook, *The Science and Art of Surgery*, urged students to accept the fact that "we cannot purchase immunity from suffering without incurring a certain degree of danger." In his 1851 textbook, one New York surgeon told students that the relief of suffering was worth the cost, even though "I know that, in urging upon the profession the *duty*, . . . of using anaesthetics, I may be instrumental in the destruction of human life."[27]

The most extreme form of pain relief at the expense of life is, of course, euthanasia. While no 19th-century American physicians openly advocated using anesthesia to take life in such cases, several went so far as to urge its use for the painless execution of condemned criminals.[28] And, as early as 1848, the surgeon in Morton's initial demonstrations, Boston's eminent John Collins Warren, published the case histories of patients for whom he had used ether to provide "euthanasia"—a painless (but not more rapid) death—in terminal cancer.[29]

The new willingness to take risks purely for the relief of suffering extended beyond the use of anesthetics. The prescription of alcohol and opiates to relieve suffering (not simply to treat disease or prevent shock) appears to have increased by the mid-19th century, particularly in surgery.[30] An even clearer indication of the new attitude was the gradual introduction of surgical operations whose only anticipated benefit was the mitigation of suffering. Thus in 1848, J. Mason Warren urged the A.M.A. to sanction operations "as a palliative" for painful incurable breast cancers. Philadelphia surgeon Henry H. Smith taught his students in 1855 to operate on such cases "not with any view of curing the patient but simply for purposes of making life pleasant and death easier."[31] During the Civil War, Silas Weir Mitchell began experiments with neurosurgery for the relief of chronic pain.[32] In each of these cases, patients were subjected to the dangers and mutilations of an operation, with little if any hope of curing an organic disease, but purely for relief. The growing legitimacy of risk taking for the relief of suffering also may be seen in the accelerating number of experiments conducted by leading conservative surgeons such as Mott and Warren, using mesmerism, freezing, compression, and other unproven or hazardous techniques to reduce the agony of surgical operations. In this experimental series, Morton's ether demonstration was neither the first nor the last.

On what basis did these physicians claim professional legitimacy for their actions? With the exception of chloroform pioneer Simpson, few of the 19th-century advocates of a higher priority for pain relief sought classical precedents for their posi-

tion. Yet, the belief that some degree of risk to life could be taken to relieve suffering did have a basis in medical tradition. One of the earliest proponents of this position was Aretaeus of Cappadocia, who in the 1st century opposed the Hippocratic ban on giving pain relievers to the terminally ill.[33] In the following century, Galen also advocated the cautious use of some potentially dangerous anodynes.[34] At various times, other ancient and medieval practitioners employed dangerous substances to relieve the sufferings of disease and as surgical anodynes. The best-known attempts involved opium, alcohol, mandragora, and the mysterious "soporific sponge." In his diligent scholarly attempt to find precedents for the professional use of anesthetics, Dr. Simpson unearthed several similar experiments with potentially dangerous painkillers. But such practices appear to have declined in number and respectability long before the 19th century. In 17th-century France, for example, a barber-surgeon who attempted to develop an herbal anodyne was fined heavily for endangering the lives of his patients.[35]

The modern revival of emphasis on the duty of doctors to relieve suffering began with Sir Francis Bacon. " . . . I esteem it the office of a physician not only to restore health, but to mitigate pain and dolors; and not only when such mitigation may conduce to recovery, but when it may serve to make a fair and easy passage," he declared in attacking Hippocratic professionalism in 1605.[36] A century and three-quarters later, the Scottish medical essayist John Gregory still had an uphill fight to legitimate the relief of suffering for the dying, against the influence of Hippocratic tradition.

> Let me exhort you against the custom of some physicians, who leave their patients when their life is despaired of, and when it is no longer decent to put them to farther expense. It is as much the business of a physician to alleviate pain, and to smooth the avenues of death, when unavoidable, as to cure diseases.[37]

Though Gregory's work was considered radical in his own day, it played an important role in influencing 19th-century efforts to expand the physician's obligation to relieve suffering.[38]

While these and other historical precedents played a role, mid-19th-century American attempts to strike a balance between the duty to cure and the duty to relieve drew most directly upon a new, therapeutically moderate approach to medicine. Calling their practice "conservative" or "rational" medicine, physicians like Austin Flint, Worthington Hooker, Oliver Wendell Holmes, and surgeons like Frank H. Hamilton promulgated a professional philosophy that carefully avoided all extremes. These self-professed "conservatives" excluded the radical excesses of Rush's heroism; they likewise rejected the therapeutic nihilism of his most extreme critics. Conservatives still retained the use of painful orthodox remedies, from bleeding to cautery, but in a limited and cautious fashion.[39]

What distinguished conservative medical decision making was its search for a moderate intermediate solution to therapeutic conflicts such as that between the duty to relieve pain and the duty to preserve life. Thus, these practitioners were willing to incur danger in order to prevent suffering, but only up to a moderate limit. As the Philadelphia *Medical Examiner* explained, "We deprecate alike the excessive enthusiasm which insists that under no possible circumstances, ether can be, or ever has been prejudicial, and the unreasonable timidity which prevents the employment of a useful agent, because, in a few cases, injurious effects have been apparently occasioned by it."[40]

## STATISTICS AND IDEOLOGY

The conservative search for a "middle course"[41] between conflicting ethical imperatives was closely tied to 19th-century advances in medical statistics, particularly the revolutionary applications of mathematics to assessments of drug safety and efficacy developed in Paris by Pierre Louis. These techniques, combining recent advances in calculus and probability theory with Bentham's utilitarian ethics, allowed physicians to measure the risks and benefits of a drug, without invoking such ethical absolutes as the traditional injunction to "do no harm." Louis and his followers taught that neither the inflicted harm done by therapeutic side effects nor the natural damage of untreated pathology was inherently preferable to the other. Rather, the physician's task was to compare directly the objective statistical magnitude of each harm regardless of its source, and act so as to maximize the overall benefit to the patient. The British scientist Sir

John Herschell captured the newness and wonder of the new therapeutic calculus in 1850.

> Men began to hear with surprise, not unmixed with some vague hope of ultimate benefit, that not only births, deaths, and marriages, but . . . the comparative value of medical remedies, and different modes of treatment . . . might come to be surveyed with the lynx-eyed scrutiny of a dispassionate analysis.[42]

This new calculus of safety formed a central tenet of American conservative professionalism. Hooker, for example, insisted upon the "accurate adjustment of remedial means to the ends to be accomplished." When deciding on the use of a dangerous drug, "the truly judicious physician is neither bewildered nor precipitate," but carefully chooses his course by measuring the benefits and risks — "this nice balancing of probabilities." Hooker's one specific illustration of this crucial process involved the decision to prescribe opium for severe pain.[43]

A medical student of 1853 put it this way: "Men of science have differed in opinion" concerning how to weigh "that most terrible of obstacles, *pain*, . . ." against "the injurious effects following the use of these valuable agents [anesthetics]. . . . Statistics can afford the only unfailing criterion and are indispensable to the formation of a judgment — they should be allowed to speak for themselves."[44] The problem thus became entirely technical. The risks and benefits of pain relievers could be measured, and the decision made according to a "rational" calculus. The physician's duty was to minimize total harm — not to make value distinctions between one type of harm and another.

By the 1850s, this mathematical approach to medical ethics enjoyed considerable professional acceptance in the United States. Thus, in the decade following Morton's ether demonstration, medical journals carried a series of statistical reports attempting to quantify the relative value of anesthetics.[45] Many of these studies suffered from a very primitive understanding of statistics. But they clearly reflected the importance of mathematics in the conservatives' attempt to choose between conflicting versions of professional duty.

Yet, as Austin Flint repeatedly pointed out, medical conservatism did not simply follow from medical statistics. Such explanations of conservatism, Flint declared, "will go only a little way. The change is one of sentiment." The desire to find a moderate course between conflicting approaches in medicine preceded acceptance of Louis's methods. Medical statistics did not create medical conservatism; rather it was because conservatives were already seeking a way to synthesize the divisive ethical and therapeutic conflicts of 19th-century medicine that they turned to statistical techniques. Conservative medicine was more than simply the result of quantitative measurement; it was an a priori ideological commitment to moderation, reunification, and synthesis in a badly divided profession. The key to understanding medical conservatism, according to Dr. Henry I. Bowditch, was the deep conviction that, in all areas of medicine, "evil is good run mad."[46]

## MEDICAL SECTARIANISM

One of the major sources of division and discord within 19th-century American medicine was the growth of a variety of alternative healing sects. At least in part as a reaction against the agonies attributed to heroic practice, many Americans turned to homeopathy, hydropathy, and other rival systems that claimed to offer a more natural, less painful route to health. Hydropaths used no "artificial" drugs or surgery—only water, steam, and ice—to assist nature in promoting healing. The key to hydropathic therapy was rigid obedience to the "natural laws" of physiology: rest, diet, and hygiene. With such natural living drugs would be unnecessary; without it they were futile.[47]

Similar to hydropathy in its invocation of nature and its roots in German romanticism, was the more popular system of homeopathy. Homeopaths employed a variety of "natural" (that is, vegetable) drugs, chosen according to the doctrine of similars. This ancient theory held that substances which produced a given symptom in a well person would cure similar symptoms in the sick. The doctrine of similars by itself could justify the infliction of at least as much suffering as in the rival practices of orthodox physicians. But homeopaths avoided the rigors of this doctrine by also teaching that the potency of their drugs increased with extreme dilution.[48]

A related source of medical dissension was the healing philosophy called by its critics "medical nihilism"—the belief that most diseases are self-limiting, and that the physician's role is to soothe suffering and allow natural recuperation. Unlike homeopathy and hydropathy, medical nihilism was never institutionalized or confined to any one formal sect.

Nineteenth-century observers traced the roots of this philosophy to the Hippocratic injunction to "do no harm," often (erroneously) rendering this credo as "primum non nocere"—*first of all*, do no harm. Medical nihilism drew on the ethical distinction between acts of omission and acts of commission, or in Victorian-era phraseology, between Art and Nature. The physician was morally responsible for the damage inflicted by medicine, but the damage passively produced by disease was blamed only on nature.[49]

Despite their differences in doctrine and organization, these alternatives to standard medical practice shared several important features: a claim to roots in classical medical ethics, a pervasive 19th-century romantic vision of nature's beneficence, and a perfectionist faith that good health was easily attainable. They also shared an intense hostility to the painfulness of heroic therapy. (These attitudes definitely did not characterize *all* 19th-century medical sects. For example, the Thomsonians practiced every bit as heroic a use of their remedies as Rush did with his.)

Patients and practitioners repeatedly cited painlessness as the major reason for choosing homeopathy over heroic practice. "Gladly would we see banished from the sick chamber the nauseous drugs, the offensive draughts, the pill, the powder, the potion, and all the painful and debilitating expedients of our present system, in favor of the mild and gentle measures of Homeopathy," declared the Boston *Christian Examiner.*[50] Just as the heroic physician's attitude toward pain was portrayed as particularly manly, homeopaths claimed that their own mildness attracted children and their mothers.[51]

The growth of conservative medicine, and the willingness of conservatives to take risks for the relief of suffering, clearly owed much to such sects. The active infliction of suffering was certainly a small part of these sects' practice (though even the use of simple water could sometimes be carried to heroic and painful extremes).[52] Competition and criticism from sectarian rivals undoubtedly helped prod mid-century physicians into abandoning the most painful aspects of heroic practice, and adopting the conservative approach to pain relievers.

But, contrary to the claims of their practitioners, these medical sects were not always less painful than their rivals. When followed strictly, their therapeutic doctrines banned clinically effective use of opium, morphine, alcohol, ether, chloroform, nitrous oxide, and most other painkillers. The practice of these alternative systems did not require the doctor to inflict much suffering but they offered little specific active relief. As Dr. Oliver Wendell Holmes pointed out, the only "natural anaesthetics" were "sleep, fainting, death."[53]

In practice, however, homeopaths and other alternative sects soon had to modify their original doctrines to allow the use of anodynes and anesthetics, largely in response to conservative physicians' adoption of these drugs. While a minority of purists led a sharp attack against this deviation, by the 1860s competition with conservative medicine forced many sectarians to accept the undiluted use of anesthetics and analgesics.[54] In short, competition encouraged *both* orthodox and alternative healers to adopt each other's least painful practices.

## SENTIMENTALISM AND SURGERY

The new willingness of conservative physicians to inflict some harm for the relief of suffering derived not only from medical ideas, but grew in part from mid-century social criticisms of professional callousness. Nineteenth-century American lay writers produced a torrent of demands for sentiment, emotion, and the expression of feelings in the practice of the professions. Yet this sentimentalist support for what later came to be called "empathy" did not always lead directly to the active relief of suffering; the connection was far more subtle and complex.

Public pressure for physicians to feel more emotional involvement with their patients grew increasingly insistent over the antebellum years. According to a typical expression of such sentiments in the *Philadelphia Bulletin,*

> Assuredly it is not a pulseless, tideless being that is desired to officiate at the couch of sickness. Rather is the man most acceptable as a physician who most approximates the feminine type; who

is kind, and gentle, and cautious, and sympathetic, and truthful, and delicately modest.[55]

One of the most caustic attacks on unfeeling surgery was Herman Melville's 1850 portrait of Dr. Cadwallader Cuticle in *White-Jacket.* Cuticle is hard, callous, and unfeeling.

> [N]othing could exceed his coolness when actually employed in his imminent vocation. Surrounded by moans and shrieks, by features distorted with anguish inflicted by himself, he yet maintained a countenance almost supernaturally calm. . . . Yet you could not say that Cuticle was essentially a cruel-hearted man. His apparent heartlessness must have been of a purely scientific origin. It is not to be imagined even that Cuticle would have harmed a fly, unless he could procure a microscope powerful enough to assist him in experimenting on the minute vitals of the creature.

But Cuticle's cold, machine-like, unemotional science is an external shell, designed to cover his real feelings — not the pangs of compassion, but his perverse and sadistic pleasure.

> Cuticle, on some occasions, would affect a certain disrelish of his profession, and declaim against the necessity that forced a man of his humanity to perform a surgical operation. Especially was it apt to be thus with him, when the case was one of more than ordinary interest. In discussing it, previous to setting about it, he would veil his eagerness under an aspect of great circumspection; curiously marred, however, by continual sallies of unsuppressable impatience.[56]

Conservative physicians endorsed such criticisms of the unfeeling practice of medicine. In 1849, Henry J. Bigelow urged curriculum reform at the Harvard Medical School in order "to reestablish a facility in the manifestation of that kindly feeling which is generally upon the surface in early youth, but which sometimes in the process of education gets embedded beneath a stratum of indifference and insensibility." Conservative spokesmen like Worthington Hooker insisted that "humane sympathies" actually exceeded technical "skill" in medical importance. In 1848, the New York surgeon Alexander H. Stevens told the A.M.A., "Our profession, gentlemen, is the link that unites Science and Philanthropy."[57]

As expressed by conservative physicians, the demand for sentiment and feeling contained more than a little elitist bias. The callousness of heroic medicine was blamed on the general decline of those genteel graces that supposedly had elevated the tone of the 18th-century professional. Elitist conservative physicians equated the lack of sensitivity in treatment with a lack of sensibility in manner. They dismissed the average 19th-century practitioner as "uncouth in his manners, vulgar and indelicate in his language, slovenly in his dress, and harsh and unfeeling in his treatment."[58] While followers of Rush had expounded the need for harshness in democratic and especially Western medicine, conservatives scorned the resulting insensitivity as a form of rustic barbarism increasingly limited to "country physicians."[59]

Mid-century romanticism, with its denunciations of scientific callousness and its appeals for more attention to feelings in medicine, played an important role in legitimating the conservative 19th-century physician's willingness to take risks for the relief of suffering. To a young medical student like John Wesley Thompson, fully imbued with the new conservatism, the surgeon's duty seemed to derive entirely from sentimentalism.

> Who can realize what is meant by intense pain and not feel himself called upon to relieve its victim? Surely no one who has a spark of sympathy within his breast. There are some who think a Surgeon, or Physician should not feel, or heed such things; but as well bid the ocean be still, or the mother forget her first-born, as to enforce such a sentiment. It is treason against humanity. . . .
> . . . [S]trange indeed would appear the creature who could boast of passing through such ordeals with the same stoicism as he would in carving a fowl at his table. . . . [U]nless he *felt* at heart, he could not be otherwise than unfit for the great responsibilities devolving upon him.[60]

But despite such gushing prose, antebellum sentimentalism by itself does not account for the conservatives' cautious willingness to take risks for the active relief of human agonies. Dr. Hooker repeatedly and emphatically insisted upon distinguishing between those sentimentalist attacks on medical callousness that sprang from a "mawkish" wallowing in misery, and true medical "benevolence," which came from "active" risk taking to relieve suffering.

It has sometimes been said that the physician, from his familiarity with scenes of distress, becomes unfeeling, and incapable of sympathizing with others. . . . True, he will not have that mawkish sensibility which vents itself in tears, and sighs, and expressions of pity, but stops short of action. . . . If he ever had any of such romantic and unpractical sensibility, he has cast it off in his actual service in the field of benevolence, into which his profession has necessarily led him. He has learned over and over, the lesson of *active* sympathy. . . . He may seem to be devoid of sympathy, as he goes to work midst scenes of suffering, without a tear, or even a sigh, performing his duties with an unblanched face, a cool and collected air, and a steady hand, while all around are full of fear, and trembling, and pity. Yet there *is* sympathy in his bosom, but it is *active*. It vents itself in the right way—in doing.[61]

## BETWEEN BENEVOLENCE AND BRUTALITY

The 19th-century cult of the sentiments originated outside medicine. It pervaded Victorian literature, art, religion, and reform, while its most popular mass exponents were the women's magazines. In this world, suffering constituted a peak of emotional sublimity.

But, as Hooker pointed out in a medical context, the relation between such sentimental rhetoric and the active relief of human suffering was quite ambiguous. To sentimentalists, pain was degrading, but suffering could be ennobling. And, although sentimentalism deeply influenced some segments of American thought, it left other parts of society unmoved. Mid-century America also witnessed the growth of a masculine cult of toughness and callousness. This antisentimental glorification of insensitivity took two very different forms: one, a reaffirmation of the traditional manly ability to endure pain; and the second, a newer, more mechanical form of indifference to suffering.

The traditional cult of manly endurance especially filled the mythology (and perhaps the reality) of the violent frontier. Americans who adopted the scarred and bullet-riddled figure of Andrew Jackson as the "symbol for an age" were responding to Old Hickory's ability to take it and dish it out. However, Jackson's Democratic party had no monopoly on such virility, as the monotonous succession of military presidents testified. But the machine age brought a new form of masculine insensitivity, more in tune with an era of commerce and technology. American commercial boosters bragged that our new indifference to the price of progress — steamboat explosions, railroad accidents, factory mutilations — enabled us to surpass the effete and decadently sensitive Europeans. In the more traditional world of Andrew Jackson, the pains of war seemed to offer the rewards of manly glory. Following the mechanical butchery of the Civil War, combat was reduced to a meaningless hell. Hardened insensitivity, not heroic endurance, seemed the appropriate response.[62]

To resolve the paradoxical nature of 19th-century social attitudes toward pain, *both* the romantic preoccupation with suffering and the antiromantic cults of hardness and insensitivity must be seen as interrelated aspects of the mid-century penchant for dichotomizing all facets of human life. Victorian social iconography divided the world into the separate and distinct spheres of: Head vs. Heart, Reason vs. Sentiment, World vs. Home, Art vs. Nature — all seen as reflections of the great division between Masculine and Feminine.[63] Although these were two antithetical worlds, the existence of each depended upon the existence of its opposite. To regard either the sentimental benevolence of Dorothea Dix or the mechanical, ruthless efficiency of William Tecumseh Sherman as uniquely characteristic of mid-century America would be to overlook the process of polarization by which each helped produce and define the other. Between romanticism and antiromanticism existed a profound Victorian dialectic of pain.

While most 19th-century Americans separated intellect and feelings, one American writer consciously set out to reverse the growing polarization of head and heart, of male and female. That poet was Walt Whitman.

While sentimentalist writers regarded pain as the brutal, physical antithesis of the spiritual and sublime, Whitman rejected all such distinctions. Physical sensations were identical with the sublime. In "Song of Myself," he wrote: "Seeing, hearing, feeling, are miracles."[64] Perfectionists tended to view pain as merely useful, an evil necessary for punishing violators of God's natural laws. Whitman upheld the natural goodness of all bodily senses in and for themselves.

> All this I swallow, it tastes good, I like it well, it
>     becomes mine,
> I am the man, I suffer'd, I was there.[65]

To live is to feel, and if living is good, then all feelings are good. Pain is a part of life; "Agonies are one of my changes of garments."[66] In "A Song of Joys," even the pangs of death are a part of life and therefore partake of joyousness.

In poetry and in life, Whitman found a powerful metaphor for this synthesis in the language and outlook of the new conservative medical ethic. The key to understanding Whitman's use of medical images is to realize that, like "Walt," 19th-century American doctors were striving to synthesize what others saw as contraries. Whitman's poetry presumed the validity of the view of medicine expressed by a New York founder of the American Medical Association, who declared medicine to be "the link that unites Science and Philanthropy."[67] For Whitman, the doctor, the surgeon, the accoucheur, the wound dresser, become the personae through whose being and language the union of benevolence and science, passive sympathy and active hardness, find expression. In "The Wound Dresser," he explained,

> I am firm with each, the pangs are sharp yet un-
>     avoidable, . . .
> These and more I dress with impassive hand
>     (yet deep in my breast, a fire, a burning flame).[68]

Medicine, like sex, unites male hardness with female benevolence.

> I do not hurt you any more than is necessary
>     for you,
> I pour the stuff to start sons and daughters fit for
>     these States. . . .[69]

In summary, conservative professionalism sanctioned taking some risks for the relief of suffering, thus marking a break with earlier medical traditions. This new departure was strongly influenced by the growth of social sensitivity to human suffering in mid-19th-century life. But the conservative approach to pain involved more than emotional sensitivity. It was a self-consciously moderate attempt to synthesize the powerful, painful remedies of heroic medicine with the milder therapies of its critics, to restore unity and consensus within a divided profession. Those physicians who followed the new doctrines of professional duty thus found themselves faced with what Hooker called a "nice balance of probabilities." For them, choices like that between the duty to relieve suffering and the duty to preserve life came to depend not on absolute deontological imperatives, but upon a moderate utilitarian measurement of the pros and cons, a calculus of suffering.

## THE ETHICS OF PROFESSIONAL DECISION MAKING

In today's world, where "cost-benefit" analysis is a profession in itself, routinely used to decide questions from drug safety to war and peace, it may be hard to imagine the extent to which the calculus of suffering constituted a major revolution in the techniques of professional decision-making in medicine. It reflected a utilitarian philosophy, a social moderation, and a numerical frame of mind, none of which was prominent in American medicine prior to the 1830s.[70] It is perhaps even more difficult for us to see any validity in alternative approaches, views like that of Charles Meigs, that "[a]ny surgical operation founded . . . on some cold and calculating computation of benefits possible, I regard as of doubtful propriety. . . . "[71] Yet a careful consideration of such criticism reveals some major difficulties unsolved by the "rational" conservative calculus.

One problem faced by conservative physicians grew out of the fact that most of the 19th-century materia medica flunked the statistical test. Thus, the objective decision-making calculus that was supposed to be an alternative to therapeutic nihilism wound up more often than not simply confirming the nihilistic position that all drugs were unsafe. Such findings may make for good science, but they don't solve the problem of the clinician who still feels a need to *do something* for sick patients.[72] Thus, even today practitioners attack the utilitarian standards of regulatory agencies like the FDA, because such rules seem to exclude drugs from the market without encouraging the development of new ones to fill the gap.

A second problem, raised implicitly by opponents of the calculus, concerned the distribution of costs and benefits. Using a commonplace example—let us say the shock of unanesthetized surgery was discovered to kill a larger percentage of patients than would be poisoned by anes-

thesia—by the calculus of conservative medicine, the physician should proceed with anesthetization. But that course would still require the poisoning of some patients. At what point does the saving of other people's lives justify the taking of even one?[73]

A related problem that deeply concerned 19th-century physicians was the level of generality at which the calculus should be applied. Should the sum of the risks from all possible uses of anesthesia be weighed against the cumulative total of benefits, to produce a simple universal rule that pain relievers should (or should not) be used? Or does the doctor also have to weigh and measure the pros and cons for each individual patient? This problem of selecting the appropriate level of individualization seriously divided mid-19th-century conservative physicians in their application of the new calculus.[74]

A final problem raised by critics of the calculus of suffering concerned the fundamental utilitarian assumption that all pains and injuries can be objectively compared in magnitude; that some common unit of measurement can be found for such things as suffering or disability. But do such units exist? For example, anesthetics can occasionally cause circulatory collapse leading to permanent brain damage. Is the mental defect that might thus result from anesthesia a bigger or smaller evil than the suffering that might result from unanesthetized major surgery? The potent antibiotic necessary to cure certain antibiotic-resistant eye infections can result in hearing loss as a side effect. How can we measure whether blindness causes more suffering than deafness? And, as another 19th-century critic asked, how can we compare the magnitude of a present pain with the suffering from a future side effect?[75]

The analytic calculus of suffering first employed by the "conservative" physicians of the mid-19th-century provided neither a value-free nor a timeless solution to the problem of weighing the relief of suffering against the avoidance of physical harm. The demands we make on physicians continue to impose such partially conflicting, even mutually contradictory, duties. And the professional values doctors adopt to reconcile and prioritize such conflicting obligations will continue to change, both reflecting and affecting the changing values and circumstances of our society.

## NOTES

This paper is adapted from a presentation to The Hastings Center's Research Group on Death, Suffering, and Well-Being, which was supported by a grant from the Arthur Vining Davis Foundations. It appeared, in somewhat different form, in the author's *A Calculus of Suffering: Pain, Anesthesia, and Utilitarian Professionalism in Nineteenth-Century American Medicine* (New York: Columbia University Press, 1985).

1   James Y. Simpson, "Account of a new anaesthetic," reprinted in *Milestones in Anesthesia: Readings in the Development of Surgical Anesthesia, 1665–1940,* ed. Frank Cole (Lincoln: Univ. Nebraska Press, 1965), p. 97.

2   Martin S. Pernick, "Medical professionalism," *Encyclopedia of Bioethics* (New York: The Free Press, 1978), III, 1028–1034.

Strictly speaking, *pain* may refer to the complex of physical and emotional effects produced by aversive sensations; *suffering* refers only to the experience of anguish and mental distress. However, 19th-century physicians rarely used the terms precisely. Therefore, in this article, especially in quotations, unless otherwise noted, the word *pain* will be used as roughly synonymous with *suffering*.

3   Quoted in James Crewdson Turner, "Kindness to animals: the animal protection movement in England and America during the nineteenth century" (Ph.D. dissertation, Harvard Univ., 1975). Turner has published a shorter version, in book form, omitting this quote.

4   Betty MacQuitty, *The Battle for Oblivion: The Discovery of Anaesthesia* (London: George G. Harrap & Co., Ltd., 1969), p. 68.

5   Markwart Michler, "Medical ethics in Hippocratic bone surgery," *Bull. Hist. Med.,* July–Aug. 1968, *42:* 298–300. On this question, however, ancient medicine was far from unanimous; see below.

6   Michler, "Medical ethics," p. 301. Hippocratic doctrine permitted the use of anodynes, but only if they could be rendered completely nonpoisonous. See Bernard Seeman, *Man Against Pain* (Philadelphia and New York: Chilton Books, 1962), pp. 57–58.

7   Celsus, *De Medicina,* translated by W. G. Spencer, Loeb Classical Library, 3 vols. (Cambridge: Harvard Univ. Press, 1935–38), III, 297; quoted in Guido Majno, *The Healing Hand: Man and Wound in the Ancient World* (Cambridge: Harvard Univ. Press, 1975), p. 355. See also Daniel de Moulin, "A historical-phenomenological study of bodily pain in Western man," *Bull. Hist. Med.,* Winter 1974, *48:* 561.

8   Stephen W. Williams, *American Medical Biography* (New York: Milford House Inc., reprint of 1845 ed., 1967), pp. 445–446.

9   Samuel Cooper, *A Dictionary of Practical Surgery* (from the 4th London ed., New York: Collins and Hannay, 1822), II, 443. For an American example, see the biography of Joseph Parrish in Williams, *American Medical Biography,* p. 435. For the similar example of Charles Darwin, see Donald Fleming, "Charles Darwin, the anaesthetic man," *Victorian Studies,* Mar. 1961, *4:* 219–236.

10   Samuel Rezneck, "A course of medical education in New York City in 1828–29: the journal of Asa Fitch," *Bull. Hist. Med.,* Nov.–Dec. 1968, *42:* 560, 561.

11   J. Collins Warren, *Influence of Anaesthesia on the Surgery of the Nineteenth Century* (Boston: privately printed, 1906), p. 4.

12   Jeffrey Berlant, *Profession and Monopoly: A Study of Medicine in the United States and Britain* (Berkeley: Univ. of California Press, 1975), p. 86.

13   *Am. J. Med. Sci.,* 1852, *23:* 453.

14   John Pearson, *Principles of Surgery* (Boston: Stimpson & Clapp, 1832), p. vii. This was the American edition of a 1788 London publication. Prior to the discovery of ether, only 15 percent of those admitted to the *surgical* wards of the Massachusetts General Hospital ever received any *operative* surgical treatment. Massachusetts General Hospital, Surgical Casebooks, Countway Library of Medicine, Boston.

15   Benjamin Rush, *Sixteen Introductory Lectures to Courses of Lectures Upon the Institutes and Practice of Medicine* (Philadelphia: Bradford and Inskeep, 1811), p. 213. Dr. Harris Coulter called this quotation to my attention.

16   For testimony as to the physical painfulness of heroic bloodletting and similar remedies, see Elizabeth Blackwell, *Pioneer Work in Opening the Medical Profession to Women* (London & New York: Longmans, Green, 1895, reprinted with a new introduction, New York: Schocken Books, 1977), pp. 41, 206. For examples of Rush's nationalistic propaganda, see Rush to John Coakley Lettsom, May 13, 1804, and Rush to John Syng Dorsey, May 23, 1804, in *Letters of Benjamin Rush,* ed. Lyman H. Butterfield, II (Princeton: Princeton Univ. Press, 1951), pp. 881, 882.

17   Anthony A. Benezet, *The Family Physician* (Cincinnati: W. H. Woodward, 1826), quoted in John B. Blake, "From Buchan to Fishbein: the literature of domestic medicine," in *Medicine Without Doctors,* ed. Guenter B. Risse, Ronald L. Numbers, and Judith Walzer Leavitt (New York: Science History Publica-

tions, 1977), p. 16. For more on American nationalism and painful medicine, see Martin Kaufman, *Homeopathy in America* (Baltimore: Johns Hopkins Univ. Press, 1971), pp. 9–11.

18  Williams, *American Medical Biography*, p. 537. Though they portrayed themselves as frontiersmen and did spend varying amounts of time in isolated rural areas while perfecting their innovations, all these men were highly trained, relatively well-traveled, and basically cosmopolitan in outlook. See also sketch of John Hart, in Williams, p. 231.

19  James Eckman, "Anglo-American hostility in American medical literature of the nineteenth century," *Bull. Hist. Med.*, Jan. 1941, *9*: 31–71; Allen O. Whipple, *The Evolution of Surgery in the United States* (Springfield, Ill.: Charles C Thomas, 1963), pp. 5, 16; *Tr. A.M.A.*, 1848, *1*: 287.

20  William Gibson, *The Institutes and Practice of Surgery* (Philadelphia, 1824) quoted in Eugene H. Pool and Frank J. McGowan, *Surgery at the New York Hospital One Hundred Years Ago* (New York: Paul B. Hoeber, Inc., 1930), p. 63.
    I do not at all mean to imply that "heroic" physicians were opposed to the *use* of anesthetics; only that they opposed risking life purely for the relief of suffering. For a typical heroic defense of anesthetics, in which the danger of their use is cited as counteracting the danger of disease from physical pain, and the use of traditional heroic remedies such as massive blistering is recommended as an anesthetic, see S. H. Dickson, "An introductory lecture, delivered before the Medical Class of Jefferson College, Philadelphia, October 13th, 1859," *Charleston Med. J. & Rev.*, 1860, *15*: 55–56, 60–62, and 33–64 *passim*.

21  Richard M. Hodges, *A Narrative of Events Connected with the Introduction of Sulphuric Ether into Surgical Use* (Boston: Little, Brown, and Co., 1891).

22  Henry K. Beecher and D. P. Todd, "A study of the deaths associated with anesthesia and surgery," *Ann. Surg.*, 1954, *140*: 2–34.

23  John Wesley Thompson, "Anaesthesia" (M.D. thesis, Univ. of Pennsylvania, Jan. 1860), p. 10. For suffering as "trivial," see Edward Clarke, "Anaesthesia in surgery" (M.D. thesis, Univ. of Pennsylvania, Jan. 1860), pp. 4–5, paraphrasing Magendie; the quote appears verbatim in S. W. Barker, "Anesthesia," *Harper's*, 1865, *31*: 457.

24  *Am. J. Med. Sci.*, 1852, *23*: 193, emphasis in original.

25  *Boston Med. & Surg. J.*, n.s., 1870, *5*: 147; *N.Y. J. Med.*, 1848, *10*: 243.

26  Edward H. Horner, "Anaesthetics" (M.D. thesis, Univ. of Pennsylvania, Feb. 1855), pp. 29–31.

27  Valentine Mott, *Pain and Anaesthetics*, 2nd ed., (Washington, D.C.: M'Gill & Witherow, 1863), p. 8; John

Erichsen, *The Science and Art of Surgery*, ed. John H. Brinton (Philadelphia: Blanchard and Lea, 1854), p. 29; C. R. Gilman, quoted in the *Am. J. Med. Sci.*, 1852, *13*: 192, emphasis in the original.

28  G. W. Peck, "On the use of chloroform in hanging," *Am. Whig Rev.*, Sept. 1848, *8*: 283–296; Henry J. Bigelow, "Execution by hanging," in *Surgical Anaesthesia: Addresses and Other Papers* (Boston: Little, Brown, and Co., 1900), pp. 376–378.

29  John Collins Warren, *Etherization: With Surgical Remarks* (Boston: William D. Ticknor, 1848), p. 70. See also Charles T. Jackson, *A Manual of Etherization* (Boston: J. B. Mansfield, 1861), pp. 101–104, in which he reprints Warren's cases and adds a few of his own; Laurence Turnbull, *The Advantages and Accidents of Artificial Anaesthesia: A Manual of Anaesthetic Agents*, 2nd ed., rev. and enlg. (Philadelphia: P. Blakiston, Son & Co., 1885), pp. 59–61; and p. 262 for active euthanasia by the S.P.C.A.

30  John Duffy, "Science and medicine," in *Science and Society in the United States*, ed. David D. Van Tassel and Michael G. Hall (Homewood, Ill.: The Dorsey Press, 1966), p. 122; Austin Flint, "Conservative medicine," *Am. Med. Monthly*, 1862, *18*: 1–24, reprinted in *Medical America in the Nineteenth Century*, ed. Gert S. Brieger (Baltimore: Johns Hopkins Univ. Press, 1972), p. 141; *Am. J. Med. Sci.*, 1852, *23*: 394; René Fülöp-Miller, *Triumph Over Pain*, trans. Eden and Cedar Paul (New York: The Literary Guild of America, Inc., 1938), p. 72; David F. Musto, *The American Disease: Origins of Narcotic Control* (New Haven: Yale Univ. Press, 1973), p. 5; Rothstein, *American Physicians*, pp. 190–194; John Harley Warner, "Physiological theory and therapeutic explanation in the 1860s: the British debate on the medical use of alcohol," *Bull. Hist. Med.*, Summer 1980, *54*: 235–257; David Todd Courtwright, "Opiate addiction in America, 1800–1940" (Ph.D. dissertation, Rice Univ., 1979); H. Wayne Morgan, *Drugs in America: A Social History 1800–1980* (Syracuse: Syracuse Univ. Press, 1981).

31  J. Mason Warren to Isaac Parrish, Mar. 28, 1848; John Collins Warren to Isaac Parrish, Apr. 30, 1848, both in Warren Family Papers, Vol. XXVI, Massachusetts Historical Society, Boston. Manuscript notes of lecture by Henry H. Smith, taken by John Hainson Rodgers, n.d., in the margins of Henry H. Smith, *Syllabus of the Lectures on the Principles and Practice of Surgery, Delivered in the University of Pennsylvania* (Philadelphia: T. K. and P. G. Collins, Printers, 1855), p. 35, located in the Special Collections, George Harrell Library, Penn State University College of Medicine, Hershey, Pa.

32  Lawrence C. McHenry, *Garrison's History of Neurology* (Springfield, Ill.: Charles C Thomas, 1969).

33 Darrel Amundsen, "The physician's obligation to prolong life: a medical duty without classical roots," *Hastings Center Rep., 8,* Aug. 1978: 27.

34 De Moulin, "Bodily pain," p. 562. However, Galen "abhor[red] more than anyone" the use of soporific drugs, presumably including most narcotics; Victor Robinson, *Victory Over Pain: A History of Anesthesia* (New York: Henry Schuman, 1946), pp. 12, 21.

35 Fülöp-Miller, *Triumph Over Pain,* pp. 21–23; Robinson, *Victory Over Pain,* p. 40. Barber-surgeons were not licensed to give *any* internal medicines, but the administration of painkillers was singled out as particularly forbidden.

36 De Moulin, "Bodily pain," p. 554.

37 John Gregory, *Lectures on the Duties and Qualifications of a Physician* (London: W. Strahan, 1772), p. 37, quoted in Laurence B. McCullough, "Historical perspectives on the ethical dimensions of the patient-physician relationship: the medical ethics of Dr. John Gregory," *Ethics in Sci. & Med.,* 1978, *5* (No. 1): 52, and 49 for the influence of Hume and Bacon.

38 Berlant, *Profession and Monopoly,* p. 88. The major spokesman for relieving the sufferings of the terminal patient in the 19th century was Thomas Percival. His thoughts on the subject appeared in close paraphrase in the American Medical Association's first code of ethics. See *Percival's Medical Ethics,* ed. Chauncey D. Leake (Baltimore: Williams & Wilkins Co., 1927), pp. 98, 221, for both.

39 Flint, "Conservative medicine"; Worthington Hooker, *Physician and Patient* (New York: Baker and Scribner, 1849, Arno Press, 1972); Oliver Wendell Holmes, *Medical Essays, 1842–1882* (Boston: Houghton Mifflin, 1891), pp. 51–65, 203, vii–xv; Jacob Bigelow, *Nature in Disease and Other Writings* (Boston: Ticknor and Fields, 1854); Percival, *Medical Ethics,* pp. 89, 183; Jacob Bigelow, *Brief Expositions of Rational Medicine* (Boston: Phillips, Sampson and Co., 1858).

40 *Philadelphia Med. Exam.,* n.s., June 1847, *3:* 380. One British text went so far as to claim that conservative surgery would have been impossible without anesthesia. The chronology clearly indicates that he put the cart before the horse; Thomas Bryant, *The Practice of Surgery* (Philadelphia: Henry C. Lea, 1873), p. 929.

41 *Am. J. Med. Sci.,* 1851, *21:* 493.

42 *Edinburgh Rev.,* 1850, *92:* 12, quoted in Richard H. Shyrock, "The history of quantification in medical science," *Isis,* June 1961, *52:* 233. On Louis and his methods, see Erwin H. Ackerknecht, *Medicine at the Paris Hospital, 1794–1848* (Baltimore: Johns Hopkins Univ. Press, 1967); William Osler, "The influence of Louis on American medicine," in *An Alabama Student and Other Essays* (New York: Oxford

Univ. Press, 1908), pp. 189–210; Ackerknecht, "Elisha Bartlett and the philosophy of the Paris Clinical School," *Bull. Hist. Med.,* Jan.–Feb. 1950, *24:* 43–60.

43 *Am. J. Med. Sci.,* 1852, *23:* 156; Hooker, *Physician and Patient,* pp. 53, 54–55, 57.

44 Charles F. Henry, "Etherization, as a surgical remedy" (M.D. thesis, Univ. of Pennsylvania, Feb. 1853), pp. 8–9, emphasis in original.

45 For a few examples, see *Am. J. Med. Sci.,* 1851, *21:* 178–183; 1852, *23:* 450–455; 1854, *28:* 13–20; *Tr. A.M.A.,* 1848, *1:* 214–221; *Penn. Hosp. Rep.,* 1868, *1:* 149–164.

46 Flint, "Conservative medicine," p. 135; Bowditch, in Kaufman, *Homeopathy,* p. 112.

47 The recent literature on sectarian medicine is extensive and of varied quality. For hydropathy, I have relied on the *Water-Cure Journal,* and the unpublished research of Prof. Regina Morantz. See also Marshall Scott Legan, "Hydropathy in America: a nineteenth century panacea," *Bull. Hist. Med.,* May–June 1971, *45:* 267–280.

48 For homeopathy, major sources include: American Institute of Homeopathy, *Proceedings; North American Journal of Homeopathy; The Hahnemannian Monthly;* Homoeopathic Medical Society of the State of New York, *Transactions;* J. G. Gilchrist, *A Syllabus of Lectures on Surgery at the Homoeopathic Medical College of the University of Michigan* (Ann Arbor: John Moore, 1877).

49 My conceptualization of the Art-Nature dichotomy was greatly enhanced by Perry Miller, *The Life of the Mind in America* (New York: Harcourt, Brace & World, Inc., 1965) and Miller, "The romantic dilemma in American nationalism and the concept of nature," *Harvard Theol. Rev.,* Oct. 1955, *48:* 239–253; Leo Marx, *The Machine in the Garden* (London: Oxford Univ. Press, 1964).

For typical attacks on "nihilism" see Holmes, *Medical Essays;* Bigelow, *Brief Expositions.* On the classical roots, see Albert Jonsen, "Do no harm: axiom of medical ethics," *Philosophy & Med.,* 1977, *3:* 27–42.

50 *Christian Exam.,* May 1842, *32:* 245–272, quoted in Kaufman, *Homeopathy,* p. 41.

51 Blackwell, *Pioneer Work,* p. 41; *Boston Med. & Surg. J.,* 1847, *36:* 128.

52 Edmund Wilson, *Patriotic Gore: Studies in the Literature of the American Civil War* (New York: Farrar, Straus, and Giroux, 1977, 1962), p. 673.

53 Holmes, "The medical profession in Massachusetts," in *Medical Essays.* To the extent that the more romantic medical sects tended toward perfectionism, they shared the complex link between perfection and martyrdom in the Christian tradition, through which suffering could be transcended by acceptance. See Matthew 5:48, 5:10–12. Through sharing the

martyrdom of Christ, the Church could become the mystical body of Christ and thus be made perfect, through suffering. Hebrews 13:3. George Fredrickson, *The Inner Civil War* (New York: Harper & Row, Publishers, 1965), p. 82; Silvan Tomkins, "The psychology of commitment: the constructive role of violence and suffering for the individual and his society," in *The Antislavery Vanguard,* ed. Martin Duberman (Princeton: Princeton Univ. Press, 1965), especially p. 274.

54  By 1865, some homeopaths were even claiming that anesthesia had originally been discovered by one of their ranks! See *Tr. Homoeopathic Med. Soc. St. N.Y.* (1865) p. 67. For the same claim, see Gilchrist, *Syllabus* (1877) p. 20.

However, the Philadelphia *Hahnemannian Monthly*, 1869, *4*: 180 claimed, "Homoeopaths are far less inclined to the use of anaesthetics than allopaths."

For a similar debate within the eclectic medical sect see the "conservative" approach adopted by P. W. Allen, *Eclectic Med. J.*, Oct. 1850, *2*: 433–438; the "heroic" defense of anesthesia in Benjamin L. Hill, *Lectures on the American Eclectic System of Surgery* (Cincinnati: W. Phillips and Co., 1850), pp. 208–209; and John King, *American Eclectic Obstetrics* (Cincinnati: Moore, Wilstach, Keys & Co., 1855), p. 506. Both the latter stress the disease-fighting aspects of ether, and recommended painful counter-irritation as preferable to anesthesia.

55  *Philadelphia Bull.*, "Female physicians," reprinted in *Water-Cure J.*, Jan. 1860, *29*: 3–4.

56  Herman Melville, *White-Jacket*, ed. Hennig Cohen (New York: Holt, Rinehart and Winston, 1967, 1850), p. 249.

57  Bigelow, "Inaugural lecture," in *Surgical Anaesthesia*, p. 226; Hooker, *Physician and Patient*, pp. 385–389, and quotation in *Am. J. Med. Sci.*, 1852, *23*: 158; Stevens' quote in *Tr. A.M.A.*, 1848, *1*: 30, quoted by Barbara Rosenkrantz, "The search for professional order in 19th century American medicine," *Proceedings of the XIVth International Congress of the History of Science* (Tokyo: Science Council of Japan, 1975), No. 4, p. 113.

58  *Boston Med. & Surg. J.*, 1849, *40*: 370, quoted in Charles Rosenberg, *The Cholera Years* (Chicago: Univ. of Chicago Press, 1962), p. 156.

59  John Duffy, *A History of Public Health in New York City, 1625–1866* (New York: Russell Sage Foundation, 1968), p. 466; Rothstein, *American Physicians*, p. 221.

60  Thompson, "Anaesthesia," pp. 8–9, emphasis in original.

61  Hooker, *Physician and Patient*, pp. 385–389, emphasis in original; see also *Am. J. Med. Sci.,* 1852, *23*: 175; *Western Lancet*, 1848, *8*: 128.

62  Lewis O. Saum, "Death in the popular mind of pre-Civil War America," *Am. Quart.,* Dec. 1974, *26*: 483–484; Daniel J. Boorstin, *The Americans: The National Experience* (New York: Vintage Books, 1967, 1965), pp. 101–104; Peter G. Filene, *Him/Her/Self: Sex Roles in Modern America* (New York: Harcourt, Brace, Jovanovich, 1975).

63  Nancy F. Cott, *The Bonds of Womanhood: "Woman's Sphere" in New England, 1780–1835* (New Haven: Yale Univ. Press, 1977), offers perceptive comments on this dichotomy, and traces its roots to before the Victorian era.

64  Walt Whitman, "Song of Myself," in *Leaves of Grass* (New York: New American Library, 1958), p. 68.

65  Whitman, "Song of Myself," p. 78.

66  Whitman, "Song of Myself," p. 79.

67  See note 57 above.

68  Whitman, "The Wound Dresser," in *Leaves of Grass*, pp. 253, 254. See also "Hospital Scenes and Persons," in *Specimen Days*, in *The Portable Walt Whitman*, ed. Mark Van Doren (New York: Viking Press, 1945), p. 508.

69  Whitman, "A Woman Waits for Me," in *Leaves of Grass*, p. 106.

70  In other areas of American society, however, the hedonistic calculus achieved earlier recognition. See Gary Wills, *Inventing America* (Garden City, N.Y.: Doubleday & Co., Inc., 1978), Ch. X, XVIII, XX, and XXIII.

71  Charles D. Meigs, *Females and Their Diseases* (Philadelphia: Lea and Blanchard, 1848), pp. 311–313. See also Charles Rosenberg, "The therapeutic revolution: medicine, meaning, and social change in nineteenth-century America," *Perspect. Biol. & Med.,* Summer 1977, *20*: 503.

72  Rosenberg, "Therapeutic revolution," pp. 503–504.

73  "It is said one death in ten thousand cases is sufficient to condemn chloroform on moral grounds." Kidd, *Manual of Anaesthetics*, p. 90.

74  The problem of applying the universal laws of biology to the individualized art of patient care has interesting parallels with the question of "rule" utilitarianism. See John Rawls, "Two concepts of rules," J. J. C. Smart, "Extreme and restricted utilitarianism," all in John Stuart Mill, *Utilitarianism,* ed. Samuel Gorovitz (Indianapolis: Bobbs-Merrill Co., Inc., 1971), pp. 175–216.

75  For present issues in health policy see The Hastings Center, "Values, ethics, and CBA in health care," *The Implications of Cost-Effectiveness Analysis of Medical Technology* (Washington, D.C.: Congressional Office of Technology Assessment, 1980), pp. 168–182. In clinical medicine see L. B. Lusted, *Introduction to Medical Decision Making* (Springfield, Ill.: Charles C Thomas, Publishers, 1968).

For the present/future issue, see *Am. J. Med. Sci.,* 1852, *23*: 394.

# 8

## The Maturation of American Medical Science

RONALD L. NUMBERS AND JOHN HARLEY WARNER

"What does the world yet owe to American physicians or surgeons?" an essayist for the *Edinburgh Review* asked contemptuously in 1820.[1] Offended Americans, unable to claim any medical heroes of their own, responded defensively by arguing that they excelled in the practice of medicine. Nevertheless, they resented their obviously dependent status in the medical sciences and yearned for the respect that would come with scientific achievement. It is time, proclaimed one patriotic surgeon in 1856, "to declare ourselves free and independent of our transatlantic brethren, as we did eighty years ago declare ourselves free and independent of the British crown."[2] In an effort to spur the medical community into action, the *Philadelphia Journal of the Medical and Physical Sciences* for several years prominently displayed the insulting Edinburgh query on its title page.

The American struggle for medical independence lasted for nearly a century after the 1820 incident. As Table 1 indicates in a crude, quantitative way, the United States continued to lag behind Europe in contributing to the medical sciences until late in the 19th century. However, the Americans overtook the English in the 1880s, the French in the 1890s, and the Germans in the 1910s. By 1920 they led the world in medical research.[3]

It is important in tracing the maturation of American medical science to distinguish between the history of the so-called basic medical sciences (e.g., anatomy, physiology, biochemistry, pathol-

RONALD L. NUMBERS is Professor of the History of Medicine and the History of Science at the University of Wisconsin, Madison, Wisconsin.
JOHN HARLEY WARNER is a Research Fellow at the Wellcome Institute for the History of Medicine, London, England.

Courtesy of Smithsonian Institution Press, from *Scientific Colonialism: A Cross-Cultural Comparison*, forthcoming, edited by Nathan Reingold and Marc Rothenberg.

ogy, and pharmacology) and the development of the clinical sciences, particularly therapeutics. The former reached maturity in the years between 1890 and 1920, when the United States created a self-sustaining institutional base for medical research. Medical therapeutics followed a much different course, achieving maturity during the last third of the 19th century, when American clinicians abandoned their insistence on a distinctively "American" practice in favor of therapies based on the principle of medical universalism. It is also important to bear in mind that even during the period when American physicians failed to keep pace with their European colleagues in using hospitals and laboratories for medical research, they not uncommonly engaged in armchair theorizing about the functions of the human body or investigated empirically the relationship between climate and

Table 1:
Numbers of Discoveries in the Medical Sciences, by Nation, 1820–1919

|          | U.S.A. | England | France | Germany |
|----------|--------|---------|--------|---------|
| 1820–29  | 1      | 12      | 26     | 12      |
| 1830–39  | 4      | 20      | 18     | 25      |
| 1840–49  | 6      | 14      | 13     | 28      |
| 1850–59  | 7      | 12      | 11     | 32      |
| 1860–69  | 5      | 5       | 10     | 33      |
| 1870–79  | 5      | 7       | 7      | 37      |
| 1880–89  | 18     | 12      | 19     | 74      |
| 1890–99  | 26     | 13      | 18     | 44      |
| 1900–09  | 28     | 18      | 13     | 61      |
| 1910–19  | 40     | 13      | 8      | 20      |

Source: Joseph Ben-David, "Scientific productivity and academic organization in nineteenth century medicine," *American Sociological Review*, 1960, *25*: 830. Based on Fielding H. Garrison's "Chronology of medicine and public hygiene."

disease. Regarded retrospectively, such activities may have contributed little to the advancement of medical science, but they were scientific nonetheless.

## THE BASIC SCIENCES

Nineteenth-century American physicians tended to attribute their meager scientific output to the relative immaturity of their country. "In the great family of enlightened nations, we are the last born," explained one doctor. "In our youth we must be sustained."[4] The United States may indeed have been a youth among nations, but, as Richard H. Shryock long ago pointed out, it lacked neither the population nor the wealth to support scientific research. By 1860 the United States claimed eight cities with populations in excess of 150,000; its per capita income exceeded that of any European nation; its industry led the world in mechanization.[5] Thus whatever the reasons for the country's failure to contribute to medical science, they did not stem from either poverty or the absence of an urban culture.

Some American physicians, embarrassed by being "the mere recipients" of European knowledge, blamed the scientific inactivity of their colleagues on the availability of foreign literature and feelings of national inferiority. Harvard's Oliver Wendell Holmes, for example, discerned a "fatal influence" to the growth of indigenous science emanating from the indolence created by the "fairest fruits of British genius and research [being] shaken into the lap of the American student."[6] The much-discussed American custom of pirating foreign works and selling them well below the cost of the original editions, which continued until the United States recognized international copyrights late in the century, encouraged this parasitical tendency.[7]

American reliance on foreign works reflected what some contemporaries diagnosed as "a morbid feeling of inferiority to our transatlantic brethren," a paralyzing fear that the humble efforts of Americans would elicit nothing but scorn from the scientific capitals of Europe.[8] Professional leaders repeatedly chastized American physicians for being slaves to foreign authority and urged them "to interrogate nature and experience more, and European opinions less," but little progress resulted.[9]

Although a proclivity for borrowing and a sense of intellectual inferiority may have contributed indirectly to America's poor record in the medical sciences, a far more basic cause was the commercial system of medical education that prevailed in the United States. Before the 19th century medical schools had traditionally stressed the dissemination rather than the production of scientific knowledge; they had frequently provided institutional homes for medical scientists, but had tended to leave organized research up to individual initiative or to scientific academies. During the first half of the nineteenth century this arrangement changed as educational reformers turned European medical schools, particularly German ones, into patrons of laboratory-based medical research. At the University of Berlin, for example, state-paid professors were expected by 1810 to conduct research as well as to teach.[10] In America most medical schools, even those nominally affiliated with a college or university, remained proprietary institutions, run for prestige and profit by ill-equipped local practitioners, many of whom could not have qualified for matriculation as medical students in Europe. Unlike most European governments, which regulated and supported medical education, the state legislatures in America granted charters virtually upon request—an estimated 457 by 1910—and allowed schools to set their own standards.[11] Such legislative liberality may have provided the expanding nation with an ample supply of medical practitioners, but it did little to promote medical science.

American medical schools derived their income almost solely from student fees, which the professors divided among themselves. This scheme virtually guaranteed mediocrity, since high standards would inevitably have reduced the number of fee-paying customers. Because medical schools generally required less of their matriculants than liberal arts colleges, they often enrolled "*the leavings of all the other professions.*" Most medical students never attended college, and some barely knew how to read and write. The college boys who did go into medicine, complained one educator, were often those "who, from various causes—ill-health, poor scholarship, bad conduct and general discouragement—fall by the wayside and after one or two years of study, leave college without a diploma."[12] In view of such conditions, it is not surprising that contemporary critics frequently identified inadequate preliminary education as the highest barrier to the cultivation of medical science in America. "Our physicians and other professional men have genius enough," observed a Boston medical journal in 1833; "their defect is in mental discipline, which was not acquired during their preparatory studies in such a degree as to make the daily acquisition of knowledge, and the habitual exercise of the mental powers, become a primary object of pursuit, and a principal source of their highest enjoyment."[13]

Students not only entered medical school ill prepared for a scientific career, they left in the same condition. In contrast to the leading European schools, which at mid-century required attendance for four years and devoted from 37 weeks (e.g., Edinburgh and Paris) to 41 weeks a year (e.g., Berlin and Pavia) to lectures, the medical school of the University of Pennsylvania, one of America's best, required only 25 weeks a year for two years; and most American schools offered annual terms of only 16 weeks. To make matters worse, American medical students until the last quarter of the century customarily repeated the same courses during their second year that they had taken during their first.[14] In 8 to 12 months of formal training they were expected to learn anatomy, physiology, chemistry, and medical botany. Instruction in the basic sciences, except for anatomy, consisted of didactic lectures. As the historian John B. Blake has pointed out, "Until late in the century, anatomy was traditionally the only laboratory course in medical school. It was, however, generally taught simply for its practical value, chiefly for surgery, and, unlike the other medical sciences, gross human anatomy had very limited potential for stimulating original research."[15] American medical students may have picked up the vocabulary of science, but unlike German students, for example, they had little opportunity to learn its methodology.

Although the quality of American medical schools and their graduates varied greatly, by and large they produced craftsmen, not scholars. "In Europe an educated physician is presumed to be an accomplished *belles lettres* and professional scholar," noted the American Medical Association's Committee on Medical Education in 1863. "In this country . . . a doctor has no special prominence,

and, because a graduate, is not therefore regarded as educated or learned."[16] (It should be noted, however, that both American physicians and foreign visitors occasionally observed that individual physicians enjoyed higher social standing in the United States than in Europe.)[17] Given their cultural environment and training, American physicians understandably valued practice above science, wealth over scholarly reputation. William Beaumont, the frontier physician-physiologist, observed these traits during a visit to New York in 1833. "The professional gentlemen of this City have quite too much personal, political and commercial business on hand to permit them to turn their attention to animal and physiological chemistry, whose high honours and rewards to them are to be the results," he wrote to a friend. "Their curiosity once gratified, they are silent and aloof from the subject."[18]

The American obsession with practice and "getting ahead" deterred even scientifically inclined physicians from engaging in research. "You will lose a patient for every experiment you make in the laboratory," one medical professor warned a student contemplating a scientific career.[19] This attitude helps to explain why the nearly 700 American physicians who studied in Paris between 1820 and 1861 failed to establish a research tradition in America. An eminent American physician, upon hearing that his Paris-trained son wished to devote several years to clinical research before entering practice, explained to his son's French mentor why he could not approve of such plans. "In this country," he wrote, "his course would have been so singular, as in a measure to separate him from other men. We are a business doing people. We are new. We have, as it were, but just landed on these uncultivated shores; there is a vast deal to be done; and he who will not be doing, must be set down as a drone."[20]

American independence in the basic medical sciences did not come until the nation's medical schools freed themselves from dependence on student fees and acquired endowments sufficiently large to allow them to raise standards for admission and provide professors with the time and facilities to undertake scientific work. Since almost no medical professorships generated sufficient income from fees to provide a decent living, American professors customarily supported themselves by practicing medicine. In fact, observed one young physician, "a professorship in a medical college is generally sought as an advertisement in acquiring practice, rather than as an opportunity for study and investigation."[21] In 1878 the president of the American Medical Association contrasted conditions in the United States, where "the names of those who have made undeniable and valuable additions to the common stock" of medical knowledge could be counted on the fingers of two hands, with those in Europe, where scientists were supported by the hundreds. Americans, he said, must recognize

> that pure science, while it is a mine of wealth to the state, cannot remunerate the investigator; that it cannot live upon itself; that those who consecrate themselves to the pursuit of it must isolate themselves from the money-getting world around them; must be relieved from all care and anxiety as to their daily bread; and must be supplied with every necessary appliance while with concentrated thought and patient toil they seek to penetrate as it were with a diamond drill the flinty barriers which separate the known from the unknown. This is particularly true of those engaged in biological research . . . .[22]

Experience in Europe demonstrated that medical schools could provide a home for science, but as long as American institutions remained primarily business enterprises, they stood little chance of attracting the necessary governmental and philanthropic assistance. The "peculiar commercial organization of medical colleges," explained John D. Rockefeller's chief philanthropic advisor, accounted for the reluctance of the wealthy to support medicine "while other departments of science, astronomy, chemistry, physics, etc., had been endowed very generously."[23] It also helped to explain the preference of American millionaires for theology over medicine. In 1890 American seminaries claimed 171 endowed chairs compared with only 5 for medical schools, and none of the latter was adequate to pay even one professor's salary. The combined capital funds of all medical schools amounted to less than a quarter million dollars, approximately 1/48 of what theological schools, with half the number of students, possessed. This disparity, grumbled one jealous physician, existed despite the fact that Edward Jenner's discovery of smallpox vaccination "saves the community more

dollars in one year than all the endowments of all the theological schools in all time."[24]

The absence of salaries and laboratories that endowments could have provided influenced not only individual careers but the general pattern of activity in the biomedical sciences. Americans, noted one physician, displayed "a bias toward systematizing and utilizing the already existing knowledge, rather than the exploration of yet untravelled routes of investigation."[25] Those with scholarly inclinations often channeled their energies into writing financially remunerative textbooks and reference works rather than conducting basic research. John Call Dalton, for example, who in the late 1840s studied in Paris with the French physiologist Claude Bernard, achieved his greatest fame as a teacher and author of texts, not as a researcher. An admiring colleague commented on this unfortunate outcome:

> This eminent physiologist is by mental constitution evidently qualified to hold the position in America which in Paris is occupied by M. Bernard. He should be exploring the dark and untravelled regions of physiology instead of leading undergraduates along its beaten track; his pen should be occupied in tracing new provinces of thought added by his genius to the ever-spreading map of discovered biological science, instead of writing text-books for students. . . . his own proclivities would lead him to produce original monographs, circumstances confine him to the systematic routine of writing a college text-book.[26]

Practicing physicians—and virtually all biomedical scientists in America until the last quarter of the century did practice medicine—found little time for systematic scientific investigation. As one medical journal pointed out, "A man, fatigued with the details of practice, and whose time is never at his own disposal, can rarely do more than keep himself acquainted with the existing condition of medical science . . . ."[27] The experience of S. Weir Mitchell, a Philadelphian who studied the physiological effects of snake venom, illustrates the difficulties facing those who combined research and practice. "It was my habit," he wrote, "to get through work at three or four o'clock; to leave my servant at home with orders to come for me if I was wanted, and then to remain in the laboratory all the evening, sometimes up to one in the morning, a slight meal being brought me from a neighboring inn."[28] As more than one investigator discovered, such self-financed research could also be expensive. William Beaumont, whose experiments on digestion in the 1820s and 1830s won international acclaim, calculated his out-of-pocket expenses at over $3,000, and he suffered less than most because his position as a salaried surgeon in the United States Army provided a steady income and considerable free time.[29]

When the first Americans began returning from German laboratories in the 1870s, they, too, experienced difficulty in finding full-time employment as scientists. One of the earliest returnees, Henry Pickering Bowditch, who in 1871 established the first laboratory for experimental physiology in the country, was able to devote full time to research and teaching only because family money supplemented his Harvard salary.[30] T. Mitchell Prudden and William H. Welch, America's pioneer pathologists, were not so fortunate. Upon returning to the United States in 1878 both reluctantly practiced medicine for a period before finding institutional homes where they could continue their research. In a letter to his sister, Welch described the frustration he experienced in trying to launch his career as a professional scientist:

> I sometimes feel rather blue when I look ahead and see that I am not going to be able to realize my aspirations in life. . . . I am not going to have any opportunity for carrying out as I would like the studies and investigations for which I have a taste. There is no opportunity in this country, and it seems improbable that there ever will be.
>
> I was often asked in Germany how it is that no scientific work in medicine is done in this country, how it is that many good men who do well in Germany and show evident talent there are never heard of and never do any good work when they come back here. The answer is that there is no opportunity for, no appreciation of, no demand for that kind of work here. In Germany on the other hand every encouragement is held out to young men with taste for science.

All these evils, he continued, derived from the fact that "the condition of medical education here is simply horrible."[31]

But even as Welch penned these words, the reformation of American medical education was beginning. Although the proliferation of substandard schools continued unabated, the best institutions were grading and lengthening their curricula to three years, requiring evidence of preliminary education, and, led by the Harvard Medical College, abandoning proprietary status to become an integral part of a university.[32] The dramatic growth of laboratory-based medical science in the latter half of the century encouraged such reforms, as did the German training of approximately 15,000 Americans between 1870 and 1914. Although only a minority of the total specialized in the basic sciences, men like Bowditch, Prudden, and Welch succeeded in transplanting the research laboratory to American soil.[33] When it became apparent that student fees alone could not support such expensive facilities, medical schools began trading proprietary autonomy for the financial security of a university connection.

A further prod to educational reform came from the state legislatures, each of which passed some kind of medical licensing act between the mid-1870s and 1900. The state licensing boards influenced medical education in two ways. First, most of them required candidates to hold a diploma from a reputable medical school, that is, one requiring evidence of preliminary education and, in some cases, offering a three-year course of study, a six-month term, and clinical and laboratory instruction. This forced any school hoping to compete for students to upgrade its curriculum, at least superficially. Second, many states, especially during the late 1880s and 1890s, revised their statutes to require all candidates, even those holding medical degrees, to pass an examination. Although some of the weaker schools quickly learned how to coach students to pass these tests, graduates from strong institutions had a much better chance of passing. Medical commercialism, observed Abraham Flexner, thus "ceased to pay."[34]

No single event contributed more to the reformation of American medical education than the opening in 1893 of the Johns Hopkins School of Medicine under the leadership of Welch. At a time when, according to Welch, no American medical school required a preliminary education equal to "that necessary for entrance into the freshman class of a respectable college," the Hopkins faculty, at the insistence of its patron, demanded a bachelor's degree.[35] Modestly following the Hopkins example, more than 20 schools by 1910 raised their entrance requirements to two years of college.[36] As

Robert E. Kohler has pointed out, this reform, more than any other, "stretched the financial resources of the proprietary school beyond the breaking point. . . . higher entrance requirements disrupted the established market relation with high schools, diminished the pool of qualified applicants, and resulted in a drastic plunge in enrollment. Medical schools could not survive on fees."[37]

Blessed with a large endowment, Johns Hopkins became the nation's first real center for medical science. In addition to creating chairs in anatomy, physiology, pathology, and pharmacology, it provided their occupants — recruited nationally — with well-equipped laboratories and salaries sufficient to free them from the burdens of practice. Before long Hopkins students were spreading across the land, similarly transforming other medical schools. "It is no exaggeration to say that the few teachers who manned these [Hopkins] departments . . . revolutionized within a single decade the status of anatomy, physiology and pathology in America," reported a national body in 1915.[38] Welch, who in 1878 despaired of ever finding employment as a pathologist, was able less than a quarter century later to write:

> Today, pathology is everywhere recognized as a subject of fundamental importance in medical education, and is represented in our best medical schools by a full professorship. At least a dozen good pathological laboratories, equipped not only for teaching, but also for research, have been founded; many of our best hospitals have established clinical and pathological laboratories; fellowships and assistantships afford opportunity for the thorough training and advancement of those who wish to follow pathology as their career . . . and as a result of all these activities the contributions to pathology from our American laboratories take rank with those from the best European ones.[39]

By the turn of the century the medical schools at Harvard, Pennsylvania, Chicago, and Michigan had joined Hopkins as major medical research centers, but the nation still lacked an institution comparable to the Koch Institute in Berlin or the Pasteur Institute in Paris. However, in 1901 the United States Congress provided funds for a national Hygienic Laboratory to investigate infectious and contagious diseases, and, more important, John D. Rockefeller, the oil magnate, donated the first of millions of dollars to create an institute that would become "the crown of medical research in this country."[40] The Rockefeller Institute for Medical Research not only freed its staff from practicing medicine but from teaching as well, allowing them to devote their entire lives to medical science. This environment brought the United States its first Nobel Prize in medicine — awarded to the French-born Alexis Carrel in 1912 — and helped to reverse the flow of medical science and scientists from west to east. Its success soon inspired the creation of other American institutes for medical research and provided a model for the Kaiser Wilhelm Gesellschaft, which opened in Berlin in 1911.[41] By 1920 snide Europeans no longer asked what the world owed to American physicians and surgeons.

## THE CLINICAL SCIENCES

In clinical medicine, which involved diagnosing and treating diseases, the process of maturation did not always parallel the transition from colonial dependence to independence that characterized the development of the basic sciences. Although Americans admired the superior clinical facilities of Europe, they commonly believed that singular circumstances in the United States demanded uniquely American responses to disease and made European knowledge suspect and in certain respects irrelevant. Thus, in areas like medical therapeutics American physicians never established a traditional colonial relationship, and they achieved maturity not by declaring independence, but by abdicating it.

The development of diagnostic tools and knowledge about morbid natural history flourished in the great hospitals of 19th-century Europe. Particularly in Paris, easy access to large numbers of diseased bodies made possible systematic clinical observation of disease processes, pathoanatomical correlation of these clinical patterns at autopsy, and statistical portraits of diseases based upon such studies. From the early 1820s, hundreds of American physicians were drawn to study in Paris both by its clinical facilities and by an environment conducive to medical research. "Merely to have breathed a concentrated scientific atmosphere like that of Paris," one physician studying in the French hospitals wrote home to Boston, "must have an effect on any one who has lived where stupidity is tolerated, where mediocrity is applauded, and where excellence is defied."[42]

Americans, however, lacked comparable institutions until late in the century, and physicians who studied in France found little opportunity at home to apply what they had learned abroad. William Wood Gerhard, who in the 1830s successfully employed Parisian methods to distinguish between typhoid and typhus fever, lamented the conditions at his hospital in Philadelphia. "I regret much the slender materials I possess and the difficulties wh[ich] seem inseparable from observation in this country," he wrote. Despite his inferior facilities for research, he optimistically expected that American physicians would place greater faith in his modest statistical studies on *American* patients than in conclusions drawn from manyfold more Parisians. Many of his countrymen nevertheless remained sceptical of his conclusions, which contradicted European opinion, until Sir William Jenner confirmed them in the 1840s.[43] American contributions to differential diagnosis and the natural history of diseases increased as the century progressed and large hospitals became common in American cities.[44]

It was in surgery that American clinical medicine attained its highest level in the eyes of both Americans and Europeans during the 19th century. Attributing their surgical skills to native mechanical ingenuity and frontier resourcefulness, Americans celebrated such pioneering work as Ephraim McDowell's 1809 operation in Kentucky for an ovarian cyst and J. Marion Sims's operation for vesicovaginal fistula, which he perfected on slave women while practicing in a small Georgia town during the 1840s. The first successful application of ether anesthesia for surgery, at the Massachusetts General Hospital in Boston in 1846, greatly inflated the American medical ego and convinced Americans that they no longer need apologize for their medical backwardness. American medical men "may not dive so deeply into abstract sciences, or linger there so long as in the old and somewhat *senile* establishments of Europe," declared one American surgeon, "but . . . as skillful operators, and practical men, they are the equals to any in the world, and second to none whatsoever."[45] Although a few exceptional achievements like the application of ether may not have warranted such

pride, surgery—and the similarly mechanical field of dentistry—did represent the most accomplished branches of clinical medicine in 19th-century America. The mechanical nature of dental and surgical therapeutics made them largely immune to arguments of American particularism, which were prominent in discussions of medical therapeutics.

The beliefs that therapeutic knowledge gained from experience with European patients and diseases might not be suitable for American practice and that therapeutic principles, unlike the tenets of the basic sciences, might not apply to all environments had deep roots in American medical thought. Although based in part on cultural nationalism, this conviction derived chiefly from the pivotal importance American physicians assigned to specificity in treating patients with different backgrounds and in different settings. Prevailing therapeutic theory stressed the necessity of tailoring therapy to the patient's age, gender, ethnicity, and habits, as well as to climate, topography, and population density.[46]

This commitment to specificity suggested, for example, that the therapeutic needs of the immigrant poor differed from those of native-born patients and, consequently, that information gained by observing pauperized Irish immigrants in a large urban hospital might be deceptive as a guide to treating middle-class private patients or even the hospitalized native-born. Thus physicians at the Commercial Hospital of Cincinnati in the mid-19th century prescribed rest for many patients "just from Ireland via New Orleans" while treating many of the other inmates with full depletive regimens of bleeding and purging.[47] A clinical lecturer at the Massachusetts General Hospital identified a phthisical woman to his students as "one of the cases of broken down health so often met with among her class";[48] another physician at that hospital, reflecting the consequences of this sort of class-specific constitution, noted that although copious bleeding and purging were appropriate for hale constitutions, hospital practice provided few opportunities to employ these remedies.[49] The notion was widespread that although active depletion might not be tolerated by degenerate urban dwellers who lived sedentary lives in vitiated surroundings, the robust farmer required a forcefully depletive therapeutic strategy.[50]

The stress on specificity fostered the notion that, because different regions of the country required distinctive therapeutic practices, physicians should be educated where they intended to practice. For example, the peculiar features of the South — its characteristic diseases, large population of Negroes, and warm climate — all argued for southern students studying medicine at southern medical schools. "Anatomy, Physiology, General Therapeutics, and Chemistry, may be studied to perfection in the Capitols of Europe and the United States," explained one proponent of this view; but, he warned, before practicing in the South such students would either have to unlearn the practical precepts their northern teachers had taught them or fail miserably in their efforts to heal the sick. In his opinion, an ill southerner would be

> better in the hands of some Planter or overseer who had long resided in this region, and who was perfectly familiar with the disease, than he would be in the hands of the ablest Physician of London or Paris, who had never practiced beyond their precincts, and who would be guided in his treatment solely by the general principles of Medicine.[51]

Just as northern therapeutic practices could be inappropriate for southerners, so too European practices might be invalid or even dangerous for Americans. Charles Caldwell, a medical professor in Louisville, Kentucky, returned from a European tour in the early 1840s to warn his classes that "the climate of London and Paris were entirely different from our own; the diet and habits of the people altogether different; and that these with other circumstances so modified the constitutions of the people and the character of the diseases, as to make the latter totally different from the diseases of this country." He expressed the common American suspicion of therapeutic knowledge generated in European clinics:

> The Hospitals of those great cities were very extensive and filled with persons laboring under great varieties of diseases; but they were from the very dregs of society[,] a class whose constitutions have been depraved by intemperance and want, and modified by vice, habit and climate until they possess no analogy in constitution or disease to any class in our own country. From this class or this kind of cases is the student of medi-

cine to derive his knowledge and experience in visiting the Hospitals of London & Paris.

Caldwell concluded that European "constitutions and diseases are so modified and so totally different from those in our country, the knowledge of Pathology and Therapeutics to be gained by visiting these hospitals can be of but little advantage to the practice of Medicine in the United States."[52]

Moreover, physicians generally believed that climate modified the influence of remedial agents on the body just as it influenced disease actions. One physician who held this view cited as his evidence "the different aspects of hyosciamus in England and Italy; of nitrite of silver in Naples and England; of the eau medicinale in Russia and France; [and] the vastly different effects of mercury in different climates."[53] If American practitioners remained "satisfied with the imbecility of European practice," they would, according to the estimate of one Boston physician, "undoubtedly lose a third or half of our patients."[54]

Americans criticized not only specific European therapies but also more general therapeutic philosophies. The therapeutic scepticism characteristic of the Paris clinical school, which argued for discarding any treatments whose clinical value had not been established by empirical observation, found an even more extreme expression in Vienna during the 1840s as therapeutic nihilism, that is, the complete rejection of therapeutic intervention in certain cases.[55] American physicians, who regarded active intervention as a crucial element in professional identity and legitimacy, found such inactive postures impractical and perhaps immoral. "The temporalizing course pursued by the French renders their therapeutics often inefficient," argued a Cincinnati practitioner, referring to the French inclination to leave the patient's cure to the healing power of nature.

> In anatomy, physiology, and pathology, they stand unrivaled; but beyond this they seem scarcely to look. Having made a *diagnosis*, the next most important matter is to prove its correctness; and as this can only be verified in the *dead body*, more enthusiasm is manifested in a post mortem examination than in the administration of medicine to cure disease. *The triumph of these physicians is in the dead-room.*[56]

As this quotation suggests, adherence to therapeutic localism did not imply a belief in the relativity of all medical knowledge. Among the medical sciences, therapeutics was largely exceptional. Although medical therapeutic knowledge did not function equally in all environments, the tenets of such basic sciences as chemistry and anatomy were universally applicable. American physicians also admitted the possibility that European therapeutics might have some applicability in the United States, but they insisted that each therapy be validated independently for the American market. Most believed, however, that therapeutic knowledge grounded upon American experience held far more promise than knowledge of foreign provenance.

In proclaiming their distrust of European clinical knowledge, American physicians assumed the burden of investigating American diseases and cures. A Kentucky student emphasized in his medical thesis the broad gap that existed between the clinical principles set forward by European medical writers and the requirements of American circumstances. Writing in the 1830s, he suggested that this

> imposes on us the greater necessity of observing for ourselves, and of culling, from among the useless rubbish of their productions, something worthy of an extensive and enlightened nation. Thus, although it has been vauntingly asked by one of their writers, "what does medicine owe to America," her sons may yet explore her wilds, and collect the materials, to rear upon the ruins of Eastern speculation, an edifice both complete and durable. [57]

The American environment provided both the opportunity and the responsibility for the reconstruction of medicine to meet American needs.

The program for medical research this emphasis on the American environment implied was avowedly localistic, drawing from a region knowledge to be applied within that region. Among the most active areas of research in early- and mid-19th-century American medicine was a species of natural historical investigation that linked together meteorological, epidemiological, and therapeutic observations. Perhaps the most original medical theses were of this genre. While most theses were merely derivative exercises, many a student elected to write an original essay based on his own investigations of the topography, climate, diseases, and

therapeutic practices of his home county. [58] Daniel Drake's massive treatise *On the Principal Diseases of the Interior Valley of North America* (1850–1854) was, in many respects, only a singularly ambitious expression of the same endeavor. [59] Studies of prevailing diseases, weather conditions, and appropriate treatments also thrived in the discussions of local medical societies, whose meetings were otherwise thin in scientific content. [60] Although American physicians did not excel in those branches of medical science that held universal interest or applications, they did actively conduct research in a sort of environmentally oriented, clinical natural history that was of considerable local import.

American allegiance to therapeutic localism and knowledge gained from direct clinical observation could be seriously challenged only during the last third of the 19th century, when a new therapeutic epistemology took its grounding in experimental laboratory science. Growing interest in this way of generating medical knowledge was both reflected in and fostered by the return from Germany of American physicians eager to exploit laboratory science as a means of transforming medical practice and elevating the status of the profession. Central to their program of reform was the idea that the laboratory was a legitimate arbiter of therapeutic knowledge.

From the early 1870s a number of prominent American physicians began arguing forcefully that the laboratory should join the bedside as an appropriate locus for the generation and validation of therapeutic knowledge. The ensuing clash between the advocates of the laboratory and the defenders of empirical clinical observation did not pit science against art, but entailed two largely incommensurable conceptions of the proper boundaries of therapeutic epistemology. For example, in the mid-1870s Alfred Stillé, a Philadelphia practitioner committed to clinical observation and environmental specificity, argued that the intrusion of laboratory science into the realm of therapeutics was presumptuous and destructive:

> The domain of therapeutics is, at the present day, continually trespassed upon by pathology, physiology, and chemistry. Not content with their legitimate province of revealing the changes produced by disease and by medicinal substances in the organism, they presume to dictate what remedies shall be applied, and in what doses and com-

binations. Their theories are brilliant, attractive and specious . . . . When submitted to the touchstone of experience, they prove to be only counterfeits. They will neither secure the safety of the patient nor afford satisfaction to the physician.[61]

Roberts Bartholow, an American enthusiast for the therapeutic promise of laboratory physiology, denounced Stillé's views to the members of a Baltimore medical society as "reactionary." "Modern physiology," he asserted,

> has rendered experimental therapeutics possible, and has opened an almost boundless field which is being diligently cultivated . . . . It is obvious that no science of therapeutics can be created out of empirical facts. We are not now in a condition to reject all the contributions to therapeutics made by the empirical method, but a thorough examination of them must be undertaken by the help of the physiological method.[62]

Bartholow and like-minded physicians rejected clinical observation as the principal way of gaining therapeutic knowledge — and as insufficient for the creation of a science of therapeutics — but they did not rule out the clinic as a source of therapeutic progress; rather, they advocated a new role for clinical observation in testing laboratory-generated therapeutic principles and practices.

The ascendance of this new view fundamentally altered the relationship between American and European therapeutics. Experimental science investigated disease processes and the practices that altered them. A tacit assumption that animated the rising vogue of vivisectional research during this period was that some fundamental tenets of physiological and therapeutic knowledge could be transferred profitably from the lower animals to man; medical scrutiny focused upon physiological processes, and it was to a certain extent irrelevant whether these processes occurred in a laboratory animal or an Irish immigrant. In this context, the heretofore crucial differentiae between northerner and southerner, immigrant and native, and American and European grew small indeed. The new experimental science, gradually taken up during the next few decades, prescribed in principle standardized treatments for diseased bodies, and considerations based on national variations (other than incidental ones) became stigmata of inferior medical practice.

Recognition of the therapeutic relevance of knowledge generated in the laboratory — abstracted from both the patient and the patient's environment — meant that therapeutic knowledge could be transferred freely between Europe and America. Thus, at the same time that American physicians acquired their own institutions for clinical research, they also freed themselves from their commitment to a distinctive "American" practice. Maturity in this context implied international reciprocity grounded upon an allegiance to medical universalism, not national independence.

## NOTES

This paper was prepared for a conference on "Scientific Colonialism, 1800–1930," held at the University of Melbourne, Australia, May 25–29, 1981. Numbers is primarily responsible for the section on the basic medical sciences; Warner, the section on the clinical sciences. The former wishes to thank Mark Shale for his research assistance. The latter gratefully acknowledges the support of NSF Grant SES-8107609, which supported part of the research for this paper.

1  [Sydney Smith], Review of *Statistical Annals of the United States of America*, by Adam Seybert, *Edinburgh Rev.*, 1820, *33*: 79.

2  S. D. Gross, "Report on the causes which impede the progress of American medical literature," *Tr. A.M.A.*, 1856, *9*: 348. On American excellence in medical practice, see, e.g., the Prospectus, *Philadelphia J. Med. & Phys. Sci.*, 1820, *1*: ix.

3  By the late 1870s Americans were publishing more articles on surgery, obstetrics and gynecology, and diseases of the nervous system than any other nationality; see Mary E. Corning and Martin M. Cummings, "Biomedical communications," in *Advances in American Medicine: Essays at the Bicentennial*, ed. John Z. Bowers and Elizabeth F. Purcell, 2 vols. (New York: Josiah Macy, Jr. Foundation, 1976), II, 731–733.

4  A. B. Palmer, "Report of the Committee on Medical Literature," *Tr. A.M.A.*, 1858, *11*: 231.

5  Richard H. Shryock, *American Medical Research: Past and Present* (New York: Commonwealth Fund, 1947), p. 28; Robert William Fogel and Stanley L. Enger-

man, *Time on the Cross: The Economics of American Negro Slavery*, 2 vols. (Boston: Little, Brown, 1974), I, 248–250; Thomas C. Cochran, *Frontiers of Change: Early Industrialism in America* (New York: Oxford University Press, 1981), p. 114.

6 Oliver Wendell Holmes and others, "Report of the Committee on Literature," *Tr. A.M.A.*, 1848, *1*: 286–287. The phrase about being "mere recipients" appears in Samuel Jackson and others, "Report of the special committee appointed to prepare 'A statement of the facts and arguments which may be adduced in favour of the prolongation of the course of medical lectures to six months,'" *ibid.*, 1849, *2*: 365.

7 See, e.g., Gross, "Report," pp. 344–346; and Alfred Stillé and others, "Report of the Committee on Medical Literature," *Tr. A.M.A.*, 1850, *3*: 181. For British reaction to this practice, see "Report on the progress of midwifery and the diseases of women and children," *Half-Yearly Abstract of the Medical Sciences*, July–Dec. 1855 (No. 22): 208.

8 Thomas Reyburn, "Report of the standing committee on medical literature," *Tr. A.M.A.*, 1851, *4*: 493.

9 Usher Parsons, "Address," *ibid.*, 1854, *7*: 48–49. For references to American physicians being "slaves" and "toadies," see S. D. Gross, "On the results of surgical operations in malignant diseases," *ibid.*, 1853, *6*: 157; and Gross, letter to the editor, *Med. Rec.*, 1868, *4*: 191. For a counteropinion, see the *Am. J. Med. Sci.*, n.s., 1857, *33*: 389–390.

10 Hans H. Simmer, "Principles and problems of medical undergraduate education in Germany during the nineteenth and early twentieth centuries," in *The History of Medical Education*, ed. C. D. O'Malley (Berkeley and Los Angeles: Univ. of California Press, 1970), p. 189; Theodor Billroth, *The Medical Sciences in the German Universities: A Study in the History of Civilization* (New York: Macmillan Co., 1924), p. 27. French medical schools only belatedly supported laboratory-based science; see Erwin H. Ackerknecht, *Medicine at the Paris Hospital, 1794–1848* (Baltimore: Johns Hopkins Press, 1967), pp. 123–126.

11 Abraham Flexner, *Medical Education in the United States and Canada* (New York: Carnegie Foundation, 1910), p. 6; Alfred Stillé, "Address," *Tr. A.M.A.*, 1871, *22*: 83; William O. Baldwin, "Address," *ibid.*, 1869, *20*: 75. On the teaching of the various medical sciences, see Ronald L. Numbers, ed., *The Education of American Physicians: Historical Essays* (Berkeley and Los Angeles: Univ. of California Press, 1980).

12 "American vs. European medical science again," *Med. Rec.*, 1868, *4*: 182–183.

13 "Medical improvement.— No. 1," *Boston Med. & Surg.*

*J.*, 1833, *9*: 92. On inadequate preliminary education, see, e.g., Stillé and others, "Report," p. 173; and N. S. Davis, "Report of the Committee on Medical Literature," *Tr. A.M.A.*, 1853, *6*: 125.

14 F. Cambell Stewart and others, "Report of the Committee on Medical Education," *Tr. A.M.A.*, 1849, *2*: 280. See also E. Giddings, "Report of the Committee on Medical Education," *ibid.*, 1871, *22*: 137.

15 John B. Blake, "Anatomy," in *The Education of American Physicians*, pp. 39–40.

16 Charles Alfred Lee, "Report of the Committee on Medical Education," *Tr. A.M.A.*, 1863, *14*: 84.

17 See, e.g., Stewart and others, "Report," p. 344; "American surgery," *Boston Med. & Surg. J.*, 1875, *92*: 21.

18 Ronald L. Numbers and William J. Orr, Jr., "William Beaumont's reception at home and abroad," *Isis*, 1981, *72*: 598.

19 S. Weir Mitchell, "Memoir of John Call Dalton, 1825–1889," National Academy of Sciences, *Biographical Memoirs*, 1895, *3*: 181. See also "The scarcity of working medical men in America," *Med. Rec.*, 1867, *2*: 277; and John S. Billings, "Literature and institutions," in *A Century of American Medicine, 1776–1876* (Philadelphia: H. C. Lea, 1876), pp. 363–364. Allegiance to medical practice helped to kill the short-lived Philadelphia Biological Society; see Bonnie Ellen Blustein, "The Philadelphia Biological Society, 1857–61: a failed experiment?" *J. Hist. Med.*, 1980, *35*: 188–202.

20 James Jackson, *A Memoir of James Jackson, Jr., M.D., with Extracts from His Letters to His Father; and Medical Cases, Collected by Him* (Boston: I. R. Butts, 1835), p. 55. On Americans in Paris, see Russell M. Jones, "American doctors and the Parisian medical world, 1830–1840," *Bull. Hist. Med.*, 1973, *47*: 40–65, 177–204.

21 Simon Flexner and James Thomas Flexner, *William Henry Welch and the Heroic Age of American Medicine* (New York: Viking Press, 1941), p. 85.

22 T. G. Richardson, "Address," *Tr. A.M.A.*, 1878, *29*: 96–97.

23 George W. Corner, *A History of the Rockefeller Institute, 1901–1953: Origins and Growth* (New York: Rockefeller Institute Press, 1964), p. 579.

24 Shryock, *American Medical Research*, p. 49. On support for theological and medical schools, see Flexner and Flexner, *William Henry Welch*, p. 237.

25 Henry F. Campbell, "Report of the Committee on Medical Literature," *Tr. A.M.A.*, 1860, *13*: 773.

26 *Ibid.*, pp. 774–775.

27 "American medicine," *Philadelphia J. Med. & Phys. Sci.*, 1824, *9*: 405.

28 Edward C. Atwater, "'Squeezing Mother Nature': experimental physiology in the United States be-

fore 1870," *Bull. Hist. Med.*, 1978, *52*: 330. Atwater emphasizes the importance of financial support for the progress of physiology.

29   Numbers and Orr, "William Beaumont's reception," p. 596. In this instance, Beaumont generously padded his expense account. On self-supporting science, see also the *Autobiography of Samuel D. Gross, M.D.*, 2 vols. (Philadelphia: George Barrie, 1887), I, 96–97.

30   W. Bruce Fye, "Henry Pickering Bowditch: a case study of the Harvard physiologist and his impact on the professionalization of physiology in America" (M.A. thesis, Johns Hopkins Univ., 1978), p. 78.

31   Flexner and Flexner, *William Henry Welch*, pp. 112–113; *Biographical Sketches and Letters of T. Mitchell Prudden, M.D.* (New Haven: Yale Univ. Press, 1927), p. 32.

32   See Martin Kaufman, *American Medical Education: The Formative Years, 1765–1910* (Westport, Conn.: Greenwood Press, 1976); and Robert P. Hudson, "Abraham Flexner in perspective: American medical education, 1865–1910," *Bull. Hist. Med.*, 1972, *56*: 545–561.

33   Thomas Neville Bonner states that "German study, especially in the basic sciences, was probably the most important factor in explaining the remarkable progress in medical studies in this country after 1870"; *American Doctors and German Universities: A Chapter in International Intellectual Relations, 1870–1914* (Lincoln: Univ. of Nebraska Press, 1963), p. 137. Robert G. Frank, Jr., Louise H. Marshall, and H. W. Magoun identify study in Germany as the "essential ingredient" in the maturation of the neurosciences; "The neurosciences," in *Advances in American Medicine*, p. 557.

34   Flexner, *Medical Education*, p. 11; Martin Kaufman, "American medical education," in *The Education of American Physicians*, p. 19.

35   Flexner and Flexner, *William Henry Welch*, pp. 219, 222–223.

36   Flexner, *Medical Education*, p. 28.

37   Robert E. Kohler, "Medical reform and biomedical science: biochemistry—a case study," in *The Therapeutic Revolution: Essays in the Social History of American Medicine*, ed. Morris J. Vogel and Charles Rosenberg (Philadelphia: Univ. of Pennsylvania Press, 1979), p. 32.

38   Richard H. Shryock, *The Unique Influence of the Johns Hopkins University on American Medicine* (Copenhagen: Ejnar Munksgaard, 1953), p. 22. See also Edward C. Atwater, "A modest but good institution . . . and besides there is Mr. Eastman," in *To Each His Farthest Star: University of Rochester Medical Center, 1925–1975* (Rochester: Univ. of Rochester Medical Center, 1975), p. 6.

39   Flexner and Flexner, *William Henry Welch*, pp. 266–267.

40   Kohler, "Medical reform," p. 53; Corner, *Rockefeller Institute*, p. 149; A. Hunter Dupree, *Science in the Federal Government: A History of Policies and Activities to 1940* (Cambridge, Mass.: Harvard Univ. Press, 1957), pp. 267–268.

41   Corner, *Rockefeller Institute*, pp. 76, 150–151; Shryock, *American Medical Research*, p. 93.

42   Oliver Wendell Holmes to his parents, Paris, Aug. 13, 1833, reprinted in John T. Morse, Jr., *Life and Letters of Oliver Wendell Holmes*, 2 vols. (Cambridge, Mass.: Riverside Press, 1896), I, 108–109.

43   William Wood Gerhard to James Jackson, Jan. 1, 1835, James Jackson Papers, Francis A. Countway Library of Medicine, Boston; Dale C. Smith, "Gerhard's distinction between typhoid and typhus and its reception in America, 1833–1860," *Bull. Hist. Med.*, 1980, *54*: 368–385. See also Ackerknecht, *Medicine at the Paris Hospital*; and Jones, "American doctors and the Parisian medical world."

44   Phyllis Allen Richmond, "The nineteenth-century American physician as a research scientist," in *History of American Medicine: A Symposium*, ed. Felix Marti-Ibañez (New York: MD Publications, 1959), pp. 142–155. On American hospitals, see Morris J. Vogel, *The Invention of the Modern Hospital: Boston, 1870–1930* (Chicago: Univ. of Chicago Press, 1980).

45   Valentine Mott, quoted in Courtney R. Hall, "The rise of professional surgery in the United States, 1800–1865," *Bull. Hist. Med.*, 1952, *26*: 234. American surgical excellence is discussed in "American vs. European medical science," *Med. Rec.*, 1869, *4*: 133–134; S. D. Gross, "American vs. European medical science," *ibid.*, pp. 189–191; and John Eric Erichsen, "Impressions of American surgery," *Lancet*, Nov. 21, 1874: 717–720.

46   For a particularly useful analysis of 19th-century American medical therapeutics, see Charles E. Rosenberg, "The therapeutic revolution: medicine, meaning, and social change in nineteenth-century America," in *The Therapeutic Revolution*, pp. 3–25.

47   Casebooks for Medical Ward Female, May 30, 1848–Mar. 7, 1850, Cincinnati General Hospital Archives, History of the Health Sciences Library and Museum, University of Cincinnati Medical Center, Cincinnati.

48   John Ware, Clinical Lectures, 1830, John Ware Papers, Francis A. Countway Library of Medicine, Boston.

49   George Cheyne Shattuck, Diary Notes on Patients, Vol. II, entry for Dec. 12, 1832, Francis A. Countway Library of Medicine, Boston.

50   "Effects of breathing impure air," *Boston Med. & Surg. J.*, 1832, *6*: 14; Northern Medical Association

of Philadelphia, "Discussion on bloodletting," *Med. & Surg. Rep.*, n.s. 1859, *3*: 271–274, 495–500, 515–521; 1860, *4*: 34–39, 486–497, 517, 518.

51 "Introductory address," *New Orleans Med. J.*, 1844, *1*: ii–iii. See also Jas. C. Billingslea, "An appeal on behalf of southern medical colleges and southern medical literature," *Southern Med. & Surg. J.*, 2nd series, 1856, *12*: 398–402; and on this concept, see John Duffy, "A note on ante-bellum southern nationalism and medical practice," *J. Southern Hist.*, 1968, *34*: 266–276, and John Harley Warner, "The idea of southern medical distinctiveness: medical knowledge and practice in the Old South," in *Science and Medicine in the Old South*, ed. Ronald L. Numbers and Todd L. Savitt, forthcoming.

52 Courtney J. Clark, Notes on the Medical Lectures of Charles Caldwell, Medical Institute of Louisville, Kentucky, 1841–1842, Courtney J. Clark Papers, Manuscripts Department, Duke University Library, Durham, North Carolina.

53 Edward H. Barton, *Introductory Lecture on the Climate and Salubrity of New-Orleans and Its Suitability for a Medical School* (New-Orleans: E. Johns and Co., 1835), p. 17.

54 Celsus, "Treatment demanded by malignant diseases," *Boston Med. & Surg. J.*, 1832, *6*: 141; "Public medical information," *ibid.*, p. 336.

55 Ackerknecht, *Medicine at the Paris Hospital*, pp. 129–138; Erna Lesky, *The Vienna Medical School in the Nineteenth Century*, trans. L. Williams and I. S. Levij (Baltimore: Johns Hopkins Univ. Press, 1976). I do not suggest by this that Viennese nihilism was fully derived from Parisian scepticism; see Erna Lesky, "Von den Ursprüngen des therapeutischen Nihilismus," *Sudhoffs Archiv für Geschichte der Medizin und der Naturwissenschaft*, 1960, *44*: 1–20.

56 Review of "Lectures on the theory and practice of physic.—by William Stokes . . . and John Bell . . . ," *Western Lancet*, 1842–43, *1*: 354–357. On American attitudes toward the healing power of nature and its associations with therapeutic scepticism, see John Harley Warner, "'The nature-trusting heresy': American physicians and the concept of the healing power of nature in the 1850's and 1860's," *Perspect. Am. Hist.*, 1977–78, *11*: 291–324. See also "Andral's medical clinic," *Western Lancet*, 1843–44, *2*: 148; John P. Harrison, "On the certainty and uncertainty of medicine," *ibid.*, 1844–45, *3*: 118; and "Modern practice of medicine," *Boston Med. & Surg. J.*, 1835, *12*: 351–352.

57 William Wood, "An inaugural dissertation on the causes of epidemics" (M.D. thesis, Medical Department of Transylvania Univ., 1834), Special Collections and Archives, Transylvania University, Lexington, Kentucky.

58 Typical of such theses are Robert H. Hanna, "An inaugural dissertation on the medical topography and epidemic diseases of Wilson County Kentucky" (M.D. thesis, Medical Department of Transylvania Univ., 1835), Special Collections and Archives, Transylvania University, Lexington, Kentucky; and Thomas Hunter, "A dissertation on the topography of south Alabama and the diseases incident to its climate" (M.D. thesis, Medical College of the State of South Carolina, 1843), Waring Historical Library, Medical University of South Carolina, Charleston.

59 Daniel Drake, *A Systematic Treatise, Historical, Etiological, and Practical, on the Principal Diseases of the Interior Valley of North America*, 2 vols. (Vol. I, Cincinnati: Winthrop B. Smith and Company, 1850; Vol. II, ed. S. Hanbury Smith and Francis B. Smith, Philadelphia: Lippincott Crombe and Co., 1854).

60 The proceedings of one such local society are recorded in the Minutes of the Union District Medical Association, Vol. I, 1867–1880, Walter Havinghurst Special Collections Library, Miami University, Oxford, Ohio.

61 Alfred Stillé, *Therapeutics and Materia Medica*, 2 vols. (Philadelphia: Henry C. Lea, 1874), I, 31. Stillé discusses the influence of such factors as climate, season, and occupation on the actions of medicines on pp. 33, 90–94. The pairing of this and the following quotation is suggested by Alex Berman, "The impact of the nineteenth century botanico-medical movement on American pharmacy and medicine" (Ph.D. dissertation, Univ. of Wisconsin, 1954), pp. 36–37.

62 Roberts Bartholow, *Annual Oration on the Degree of Certainty in Therapeutics* (Baltimore, 1876), pp. 12–14. For an assessment of the relationship between experimental physiology and therapeutics in the mid-19th century, see John Harley Warner, "Physiological theory and therapeutic explanation in the 1860s: the British debate on the medical use of alcohol," *Bull. Hist. Med.*, 1980, *54*: 235–257; and *idem*, "Therapeutic explanation and the Edinburgh bloodletting controversy: two perspectives on the medical meaning of science in the mid-nineteenth century," *Med. Hist.*, 1980, *24*: 241–258.

# EDUCATION

America's first medical school opened in Philadelphia in 1765. Prior to that time, colonials who wanted to become physicians either studied in Europe or, more commonly, served a brief apprenticeship with a local practitioner. Even after the advent of formal medical education the apprenticeship remained the primary means of obtaining clinical experience, supplementing the lectures available in schools.

By 1800 Columbia, Harvard, and Dartmouth also had established medical departments, and within a few decades medical schools were flooding the country. Although some continued to affiliate with colleges or universities, most of the new schools were run by private groups who cared more about profits than pedagogy. The typical mid-century institution had five or six nonsalaried professors, usually physicians, whose income depended on how many lecture tickets they could sell. Each term lasted only three or four months and consisted of perhaps half a dozen courses, ranging from anatomy to the theory and practice of medicine. To graduate with an M.D. degree, students attended the same lectures for two terms and — at least in theory — completed an apprenticeship.

Efforts to improve this dismal situation, described by Edward C. Atwater and Robert P. Hudson, culminated in Abraham Flexner's 1910 exposé, which hastened the closing of the most wretched schools. The institutions that survived into the 1920s offered a four-year, graded curriculum, usually divided between the basic sciences (e.g., anatomy, physiology, and biochemistry) and practical experience in the clinic or hospital. Unlike times past, when reading and writing were virtually the only skills required for admission, students now had to attend college for at least two years before admission.

As medicine grew more and more complex in the 20th century, medical educators found it increasingly difficult to squeeze into four years all the clinical training a physician or surgeon would need to practice medicine effectively. Thus in the 1910s schools and state licensing boards began requiring an additional year of internship in a hospital. But even this proved insufficient training for some specialties, and by the 1920s and 1930s a number of physicians were continuing to train for several years after the internship in postgraduate residency programs, specializing in fields such as ophthalmology, obstetrics, and orthopedic surgery. After World War II it became customary for all but general practitioners to study medicine for about eight years before engaging in independent practice.

Until shortly before the Civil War, American medical schools admitted only white males, but this barrier fell under the influence of the antebellum abolitionist and feminist movements. Elizabeth Blackwell in 1849 became the first American woman to earn a medical degree. Women made rapid strides in separate as well as coeducational medical schools during the late 19th century — only to fall back again in the 20th. Between 1910 and 1960, few medical schools had enrollments of more than 5 percent women, and they admitted an even smaller percentage of minority students. But once again social ferment forced these schools to reevaluate their admission policies, and by the mid-1970s almost one-fourth of entering students were women and one-eighth represented various minority groups.

# 9

## Touching the Patient: The Teaching
## of Internal Medicine in America

### EDWARD C. ATWATER

"By an application of the science of acoustics to diseases of the chest, we are now enabled to pronounce with unerring precision upon the nature, location, and extent of diseases of the circulatory and respiratory organs, which less than half a century ago were veiled in impenetrable darkness and obscurity." So said the president of the Medical Society of the State of New York to those assembled for the annual meeting of the organization in 1854.[1] Exaggerated as the claim may be, it is hard for us who take for granted the methods of physical examination to appreciate the changes that occurred in medicine in the four decades before the American Civil War.

At the beginning of the 19th century there was no stethoscope, no clinical thermometer, no percussion hammer, no ophthalmoscope, no sphygmomanometer, and no useful microscope. Though Hippocrates had described the succussion splash of pleural or cavitary effusion more than 2,000 years earlier and Leopold Auenbrugger's work on percussion had appeared in 1761, they were generally ignored. In fact, the known methods of physical examination, including direct auscultation by placing the ear on the chest wall, were seldom used or mastered technically; and the significance of the information that could be obtained by such means was obscure. Beyond superficially inspecting a patient and perhaps feeling the pulse, the American physician devoted little time to physical examination.[2]

EDWARD C. ATWATER is Associate Professor of Medicine and the History of Medicine at the University of Rochester Medical Center, Rochester, New York.

Reprinted with permission from *The Education of American Physicians: Historical Essays*, edited by Ronald L. Numbers (Berkeley: University of California Press, 1980), pp. 143–174.

Nor did he attempt to reconstruct the natural history of the patient's illness in any systematic way.

He knew little about what went on within the body, in health or disease. The nature of some functions could be inferred from anatomical knowledge, obtained by dissecting cadavers. However, physiology was in its infancy, and vivisection, later its fundamental technique, was not yet employed. Though Giovanni Morgagni had demonstrated toward the end of the 18th century that disease usually produced distinctive changes in specific organs, it was not possible to identify or evaluate these changes in the living patient. Physicians continued to deal with disease and treatment largely in a priori philosophical terms, referring to fever as a disease and unbalanced humors as a cause.

By the end of the 19th century physical examination was a highly sophisticated method with an array of bedside instruments. The perfection of the microscope made it possible to go from the organ pathology of Morgagni and the tissue pathology of Xavier Bichat to the cellular concepts of Rudolf Virchow, and the later introduction of the oil immersion lens greatly aided the development of microbiology. The discovery of anesthesia made vivisection practical, thereby providing the physiologist with his most important tool. The microscope and developments in chemistry made it possible to study the morphological and molecular elements of body fluids. All of these advances contributed to the practice of medicine generally. But it was application of the stethoscope, more than anything else, that made internal medicine a separate discipline.

Internal medicine, like most specialties, acquired a separate identity as a result of new technology that required specialized training. The need to learn the methods of physical diagnosis, particularly use of the stethoscope, made individualized bedside teaching necessary and the previously popular grand walking round and the clinical lecture inadequate. Once proficiency in the use of certain tools became essential, the method of giving clinical instruction had to change from a passive to an active one.[3]

It was not until the 20th century, however, that undergraduate instruction at American medical schools regularly included practical clinical training and medical students routinely examined patients carefully and recorded the details of their illnesses. The reasons for this delay were economic and social as well as technological. In order to provide such training there had to be hospitals where large groups of patients could be examined under supervision, a situation that did not exist generally until the end of the 19th century. Financial subsidies for medical education were also necessary so that class size could be limited and sufficient faculty provided for individual bedside instruction. Course length had to be increased in order to provide time for clinical instruction. Once these prerequisites were available, the individualized teaching method, called the clinical clerkship, became virtually universal. It has remained the fundamental way of teaching internal medicine.

The "internal" concept itself reflected the fact that the techniques of physical examination, especially auscultation and percussion, made it possible to examine the "inside" of a patient from the outside. In contrast to this, surgery still dealt almost exclusively with the then "external" problems of orthopedics, urology, and superficial tumors. With the coming of anesthesia, asepsis, and the surgical invasion of the body at the end of the century, the surgeon became, in fact, the internist, but the contrary usage was by then established.

The term *internal medicine* came into general use late in the 19th century. Before then the great body of medicine, from which surgery and obstetrics had already been separated, was known as physic and its teachers as professors of the theory and practice of physic. The founding of a Society for Internal Medicine in Berlin in 1881, the holding of the first Congress of Internal Medicine in Germany in 1882, and the organizing of the Association of American Physicians in 1885 officially introduced the new term.

In the evolution of the teaching of internal medicine several themes are important: the introduction of a special technology, the development of hospitals for teaching, the delay in providing individual clinical experience for the undergraduate until financial subsidies made it possible to limit class size and increase the number of faculty, and the more recent effect of specialization and graduate training programs on undergraduate clinical instruction.

## THE TECHNOLOGY OF INTERNAL MEDICINE

Following the publication of the *Traité de l'auscultation médiate* by René-Théophile-Hyacinthe Laennec in 1819, in which the author described the use of his stethoscope for studying the acoustics of the respiratory and cardiovascular systems, diagnosis became a science. Laennec's contribution was not merely the device that made his observations more precise but also the care with which he made his examination and the way he interpreted his data in terms of anatomical change. By associating particular sounds with structural abnormalities later found at autopsy, it was possible to predict or describe what was occurring internally in organs hidden from view in the living patient.

Unlike Auenbrugger's long-obscure work, Laennec's was soon well known.[4] In 1820 a translation of a French review appeared in an American journal,[5] and the following year an American physician wrote that "the continued use of this instrument has satisfied us more and more of the benefits which may be attained by it." He added, however, that it would take a lot of hard work and practice.[6] Laennec's book itself was published in Philadelphia in 1823, two years after the appearance of an English translation in London. By 1839 there had been 19 printings in French, German, Italian, and English, four of them in the United States.[7]

In 1824 John Bell, a Philadelphian who had studied with Laennec, published the first American work on the subject of stethoscopy, entitled "Some General Remarks on the Use of the Stethoscope, as an Aid in Forming a Correct Diagnosis of Diseases of the Lungs, Together with Some Observations on the Symptom Called by M. Laennec, Pectoriloquy."[8] That same year, a 22-year-old medical student, Edmund Strudwick of North

Carolina, published some reports that included stethoscopic examination of patients he had cared for on the wards of the Philadelphia Almshouse.[9] Soon American publishers were providing a succession of French and English works on stethoscopy, the former usually translated by Americans who had studied in Paris.[10] Two men, Samuel Jackson, attending physician at the almshouse in Philadelphia, and James Jackson, Hersey Professor of the Theory and Practice of Physic at Harvard, were major sponsors in introducing stethoscopy to America,[11] probably because each of them had students who studied in Paris and returned as "apostles of the school of observation."[12]

The older men found the new technique difficult. James Jackson acknowledged his ears were "old and were not trained early. . . . [Oliver Wendell] Holmes has attended to auscultation more than any other of my (recent) pupils and I often call on him to help me with my ears." To his son he wrote that he did not expect to master the stethoscope, "yet I expect you to do it. It is incomparably easier for you than for me."[13] The senior generation did recognize the instrument's importance. Jackson's colleague, the versatile Jacob Bigelow, wrote in 1839 that "the discoveries of Laennec . . . have constituted the most important acquisition which medical science has received during the present century."[14]

Between 1820 and 1860 almost 600 young American physicians studied in Paris hospitals, especially with P. C. A. Louis, who, after the death of Laennec in 1826, became one of the most popular teachers of the new medicine.[15] From these students came a generation of leaders of the medical profession in America. William W. Gerhard of Philadelphia and Henry I. Bowditch of Boston both wrote books on physical diagnosis that became classics, and Oliver Wendell Holmes won a Boylston Prize for his essay on physical examination of the chest. Caspar Pennock and Edward Mott Moore did early experimental work attempting to correlate physiological function with physical signs in living animals.[16] William Pepper, Alfred Stillé, and George C. Shattuck became leading figures at the University of Pennsylvania and at Harvard.

The students of Louis learned more than auscultation. Some of them also organized a Society for Medical Observation in 1832 and asked Louis to preside. Their purpose was to improve their own abilities as clinical observers by taking a detailed history from the patient, performing a meticulous physical examination, and discussing the findings in patho-physiologic terms. Their group met weekly, with each student in turn presenting a case he had prepared.

> The members were arranged around a table that occupied three sides of the room, and each person had paper and pen or pencil before him. He was prepared . . . to note the most trivial omission or a too inconsiderate deduction made by the reader. Each subsequently criticized the paper from these notes. This was done in the keenest manner. Louis, as President, summed up the result of the meeting by not only criticizing the reader, but also his critics' remarks.

There were no petty quarrels or personal attacks, but also no sentimental delicacy. All of this was described by Louis in "An Essay on Clinical Instruction," in which he noted modestly that the methods of observation used were "more exact than those of former periods, but less rigorous than those which will succeed."[17] His prediction proved correct.

In the decades that followed, the convenience and precision of physical diagnosis increased. The most notable improvement in the stethoscope was the semiflexible binaural model made popular by George P. Cammann of New York City in 1851, which remained the standard instrument in this country until the development of the combination bell and diaphragm by the Boston engineer R. C. M. Bowles at the end of the century. In 1851 Hermann von Helmholtz elaborated the principle of the ophthalmoscope. The thermometer was adapted to clinical use in the 1870s, when Carl Wunderlich and others began recording temperatures on graphs and using the patterns in a practical way. The explanation of the reflex arc by Wilhelm Erb and Carl Westphal brought the percussion hammer into neurology after 1875. In 1896 the application of an inflatable bladder made the sphygmomanometer—the last of the major tools of bedside examination—practical for the first time. Significant improvements in the achromatic microscope made it possible to examine blood smears and urine sediments.[18]

In addition to these innovations, physicians began applying the stethoscope to acoustical phe-

nomena of the body other than those of respira-
tion. The French surgeon Jacques Lisfranc found
that the crepitus produced by movement of fractured bones and the grating sound made by a
catheter rubbing against a bladder stone was diag-
nostically useful.[19] Cardiac murmurs and extra-
thoracic vascular bruits were also identified. Since
many of these conditions were amenable to treatment, the stethoscope was of more varied usefulness in the days before the development of radi-
ography.

As early as 1855 an English manual appeared
in the United States outlining the method of collecting and recording historical data still in use
today. It described not only percussion and auscultation, but also abdominal, neurological, and
psychiatric examinations, and the use of the opthal-
moscope, the speculum, and the spirometer. Also
included were instructions for performing microscopic and chemical tests on blood and urine. By
the mid-1860s the manual was appearing on the
recommended reading lists of at least two medical
schools, Harvard and Vermont.[20]

By the eve of the Civil War Austin Flint, probably the most prominent American internist of his
generation, had become the leading exponent of
teaching auscultation. For this his peers dubbed
him "the American Laennec." Between 1850, when
he published his first "Contributions to the Study
of the Physical Diagnosis of Diseases of the Chest"
in the *Buffalo Medical Journal*, and his death in 1884,
Flint wrote seven major works dealing with physical diagnosis, including the first American classic
on cardiac disease, a description of the murmur
which bears his name, and a textbook that appeared in its ninth edition 41 years after his death.[21]

By the end of the 19th century the technical
methods of internal medicine had been developed.
It was possible to examine a patient at the bedside
and to learn from the outside much about what
was occurring inside. But if physical examination
made medicine more precise, it also made it more
difficult. As James Jackson, Jr., wrote to his father
from Paris, "If Laennec has added an important
aid to our insufficient means of exploring diseases
of the chest, he has, at the same time, rendered
the study of those diseases more difficult, more laborious I would say, to the learner."[22]

Most American physicians who learned physical diagnosis did so on their own initiative, and

it would be wrong to assume that the methods
were in general use in the 19th century. More important, they were not consistently a part of undergraduate medical education in the United States
until the 20th century. Gerhard attributed this
deficiency to "the small number of observers who
[were] interested in prosecuting medicine as a science, with but a slender expectation of ultimate
pecuniary reward." Describing what he called "the
profitless pursuits of medical science," Gerhard predicted that such would always be the case in a society in which "commerce and manufactures offer
large rewards for the employment of capital, and,
indirectly, rather obstruct pursuits in which an immediate advantage is not presented."[23]

Had Gerhard lived to the end of the 19th century, when the fruits of commerce and manufacturing began to benefit medical education in the
form of endowments, he would have seen himself
contradicted. With the subsidization of medical
education, it became possible to provide the expensive individual instruction needed to train
students in the use of the tools and techniques of
internal medicine.

## THE HOSPITAL:
## A CLINICIAN'S LABORATORY

Before the methods of bedside physical examination were available, the ambulatory medical apprenticeship had often provided satisfactory clinical experience, as William Beaumont, who later
became famous for his studies of digestion, attested. Beaumont's preceptor in rural Vermont put
his young apprentice in "charge of many of his patients during his calls elsewhere."[24] When it became necessary to master precise techniques like
stethoscopy, however, the occasional and often solitary bedside experience of the apprentice, though
it might stimulate self-reliance, could not provide
proper instruction. The hospital, which brought
together large groups of patients, made it possible
to do many examinations sequentially and to repeat the examinations periodically. It also attracted
to its staff those men who especially wanted to
teach. The hospital provided the laboratory for
systematic clinical training, and the appearance of
this institution was one of the prerequisites to any
major change in the clinical curriculum.

Teaching was, almost without exception, one of

the reasons physicians gave for promoting hospitals.[25] But using the hospital for teaching was not always easy. Throughout most of the 19th century only the poor sought hospital care, and the attending physician offered his services free in return for the privilege of bringing medical students with him on his rounds.[26] Inevitably, conflicts arose regarding the rights of patients to competent care and personal privacy, the need to provide training for inexperienced students, and the effort to conserve public funds by accepting the free service of physicians. The emphasis usually fluctuated. In prosperous times politicians talked about the dignity of the poor, while in times of recession they were only too glad to allow teaching in return for free professional care. Misunderstandings between the professional staff, both physicians and students, and the hospital managers and administrators compounded the problem. None of the early hospitals was exempt.

When seeking tax funds, the promoters of the Massachusetts General Hospital found it necessary to reassure the legislature that there was no intention "to give to students in medicine an opportunity to experiment, at the expense of the feelings, health, and lives of the poor patients." A few years later the managers of the same institution announced that

> pupils are not to remain at the Hospital longer than is absolutely necessary for the visits. They are not to converse with the patients or nurses. During operations and while in the wards they are to abstain from conversation with each other; they are not to walk about; nor in any other way to disturb either the medical officer, or the patients. . . . In all cases, in which it will be proper for the pupils to make any personal examination of a patient, such as feeling the pulse, examining a tumor, etc. an intimation to that effect will be given them by the physician or surgeon. It must be obvious that the greatest inconveniences must arise, if such examinations were commonly made by the pupils.

This feeling apparently still existed in 1846 when the managers, responding to a proposal to move the medical school adjacent to the hospital, stated "that they cannot perceive any advantage to this institution to arise therefrom."[27]

In Philadelphia, the Guardians of the Almshouse at Blockley stated that their concern for medical teaching did "not predominate over the interest we feel in the discharge of duty towards the poor, as their legal Guardians," and they worried "whether it is consistent with our duty toward these unfortunate inmates of the Hospital to place them in [the] charge of mere novices who never had a case before entering its wards."[28]

In the 70 years before the Civil War this institution, later known simply as Blockley Hospital and generally considered the finest teaching hospital of that day, was partially or entirely closed to student activity for more than one-third of the time as a result of these conflicts. On June 30, 1845, for example, a cockroach crawled onto the dining room table where the resident physicians were eating; the residents demanded to be served at the matron's table and, on being refused, walked out. The board of managers was only too happy to replace them all with one full-time resident physician at a salary of $1,800 a year and three consultants—medical, surgical, and obstetrical—at $100 each. They abolished the entire teaching hierarchy of voluntary attending physicians, resident physicians and students, and Blockley ceased to function as a teaching hospital for nine years.[29] Commenting on this problem, one observer wrote that "very seldom, indeed, is there a cordial harmony between hospital managers and resident physicians. The exercise of power is as dear to the one as intolerance of it is natural to the other. The one lacks sympathy and the other humility."[30] This was later expressed even more strongly by another professor who wrote "that among the governors of the institution there must have been then, as there usually have been since, individuals who had attained the last possible degree in the way of being asses."[31]

Another problem was the disproportionate number of students to patients. As late as 1873, when the first hospital survey was made in the United States, there were fewer than 20,000 general hospital beds, many of which were not near a medical school.[32] At the same time there were 10,000 medical students in America. Though Blockley Hospital provided close to 8,000 patients a year in the 1850s for the 650 or so medical students in Philadelphia, the burden of clinical teaching fell upon the facilities of the Pennsylvania Hospital, with only 1,000 patients, during prolonged periods. Most other cities were even less fortunate. In the 1840s the Massachusetts General Hospital had only about 400 patients a year, while there were 90 medical students at Harvard.

It was physically impossible to provide individual clinical experience until the number of students was reduced, the number of patients increased, and more sympathetic administrators were appointed.[33] It is not surprising that in 1849 the American Medical Association's Committee on Medical Education reported that only 9 of 35 American medical schools required *any* hospital experience for a diploma.[34]

A few schools attempted to gain control of some nearby hospital beds or to establish hospitals of their own, but these efforts were generally unsuccessful.[35] In the late 1850s New York Medical College, founded in 1850 with a commitment to implement the educational reforms proposed by the American Medical Association, operated a charity ward of 27 beds in the school building for the express purpose of teaching. But this experiment did not survive. It was not until later in the century that the University of Michigan (1869) and the University of Pennsylvania (1874) established clinical facilities under school control.[36]

In the meantime another solution, the college clinic, became popular. This was essentially a dispensary, similar to the later outpatient department or neighborhood health center. Philadelphia had a dispensary as early as 1786, and New York, Boston, and Charleston each established one in the early part of the 19th century. But even here there were frequent conflicts between physicians and managers over student activities. At the Boston Dispensary in 1827 the visiting physicians defended their action in allowing students to prescribe on the grounds that it was good practical experience and pointed out that student fees were the only recompense the physicians had for their professional services. They denied that students experimented on patients. The matter was resolved (and the real nature of the managers' concern clarified) when it was agreed that the apothecaries would instruct the students once a week to acquaint them "with the price of medicine."[37]

In spite of such difficulties, the medical profession defended the usefulness of dispensaries for teaching. In 1834 a physician at the Medical College of Ohio called service in a dispensary "a most desirable opportunity for acquiring a large fund of useful practical knowledge," but he was careful to emphasize the benefit the public might expect, especially in the case of "a dispensary maintained by the voluntary contributions of the poor, while in health," since this would reduce dependency among sick paupers.[38]

By the 1840s many medical schools were organizing their own dispensaries in order to avoid the problem of unsympathetic managers. In Philadelphia, "where hospital privileges had been so much restricted as to be of little service to the winter students," the popularity of dispensaries grew, especially after the more appealing name of "clinique" was substituted for "dispensary." A veritable "clinique epidemic" broke out and quickly spread to other cities.[39] In the winter of 1846, though there were 600 to 700 medical students in New York City, one professor found the hospitals forsaken for the cliniques and reported that "it was a rare thing to see the face of a single student in any of [his] wards during the whole of [his] attendance." In his address to the students at the opening of the medical school session that year he pleaded for practical medical education in a hospital, stressing the liberality of the New York Hospital regarding the needs of students.[40] In Philadelphia the professors soon gave up the dispensaries and instead provided hospital tickets at their own expense for senior students.

The fundamental problem remained, however. Many schools offered no clinical opportunities, and those that did put little pressure on the students to make use of them. When Nathan Davis published his history of American medical education in 1851, he reported that only 16 of the 37 active medical colleges were near clinical facilities and that almost one-half of those who graduated from American schools had no "genuine bed-side instruction whatever."

> How many of the thousand students who annually congregate in Philadelphia, or of the seven hundred who spend their winter in New York, are daily found studying with care the most important of all subjects, viz.—clinical medicine and surgery, at the bed-side, in the capacious hospitals of those cities? I speak from personal observation, when I say that not one in twenty are found paying attention to these things.[41]

It was a problem of too many students, too few teachers, too little time, and too few patients.

Hospitals became more common in the latter half of the century, when large-scale urban poverty began to appear in small inland industrial cities and care of the sick poor became a serious problem. The need for the federal government to provide care for wounded or sick soldiers during and immediately after the Civil War created an even greater demand for hospital beds. With the coming of aseptic surgery at the end of the 19th century, hospital facilities increased rapidly and, as a result of the endowment of medical education by philanthropists, it became possible to reduce the size of medical school classes. At Johns Hopkins, for example, there were fewer than 50 students in a class and about 3,400 patients hospitalized in 1897. During the first quarter of the 20th century the number of hospital beds in the United States tripled while the number of medical students dropped by half. With an adequate setting in which to teach the new methods of internal medicine, an effective means of instructing undergraduates in clinical medicine finally evolved.

## CLINICAL INSTRUCTION
## IN THE 19TH CENTURY

The style of early American clinical teaching came from Scotland. Most American physicians who studied abroad in the late 18th century went to Edinburgh. Men like Benjamin Rush, William Shippen, Adam Kuhn, Caspar Wistar, Philip S. Physick, John Morgan, and Samuel Bard were all products of the Scottish school, and it is not surprising that the traditions of that institution influenced the character of early collegiate education in the United States.[42]

The method of clinical teaching used at Edinburgh and in most English-speaking schools was the grand walking round, in which the professor, followed by an entourage of students, stopped successively at the bedsides of several patients. The professor questioned the patient in a loud voice, and a senior student chosen for the purpose repeated, in an equally loud voice, the patient's answers. The professor made appropriate comments on diagnosis, prognosis, and treatment before moving to the next patient. Wrote a student of the period:

> It is no easy task; it requires an exertion almost stentorean to render this conversation between the physician and his patient audible by the most distant members of the class; while the impossibility of seeing the patient, obliges all who are not in his immediate vicinity to trust solely to their ears for information.[43]

Until the early 19th century, in Europe at least, the professor's remarks were rendered in what passed for Latin. The experience was hardly conducive to student participation or to acquiring proficiency in the care of patients.

An abundance of firsthand descriptions makes it clear that the few American schools with hospital facilities universally used this teaching method. Typical is Asa Fitch's account of his winter medical course in New York City. Each day he spent seven hours in lectures and one visiting the wards of New York Hospital with the attending physician. He reported that there were so many students on the round that it was "impossible to make any improvement by attending here. However I crowded around with the rest and saw all I could."[44] The typical student paid a fee of about ten dollars for a hospital ticket, which entitled him to attend the rounds, usually held twice a week. The proceeds went to the hospital, and in the early days most schools with hospital facilities required attendance.

When classes grew to several hundred students —the University of Pennsylvania had over 400 by 1810 and Jefferson had over 300 by the middle 1830s—it was necessary to substitute the clinical lecture in an amphitheatre for the walking round on the ward. Medical leaders touted the clinical lecture highly. Edward Delafield told medical students in 1837 that it "will prove to be the best possible means of preparing you by engaging yourselves in the treatment of disease."[45] Critics observed that this was making a virtue of necessity. "Except that the [clinical] lecture is made more imposing by the subject of it being present, and possibly the students' attention to the case being fastened by the display," said members of one unsympathetic hospital board, "we know of no benefit which can accrue from it which would not equally result from the case being lectured on in the absence of the patient, from the notes of the physician, which form, in reality, the basis of the lecture."[46] Even country schools could provide this type of experience by using ambulatory patients.

Some medical educators recognized the faults

of the clinical lecture. Not only did the lecturer tend, then as now, to describe the unusual,[47] but also he provided no continuity to his instruction. "What idea has a man of typhus fever who has seen a case once and then only for the space of five minutes?" asked a professor in 1844, adding that there was "no hospital in America which furnishes a sufficient clinic to any other pupils than those which reside within its walls." The most important matter, he continued, is constant access to the bedside. "One case, however slight, thus studied, is worth a hundred seen at long intervals, and worth a thousand seen once from the benches of the amphitheatre, then sent away and never heard of more. The student should also be allowed to take part, from time to time, in the treatment of the sick."[48]

Despite these criticisms, the large clinical lecture prevailed as late as 1890 in most schools, including the country's most prestigious, the University of Pennsylvania. "The old type of lecture system was in full flower," recalled one student.

> We were lectured to from nine in the morning until six at night, [he wrote] although by four o'clock the saturation point had been reached and we were far too sleepy to comprehend what was said to us. . . . [We also had] what were called clinical lectures in the pit of a huge amphitheater. The patient would be brought in and the several hundred students on the benches could see him, but they learned very little in a practical way from that kind of exercise. It really made no difference what ailed the patient; the professor could use him as text for almost any disease and we would be none the wiser. Occasionally we were taken into the wards . . . but I cannot recall that I examined more than two or three cases in my entire course.[49]

A student who graduated from the College of Physicians and Surgeons in New York in 1890 had similar recollections. "During the last two years," he said, "we had a few clinical lectures in the Vanderbilt Clinic, but we never came within a mile of touching a patient." It was common for students to graduate from even the best schools without ever examining a patient.[50]

At first this was not a serious drawback since students were still expected to get their clinical experience during a three-year apprenticeship with a hometown preceptor. Since antiquity the apprenticeship had been the fundamental means of professional replication, and it was required by law in the early 19th century. The early American medical schools merely supplemented this training by providing lectures to cope with a rapidly expanding (as it seemed even then) body of knowledge.

Over the years emphasis on lectures grew, stimulated especially by state legislatures which, hoping to encourage attendance at the lectures, gave medical school diplomas equal legal status with the licenses hitherto issued exclusively by county medical societies. The societies, of course, were strict, since each new licensee was a professional colleague and an economic competitor. The schools, whose fame and income came from large numbers, were lenient. It is not surprising that the apprenticeship dwindled and, with it, clinical training. Though the three-year apprenticeship remained a requirement of American medical schools until late in the 19th century, it had long since become a formality, often amounting to little more than the preceptor lending the student a few books and his name as sponsor. The student was left without clinical training, since the schools could not provide it; and undergraduate medical education became didactic and passive.

Significant clinical training for most American physicians came in one of two ways. Some went abroad for a year or two after graduating, and others, especially after the Civil War, served as house officers in a hospital, almshouse, or asylum. But for most, practical learning came by trial and error on their first patients. The reasons were simple: too many students, too few patients, too few teachers, too little time. Lectures were given from 9:00 to 12:30 and from 3:00 to 6:00, so that even where hospitals were available there was no time for bedside medicine. One solution, proposed in 1851 by Nathan Davis, was to lengthen the term from four months to nine or ten months, reduce fees so that more students could attend schools with hospital facilities, and limit lectures to four hours a day, leaving two hours for practical training, including dissection, clinical medicine, surgery, and, "of course, physical diagnosis."[51] In 1859 Davis experimented with two five-month graded terms at Lind University, but it was over three decades before Harvard adopted a four-year graded curriculum with terms of nine months.

Extending the medical course from a total of 8

or 9 months to 36 months had at least two important effects: it increased curriculum time fourfold, providing time for clinical teaching, and it segregated students into graded courses, reducing the size of classes. By the end of the 19th century the techniques of bedside clinical medicine had been developed, hospitals where these methods could be taught effectively had come into existence, and the course had been made sufficiently long to include clinical training. Further reduction of the number of students, provision of salaries for clinical teachers, and collegiate control of hospitals were yet to be established.

## THE STUDENT TOUCHES THE PATIENT

It was not until the 20th century that undergraduate medical students in America had much personal contact with patients. Bedside instruction of individual students existed in Hippocratic times and during the Renaissance at Padua, but it did not survive or spread from there. Its modern ancestry can be traced to the University of Leyden, where in 1630 students were required to examine patients and commit themselves to a diagnosis and plan of treatment. Pupils of Hermann Boerhaave carried this tradition to Vienna and later to Germany.[52]

At the University of Berlin in the early 19th century the professor of clinical medicine held daily teaching clinics in which students examined ambulant patients while their classmates sat around a large table. The examining pupil declared aloud, in Latin, "his diagnostic, prognostic, and *methodus curandi*," after which the professor questioned him further and the student prepared a prescription, which his instructor signed. The patient returned daily "to be examined in the same way by the same pupil, until the cure be completed." If the patient was unable to attend, the student made a house call. This experience was required for graduation.[53] At another Berlin institution the patient was put under the immediate management of a fourth-year "outdoor pupil" who interrogated and examined him and decided upon a diagnosis and treatment.[54]

Robert Graves of Dublin introduced this German system to the English-speaking world. He had traveled on the continent for three years prior to his appointment in 1821 as professor of medicine and physician at the Meath Hospital. In his first lecture as professor the 24-year-old Graves proposed to replace the Edinburgh grand round system of clinical education, then used at Dublin, with the German clinical clerkship method. Said Graves to the students:

> You come here to convert theoretical into practical knowledge. . . . The human mind is so constituted, that in practical knowledge its improvement must be gradual. Some become masters of mathematics, and of other abstract sciences, with such facility, that in one year they outstrip those who have laboured during many. It is so, likewise, in the theoretical parts of medicine; but the very notion of practical knowledge implies observation of nature; nature requires time for her operations; and he who wishes to observe their development will in vain endeavor to substitute genius or industry for time . . . therefore . . . a certain portion of each day should be devoted to attendance at a hospital. . . . Students should aim not at seeing many diseases every day . . . no, their object should be constantly to study a few cases with diligence and attention; they should anxiously cultivate the habit of making accurate observations.[55]

After a decade of experience with the clerkship method Graves was able "strongly to recommend the method of instruction pursued in Germany," regretting only that it had not become more generally accepted.

By the 1830s even Americans were commenting on the German system.[56] Reynell Coates, speaking in Philadelphia about 1835 on the defects of American medical education, noted that "clinical instruction [is] regarded as a thing of almost no importance!" Hospital rules were designed to exclude students "except for two short hours upon two mornings in the week!" Coates felt that only in Germany was the student properly taught. Who in America, he asked, excluding the trivial number of house pupils, "has enjoyed the privilege of genuine, thorough observation, upon a single case within their wards, before he sallies forth, with licence to commence his medical career and claim the confidence of the public?"[57]

Another professor, James Conquest Cross of Louisville, proposed that the term be 50 percent longer, that not just one, but all professors give clinical instruction, and that classes be divided into small groups so that every student would . . . be enabled, to hear and see all that he could wish. . . . At every visit the professor should spend two or three hours, and even longer if necessary. The student must be taught the "use of his eyes, his ears, and his hands." . . . Every pupil should be presented with a stethoscope . . . and the professor should patiently stand by the bedside while he is listening.[58]

A few undergraduate students received clinical experience as institutional residents, apprenticed to hospitals instead of to individual physicians and instructed by the attending physicians. However, hospitals soon showed a preference for more experienced help, and after 1814 at New York Hospital and 1824 at Pennsylvania Hospital, for example, such "house physicians" were always graduates.[59] Only a few institutions, such as the Baltimore Infirmary, opened in 1823, continued to have undergraduates as resident pupils. In this infirmary, five students were personally responsible for patients. The attending physician

is to be present at all important operations of surgery and if he does not operate himself, assigns the cases to the students, viz: obstetrical cases alternately, commencing with the senior student; at which only two students shall be present. In difficult cases, the attending physician is to direct in presence of all the students,[60] all other surgical operations alternately—the senior taking always the first of each class of such operation.

Patients were assigned in rotation to the students, who cared for them "until the case is decided."[61]

By the 1840s some schools were beginning to provide individual clinical experience. One of these, at least for a while, was the Medical College of Ohio in Cincinnati. During the session of 1841/42 the faculty included a professor of physical diagnosis and pathological anatomy, fresh from a year in the hospitals of Paris, who attended at the hospital each morning for one hour before lectures began and gave practical bedside instruction to groups of ten students.[62]

By the middle 1840s Harvard was offering students "an opportunity of visiting all the cases, and of observing and learning the symptoms and treatment of each case, and particularly of the exploration of the body, for the PHYSICAL SIGNS of disease, by *palpation, auscultation* and *percussion*." By 1857 it was possible for students to "investigate disease for

themselves, and study it minutely." After 1846 the older students at Harvard met "once a week for the reading of cases and for criticisms thereupon" as a Society for Medical Observation, modeled after the one founded 25 years earlier in Paris.[63]

About half of the students at Harvard also attended the private Tremont Street Medical School, which provided instruction from March until November when the medical college was not in session. From its start in 1838 until 1858, when Harvard formally recognized it as the second or summer semester of an extended curriculum, the school was in reality part of that institution. The official medical school announcement for 1855/56 even promoted it. Tremont was, in effect, a group preceptorial run by members of the Harvard faculty who took their private students into the wards of the Massachusetts General Hospital in the summer as they did all Harvard students in the winter. Particular attention was paid "to auscultation, percussion and all physical signs in connection with diseases of the chest and abdomen." Students also learned chemical and microscopic analysis of blood and urine.[64] At least three other private schools in the Boston area offered similar instruction. At the United States Marine Hospital in Chelsea, where Henry I. Bowditch taught, students were permitted "to examine and make records of all the cases."[65]

Such extramural training was common in many cities, though perhaps not as comprehensive as in Boston. Many professors had large groups of students to whom they gave private instruction, in addition to their public lectures in the medical school. In these smaller groups a more active experience was possible for the student.[66]

At the University of Michigan in the late 1850s a "full two hours each day (except Sundays) were spent by the students in examining, immediately under the direction of their instructors, the patients in the hospital." These students had learned the normal sounds by practicing on each other, and were expected to learn about the evolution of physical changes by reexamining patients periodically.[67]

Despite these early efforts, it was Erasmus Darwin Fenner, professor of medicine, dean, and leading light of the New Orleans School of Medicine,[68] who really introduced the clinical clerkship to America. In his introductory address at the opening of the new school in November 1856, Fenner cited Graves's statement that a student should observe patients daily throughout the course of their illnesses and should do so during the whole period of pupilage. This could be done only in a hospital, and the new school was directly opposite the Charity Hospital. *Every one* of the seven professors on the faculty was to give clinical instruction there daily until 10:30 A.M., when lectures began.[69]

The next year Fenner published a detailed description of the New Orleans plan.

> The course of qualification preparatory to entering upon the practice of medicine hitherto pursued by nine-tenths of the medical students in this country, has been, to read a textbook on each of the different branches, to hear two courses of lectures, occasionally walk through the wards of a hospital, where he may see a Professor prescribe for a number of patients or perform a surgical operation, then be able, when questioned, to repeat a respectable amount of what he has read in books or been told by his teachers, and he obtains his diploma. Under such a system of instruction, experience is only to be acquired at a considerable expense of human life. . . . I think I may safely say that previous to the present day, nothing like a systematic course or plan of clinical instruction has been adopted by any of the Medical Colleges in the United States.[70]

At New Orleans the student received a printed ticket containing spaces to record data identifying the patient by location, name, age, nativity, vocation, diagnosis, duration, and outcome. This he pasted in his notebook. In addition, he was given a list of questions to ask regarding the duration of the illness, symptoms, course, previous therapy, and present state including a review of systems. He was also to record the patient's appearance and any abnormal findings on physical examination: "Note the Chest symptoms — breathing, cough, pain[,] physical signs. Note the Heart, sounds of. Note the Pulse, number and character of." From these data the student was expected to write a "connected narrative," to be read to the professor on rounds. If the patient died, an autopsy was performed before the class after the professor predicted what the findings would be.[71]

Several factors were essential to the success of this innovation. The faculty, which soon grew from seven to ten men, *all* gave bedside instruction. The

term was lengthened from four to five months so there were fewer lectures per day and more time for clinical activities, and the school was adjacent both to a dispensary and to Charity Hospital, which cared for 15,634 patients in 1849. With well over 2,000 deaths a year and the most liberal autopsy laws in the United States, New Orleans had clear advantages for training physicians.

Where did Fenner get the idea? In his introductory address he said that the faculty had "adopted a course of clinical instruction very much like that pursued in Germany, where this branch is taught better than anywhere in the world."[72] The next year he stated that the plan was "much the same as that pursued in the General Hospital of Vienna, which was introduced into the Meath Hospital, of Dublin, by Dr. Graves, in 1821, and has been continued there ever since, with entire satisfaction."[73] Possibly it was through contact with his friend John Y. Bassett, who had studied in Dublin and who was a regular contributor to a journal edited by Fenner, that the idea came.[74]

Such clinical instruction proved popular, and the New Orleans School of Medicine prospered until closed by the Civil War. Its enrollment increased from 76 to 216 in the first four years, at the end of which it was the seventh largest school in America. The school reopened after the war, but it soon fell victim to bad times, made worse by Fenner's death in 1866.[75]

Though more than two decades passed before William Osler successfully established a clinical clerkship program at Johns Hopkins, individual clinical instruction became more common during the 1870s and 1880s. The Syracuse catalogue stated that "students will be required to examine cases and report them before the class." Rush Medical College offered individual clinical instruction in 1879, and students were "specially drilled in the methodical examination of patients [and] the taking of histories." At the Chicago Medical School, predecessor of Northwestern, a distinguishing feature was individual bedside instruction in small groups and student contact with patients.[76]

But none of these experiments was the same as the experience at New Orleans or Hopkins. Osler, like Fenner, had been influenced by the methods of the European medical schools. His first preceptor in medicine, James Bovell, had been a student of Graves and of William Stokes,[77] as were three of his teachers at McGill in the early 1870s. The bedside instruction at the Montreal General Hospital at that time, Osler later recalled, "was excellent and the clerking a serious business." Later, while studying physiology in London, he was impressed by "the admirable English system, with the ward work done by the student himself the essential feature." Afterward, when he went to Berlin, he saw the students examine, explain, and follow—"day by day"—the cases to which they were assigned.[78]

Osler became professor of medicine at the University of Pennsylvania in 1884, but it was not until he reached Hopkins that he found his classes small enough to establish a clerkship system at an American school. At Pennsylvania in 1890, a clinical class had around 130 students, at Hopkins about 25. It was for this clerkship that Osler wished especially to be remembered, saying, "I desire no other epitaph . . . than the statement that I taught medical students in the wards, as I regard this as by far the most useful and important work I have been called upon to do."[79]

The plan established at Hopkins in the middle 1890s—and adopted by most schools in the 20th century—included wardwork, "in which the students, acting as clinical clerks, will be assigned beds and take the histories of new cases as admitted, and be responsible (under the direction of the house physician and the first assistant) for the ward notes. . . . The student will make the visit with Professor Osler on three days of the week at 9:00 A.M., and in this way will be enabled to study in a routine manner the progress of the cases."[80] During the third year the 22 students "arranged their chairs informally in a semicircle around a rattan couch for the patient and a plain deal table with Osler sitting beside it." One of the students made the examination. Osler stressed order and thoroughness, emphasizing inspection, and then proceeding to palpation, percussion, and auscultation. Students recalled that "until we had gained all the information possible by one method, we were forbidden to pass on to the next." Like the great Louis, Osler also emphasized the careful recording of data.[81]

Though the clinical clerkship may not have been Osler's idea, it was he who established it firmly in the American scene. That he was able to do so was a consequence of his times. Medical school

endowments made it possible to pay professors, restrict class size, and establish clinical facilities under faculty control. Johns Hopkins was the first school to do all these things.

Other schools gradually followed suit.[82] The experience at Western Reserve, one of the first to do so, gives some idea of the trend. The school offered its first clinical clerkships in 1901. By 1907 the class was being assigned to wards in small groups. Between 1910 and 1923 the total amount of formal instruction rose from 1,052 to 1,788 hours with the didactic portion declining from 32 percent to 6 percent. Perhaps most striking was the threefold increase in the time for clinical clerkships, from 250 hours in 1913/14 to 800 hours in 1916/17.[83] At the 37th annual meeting of the Association of American Medical Colleges in 1926, it was reported that "ward clerkships . . . have been instituted in all medical schools."[84] Only two years later Northwestern claimed to be the first school to appoint a supervisor of clinical clerks.[85]

As the 19th century progressed, individual bedside experience—laboratory experience in the clinical sciences, so to speak—became a necessity. The need to take a careful systematic history of a patient's illness, to examine his body, and to draw diagnostic and prognostic conclusions by relating the data collected to the practice of medicine could not be avoided. No amount of talent or inspiration could replace time and practice in acquiring this ability.

The hospital provided an ideal clinical arena. But until the number of beds increased and the number of medical students decreased, it was impossible for each student to have an active experience. Without financial subsidies it was not practical to limit class size or to have sufficient faculty to supervise the student at the bedside and adequately to protect the rights and safety of the patient.

## GOODBYE, DR. OSLER

The clinical clerkship was almost universally established by the 1930s and became the fundamental way of teaching internal medicine.[86] At first, the lecture continued to be the principal mode of conveying information. On the wards the student was not welcomed but tolerated, partly for his service as a paramedical domestic who did "scut" work; he was hardly an integral part of the "team." In the 1930s at Columbia-Presbyterian Hospital in New York, for example, clerks were not allowed on the wards during rest hours from noon until 2:00 or after 8:00 in the evening. Gradually, after 1950, lectures and other nonward activities became fewer, the clerk's responsibility for his assigned patients became greater, and his place in patient care became more secure.

Changes have occurred in the past 50 years, some intentional, but many of the most important ones not. Most medical schools introduced curricular variations, such as changes in the timing and duration of the clinical clerkships, including contact with patients in the first two years, but these modifications had limited effect, their extent often restricted by the "territorial imperatives" of other medical school disciplines.[87] Preclinical departments usually resisted encroachments on any time that had become established as part of a sacred progression, raising in their defense the specter of the scientifically illiterate student of the 19th century who, in fact, had become almost extinct among medical school matriculants.

Attempts to design interdisciplinary courses, whether on a cellular, regional, or social level, were often unsuccessful, partly because of the departmental political structure of medical schools. Also, while it became increasingly common for clinicians to be conversant with basic science, the lack of comparable clinical sophistication among the full-time basic science teachers put them at a disadvantage.

The growing demands of inpatient service all but smothered efforts to provide or maintain effective experience with ambulatory patients, whether of a comprehensive or a limited type. While there was greater emphasis on the psychosocial aspects of illness in many schools, the ambulatory patient who sought care in clinics used for teaching students frequently had disabling social problems which could be neither disentangled from the medical sickness nor resolved in a brief visit by pharmacologic means. The clinic patient was unreliable in keeping his appointments, and was often less observant and less able to convey to the physician what might have been apparent if seen in the home setting. The hospitalized patient offered easy continuity and a more efficient use of professional time and became the focus of teaching medicine.

Probably the most significant intentional change in the undergraduate clinical curriculum was the introduction of electives. This innovation was an attempt to alleviate curricular rigidity. The Commission on Medical Education, which functioned in the late 1920s, urged such flexibility, at the same time warning against "the dangers of superficial, undisciplined training, lack of unity in courses, dissipation of energy, and too early endeavors towards specialization," which would occur if the student was unaccustomed to independence or lacked adequate guidance.[88] As late as 1950, however, a survey of medical education found only four schools that had introduced substantial amounts of elective time into the clinical years.[89] At Harvard, for example, there was no elective time in the third year and only one to three months in the fourth year.

This situation changed drastically in the 1960s and 1970s, partly in response to student demands and partly in recognition of the fact that students were entering medical school well — but variously — prepared. However, the effect of electives on clinical training was different from their effect on instruction in the laboratory sciences. It was one thing to offer the student choices and exemptions in theoretical laboratory courses in which he might already have had considerable experience, but quite another to do so in the practical clinical years for which he had no previous training. Furthermore, as subspecialization in medicine developed, an increasing proportion of clinical electives were of a specialized type which often failed to provide the undergraduate adequate supervision by house officers or comprehensive involvement with patients. The Commission's fear was realized.

The most fundamental changes in undergraduate clinical instruction were unintentional and occurred quite independently of curricular manipulation. They involved the relationships between student, patient, and teacher and resulted mainly from the increasing complexity of diagnostic and therapeutic technology, and the expansion of hospital facilities and financial support for medical education, to say nothing of broad changes in society generally. Universities and medical schools established control over major teaching hospitals. These institutions became sophisticated laboratories rather than infirmaries with nurses, as the hospitals of the 19th and early 20th centuries had been. Technicians instead of physicians and students increasingly filled diagnostic and therapeutic functions. Full-time teacher-investigators replaced practitioners as clinical teachers. As an increasing proportion of the population had hospital insurance, it became necessary to use private patients for teaching. The patient was sicker but usually stayed a shorter time. Frequently, his problems were so complicated that the junior student was unable to have significant involvement in his care. Consequently the student often had a briefer and more superficial relationship with the patient, had less personal responsibility for him, and had less opportunity to perfect his own abilities.

As the 20th century progressed and technology became more complicated, specialized postdoctoral training became more important. Consequently, the student shared the patient and the experienced teacher with a growing number of house officers, trainees, fellows, and junior faculty specialists, to say nothing of paramedical students such as nurse practitioners. On the medical service of the University of Rochester's Strong Memorial Hospital, for example, the patient-intern ratio fell from 18:1 to 12:1 and the patient-assistant resident ratio from 25:1 to 12:1 between 1955 and 1975. The number of senior residents, trainees, and fellows more than doubled in a dozen years, and the number of medical students in a class rose from 72 to 97. Yet the number of hospital beds remained the same, partly as a result of community planning efforts to control rising hospital costs.

Diagnostic and therapeutic tests that were performed away from the patient's room and by people other than the student occupied an increasing portion of the patient's hospital stay and further limited the student's involvement with the patient. In five years since 1970 the total number of radiographic, nuclear, and electrodiagnostic examinations (excluding electrocardiograms) at Strong Memorial Hospital increased 33 percent. Academic expectations, fear of litigation, high fixed costs of maintaining complex technical appliances, and the incentive of a procedure-oriented insurance system encouraged maximum use of tests and drowned out pleas for restraint. Such tests added about 30 percent to the patient's hospital bill, and were a substantial source of income to hospitals.[90]

The most important change in undergraduate teaching of clinical medicine was the gradual replacement of the practitioner by the specialized full-time investigator as the student's professional model. When William Osler left Johns Hopkins Medical School in 1905 he predicted that the full-time system would soon include the clinical faculty as it did already the preclinical teacher. He was strong in his opposition to this. "The primary work of a professor of medicine in a medical school is in the wards . . . to turn out men who know how to handle the sick," wrote Osler.[91] The new system, he thought, would produce "a set of clinical prigs."[92] Though his judgment seems harsh, there is no doubt that the present teachers of medicine are quite different from those of the past, partly because of new and more complicated therapeutic techniques such as cardiac surgery, renal dialysis, assisted ventilation, musculoskeletal reconstruction, and cancer chemotherapy, all of which require subspecialization.

Though the full-time teacher had an established position prior to World War II, the teaching role of the practitioner did not diminish drastically until after the war. The full-time teacher of preclinical subjects became increasingly common toward the end of the 19th century, especially after Johns Hopkins put its entire preclinical faculty on salary in 1893. But the full-time clinical teacher did not begin to appear until the time of World War I at that same institution. Serious doubts that the nonpractitioner could teach the practice of medicine and the economic realities of the Depression initially checked the early proliferation of the full-time faculty member. After World War II full-time clinical faculties expanded rapidly under the stimulus of federal support to research. Between 1955 and 1975 the full-time senior faculty in the Department of Medicine at the University of Rochester increased from 14 to 67 physicians. During the same period the percentage of practitioners on the part-time faculty who served annually as attending physicians on the wards of that school's medical service declined from 50 to less than 15. The practitioner of medicine gradually played a smaller role as teacher, and medical education itself became a medical specialty.

The centripetal force of modern technology made inevitable the loss of the practitioner as a model for the student and has tended to drive the teacher from the bedside to the chalkboard.[93] At the end of the 19th century the physician himself was able to perform virtually all of the diagnostic techniques at the bedside. By the middle of the 20th century this was no longer true and was rapidly becoming less so.

Other factors further diminished the influence of the practitioner as a teacher. After the 1960s students and house officers were less dependent on the hospital. Often married, they spent less time within the walls, ate fewer meals in the cafeteria, and were less interested in older physicians for social contact with the outside world. Another major educational experience was lost as a result of this. By 1975 undergraduate and house officer contact was largely restricted to the full-time clinical specialist while he made his daily ward round with an entourage of junior colleagues who themselves tended to isolate the senior man from direct student contact.

Though clinical medicine has changed considerably in recent decades, the clinical clerkship remains the most satisfactory method of instruction. In the words of one observer, "It is never behind the times."[94] It requires much smaller classes than instruction by lecture, it requires a substantial number of patients who are sick but not too sick, it requires teachers who are comfortable at the bedside and who have the time and knack for teaching. Each of these prerequisites is to some degree in jeopardy today. The demand for more physicians has led to larger classes, the patients in teaching hospitals are often sicker and dependent on complicated technological devices for survival, the clinical teacher is required to practice medicine increasingly as a means of support so that he is, in effect, again being called upon to subsidize clinical medical education as he was throughout the 19th century. Nevertheless, the clerkship seems secure in the foreseeable future.

## NOTES

Mr. Philip Weimerskirch, history of medicine librarian at the Edward G. Miner Library of the University of Rochester School of Medicine and Dentistry, found many useful source materials; and Miss Sandra Markus, interlibrary loan librarian, was able to obtain for me many materials not available locally. Useful suggestions came from Drs. Lawrence A. Kohn, Donald G. Anderson, and William L. Morgan, Jr.

1 Jenks S. Sprague, "Annual address," *Trans. Med. Soc. St. N.Y.,* 1854: 17.

2 Dr. Edward A. Holyoke, well-known teacher and physician of Salem, Massachusetts, was an exception. He used direct auscultation in 1793 on a 53-year-old man to diagnose empyema with bronchopleural fistula. An autopsy proved him correct ("Auscultation in Boston in 1793," *Boston Med. & Surg. J.,* 1858, *58:* 83–84).

3 John Ware, who later succeeded James Jackson as Hersey Professor of Theory and Practice of Physic at Harvard, drew attention to this fact in one of his clinical lectures as early as 1835. In clinical attendance, he said, the student must not be passive. Learning physical signs is a slow process except in a hospital with instruction (Ware Papers, Box 2, Francis A. Countway Library, Harvard Medical School, Boston).

4 Hippocratic authority and the fact that Auenbrugger had no students to spread the word delayed acceptance of the "New Invention" (Bernhard J. Stern,

*Social Factors in Medical Progress* [New York: Columbia Univ. Press, 1927], p. 52). On the other hand, Laennec and those who followed him were active teachers.

5 *Am. Med. Rec.,* 1820, *3:* 534–546.

6 *N. Eng. J. Med. & Surg.,* 1821, *10:* 132–156, 265–293, quotation on p. 293.

7 Henry R. Viets, "'De l'auscultation médiate' of Laennec," *Arch. Surg.,* 1929, *18:* 1280–1297.

8 *N.Y. Med. & Phys. J.,* 1824, *3:* 268–281. Only four Americans are known to have studied with Laennec. Another one of them, Samuel George Morton (M.D., Univ. of Pennsylvania, 1820) wrote what William Osler later called "the earliest and one of the best books on phthisis written in America."

9 Edmund Strudwick, "Remarks on the stethoscope in relation to phthisis pulmonis," *Philadelphia J. Med. & Phys. Sci.,* 1824, *8:* 33–52. The Almshouse was predecessor of the famous Philadelphia General Hospital at Blockley, Pennsylvania.

10 Martinet, 1827; Collin, 1829; Williams, 1830; Meriadec Laennec, 1832; Rouanet, 1833; Louis, 1834; Raciborski, 1839; Hope, 1842; Walshe, 1843.

11 Austin Flint, recalling his medical student days at Harvard in 1832, said that James Jackson "was earnestly engaged in the subject of physical exploration. He never failed to carry the stethoscope during his hospital visits, and the signs of cardiac and pulmonary diseases entered largely into his clinical instructions" (Austin Flint, "The life and labors

of Laennec: an introductory address delivered at the New Orleans School of Medicine, Nov. 14, 1859," *New Orleans Med. & Hosp. Gaz.*, 1859, 6: 736–756; see also W. W. Gerhard, *On the Diagnosis of Diseases of the Chest* [Philadelphia: Key and Biddle, 1836], p. xi). Claims of priority for introducing stethoscopy were made by others. A Philadelphia physician wrote that "the stethoscope was introduced into Philadelphia within somewhere about the year of its first publication and that it has been used ever since that time without interruption." A New Englander responded that he had obtained a stethoscope and an 1819 edition of Laennec from France as soon as it had been possible, adding, "I have ever since been as constant to my stethoscope as a Dutchman to his pipe or an Englishman to his umbrella" (see the introduction to Victor Collin, *Manual for the Use of the Stethoscope: A Short Treatise on the Different Methods of Investigating the Diseases of the Chest*, trans. W. N. Ryland [Boston: B. Perkins, 1829]).

12  William Osler, "Memoir of Alfred Stillé," *Tr. Coll. Physicians Phila.*, 3rd series, 1902, 24: lviii–lxxi, quotation on p. lxi.

13  Letter to H. I. Bowditch, then studying in Paris, quoted in George R. Minot, "James Jackson as a Professor of Medicine," *New Eng. J. Med.*, 1933, 208: 254–258, quotation on pp. 256–257. James Jackson Putnam, *A Memoir of Dr. James Jackson* (Boston and New York: Houghton, Mifflin, 1905), p. 331.

14  Jacob Bigelow, "Brief rules for exploration of the chest, in diseases of the lungs and heart," *Boston Med. & Surg. J.*, 1839, 20: 357–369, 373–378, 389–394, quotation on p. 357.

15  The literature on this subject is extensive: William Osler, "Influence of Louis on American medicine," *Johns Hopkins Hosp. Bull.*, 1897, 8: 161–167; Walter R. Steiner, "Some distinguished American medical students of Pierre-Charles-Alexandre Louis of Paris," *Bull. Hist. Med.*, 1939, 7: 783–793; Guy Hinsdale, "The American medical argonauts: pupils of Pierre Charles Alexandre Louis," *Tr. Coll. Physicians Phila.*, 1945–1946, 13: 37–43; Russell M. Jones, "American doctors in Paris, 1820–1861: a statistical profile," *J. Hist. Med.*, 1970, 25: 143–57; Russell M. Jones, "American doctors and the Parisian medical world, 1830–1840," *Bull. Hist. Med.*, 1973, 47: 40–65.

16  W. W. Gerhard, *On the Diagnosis of Diseases of the Chest*; Henry I. Bowditch, *The Young Stethoscopist; or, the Student's Aid to Auscultation* (New York: J. and H. G. Langley, 1846); Oliver W. Holmes, "On the utility and importance of direct exploration in medical practice," in *Boylston Prize Dissertations for the Years 1836 and 1837* (Boston: Little and Brown,

1838), pp. 245–371; Caspar Pennock and Edward Mott Moore, *Report of Experiments on the Action of the Heart, Read Before the Pathological Society of Philadelphia, Oct. 28 to Nov. 4, 1839* (Philadelphia: Merrihew and Thompson, 1839). A typical experiment consisted of rendering a ram unconscious with blows on the head, inserting a bellows through a tracheotomy, opening the chest and placing a stethoscope directly on the heart in an attempt to relate the heart sounds with the observed muscular contractions.

17  [Henry I. Bowditch], "Louis and his contemporaries," *Boston Med. & Surg. J.*, 1873, 87: 292–295, quotation on p. 293. P. C. A. Louis, *An Essay on Clinical Instruction*, trans. Peter Martin (London: S. Highley, 1834), p. 2.

18  See S. Weir Mitchell, "An early history of instrumental precision in medicine," *Tr. Cong. Am. Phys. & Surg.* 1891, 2: 159–198; Kenneth D. Keele, *The Evolution of Clinical Methods in Medicine* (Springfield, Ill.: Charles C. Thomas, 1963).

19  "Employment of the stethoscope in practice," *Med. Recorder*, 1824, 7: 432–433.

20  Thomas H. Tanner, *A Manual of Clinical Medicine and Physical Diagnosis* (Philadelphia: Blanchard and Lea, 1855). This book was among those recommended to students in the Harvard catalogue for 1867/68, and in the University of Vermont catalogue for 1866/67.

21  Austin Flint, *A Practical Treatise on the Diagnosis, Pathology and Treatment of Diseases of the Heart* (Philadelphia: Blanchard and Lea, 1859); idem, "On cardiac murmurs," *Am. J. Med. Sci.*, n.s., 1862, 44: 29–54; idem, *A Manual of Physical Diagnosis*, 9th ed. (Philadelphia and New York: Lea and Febiger, 1925).

22  James Jackson, *Memoir of James Jackson, Jr., M.D., Written by his Father, with Extracts from His Letters . . .* (Boston: Hilliard, Gray, 1836), p. 109.

23  Quoted in Lawrason Brown, *The Story of Clinical Pulmonary Tuberculosis* (Baltimore: Williams and Wilkins, 1941), p. 177.

24  Jesse S. Myer, *Life and Letters of Dr. William Beaumont* (St. Louis, Mo.: C. V. Mosby, 1912), p. 27.

25  Samuel Bard, *A Discourse on Medical Education* (New York: C. S. Van Winkle, 1819); Daniel Drake, *An Inaugural Discourse on Medical Education* (Cincinnati: Looker, Palmer and Reynolds, 1820); Connecticut Senate Committee Report in Pliny A. Jewett, *Semi-Centennial History of the Gen'l Hospital Society of Connecticut* (New Haven: Tuttle, Morehouse and Taylor, 1876), p. 29; James Jackson and John C. Warren, *Circular Letter to Benevolent Citizens of Boston, August 20, 1810*, report in N. I. Bowditch, *A History of the Massachusetts General Hospital*, 2nd ed. (Boston, 1872), pp. 3–9 n.

26  D. G. Thomas, "History of the founding and development of the first hospitals of the United States," *Am. J. Insanity*, 1867, *24*: 130–154.

27  R. Sullivan, *Address Delivered Before the Governor and Council, Members of the Legislature and Other Patrons of the Massachusetts General Hospital at King's Chapel, Boston, June 3, 1819* (Boston: Wells and Lilly, 1819); T. F. Harrington, *The Harvard Medical School*, 3 vols. (New York and Chicago: Lewis, 1905), II, 582–583; Bowditch, *A History of the Massachusetts General Hospital*, p. 197.

28  Quoted in William S. Middleton, "Clinical teaching in Philadelphia Almshouse and Hospital," *Med. Life*, 1933, *40*: 191–200, 207–225, quotation on p. 215.

29  W. S. Middleton, "Clinical teaching," pp. 215–216; D. G. Thomas, "History of the founding and development," p. 113.

30  Alfred Stillé, quoted in W. S. Middleton, "Clinical teaching," p. 215.

31  John Chalmers DaCosta, "The old Blockley Hospital: its characters and characteristics," in *Selections from the Papers and Speeches of John Chalmers DaCosta, M.D., LL.D.* (Philadelphia: W. B. Saunders, 1931), p. 159.

32  Joseph M. Toner, "Statistics of regular medical associations and hospitals of the United States," *Tr. A.M.A.*, 1873, *24*: 285–333.

33  For comparison, today there are 24,000 inpatients a year at the University of Rochester's Strong Memorial Hospital and 200 medical students in the clinical classes, a 120 to 1 ratio. In addition, four other affiliated hospitals are used for teaching purposes.

34  "Report of the Committee on Medical Education," *Tr. A.M.A.*, 1849, *2*: 257–352. The nine schools were Harvard, University of Pennsylvania, Jefferson, Pennsylvania College, University of Maryland, University of Louisville, Rush, St. Louis University, and the University of Louisiana—all schools in large cities where there were hospitals.

35  George W. Corner, *Two Centuries of Medicine* (Philadelphia: Lippincott, 1965), pp. 88–89; *Auburn (New York) Free Press*, Jan. 21, 1829; *Deed of Trust from Lyne Starling to Robert W. McCoy and Others . . .* (Columbus, Ohio: William B. Thrall, 1847). This school was an ancestral component of Ohio State Medical School.

36  Abraham Jacobi, "The New York Medical College, 1782–1906," *Ann. Med. Hist.*, Dec. 1917, *1*: 368–373, quotation on p. 371. Richard M. Doolen, "The founding of the University of Michigan Hospital: an innovation in medical education," *J. Med. Educ.*, 1964, *39*: 50–57.

37  *A History of the Boston Dispensary*, comp. by one of

38  Thomas D. Mitchell, *The Annual Oration of the Ohio Medical Lyceum* (Cincinnati: Truman, Smith, 1834), p. 15.

39  It was claimed by William H. Rideing, "Medical education in New York," *Harpers Magazine*, 1882, *65*: 668–679 (quotation on p. 669), that Valentine Mott founded the first "clinique" in America at the medical department of the University of New York in the 1840s.

40  John Watson, *A Lecture on Practical Education in Medicine* (New York: J. and H. G. Langley, 1846).

41  Nathan S. Davis, *History of Medical Education and Institutions in the United States* (Chicago: S. C. Griggs, 1851), pp. 166, 221, 217.

42  See Francis R. Packard, *History of Medicine in the United States*, 2 vols. (New York: Paul B. Hoeber, 1931); *Ann. Med. Hist.*, n.s., 1932, *4*: 219–244. A more extensive bibliography appears in *Bull. Hist. Med.*, 1973, *47*: 40.

43  Robert J. Graves, "On clinical instruction; with a comparative estimate of the mode in which it is conducted in the British and Continental schools," *London Med. Gaz.*, 1832, *10*: 401–406, quotation on p. 403. This talk had been given by Graves in 1821 as an introductory lecture. Latin was abandoned at Dublin in the early 1830s.

44  Samuel Rezneck, "A course of medical education in New York City in 1828–29: the journal of Asa Fitch," *Bull. Hist. Med.*, 1968, *42*: 555–565, quotation on p. 559. See also William D. Hoyt, Jr., "A young physician prepares to practice medicine, 1796–80," *Bull. Hist. Med.*, 1942, *11*: 582.

45  Edward Delafield, *Introductory Address to the Students in Medicine of the College of Physicians and Surgeons of the University of the State of New York* (New York: Scatcherd and Adams, 1837), p. 33.

46  Quoted in J. A. DaCosta, "The old Blockley Hospital," pp. 159–160.

47  Robley Dunglison, *The Medical Student* (Philadelphia: Carey, Lea and Blanchard, 1837), p. 165.

48  Henry S. Patterson, *Lecture Introductory to the Course of Materia Medica and Pharmacy* (Philadelphia: W. S. Young, 1844).

49  David Riesman, "Clinical teaching in America, with some remarks on early medical schools," *Tr. Coll. Physicians Phila.*, 4th series, 1939–1940, *7*: 89–110, quotation on p. 100.

50  Lewis A. Conner, quoted in James A. Harrar, *The Story of the Lying-in Hospital of the City of New York* ([New York]: Society of the Lying-in Hospital, 1938), p. 75. Statements to this effect may be found in J. Marion Sims, *The Story of My Life* (New York: D. Appleton, 1884) p. 139, and Henry M. Thomas,

the board of managers (Boston: J. Wilson and Son, 1859), pp. 98, 106.

"Some memories of the development of the medical school and of Osler's advent," *Johns Hopkins Hosp. Bull.*, 1919, *30*: 185–189, quotation on p. 187.

51 Nathan S. Davis, *History of Medical Education and Institutions*, pp. 218–219, 225.

52 Theodor Puschmann, *A History of Medical Education* (1891; reprint ed., New York: Hafner, 1966), pp. 410–412; Theodor Billroth, *The Medical Sciences in the German Universities* (New York: Macmillan, 1924), p. 32. A more detailed examination of the Dutch origins of bedside instruction appears in Evert C. Van Leersum, "Contribution to the history of the clinical instruction in the Netherlands," *Janus*, 1926-1927, *30-31*: 133–151.

53 T. F. Andrews, "An account of the medical institutions of Berlin," *Am. Med. Rec.*, 1823, *6*: 471–486, quotation on p. 475.

54 *Ibid.*, p. 479; Joseph Leo-Wolf, "Medical education in Germany," *Am. Med. Rec.*, 1828, *13*: 481–490.

55 R. J. Graves, "On clinical instruction," pp. 401–403. One of America's early clinical professors, Dr. Thomas Bond of the Pennsylvania Hospital, made similar observations years before this. "Language & Books alone," he said at the start of his lectures in the hospital, "can never give him [the student] Adequate Ideas of Diseases. . . . For which reasons Infirmaries are Justly reputed the Grand Theatres of Medical Knowledge. There, the Clinical professor comes in to the Aid of Speculation & demonstrates the Truth of Theory by Facts" (quoted in Thomas G. Morton, *The History of the Pennsylvania Hospital*, rev. ed. [Philadelphia: Times Printing House, 1897], p. 463).

56 T. F. Andrews, "An account of the medical institutions"; Reynell Coates, *Oration on the Defects in the Present System of Medical Education in the United States* (Philadelphia: James Kay, jun. and Brother, [1835?]).

57 Coates, *Oration on the Defects*, p. 24.

58 James Conquest Cross, *Thoughts on the Policy of Establishing a School of Medicine in Louisville* (Lexington: N. L. Finnell, 1834), pp. 90, 91.

59 At the Massachusetts General Hospital "house pupils," as they were known, were graduates of the Harvard Medical School from the time the hospital opened in 1821. See *128th Annual Report of the Society of the New York Hospital* (New York and Albany: Wynkoop Hallenbeck Crawford, 1899); George Bacon Wood, *An Address on the Occasion of the Centennial Celebration of the Founding of the Pennsylvania Hospital* (Philadelphia: T. K. and P. G. Collins, 1851); Grace W. Myers, *History of the Massachusetts General Hospital* (Boston, [1929?]).

60 Such training in midwifery was rare, at least in the North. When introduced by Dr. James P. White at Buffalo Medical College in 1851, it led to public

consternation and a lawsuit. See Oliver P. Jones, "A bench mark for the obstetric history of the United States," *Obst. & Gynec.*, 1974, *43*: 784–791.

61 *Report of a Committee Appointed by the Guardians for the Relief and Employment of the Poor of Philadelphia, etc., To Visit the Almshouses of Baltimore, New York, Boston, and Salem, Nov. 1833* (Philadelphia: W. F. Geddes, 1834), p. 11.

62 *Annual Catalogue of the Officers and Students of the Medical College of Ohio: Session 1841-42* (Cincinnati: L'Hommedieu, 1842), with an additional circular appended, p. 5.

63 Harvard University, *Catalogue of Students Attending Medical Lectures in Boston, 1844-45, with a Circular of the Faculty* (Boston: D. Clapp, Jr., 1845), p. 12; Harvard University, Medical Department, *Announcement of the Medical Course, Commencing on the First Wednesday in November, 1857* (Boston: David Clapp, 1857), p. 8; Harvard University, Medical Department, *Announcement of the Medical Course, Commencing on the First Wednesday in November, 1861* (Boston: David Clapp, 1861), p. 6.

64 *Catalogue of the Past and Present Students of the Tremont Street Medical School* (Boston: David Clapp, 1855), p. 9.

65 Advertisement in the *Boston Med. & Surg. J.*, 1840, *22*: 308.

66 See, for example, Douglas Guthrie, *Extramural Medical Education in Edinburgh* (Edinburgh and London: E. and S. Livingstone, 1965); William Williams Keen, "The history of the Philadelphia School of Anatomy and its relation to medical teaching," in *Addresses and Other Papers* (Philadelphia and London: W. B. Saunders, 1905); James A. Harrar, *The Story of the Lying-in Hospital*, p. 30.

67 Letter from Alonzo B. Palmer to Zina Pitcher, Dec. 7, 1857, *Peninsular J. Med. & Collateral Sci.*, 1858, *5*: 400–402; "Report of a clinical lecture by Dr. Palmer to the clinical class at St. Mary's Hospital — tuberculosis," *ibid.*, 1857, *5*: 225–232.

68 Not to be confused with the older University of Louisiana Medical Department, later Tulane, this school boasted a remarkable faculty which included Austin Flint.

69 E. D. Fenner, "Introductory lecture," *New Orleans Med. News & Hosp. Gaz.*, 1856, *3*: 577–600, quotation on pp. 598–599.

70 E. D. Fenner, "Remarks on clinical medicine," *New Orleans Med. News & Hosp. Gaz.*, 1857, *4*: 458–472, quotations on pp. 458, 467.

71 *Ibid.*, pp. 468–469.

72 E. D. Fenner, "Introductory lecture," p. 599.

73 E. D. Fenner, "Remarks on clinical medicine," p. 470. The announcement of the school the year before stated that "the plan [of clinical instruction to

be] adopted will be that which has been found so eminently successful in the hospitals of Paris. This is founded on the great truth: that observation in medicine, to be profitable, must be complete . . ." (see Harold Cummins, "Formal medical education in New Orleans, 1834–," *Bull. Med. Lib. Assn.,* 1941–1942, *30*: 300–308, quotation on p. 307). Members of the Paris School, especially Louis, used the same techniques as in Berlin and Dublin, but only graduate students were exposed to them.

74  David Riesman, "The Dublin Medical School and its influence upon medicine in America," *Ann. Med. Hist.,* 1922, *4*: 86–96. Riesman found records of only four Americans who studied with Graves and Stokes in Dublin. The first was John Y. Bassett. Fenner published *Southern Medical Reports* (1849–1851), which included several papers by Bassett, and it was these papers which later stimulated Osler to write his famous biographical essay, "An Alabama Student." See William D. Postell, "Erasmus Darwin Fenner and the beginnings of medical literature in Louisiana," *Ann. Med. Hist.,* 3rd series, 1941, *3*: 297–305. See also David C. Elkin, ed., *The Medical Reports of John Y. Bassett, M.D., the Alabama Student* (Springfield: C. C. Thomas, 1941), p. 69.

75  A. E. Fossier, "History of medical education in New Orleans from its birth to the Civil War," Part II, n.s., *Ann. Med. Hist.,* 1934, *6*: 427–447.

76  *Fourth Annual Announcement of the College of Medicine of Syracuse University 1875–76* (Syracuse: William L. Rose, 1875), p. 8; *Thirty-Seventh Annual Announcement of Rush Medical College, Chicago, for the Session of 1879–80* (Chicago: Bulletin Printing Co., 1879), p. 11; *Twenty-Fourth Annual Announcement of the Chicago Medical College, Session of 1882–83* (Chicago, 1882), p. 5. The medical department of the University of California provided a similar, if less detailed, experience in the early 1870s. "A patient is placed in charge of a senior student, and by him examined, a diagnosis and prognosis given, together with his views of treatment, in the presence of the class. . . . Every student, thus detailed, is expected to keep a complete history of the case" (*Biennial Report of the Regents of the University of California for the Years 1873–75,* p. 94). I am indebted to Dr. Gert Brieger for bringing this evidence to my attention.

77  See *Dictionary of Canadian Biography,* Vol. X, ed. Marc LaTerreur (n.p.: Univ. of Toronto Press, 1972), pp. 83–84.

78  William Osler, "An address on the medical clinic: a retrospect and forecast, delivered before the Abernethian Society, St. Bartholomew's Hospital, London, Dec. 4th, 1913," *Brit. Med. J.,* 1914, *1*: 10–16, quotations on p. 10.

79  William Osler, *Aequanimitas,* 3rd ed. (Philadelphia: Blackiston, 1943), p. 390.

80  Alan M. Chesney, *The Johns Hopkins Hospital and Johns Hopkins University School of Medicine: A Chronicle,* 3 vols. (Baltimore: Johns Hopkins Press, 1943–63), II, 130.

81  *Ibid.,* pp. 127–129. Recollections of Walter R. Steiner, Joseph H. Pratt, and Percy M. Dawson. See also Lewellys F. Barker, "The teaching of clinical medicine," *Proc. A.A.M.C.,* 26th Annual Meeting, Chicago, Feb. 8, 1916, pp. 43–57.

82  Harvard instituted clerkships in 1913. See James Howard Means, "The teaching of medicine in the Massachusetts General Hospital," *Harvard Med. Alumni Bull.,* Oct. 1934: 1–5.

83  Frederick C. Waite, *Western Reserve University Centennial History of the School of Medicine* (Cleveland: Western Reserve Univ. Press, 1946), pp. 393–394.

84  John W. Moore, "Clinical clerkships in medicine: student unit system," *Bull. A.A.M.C.,* 1927, *2*: 136–139, quotation on p. 136.

85  Fred C. Zapffe, "The clinical clerk system at Northwestern University Medical School," *Bull. A.A.M.C.,* 1928, *3*: 41–46.

86  Council on Medical Education and Hospitals, *Medical Education in the United States, 1934–1939* (Chicago: American Medical Association, 1940), pp. 173–174.

87  A good summary of curricular changes may be found in Vernon W. Lippard, *A Half-Century of American Medical Education: 1920–1970* (New York: Josiah Macy, Jr., Foundation, 1974), pp. 8–27.

88  *Final Report of the Commission on Medical Education* (New York: Office of the Director of the Study, 1932), p. 230.

89  John E. Deitrick and Robert C. Berson, *Medical Schools in the United States at Mid-Century* (New York: McGraw-Hill, 1953), pp. 235–236, 242–243.

90  Paul F. Griner and Benjamin Lipzin, "Use of the laboratory in a teaching hospital: implications for patient care, education and hospital costs," *Ann. Intern. Med.,* 1971, *75*: 157–163. By 1976 several states were refusing to accept automatic rises of per diem patient costs, thus limiting the profit from increased laboratory utilization.

91  William Osler, "The coming of age of internal medicine in America," *Int. Clinics,* 25th series, 1915, *4*: 4.

92  William Osler to Ira Remsen, quoted in Alan M. Chesney, *The Johns Hopkins Hospital,* III, 180.

93  Anne R. Somers, "Conflict, accommodation, and progress: some socioeconomic observations of medical education and the practicing profession," *J. Med. Educ.,* 1963, *38*: 466–478.

94  Lippard, *A Half-Century of American Medical Education,* p. 11.

# 10

## Abraham Flexner in Perspective: American Medical Education, 1865–1910

### ROBERT P. HUDSON

The Flexner report of 1910[1] justifiably stands as a monument in the reform of American medical education. Yet there is much in the report itself to suggest that Flexner's contribution was not so much revolutionary as catalytic to an already evolving process. The present study reassesses Flexner's impact, but only peripherally. The principal aim rather is to sketch in some of the pertinent social and educational trends during the half century between the end of the Civil War and Flexner's genteel thunderbolt.[2]

The Civil War abated only temporarily the spread of proprietary medical schools. This spread, it should be remembered, was malignant less because it produced too many physicians and more because the ensuing competition for students diluted the already limited resources and eroded academic standards.[3] Plumpers for reform who had sounded their monotonous litanies in the quarter century after the founding of the American Medical Association were by 1870 generally pessimistic. They not only appeared to agree with John Shaw Billings that "it does not pay to give a $5000 education to a $5 boy,"[4] but by now they had despaired of doing anything about either education or the boy.

Still defeatism was not universal. A few observers thought they saw glimmers of improvement both in the quality of incoming students and in the educational process itself.[5] These disparate views can be made at least comprehensible. Part of the improvement was purely on paper. Medical school catalogues became increasingly imaginative as

ROBERT P. HUDSON is Professor and Chairman, Department of the History and Philosophy of Medicine, University of Kansas Medical Center, Kansas City, Kansas.

Reprinted with permission from the *Bulletin of the History of Medicine*, 1972, *56*: 545–561.

competition for students grew ever more heated. The catalogues of around 1880 contained few stipulations which could be described as non-negotiable. Most medical colleges specified, for example, that applicants must have a high school diploma or its "equivalent." Flexner, with characteristic candor, disposed of the equivalent as "a device that concedes the necessity of a standard which it forthwith proceeds to evade."[6]

There can be no serious disagreement with Shryock's conclusion that American medical training remained "relatively inferior" during the two decades following the Civil War.[7] But it was a complex period, one in which entrenched mediocrity and rising reform coexisted. While new schools continued to pop up with the discouraging persistence of dandelions, worthier seeds were sprouting. These early improvements, though they frequently interlocked, can be considered under three headings: admission requirements, medical school curricula, and postgraduate training.

The 35 years before the turn of the century saw something of a revolution in higher education in America. The public, which previously saw little utility in education, began to change its mind. This new attitude was reflected in the state's perception that it had an obligation to make educational opportunities more accessible to the masses. The 1862 Morrill Act not only initiated the land grant university movement, but indirectly gave rise to a new institution, the public high school. These multiplied so rapidly that by 1892 their enrollment surpassed that of the academies.[8] Thus premedical education of improved quality became generally available during the period under consideration.[9] Even though compulsory education reportedly existed in only seven states by 1896,[10] the fact remains

148

that the opportunity at least for better premedical preparation expanded rapidly in the post-bellum decades.

The question remains — did more students bound for medical studies during this time take advantage of their new opportunities? [11] A precise answer in numerical terms is not possible. There is evidence that students increasingly pursued premedical training of steadily improving quality, and that medical colleges upgraded their entrance requirements both on paper and in fact. But the case should not be overstated. The situation was characterized by a spectrum rather than by uniformity, and most students still received inferior premedical training. The Johns Hopkins required an academic degree from the outset (1893) but by 1906 the Council on Medical Education of the American Medical Association was still recommending only a minimal one year of college for medical school admission. [12]

Still trends slowly pushed toward higher standards. John Rauch, a champion of reform in Illinois, reported that the number of medical colleges exacting certain specified educational requirements for matriculation was 45 in 1882, 114 in 1886, 117 in 1889 and 124 in 1890. [13] Of the 155 schools Flexner surveyed, 16 required two years of college and 6, which demanded only one year, were scheduled to go to a two-year requirement in 1910. [14] Among these 16 schools, 1,850 students had satisfied the two-year requirement as of 1908–1909. [15] By way of balance it should be recalled that in 1910 some 50 medical colleges demanded for admission only a high school education or the much abused equivalent. [16]

One of the most significant features of the decades under study was that many aspiring physicians fashioned educational programs superior to those dictated by law or custom. This held true for collegiate preparation as well as medical and post-graduate training. Regarding premedical studies evidence of this is found in an analysis of the 1,513 physicians in the *Dictionary of American Medical Biography* (*D.A.M.B.*) who took their medical training in 19th-century America. A surprising 607 or some 40 percent of these men earned predoctoral degrees before beginning medical studies. Another 430 had education beyond grammar school but short of a degree. [17]

By definition men selected for inclusion in the *D.A.M.B.* are not representative of the general physician population. Still, if properly qualified, the figures have value. For one thing the 1,513 physicians may be more representative than they appear at first glance. In the 19th century America did not produce fifteen hundred physicians who distinguished themselves by scientific or literary contributions to medicine. Deciding just why a given physician was selected for inclusion in the *D.A.M.B.* was imprecise at best, but in this study 531 were included apparently because they achieved excellent reputations in medical practice and nothing more. These men must have differed little from many others who were not selected by editors Kelly and Burrage.

Two other features of the *D.A.M.B.* study apply to the question at hand. The average age at which the 607 men took their predoctoral degree increased from 19.5 years in the first decade to 21.1 in the last. There are several possible explanations for this, but the most reasonable is that as the century progressed these students undertook more college preparatory work or a longer collegiate program or both.

Finally in the *D.A.M.B.* the percentage of men earning a predoctoral degree increased steadily decade by decade. In the seventh decade the figure was 46.9 percent and by the tenth, 63.4 (that is 63.4 percent of all men completing medical training in the tenth decade had earned a predoctoral degree). In short both the quality of premedical education and the number of men pursuing predoctoral degrees increased as the century progressed. Putting aside the question of representativeness, the *D.A.M.B.* sample was itself improving with time.

The 45 years encompassed in the present study saw a persistent though phlegmatic upgrading of the formal medical curriculum as well. The process involved the teaching of laboratory medicine as well as the length and content of clinical training. Before the Civil War medical studies centered about a preceptorship (nominally three years in length, but steadily diluted in practice during our period) and two lecture courses of some three months duration. The lecture courses were ungraded and the second was identical to the first — tedium compounded. Earlier requirements for Latin and the M.D. thesis were by now defunct, and since students were assessed a diploma fee final examinations rarely took a scalp. Even the rule that medical graduates must be 21 years of age was widely ignored.[18]

Throughout the first four post-bellum decades basic science teaching, with few exceptions, remained the domain of practicing physicians. In the earlier decades of the 19th century these men generally had no formal basic training beyond their own medical school experience. This too began changing as the 20th century approached. Laboratory medicine (along with laboratory science generally) was scantily taught prior to the Civil War,[19] but increased thereafter with the period of rapid development beginning between 1890 and 1895.[20] During this time the number of nonmedical graduate students rose "with astonishing speed."[21] These men formed the pool from which specialized basic science teachers eventually came, but by Flexner's time the appointment of Ph.D. teachers in medical schools was still an innovation to be "watched with interest."[22] Widespread support of basic research in America was spurred by the impressive practical successes of German science. The movement was well under way by 1900 and was bound to contribute to the favorable reception accorded Flexner's recommendations.

With a few significant exceptions[23] clinical teaching prior to 1865 took place in the crowded formality of classrooms and amphitheaters. Riesman scored the principal defect of the method when he said of his own experience at Pennsylvania, "It really made no difference what ailed the patient; the professor could use him as text for almost any disease and we would be none the wiser."[24] Even in medical schools with affiliated hospitals the situation could be deceptive. Norwood could justly say of Philadelphia schools, "What appears to be a formidable array of clinical material was in reality not always made available for clinical teaching."[25]

But again improvement was under way. After the Civil War a growing number of medical colleges graded the curriculum[26] and extended its length. Those who opposed stretching the term argued that a six-month session was "preposterous, in violation of all laws of health, physical or mental. . . ."[27] As always in this situation it is difficult to sort out true convictions from the economic incentives that in fact dominated many actions by proprietary professors. In any event the transition was far from painless. The University of Pennsyl-

vania attempted a six-month course of study as early as mid-century, but had to abandon the experiment when competing schools refused to fall in line.[28]

Between 1800 and 1830 the lecture term generally remained at 13 weeks.[29] By 1882, 42 schools reportedly required courses of six months or more and by 1890 the figure was 76.[30] Improvement continued so that by 1910 practically all schools offered four years of graded instruction although the number of months required each year continued to vary.[31]

Despite the many defects of the American M.D. degree program at this time, a physician must have been better prepared for practice by earning a degree than by the simple process of self-ordination. Another bit of positive evidence appears in the *D.A.M.B.* study where the number of men earning medical degrees increased consistently in the three decades after the Civil War.[32]

For the more affluent student of this period two domestic postgraduates experiences were available —house staff training and postgraduate clinics. The latter came on the scene relatively late; the New York Polyclinic, for example, opened its doors in 1882.[33] A few of these clinics flourished, but generally they never attained the prestige of their European counterparts. To Flexner the earlier clinics were nothing more than "undergraduate repair shops,"[34] though this is less an indictment than Flexner may have intended, because a measure of repair was needed. Still the postgraduate clinic was not as important for our purposes as house staff training. The clinics rather quickly settled on imparting the technical skills of a specialty, and were not looked to as a source of broad clinical training.

Insofar as it helped remedy the deficiencies of formal clinical instruction the role of postgraduate hospital training[35] has been underestimated. The situation is inevitable if one thinks only in terms of formal internships and residencies as they exist today. In the pre-Flexnerian period house staff training was arranged more or less informally, and there is evidence that such personal arrangements were not rare. As early as 1914 an internship was made requisite to licensure in Pennsylvania,[36] and in that same year the American Medical Association published its first list of approved internships plus a list of 95 hospitals offering specialty training.[37] Even more striking is the report that a year or two earlier 70 percent of the nations' medical graduates elected an internship.[38] Of the 1,513 physicians in the *D.A.M.B.* sample 248 took some form of house staff training. In the first decade of the 19th century the figure was only 1.6 percent, for the seventh decade, 20.2 percent, and by the last decade, 43.9.[39]

In part the importance of house staff training in improving physical education during this time has been understressed because the movement arose spontaneously and informally with no visible external crusade such as that directed against the undergraduate curriculum by the American Medical Association and others from mid-century on. Hospitals were growing in numbers and practitioners needed resident physicians. At the same time medical graduates were increasingly aware of their inadequate clinical skills. The two needs met quietly in a symbiotic relationship which was well established and which had most of the characteristics of modern house staff training by the time Flexner came along.

The third postgraduate option open to American students was medical training abroad. Remembering that students were under no legal compulsion to undertake such a costly venture, the numbers involved are mildly staggering. Bonner estimated that some fifteen thousand visited Germany and Austria alone in the period 1870–1914.[40] In the *D.A.M.B.* study 372 (24.6 percent of the 1,513 subjects) went abroad within five years after completing their American medical training. Only 14.8 percent did so in the first decade, a figure that rose to 24.6 percent in the seventh decade and 36.6 in the tenth.[41]

It could be argued and correctly that this amazing European exodus merely underscored the inadequacy of clinical opportunities at home. Yet the larger significance is that they *did* go abroad, most of them presumably intent on improving their medical proficiency. Each wave of returning students evangelized a new group which in turn came back impressed with what medical training could and should be like. The influence of these European-trained men in abetting eventual reform is impossible to assess quantitatively, but undoubtedly it was greater than observers appreciated at the time. When the Johns Hopkins University opened a medical school along German lines, J. S. Billings feared it would be many years before the

school could hope to graduate a class of 25. The first class graduated only 15, but two years later the figure was 32.[42]

Field points out that 16 of the 28 founding members of the American Physiological Society (1887) were trained in Germany and four others had studied in England or France. The group included a number of men who later led the battle to reform medical education in this country, such names as H. P. Bowditch, W. H. Howell, H. N. Martin, C. S. Minot, William Osler, and William Welch.[43] It is reasonable to conclude that the fifteen thousand or so men who saw German medical education firsthand must have been a powerful, though never organized, influence supporting Flexner's efforts of 1910 and thereafter.

It was Welch who summarized the period by saying "The results were better than the system."[44] He was right, and in part the results were better than the system because an increasing number of students forsook the system to create a system of their own. In assessing the status of American medical education before Flexner it is important to look beyond the extant degree requirements and consider the finished product as well. While the majority continued to settle for the prevailing mediocrity, a growing number of young physicians around the turn of the 20th century voluntarily supplemented their formal medical education with undergraduate collegiate preparation, house staff training, and study abroad. During the same period certain social forces began to be felt, and these too contributed to the catalytic effect of the implacable little schoolmaster from Louisville. Among the external forces were organized medicine, state licensing boards, and the improbable educational experiment made possible by Baltimore businessman Johns Hopkins.

The two principal medical organizations involved were the American Medical Association (A.M.A.) and the Association of American Medical Colleges (A.A.M.C.). From its inception in 1846 to the end of the century the A.M.A. battled for reform with little visible effect. Lacking any legal bite the A.M.A. sought to work by moral suasion alone. A main reason for its failure is found in the structure of the A.M.A. itself. From the outset the A.M.A.'s architects faced an organizational dilemma. If physician-owners of proprietary schools were to be induced to join a national organization which strongly favored educational reform, they would have to be offered greater voter representation than their numbers would dictate. On the other hand, of course, giving the medical schools too large a voice would block any chance for reform. The founders attempted a compromise which was doomed from the beginning. Only about a third of the eligible medical schools were present at the A.M.A.'s organizational convention in 1846.[45] From 1847 to 1852 medical college representation fell from 59 to 39 while medical society membership increased from 178 to 226.[46] The rift grew so wide that in 1853 there was an attempt to eliminate medical college delegates altogether.[47] Thus a town-gown split was all but assured by the A.M.A.'s original constitution, though it is difficult to imagine any scheme that would have satisfied the contending factions. Perceiving that the A.M.A. was essentially powerless, the physician-professors refused to participate and thus were free to ignore the A.M.A.'s exhortations. The best that can be said for the A.M.A. before 1900 is that its monotonous editorial lamentations did keep the matter somewhere in the far reaches of the profession's conscience. So frustrated did matters become in reality that at one time the A.M.A. entertained such now-startling possibilities as federal legislation and a national medical college.[48]

In 1904 the A.M.A. formed a permanent Council on Medical Education and from that point on its voice began to be heard. Staffed originally with a group of outstanding men, the council periodically inspected medical schools and began a rating system of A (worthy), B, and C (hopeless). Their reports were broadcast and the ensuing publicity undoubtedly contributed to the closure or merger of 29 schools between 1906 and Flexner's report[49] four years later.

In 1908 the council helped enlist Carnegie Foundation support for Flexner's survey and made available to him data accumulated from the council's previous investigations.[50] Dr. N. P. Colwell, secretary of the council, accompanied Flexner on several inspection trips, and, although Colwell's reports had to be couched "cautiously and tactfully,"[51] his medical insights must have proved helpful to Flexner. When it came time to write, Flexner, with his independent status, was free to put down with brutal objectivity many of the findings Colwell had felt free only to mutter about.

During the years after 1846 the disabling internecine problems of the A.M.A. became apparent to a small number of reform-minded men in the ranks of medical education itself. Responding to an organizational call on June 2, 1876, representatives from 22 medical colleges met to consider the possibility of reform from within. The following year they organized as the American Medical College Association.[52] Their laudable idealism soon came to grief. In 1880 the A.M.C.A. voted to require three years of medical training with at least six months of each year in a "proper medical college." Within two years ten schools withdrew, including several of the better founding colleges, and the organization collapsed. A successful reorganization took place in 1890 and from then on the pace of reform picked up. By 1896 the renamed Association of American Medical Colleges could report that 55 of the nation's 155 medical colleges were "cooperating," which meant at least nominal adherence to the higher self-imposed standards of A.A.M.C. members.[53] This, it should be recalled, at a time when even catalogue adherence to higher standards placed a school at a real disadvantage in the fierce competition for students.

The overriding importance of the A.A.M.C.'s early years was that at last reform was stirring within the proprietary system itself. Educators themselves now admitted at least that a mess existed. Earlier A.A.M.C. standards, while not always met by member schools themselves, created something of a self-fulfilling prophecy. The fact that a number of schoolmen could now organize for reform finally cracked the solid front presented by proprietary professors for most of the century. As its power and prestige grew the A.A.M.C. demanded a series of higher standards from its member colleges, and in 1905 the Confederation of State Medical Examining and Licensing Boards adopted the A.A.M.C.'s standard curriculum. From this point on the story became one of increasingly effective cooperation between the A.A.M.C., the A.M.A., and a new force, state legislatures, intent upon revitalizing medical practice acts.

During the early 19th century licensure was under some measure of legal control in most states of the Union. Regulatory mechanisms variously involved medical societies, medical schools, and governing boards of universities. Around 1830 licensure laws began to be repealed and by 1850 legislative control of medical licensure was practically nonexistent.[54] The anarchy that characterized American medicine from 1830 to 1875 came about for a number of reasons which cannot be detailed here. In general, abandonment of medicine by the state paralleled the rise of medical sects and indeed in the judgment of Reginald Fitz the spread of Thomsonianism was "the first serious blow to the regulation by the State of the practice of medicine. . . ."[55]

To put the matter perhaps too simply, public dissatisfaction with the heroic therapy of regular physicians coupled with widespread confusion over the conflicting claims of some two dozen different medical sects led legislators to withdraw legal sanctions from all the contending parties. A nadir of sorts was reached in 1838 when Maryland made it legal for any citizen of that state to charge and be paid for medical services.[56]

In medical practice absolute freedom can corrupt as thoroughly as absolute power, and in truth the two become effectively synonymous. N. S. Davis, whose prescience becomes more remarkable with time, resolved at the first convention of the A.M.A. that licensing be placed in the hands of a single independent state board in each state.[57] Not surprisingly the resolution failed and by 1860 editorialists such as Stephen Smith had given up hope for state control and tossed the matter back to the A.M.A.[58] By 1875 the chaos could not be ignored any longer. The process of repeal reversed itself and states began writing new laws controlling licensure and practice. New York was in the vanguard, and the story there in many ways exemplifies the complex seesaw evolution of legislative attempts at controlling medical licensure.[59] By 1894 Fitz reported that all states except New Hampshire and his own Massachusetts had laws regulating medical practice.[60] Although these laws varied in their inherent worthiness as well as the energy with which they were prosecuted, Fitz concluded that "to them, more than any one cause, is due the difference which exists between the condition now [1894] and in 1870."[61]

The state licensing boards created by this new wave of legislation confederated and finally there existed a national organization invested with the power that for years the A.M.A. and A.A.M.C. could only sigh after. To Flexner's eye the state boards of 1910 left much to be desired — their continued loose interpretation of his *bête noire*, the "equivalent," for example — but he wisely perceived that the legal approach held the best hope for reform. "The state boards," he said, "are the instruments through which the reconstruction of medical education will be largely effected."[62]

Viewed in terms of the ground they plowed for Flexner, legislative reforms after 1870 were far more significant than their immediate success in eliminating diploma mills, quacks, and ignorant but sincere sectarians. The new laws reflected a wholly new national attitude. No longer was the scene dominated by fears of class legislation, by the pervasive attitude of *laissez-faire*, or Herbert Spencer's version of social Darwinism which made the patient responsible for his own folly when he chose his physician unwisely.[63] The confused lawlessness of 1830–1870 had by now convinced the populace and their lawmakers that some degree of state regulation was both proper and necessary.

Other factors contributed. Regular medicine emerged as genuinely superior to its sectarian competition, which was handicapped by a simplistic, usually unitarian, approach to disease causation and therapy. Whatever its faults regular medicine retained the capacity for change, a trait that allowed it to accommodate the remarkable advances of European medicine, albeit at times with some chauvinistic delays. The regulars could scarcely claim a jockey's role in medicine's late 19th-century emergence as a science, but at least they backed the right horse. Nationalistic elements remained, but by Flexner's time the profession and the public generally accepted the superiority of German science.

The next step was eminently reasonable. If the fruits of German medical science could be imported into this country, why not the educational system that underpinned it all? Indeed the process had begun as far back as 1876 in the hands of a few visionary men and a Baltimore merchant who was wise enough to avoid all restrictive adjectives when he endowed a new type of American university.[64] The Hopkins' story is too well known to need retelling here.[65] The fact that the Johns Hopkins medical school succeeded almost two decades before the Flexner report testifies that American attitudes toward medical education had changed drastically between 1865 and 1893. True, a number of proprietary schoolmen refused to see the message on the wall, but by 1910 the writing was plainly there.

A final force deserves mention, that of economics. The same free marketplace which originally encouraged the wild growth of medical schools had begun to take its toll. Supply now exceeded valid demand, and as Flexner wryly remarked, "Nothing has perhaps done more to complete the discredit of commercialism than the fact that it has ceased to pay. It is but a short step from an annual deficit to the conclusion that the whole thing is wrong anyway."[66]

Indeed commercialism had ceased to pay. Flexner found that during the single year prior to his report a dozen schools had collapsed and "many more are obviously gasping for breath."[67] Had this attrition rate prevailed consistently it would more than have accounted for the decrease in schools from a 1906 peak of 161 to the 100 or so surviving in 1915.[68]

Thus the tide of reform was running heavy by 1910. Flexner himself observed that "there is no denying that especially in the last fifteen years, substantial progress has been made."[69] Yet none of this need detract from Flexner's renowned contribution.[70] There is no doubt but that his meticu-lously documented survey shocked the nation and hastened the closing of a number of marginal schools. But that was not his chief bequest. The sorry state of America's medical schools was no secret before 1910. His enduring legacy derived from what he accomplished quietly after the sensation created by his report had subsided. Largely due to Flexner's efforts John D. Rockefeller donated almost fifty million dollars to improve the nation's medical schools through the ministrations of the General Education Board. Within a few years a fine new school was established at the University of Rochester and major overhauls had been financed at schools such as Iowa, Cornell, Vanderbilt, and Washington at St. Louis. Nor did the tide stop there. As Flexner and members of the General Education Board anticipated, state rivalries erupted around the few schools selected for financial assistance.[71] Many of these states, when they failed to secure philanthropic help, took upon themselves the long-neglected fiscal responsibility for training their own physicians. Thus Flexner is properly remembered not so much for the fire he set as for his blueprint of the new structure which was to rise from the ashes.

## NOTES

1 A. Flexner, *Medical Education in the United States and Canada* (New York: Carnegie Foundation, 1910).

2 Elements of the story appear in chapters by W. F. Norwood and J. Field in *The History of Medical Education*, ed. C. D. O'Malley, U.C.L.A. Forum Med. Sci. No. 12 (Los Angeles: Univ. of California Press, 1970), pp. 463–499 and 501–530.

3 N. S. Davis calculated that physicians and population had increased *pari passu* in the 35 years prior to 1876. *Contributions to the History of Medical Education and Medical Institutions in the United States of America 1776–1876* (Washington, D.C.: Government Printing Office, 1877), pp. 41–42. Davis makes no mention of men entering practice without degrees. Stern agreed when he estimated one physician for 572 persons in 1860 and one for 578 persons in 1900. B. J. Stern, *American Medical Practice in the Perspectives of a Century* (New York: Commonwealth Fund, 1945), p. 63. Stern is quoting the *Eighth Census* (Washington, D.C., 1860), pp. 670, 677. Flexner, *Medical Education*, p. 14, concurred in Stern's figures, but argued that the ratio was too great. Cur-rent thought would tend to support Flexner, but transportation and distribution of physicians would demand a higher ratio for the last part of the 19th century.

4 F. H. Garrison, *John Shaw Billings: A Memoir* (New York: Putnam's, 1915), p. 256.

5 Samuel Chew, generally inclined to the rosy view, said, "A favorable change has already taken place. The number of well educated young men who engage in the study of medicine is every year increasing." *Lectures on Medical Education* (Philadelphia: Lindsay and Blakiston, 1864), p. 136. The bulk of contemporary editorial opinion of course was distinctly pessimistic.

6 Flexner, *Medical Education*, p. 30.

7 R. H. Shryock, "Public relations of the medical profession in Great Britain and the United States: 1600–1870," *Ann. Med. Hist.*, 1930, n.s. *2*: 327.

8 T. R. Sizer, *Secondary Schools at the Turn of the Century* (New Haven: Yale Univ. Press, 1964), p. 4.

9 R. F. Butts summarized the trends in higher American education during the 19th century as follows:

growth of large elective curricula, broadening of the traditional B.A. degree, rise of the German ideal of the university, increase in teaching of science and technology, decline of the notion that intellectual discipline could be honed only on the classics, increasing secularism, greater personal freedom for students, and opening college to all classes including women. *A Cultural History of Education* (New York: McGraw-Hill, 1947), pp. 519–521.

Flexner, speaking of the South, which lagged behind the rest of the nation in this regard, described the scene as an educational "renaissance." *Medical Education*, p. 40. He reported some 300,000 students enrolled in public high schools in 1910 and about 120,000 (males) in colleges of the North and West as of 1908, excluding preparatory and professional students. *Ibid.*, p. 42.

10  F. V. N. Painter, *A History of Education* (New York: Appleton, 1898), p. 322.

11  On the negative side McIntire surveyed 222 New Jersey and Pennsylvania physicians in 1882 and found 178 with no collegiate preparation at all. Unfortunately he does not indicate how many of his sample took their medical training before the Civil War. C. McIntire, Jr., *The Percentage of College-Bred Men in the Medical Profession* (Philadelphia: American Academy of Medicine, 1883), pp. 3–6.

12  M. Fishbein, *A History of the American Medical Association: 1847–1947* (Philadelphia: Saunders, 1947), p. 243.

13  J. H. Rauch, *Report on Medical Education, Medical Colleges and the Regulation of the Practice of Medicine in the United States and Canada 1765–1890* (Springfield: Illinois State Board of Health, 1890), pp. iii–iv.

14  Flexner, *Medical Education*, p. 28.

15  *Ibid.,* p. 46.

16  *Ibid.,* p. 29.

17  H. A. Kelly and W. L. Burrage, eds., *Dictionary of American Medical Biography* (New York: Appleton, 1928). The study is by R. P. Hudson, "Patterns of medical education in nineteenth century America" (Unpublished essay for the M.A. degree, The Johns Hopkins University, 1966). The section dealing with premedical education is on pp. 23–34. This study will be referred to several times in the present paper, so a *caveat* is in order. The *D.A.M.B.* analysis is essentially statistical. This demanded the employment of certain arbitrary definitions and categories which are carefully spelled out in the essay. These should be consulted firsthand before any figures or conclusions from the study are used. The analysis included the reasons individuals were included in the *D.A.M.B.*, patterns of premedical, medical, and postgraduate education decade by decade, patterns of age, the influence of economic factors, effects of

father's occupation and marriage, and educational patterns of the various specialties.

18  W. F. Norwood *Medical Education in the United States Before the Civil War* (Philadelphia: Univ. of Pennsylvania Press, 1944), p. 406, states that the requirement for an attained age of 21 "seems to have been the only general regulation that was not grossly violated at some time during the decades covered by this survey." However the *D.A.M.B.* study revealed that 100 of the 1,513 men earned the M.D. degree before the age of 21. Hudson, "Patterns of medical education," p. 46. See also H. B. Shafer, *The American Medical Profession 1783 to 1850* (New York: Columbia Univ. Press, 1936), p. 82, and the implication of Daniel Drake's plea in *Practical Essay on Medical Education and the Medical Profession in the United States, 1832* (as reprinted in Baltimore by the Johns Hopkins Press, 1952), p. 57.

19  R. Hofstadter and C. D. Hardy, *The Development and Scope of Higher Education in the United States* (New York: Columbia Univ. Press, 1952), p. 20. The authors refer to W. P. Rogers, *Andrew D. White and the Modern University* (Ithaca: Cornell Univ. Press, 1942), pp. 23–29, and D. J. Struik, *Yankee Science in the Making* (Boston: Little Brown, 1948), chs. VI, X.

20  This is the estimate of R. M. Pearce, "An analysis of the medical group in Cattell's Thousand Leading Men of Science," *Science*, 1915, n.s. *42*: 264. Flexner dated the beginning of improved laboratory teaching at 1878, when Francis Delafield and William H. Welch opened clinical laboratories at the College of Physicians and Surgeons (N.Y.) and Bellevue Hospital Medical College respectively. *Medical Education*, p. 11.

21  Figures given are 198 in 1871, 2,382 in 1890 and 9,370 in 1910. Hofstadter and Hardy, *Development and Scope of Higher Education*, p. 64.

22  Flexner, *Medical Education*, p. 72.

23  Probably because of its French connections New Orleans apparently had a genuine go at bedside teaching as early as the 1850s. Speaking of his New Orleans School of Medicine in 1857, D. W. Brickell said flatly, "Six, out of ten, of us give *daily* bed-side instruction in the great Charity Hospital. . . ." *New Orleans Med. News & Hosp. Gaz.*, December 1857, *4*: 601. See also A. E. Fossier, "History of medical education, in New Orleans from its birth to the Civil War," *Ann. Med. Hist.*, 1934, n.s. *6*: 432. For the French influence see R. Matas, *The Rudolph Matas History of Medicine in Louisiana*, ed. J. Duffy (Louisiana State Univ. Press, 1962), II, 237–268. Norwood appears to accept the New Orleans claim. *Medical Education . . . Before the Civil War*, p. 370.

Abraham Jacobi reportedly initiated bedside

pediatrics teaching in New York in 1862. *The American Pediatric Society 1888–1938* (Privately printed, 1938), p. 4. According to Shryock, Jacob Da Costa began bedside teaching at Jefferson around 1870. "Medicine in Philadelphia during the nineteenth century," *Bull. Soc. Med. Hist. Chicago,* 1948, 6: 70. On the other hand, Osler maintained that as of 1890 there was "not a single medical clinic worth the name in the United States." W. Osler, "The coming of age of internal medicine in America," *International Clinics,* 1915, 4: 3.

24  D. Riesman, "Clinical teaching in America with some remarks on early medical schools," *Tr. Coll. Physicians Phila.,* 1939, 3rd series, 7: 109.

25  Norwood, *Medical Education . . . Before the Civil War,* p. 107.

26  Credit for the first graded curriculum is difficult to assign. To be answered the question must be put with precision. Who first advocated grading the curriculum? Where was it first attempted? Was it optional or required? Where did it first take hold? See F. C. Waite, "Advent of the graded curriculum in American medical colleges," *J. Assn. Am. Med. Colls.,* 1950, 25: 315–322.

27  Quoted by Brickell, *New Orleans Med. News & Hosp. Gaz.,* December 1857, 4: 599.

28  J. Carson, *A History of the Medical Department of the University of Pennsylvania* (Philadelphia: Lindsay and Blakiston, 1869), p. 172.

29  Shafer, *American Medical Profession,* p. 51.

30  Rauch, *Report on Medical Education,* p. iv.

31  Flexner, *Medical Education,* pp. 10–11.

32  In the *D.A.M.B.* sample (n. 17) subjects were categorized as degreed, nondegreed, and delayed, meaning the man earned a degree but only after he had begun medical practice. Forty-eight were delayed, and 68 nondegreed. The remaining 1,397 earned medical degrees before practising. In the first decade only 55.7 percent earned the M.D. Figures for the last four decades were 96.0, 99.4, 100, and 100 respectively. All figures excluded honorary and *ad eundem* degrees. Hudson, "Patterns of medical education," p. 53.

At the other extreme Norwood states that two-thirds to three-fourths of medical school matriculates did not remain to take the degree, implying that they entered practice without ever earning the M.D. *Medical Education . . . Before the Civil War,* p. 432. This estimate strikes me as too dismal. It was based on a "sampling of school circulars and catalogues and contemporary literature." The use of catalogues and circulars for this purpose is particularly precarious, since many students wisely took the second lecture course at a different school from the first. Such students would appear

in successive catalogues as dropouts rather than transfers.

33  T. E. Keys, "Historical aspects of graduate medical education," *J. Med. Educ.,* 1955, 30: 260. As Keys makes clear, this was not the first attempt at graduate medical education in America.

34  Flexner, *Medical Education,* p. 174. Flexner summarizes postgraduate schools as of 1910 on pp. 174–177.

35  House staff training is used here to cover all hospital-based clinical training taken after the medical degree. So used, the term must be approached with caution, because terminology describing hospital training shared the general educational confusion of the time. See, for example, *Graduate Medical Education* (Chicago: Univ. of Chicago Press, 1940), p. 98. The terms "resident" and "resident physician" have a tortuous history dating back at least 125 years. *Ibid.,* p. 97. The earliest hospital training programs centered around medical students who were called resident students. They were outgrowths of the indenturing practice such as that initiated in 1773 at Pennsylvania Hospital. Beginning in 1820 at City Almshouse of Philadelphia, house pupils were required to pay a fee and were dignified by the title of house physician or house surgeon. By 1823 a candidate for this position had to be a medical graduate. Norwood, *Medical Education . . . Before the Civil War,* p. 49. The following year the same held true of Pennsylvania Hospital, and a similar evolution occurred elsewhere. T. Morton and F. Woodbury, *The History of the Pennsylvania Hospital 1751–1895* (Philadelphia: Times Printing House, 1895), p. 480.

For most of the 19th century "interns" were medical students, the equivalent of the early hospital pupils. To illustrate, in 1880 the Board of Trustees of Charity Hospital in New Orleans decided that interns must have one year of medical study before appointment. A. E. Fossier, "The Charity Hospital of Louisiana," reprinted from *New Orleans Med. & Surg. J.,* May–October 1923, 75–76: 38. As applicants for the position of intern gradually were required to be physicians, hospital pupils came to be known as externs, and in 1892 we find the two working side by side "without any official friction." *Ibid.,* p. 43. The Philadelphia and New Orleans examples are not offered as precise for other geographical situations, but rather to provide illustrations of the confusion that followed the evolution of hospital training positions.

The term "internship" reportedly first appeared about the time of the Civil War. *Graduate Medical Education,* p. 31. The word gained distinction only slowly and did not achieve its modern meaning until about 1914. From the end of the Civil War to the end of the century, however, "intern" continued to be used interchangeably with "resident" and "resident physician." Today's highly standardized residency program was patterned on the German system and formalized by William Halsted at the Johns Hopkins at the beginning of the 20th century. See W. S. Halsted, "The training of the surgeon." *Johns Hopkins Hosp. Bull.,* 1904, *15*: 271 ff. The current use of the word "resident" followed.

36  Fishbein, *A History of the American Medical Association,* p. 899.

37  *Ibid.,* p. 899-900.

38  *Ibid.,* p. 899. The source of this figure is not given and it is difficult to know if the year referred to is 1912 or 1913.

39  Hudson, "Patterns of medical education," p. 108.

40  T. N. Bonner, *American Doctors and German Universities* (Lincoln: Univ. of Nebraska Press, 1963), p. 23.

41  Hudson, "Patterns of medical education," p. 88. The five-year limitation was imposed in an attempt to eliminate the large number of physicians who toured Europe after years of successful practice.

42  Flexner, *Medical Education,* p. 46.

43  O'Malley, *History of Medical Education,* p. 504. Field apparently surveyed the founders' biographies in W. J. Meek, W. H. Howell, and C. W. Greene, *History of the American Physiological Society Semicentennial 1887-1937* (Baltimore, 1938).

44  Flexner, *Medical Education,* p. 10, quotes Welch, "Development of American medicine," *Columbia Univ. Quart. Suppl.,* December 1907.

45  N. S. Davis, *History of the American Medical Association* (Philadelphia: Lippincott, 1855), p. 37.

46  *Ibid.,* p. 117.

47  *Ibid.,* p. 115.

48  Dr. William Baldwin, president of the newly formed Association of American Medical Editors, suggested federal legislation in an address to the A.M.A. in 1869. Fishbein, *A History of the American Medical Association,* p. 79. A resolution supporting the establishment of a national school of medicine was introduced at the 1870 meeting of the A.M.A. (*Tr. A.M.A.,* 1870, *21*: 37-39), and the idea was revived in his presidential address of 1876 by J. Marion Sims. *Ibid.,* 1876, *27*: 94-95.

49  See O'Malley, *History of Medical Education,* pp. 507-508. Of 140 schools visited by the Council on Medical Education and reported to the A.A.M.C. in 1910, 68 were rated A, 38 B, and 34 C.D.F. Smiley, "History of the Association of American Medical Colleges, 1876-1956," *J. Med. Educ.,* 1957, *32*: 520.

50  H. S. Pritchett in Flexner, *Medical Education,* p. viii.

51  A. Flexner, *An Autobiography* (New York: Simon and Schuster, 1960), p. 74.

52  This story can be found in Smiley, "History of the Association of American Medical Colleges."

53  In the earlier years the A.A.M.C. had difficulty mounting a vigorous leadership role. Their higher standards usually were adopted only after a number of schools had led the way. In 1900 premedical requirements were upgraded, but the A.A.M.C. did not insist that member colleges require three years of collegiate preparation until 1952. *Ibid.,* p. 523. By 1904 66 member schools reported a required four-year medical curriculum with terms ranging from six to nine months. *Ibid.,* p. 518.

54  R. H. Fitz, "The legislative control of medical practice," *Med. Comm. Mass. Med. Soc.,* 1894, *16*: 306-307. Fitz's account is perhaps the best to come from the contemporary scene. To his mind, laws regulating medical practice were unpopular because (1) they were considered class legislation, (2) legislators suspected the motives of regular physicians, (3) the populace believed every person had a right to choose his own medical attendant, and (4) regular physicians themselves objected, out of a belief that the very act of regulating irregulars would exert a protective influence upon them. *Ibid.,* pp. 282 ff.

55  *Ibid.,* pp. 301-306. Fitz saw Thomsonianism as paving the way for homeopathy, "which proved to be the more effectual agent in annulling the licensing of physicians."

56  *Ibid.,* p. 306.

57  Davis, *History of the American Medical Association,* p. 35.

58  "What shall be our title?" *Am. Med. Times,* July 28, 1860, p. 63. The editorial is unsigned, but in a personal communication Gert Brieger expressed his conviction that Smith was the author.

59  J. B. Bardo, "A history of the legal regulation of medical practice in New York State," *Bull. N.Y. Acad. Med.,* 1967, *43*: 924-949. Bardo's narrative is revealing in that it shows the difficulties encountered in efforts at regulating licensure when neither the state, the medical schools, nor the profession had clear-cut legal backing. In 1684 New York law prohibited medical practice without the "consent of those skillful" in it. In 1760 specified magistrates were empowered to examine and license, and in 1797 the magistrates could license by endorsing a preceptor's certificate. An 1806 law made the medical profession responsible through state and local medical societies. Three years later the University of the State of New York could authorize colleges to issue the M.D. degree, which was then a license to practice as well. By 1872 the Regents could appoint a board of examiners, which again made licensure a state function. In 1880 medical societies were divested of any licensing function, and by 1890 the M.D. degree no longer conferred automatic licen-

sure, which was now solely in the Regents' hands. To insure professional input, Boards of Medical Examiners were created, one each for regular practitioners, homeopaths, and eclectics. In 1893 existing laws were brought together as part of a Public Health Law and in 1907 the three separate boards were made one. At no point in this long evolution did enforcement of a law necessarily follow its enactment.

60  Fitz, "Legislative control," pp. 294, 313.

61  *Ibid.*, p. 315.

62  Flexner, *Medical Education,* pp. 167–173.

63  Spencer is quoted as saying, "Unpitying as it looks, it is best to let the foolish man suffer the appointed penalty of his foolishness. For the pain—he must bear it as well as he can; for the experience—he must treasure it up and act more rationally in the future." *Social Statics,* 1851, p. 373, quoted in Fitz, "Legislative control," p. 284.

64  A. Flexner, *Daniel Coit Gilman: Creator of the American Type of University* (New York: Harcourt, Brace, 1946), p. 35.

65  *Ibid.*, and especially R. H. Shryock, *The Unique Influence of the Johns Hopkins University on American Medicine* (Copenhagen: Munksgaard, 1953).

66  Flexner, *Medical Education,* p. 11.

67  *Ibid.*

68  The figures are from *The General Education Board* (New York: General Education Board, 1915), p. 161.

69  Flexner, *Medical Education,* p. 10.

70  In some current circles it has become fashionable to criticize Flexner for the nationwide adoption of the Hopkins' plan—for what has come to be called the tyranny of the four-year lockstep curriculum. This is akin to holding Galen responsible for the 1500 years his doctrines influenced medical thought after his death. Worse, it ignores Flexner's own unequivocal caveat, "In the course of the next thirty years needs will develop of which we here take no account. As we cannot foretell them, we shall not endeavor to meet them." *Medical Education,* p. 143.

71  This story is told in Flexner, *An Autobiography.* See esp. pp. 178 ff.

# WOMEN AND MEDICINE

Although women had practiced medicine informally for millennia, when they sought formal medical training within male institutions in the United States in the middle of the 19th century, they frequently met with rejection. Elizabeth Blackwell received an M.D. degree from Geneva Medical College in New York in 1849, the first awarded to a woman in the United States, but many women who tried to follow in her footsteps were rebuffed. Women responded to their exclusion by forming their own medical institutions, including seventeen all-female medical schools in the nineteenth century. Because of the need for additional clinical experience, in 1862 Dr. Marie Zakrzewska opened the New England Hospital for Women and Children in Boston, which trained hundreds of women physicians while providing care for poor women and children.

Many 19th-century women who chose medicine as a career did so in the belief that they could make a unique contribution to the field. As Regina Morantz shows here, women's struggle to enter medicine was helped by their traditionalist argument that women's nurturant talents could enhance the healing process. Not only could women physicians utilize their natural female behavior, they could also form the "connecting link" between women's domestic lives and the scientific world of medicine.

Virginia Drachman documents both the successes and the pitfalls of women's separate institutions in her account of the New England Hospital. The pioneer generations of women in medicine discovered that younger women, coming into the profession after places for women were relatively secure, brought very different needs and expectations and harbored complaints about the founders. As women made rapid strides in separate medical institutions, their successes led many male institutions to open their doors to women. The greatest breakthrough came in 1893 when the Johns Hopkins University School of Medicine accepted $500,000 in contributions from women patrons—along with the stipulation that women students be admitted equally with men. By 1910 over 9,000 women (6 percent of the total) were practicing medicine in the United States, and in some cities, such as Boston and Minneapolis, almost 20 percent of practitioners were women. Ironically, most all-female medical schools, believing that the admission of women to male schools had allowed women to enter the mainstream of medicine, closed at the very height of their success.

Women soon learned, however, that their welcome in coeducational institutions was limited, and in the years between 1910 and 1965, few medical schools enrolled more than 5 percent women. The sole remaining female school, the Woman's Medical College of Pennsylvania, which became coeducational in the 1970s, trained one-third of the women medical graduates during the first half of the 20th century. Not until the 1960s, when federal guidelines pressured medical schools to accept more women, did the numbers rise again to their 19th-century standings. In 1984, 28 percent of the medical school graduates in the United States were women.

# 11

## The "Connecting Link": The Case for the Woman Doctor in 19th-Century America

### REGINA MARKELL MORANTZ

Little more than a decade before the Civil War, Elizabeth Blackwell, daughter of a prominent reform-minded family, achieved notoriety by becoming the first woman to earn a medical diploma in the United States. Soon after she received her degree in 1849, Geneva Medical College, a small regular institution in upstate New York, closed its doors to women. Undaunted, women continued to seek medical training. Within two years, three female students at the eclectic Central Medical College in Syracuse — the first coeducational medical school in the country — gained medical licenses.

In Philadelphia a group of Quakers led by Dr. Joseph Longshore pledged themselves to teach women medicine and established the Woman's (originally Female) Medical College of Pennsylvania in 1850. The following year eight women graduated in the first class. A Boston school, founded originally by Samuel Gregory in 1848 to train women as midwives, gained a Massachusetts charter in 1856 as the New England Female Medical College. Here Marie Zakrzewska, former medical associate of Elizabeth Blackwell, early female graduate of the Cleveland Medical College, and the influential founder of the New England Hospital for Women and Children, came to teach in 1859.

Meanwhile, in New York the Homeopathic New York Medical College for Women, established in 1863 by still another early graduate, Clemence Lozier, enjoyed such success that by the end of the decade it had matriculated approximately 100 women. Five years later Elizabeth Blackwell, now joined in practice by her sister Emily, also a gradu-

REGINA MARKELL MORANTZ-SANCHEZ is Associate Professor of History at the University of Kansas, Lawrence, Kansas.

ate of Cleveland, opened the Women's Medical College of the New York Infirmary.

By 1870 a handful of medical schools, both orthodox and sectarian, accepted women on a regular basis. In fact, over 300 women had already graduated, though mostly from sectarian institutions. Several of these women founded dispensaries in New York, Boston, and Philadelphia to offer needed clinical training to the increasing numbers of female colleagues. Of course, opportunities for women in medicine remained circumscribed, for throughout the century the majority of institutions barred them from attendance. Nevertheless, the ranks of female physicians grew: by 1900 their numbers reached an estimated 7,387.[1]

Women entered the medical profession as part of a broader 19th-century movement toward self-determination in which all reformist women, from conservative social feminists to radical suffrage advocates, played a significant part. Like many members of their sex, women doctors sought to examine and redefine the concept of womanhood to fit the changing demands of a complex, industrializing society. Furthermore, the move to educate women in medicine grew out of the antebellum health reform crusade. Abolitionists, peace advocates, temperance reformers, and women's righters participated in the drive to improve the nation's health, and middle-class women were particularly active in health and dietary reform in these years.[2]

Indeed, medicine attracted more women votaries in the 19th century than any other profession except teaching. Female physicians took seriously their role in health education. For many, medical training appeared the logical outcome of their prior interest in health issues. Borrowing arguments from the health reformers, they emphasized the importance of giving information on hygiene and physiology to all women. Women's new and central role in family life made systematic knowledge imperative. Female physicians, as teachers and clinicians concerned with such issues, would be essential to improving the health and nurturing the expertise of all women.

Although they remained a small minority, women doctors were conspicuous because they violated 19th-century norms of female behavior. Consequently they became the focus of a vigorous controversy over women's proper role in and relationship to public and private health. Whereas amateur female instructors of physiology could be dismissed as objects of public ridicule, professionally trained women doctors were entirely another matter. By the end of the 1860s protests against them mounted from within the profession, forcing them and their supporters to refine and elaborate an ideology to defend their cause.

The arguments with which they chose to justify themselves revealed women physicians both as ideological innovators and as daughters of their century. Sharing this role with other women of their generation who sought an expansion of their activities, their ideas fell well within the mainstream of feminist thinking. Their ideology served a dual purpose. As self-explanation it enabled them to convey to the world what they hoped to accomplish and why. By their use of ideas they attempted to place themselves in cultural and historical perspective. Yet their ideology also exerted a powerful influence on the way they perceived reality, shaping that perception and giving it meaning within the context of Victorian values.

This essay examines the means by which women physicians justified their role in the 19th-century health revolution. Because their arguments deviated only slightly from those of others favoring a more active place for women in society, such an investigation illustrates how similar groups of 19th-century women came to grips with their culture. The reasoning of women physicians was often brilliant and effective, and their practical work extremely important. Yet their ties to 19th-century values also impaired their vision. Only a handful of them understood the ways in which a self-limiting conception of their potential contribution hampered their progress within the profession.

I

The opponents of medical education for women deserve attention first because their objections fixed the context of the debate. Women doctors remained sensitive to criticism, realizing that professional opposition reached far beyond ideology in its implications, sharply curtailing their opportunities to study and practice.

Most doctors were traditionalists who shared the same ambivalence towards women's role that dominated 19th-century American culture. Placing women on a pedestal and cementing them firmly within the confines of the home, they justified an emotional preference for sequestered women by making them the moral guardians of society and the repositories of virtue. Fearing that women who sought professional training would avoid their childrearing responsibilities, they reminded their colleagues in overworked metaphors that "the hand that rocks the cradle rules the world." Woman, argued a spokesman, held "to her bosom the embryo race, the pledge of mutual love." Her mission was not the pursuit of science, but "to rear the offspring and ever fan the flame of piety, patriotism and love upon the sacred altar of her home."[3]

Rational legitimation of the female role often veiled less rational preferences: the home represented for 19th-century Americans a refuge from an immoral and often brutalizing world. A woman who dared to move beyond her sphere was "a monstrosity," an "intellectual and moral hermaphrodite." Nevertheless, insisted Dr. Paul de Lacy Baker, women controlled society, government, and civilization through the "home influence." Home was

the place of rest and refuge for man, weary and worn by manual labor, or exhausted by care and mental toil. Thither he turns him from the trials and dangers, the temptations and seductions, the embarrassments and failures of life, to the one spot beneath all the skies where hope and comfort come out to meet him and drive back the demons of despair that pursue him from the outside world. There the sweet enchantress that rules and cheers his home supports his sinking spirits, reanimates his self-respect, confirms his manly resolves and sustains his personal honor.[4]

While revering the purity and repose of the home, doctors, like other Victorians, feared the animal in man and dwelt on the significance of female moral superiority in curbing man's most brutal instincts. Woman's venturing out into the world would bode ill for civilization, for women kept men respectable. In copying men, they ran the risk of demoralizing both sexes. Men, confessed Dr. J. S. Weatherly to his colleagues, were "little less than brutes," and "where men are bestialized, women suffer untold wrongs." Woman's great strength and safety, he concluded, was in the institution of marriage, and "everything she does to lessen men's respect and love for her, weakens it, and makes her rights more precarious; for without the home influence which marriage brings, men will become selfish and brutal; and then away go women's rights." [5]

Traditionalists also worried that teaching women the mysteries of the human body would affront female modesty. "Improper exposures" would destroy the delicacy and refinement that constituted women's primary charms. Men recoiled at the thought of exposing young women to the "blood and agony" of the dissecting room, where "ghastly" rituals were performed. [6]

Despite the popularity of this defense of female delicacy, traditionalists compromised their case when they admitted that women's ready sympathy made them excellent nurses. Praising Florence Nightingale's achievements in the Crimea, they credited them primarily to her ignorance of scientific medicine. Medical education, they argued, would surely have hardened her heart, leaving her bereft of softness and empathy. [7]

Supporters of female education quickly discovered, however, that respect for Victorian delicacy could work in their favor. Was the mother who nursed her family at the bedside ever shielded from the indelicacies of the human body? they asked. Furthermore, if the issue was female modesty, then why should men — even medical men — ever be allowed to treat women? As the use of pelvic examinations became part of ordinary practice, male physicians posed a greater threat to feminine delicacy than women practitioners. Indeed, many supporters of medical training for women were conservative champions of female modesty. [8] Though the arguments of these supporters were extremely persuasive within the context of Victorian values, traditionalist physicians continued throughout the century to object to training women on the grounds of Victorian delicacy.

Some male physicians alleged other unsuitable character traits against women besides their innocence. Many agreed that Nature had limited the capacity of women's intellect. They were impulsive and irrational, unable to do mathematics, and deficient in judgment and courage. Their passivity of mind and weakness of body left them powerless to practice surgery. And if these disadvantages were not enough, there remained the enigmatic side of the female temperament. Dependent, "nervous," and "excitable," women, "as all medical men know," were subject to hysteria over which they had no control. "Hysteria," regretted J. S. Weatherly, M.D., "is second Nature to them." [9]

Because at least some women physicians in the 19th century received inferior training, doctors often mistook poor preparation for innate ignorance. On this point critics were most disingenuous. The issue became particularly controversial as local and national medical societies began to debate the admission of female members in the 1870s and 1880s. Though circular, the reasoning seemed incontrovertible — at least for a time. First-rate regular medical schools barred women from attendance. Meanwhile opponents unfairly stigmatized the women's medical colleges as either irregular or of poor quality. While denying them access to the kind of education they could approve, critics held their alleged inferior training against them, often refusing to consult with women physicians and ostracizing male practitioners who did. The final irony was that a fair number of medical women received excellent training in the 19th century. A comparative study of curriculum and clinical offerings in several 19th-century medical schools suggests that the women who earned their diplomas from the New York Infirmary and the Woman's Medical College of Pennsylvania were exposed to a vigorous, demanding, and comparatively progressive course of study. [10] Self-conscious of their need for proper preparation, other women sought postgraduate training in Europe.

Probably much of the grumbling over inferior training arose out of disgust for the multiplication of proprietary schools in the 1830s and 1840s and the resulting sharp increase in the number of practitioners. Some physicians complained of the possibility of increased economic competition if women were admitted to study. Such concern dissipated toward the end of the century when women doctors appeared to segregate themselves in certain specialties. What remains most striking about this objection, however, is that it took for granted not only women's ability to practice medicine, but also their ready acceptance by the public.[11]

Rejecting many of the preceding arguments, an increasingly influential group of medical men preferred instead to take a more scientific posture. Rallying around Harvard professor E. H. Clarke's book *Sex in Education: A Fair Chance for Girls*, published in 1873, they based their case against women entirely on the predominating negative influence of their biology. When they chose to emphasize the debilitating and still mysterious effects of menstruation, traditionalists were indeed effective. Physicians knew little about the influence of women's periodicity, and the culture treated menstruation as a disease.[12] Reasoning that only rest could help women counteract the weakness resulting from the loss of blood, complete bedrest was commonly prescribed. Thus even if opponents appeared willing to concede women's intellectual equality—and many were prepared to do so—women's biological disabilities seemed insurmountable.[13] Since menstruation incapacitated women for a week out of every month, could they ever be depended on in medical emergencies?

Female physicians helped to dispel doubts about the effects of menstruation in their own professional lives. A few investigated the problem scientifically. Outraged by the influence of E. H. Clarke's book, the feminist community in Boston cast about for a woman doctor with the proper credentials to call its thesis into question. In 1874 women gained a public forum when Harvard announced that the topic for its celebrated Boylston Essay would be the effects of menstruation on women. Writing to Dr. Mary Putnam Jacobi in 1874, C. Alice Baker urged her to take up the "good work," and "win credit for all women, while winning for yourself the Boylston Medical Prize for 1876." Jacobi met the challenge; and her pioneering essay, "The Question of Rest for Women During Menstruation," which, to the opposition's chagrin, won the esteemed prize, was exemplary in its modern statistical methodology. Her conclusion, that there existed "nothing in the nature of menstruation to imply the necessity, or even the desirability, of rest for women whose nutrition is really normal," directly challenged conservative

medical opinion.[14] Despite widespread respect for her paper, it failed to convince many physicians, and the debate continued into the 20th century.

In the realm of emotion, of course, apologists for women's sphere needed to be neither scientific nor consistent; they offered arguments for female inferiority, vulnerability, and dependence alongside claims for their moral superiority and responsibility. After all it was they who molded the life of future generations and spent tireless hours tending the sick long after the physician had retired from his daily rounds. Nineteenth-century society never did come to terms with this Manichean image of women, at least not until female physicians and other social feminists exploited the contradictions in the ideal and forced a reconciliation of the two extremes. In the process they created a new image for their sex and a broader definition of woman's sphere.

## II

Women physicians argued within the context of the shared values of 19th-century culture. They and their male supporters took seriously the idea of their moral superiority and their ability as natural healers, embracing 19th-century definitions of feminine qualities intact. With intelligence and skill they made Victorian ideology yield to them and used these notions to justify seeking medical education.

One example of their subtle use of the value structure has already been noted: their reversal of the "delicacy" argument. Defending the "propriety of entrusting feminine life to feminine hands," they denounced exclusive male attendance to women's ailments as an outrage against female modesty pernicious to the "social and moral welfare of society."[15] Elizabeth Blackwell called it an "unnatural and monstrous arrangement" that women had "no resort but to men, in those diseases peculiar to themselves." Were the "methods of modern medicine quietly received and passively submitted to," she claimed, "it would indicate a terrible deficiency in some of the most important elements of womanly character." Here medical science clashed with morality, in the demand that to preserve morality women be taught science.[16]

Female physicians did not quarrel with the concept of separate spheres for men and women, though they meant something quite different from their opponents when they spoke of "woman's sphere." They sought an altogether novel definition of "femaleness." Examining the ethical implications of scientific methods for medicine and society, they claimed for women the task of integrating Science and Morality.

A glance at the titles of the popular health manuals of the period reveals the pervasiveness of the concept of Woman as Healer.[17] In response to these widespread assumptions, traditionalists had glorified women's abilities as nurses, while denying them the right to become physicians. Supporters of medical training for women were outraged by such logic. "Is not Woman man's Superior?" asked Dr. J. P. Chesney of Missouri. "It is an idea extremely paradoxical," he continued, "to suppose that woman, the fairest and best of God's handiwork, and practical medicine, a calling little less sacred than the holy ministry itself, should, when united, become a loathsome abomination . . . from which virtue must stand widely aloof." If the traditionalists' own logic were applied consistently, he noted, "men would long ago have been banished from obstetrics."[18]

Zealously cataloguing women's past contributions to healing, supporters of female medical education argued that women needed the tools of modern medicine. Women *would* attend in the sickroom, and instinct and sympathy were not sufficient as advances in medical therapeutics rendered folk medicine ineffective. "It has begun to occur to people," observed Dr. Emmeline Cleveland of the Woman's Medical College of Pennsylvania in 1859, "that perhaps the fullest performance of her own home duties" required of woman "a more extended and systematic education . . . especially in those departments of science and literature which have practical bearing upon the lives and health of the community."[19]

Women doctors and their allies frequently echoed Victorian sentimentality over womanly attributes. Like their opponents they constantly connected womanhood with the guardianship of home and children. Women were morally superior to men, claimed Elizabeth Blackwell, because of the "spiritual power of maternity." The true physician, male or female, she argued, "must possess the essential qualities of maternity."[20]

Medical training was necessary for scientific motherhood. Ignorance of their own bodies and poor training in child management were taking their toll on American mothers and offspring alike. "What higher trust could be dedicated to the wife and mother," asked Dr. Joseph Longshore in his introductory lecture to the first class at the Woman's Medical College of Pennsylvania, "than guardianship of the health of the household?" His colleague Emmeline Cleveland, a brilliant gynecological surgeon, affirmed the necessity of giving to all women knowledge of the human body. She reminded her students that their high vocation was "as nature's appointed guardians of childhood and youth," that as mothers and teachers they would "become the conservators of public health and in an eminent degree responsible for the physical and moral evils which afflict society."[21]

Medical women like Cleveland intended to play a central role in the elevation of their sisters. As science was brought to bear on domestic life, women physicians would become the "connecting link" between the science of the medical profession and the everyday life of women.[22] To accomplish this purpose, each of the female medical schools offered courses in physiology and hygiene to nonmatriculants, who were often mothers and teachers hoping to gain knowledge in health education.

When critics charged that medical training was wasted on women who would eventually marry and have children, female physicians responded by pointing out that medical knowledge was important for any woman, even if the skills acquired would not be used to practice. Competence in medicine made women better mothers. Others were bolder, displaying the temerity that helped to expand society's conception of woman's role: they saw no necessary conflict between motherhood and general practice. This recognition of the possibility of combining marriage and career marked a radical departure from 19th-century thinking. "A woman can love and respect her family just as much if not more," asserted Dr. Georgiana Glenn, "when she feels that she is supporting herself and adding to their comfort and happiness." Dr. Mary Putnam Jacobi agreed. Conceding that marriage complicated professional life, she nevertheless felt that "the increased vigor and vitality accruing to health women from the bearing and possession of children, a good deal more than compensates for the difficulties involved in caring for them, when professional duties replace the more usual ones, of sewing, cooking, etc."[23]

The social Darwinism of the post-Civil War period enabled traditionalists to reiterate their prejudices with the finality of scientific truth. Little changed in the controversy over female physicians besides the language of the debate. Scientific rationalism predominated by the 1880s, with evolution and eugenics mustered in defense of both sides. Critics of women doctors made pessimistic pronouncements that female higher education would be biologically destructive of the race.[24] Female physicians countered with measured optimism. They depicted themselves as living examples of the transition to higher life forms. Yet they also remained suspicious of prevailing trends, especially the frivolous pursuits of leisured women. Warning that the increased leisure accruing from technological advances demanded that women be given noble work to do, they urged society to check the notorious aimlessness of the civilized woman's life. Women's boredom was notorious: "For one case of breakdown from overwork among women," quipped Dr. Ruffin Coleman, "there are a score from ennui and sheer inanation from doing nothing."[25]

Along with most American scientists of the period, physicians accepted the neo-Lamarckian concept of the inheritance of acquired characteristics. Women doctors drew the logical object lesson: if mental as well as physical characteristics were inherited, the race would steadily improve only if women could uplift themselves. Their arguments remained a warning as well as a prophecy: Hold back your women—your mothers—and you retard the race.[26]

Medical women also insisted that they had special contributions to make to the profession. Feminization could enhance the practice of medicine, which concentrated on the eradication of suffering. Association with female colleagues would "exert a beneficial influence on the male." Combining the best of masculine and feminine attributes should raise medical practice to its highest level.

Occasionally supporters carried the implications of this reasoning even further. Female physicians expected to challenge heroic therapeutics directly. As the "handmaids of nature," women would place greater value on the "natural system of curing diseases . . . in contradistinction to the pharmaceu-

tical." They would promote a "generally milder and less energetic mode of practice." "The Past," claimed the health reformer Mary Gove Nichols, "with the lancet, and poison, and operative surgery, did not insult woman by asking her to become a physician; and the Past has not asked her to become a hangman, general or jailer. We may well excuse all believers in Allopathy, if they judge woman unfit for the profession."

Many women physicians did spurn heroic medicine. The husband of Hannah Longshore, the first female physician to establish a practice in Philadelphia, recorded the following in a biographical sketch of his wife:

> The Woman's Medical College claimed to be an entirely regular or old school institution and its faculty had a testimony to bear against homeopathy and eclecticism or in any irregularity of its graduates from the established old school practice. But many of its alumni [sic] discovered that the growing aversion to large doses of strong and disagreeable medicine among the more liberal and progressive elements in society and that many intelligent woman had become tinctured with the heresy of Homeopathy and gave a preference to the physician who would prescribe or administer their milder and pleasant remedies, and especially for the children who would take their medicines voluntarily. This discovery led the woman doctor to an investigation of their remedies and theories of therapeutics and to partial adoption of their remedies and methods of treatment. This conformity to the demands for mild remedies gave the women doctors access to many families whose views were in accord with the reform movements that recognized the growing interest in enlarging the sphere of woman. The woman doctors who saw that the door was opening for this reform of regular practice and prepared themselves accordingly were the first to get into successful business.

Marie Zakrzewska, who, as founder of the New England Hospital for Women and Children in Boston, earned the respect of even the most stubborn members of the male opposition, also remained skeptical of heroic dosing. In a letter to Elizabeth Blackwell she confessed that her whole success in practice was based on the cautious use of medicine, "often used as Placebos in infinitesimal forms." "In fact," she wrote, "I have the reputation among my large clientele, men, women, and children as giving hardly any medicine but teaching people how to keep well without it. This subject is a large theme and I am thankful from the innermost of my emotions . . . that nobody has ever been injured, if not relieved by my prescriptions."[27]

In keeping with this interest in prevention rather than cure, friends claimed that women physicians would become zealous advocates of public health and social morality. Emmeline Cleveland noted that women were naturally altruistic, while Elizabeth Blackwell expected her female colleagues to provide the "onward impulse" in seeing to it that human beings were "well born, well nourished, and well educated." Dr. Sarah Adamson Dolley urged women doctors to bring to the profession their "moral power." "Educated medical women," wrote Dr. Eliza Mosher, of the University of Michigan, "touch humanity in a manner different from men; by virtue of their womanhood, their interest in children, in girls and young women, both moral and otherwise, in homes and in society." Most of their male supporters agreed. Dr. James J. Walsh admitted that men did not recognize their social duties as readily as women. "Therefore," he confessed, "I have always welcomed the coming into the medical profession of that leaven of tender humanity that women represent."[28]

### III

It is possible to claim that women doctors made their arguments, not necessarily because they believed them, but because they sensed the pervasiveness of traditional ideas about woman's sphere. Their rhetoric, as well as that of other feminists, has been interpreted as a calculated and well-planned offensive designed to challenge 19th-century assumptions with familiar ideas. Yet women physicians sincerely believed that they were different from men and that they had their own special contribution to make to society. Of course many of them realized the expediency of their case, especially because it did not wholly challenge traditional assumptions. Yet the desire to educate women in medicine remained part of 19th-century social feminism, a movement with roots in antebellum reform and nurtured in an atmosphere of perfectionist concern with the revival of moral values. Female physicians were not the only group of women to seek a broadening of women's role by expanding the notion of separate spheres.

Certainly many women chose a career in medicine for more private reasons than the belief in their own special female abilities. Many probably saw medical practice as a lucrative means of self support. But whatever their personal motives, such women belonged to a movement that justified itself in larger terms, and they gained their self-image from the social context in which they acted. After wishing the New York Infirmary graduating class of 1899 financial success—"we are always glad to hear of a woman's making money"—Dean Emily Blackwell urged her students to remember that "there are other kinds of success that . . . we hope you will always consider far higher prizes." These, she continued, were "the consciousness of doing good work in your own line, of being of use to others, of exerting an influence for right in all social and professional questions." Readily conceding that her students "doubtless all entered upon medical study from individual motives," she hoped that they had learned "that the work of every woman physician, her character and influence, her success or failure, tells upon all, and helps or hinders those who work around her or come after her."

Forty years earlier, a younger Emily Blackwell confided similar sentiments to her diary when she thanked God that she was only 25 and not yet too old to commence a life's labor full of "great deeds." Newly decided on a medical career, she prayed that at life's close God would grant her the ability to look back on a "woman's work done for thee and my fellows." Opportunities were then appearing for women to live a "heroic life," and Emily desperately wished to avail herself of them.[29]

Victorian ideology, then, was not entirely repressive to women. On the contrary, courageous individuals hoping to move out of the home could use the ideology for their own ends, and in a way consistent with their acceptance of prevailing values. The glorification of woman's moral power was their most potent weapon. Taking refuge in the concept of female superiority, they provided future generations of women with an imperfect but essential stepping stone on the route to sexual equality.

While both sides in the debate claimed to be seeking moral progress and civilization's advancement, female physicians, in their commitment to using women's abilities systematically and scientifically, diverged fundamentally from their conservative opponents. Women doctors hoped to reform society by feminizing it, a task which required the professionalization of "womanhood." Acknowledging that their goals required a broader interpretation of woman's sphere, they felt this a small price to pay for a morally righteous and civilized America.

Nineteenth-century women doctors never drifted out of touch with the mainstream of Victorian ideology. As proponents of the gradual expansion of women's role, they perceived gradual change to be the only kind the public would tolerate. Slowly they succeeded in creating a positive image for the female physician. A minority proved that wives and mothers could handle a professional career. Their inevitable interaction with male colleagues eventually convinced many critics that women could be competent doctors and still maintain their femininity.

Female physicians confined themselves to feminine specialties—obstetrics and gynecology in the 19th century, pediatrics, public health, teaching, and counseling later on. Such specialization was not due solely to resistance from male professionals, although women doctors occasionally blamed discrimination. Women practitioners gravitated to these specialties because they were conscious of their "special" abilities. They concerned themselves with the health problems of women and children because they hoped to raise the moral tone of society through the improvement of family life.

Doubtless for some unmarried women physicians, the practice of obstetrics or pediatrics gave them vicarious fulfillment from an intimate involvement in the primary events of the female life cycle, while freeing them from traditional Victorian marriage. Recently, historians have explored the female support systems that existed throughout the 19th century.[30] Many women physicians gravitated to feminine specialties—in fact, to medicine itself—out of a desire to perpetuate these support systems. Mothers, they argued, would more readily discuss their problems with women doctors because male physicians did not have "the patience to deal with the anxieties, ignorance, and frequent terrors of women who are often overwhelmed by some misunderstood condition in themselves or in their children." During the sensitive period of gestation, a woman needed someone whom she could approach "without reserve," and from whom she could get "a woman's sympathy." "Being women as well as physicians," acknowledged Dr. Florence B. Sherbon, president of the Iowa State Society of Medical Women, "we share with our sex in the actual and potential motherhood of the race. Being women we make common cause with all women. . . . And being women and mothers, our first and closest and dearest interest is the child. . . ."[31]

Such arguments naturally had limitations. Confining themselves to women's concerns circumscribed women physicians' professional influence. A few even willingly advocated an informal curtailment of their medical role, hoping to gain support by taking themselves out of competition with men.[32] But the more perceptive disdained this approach. Such women converted early to the modern and empirical world of professional medicine, and their first love was science. Often uneasy in the moralistic world of their medical sisters, they exhibited a toughness and clarity of vision which set them apart from those women who used medicine primarily as a moral platform. Physicians like Mary Putnam Jacobi and Marie Zakrzewska insisted from the beginning that medical women need be of superior mettle. Fearing that specialization in diseases of women and children would mean a loss of grounding in general medicine, they warned that women would be justly relegated to the position of second-class professionals. Eventually their performance even within their specialty would become second-rate. If women were to succeed in medicine, they asserted, they had to be thoroughly trained.[33] Despite their predictions, specializing remained popular throughout the 19th century and into the next because it provided advantages in blunting the resentment of male colleagues.

The emphasis female physicians placed on the mother's child-rearing responsibility also reflected and reinforced social values which would present future problems. As more married women entered the work force, acute ideological conflicts arose to hamper the development of alternative methods of child-rearing. When Charlotte Perkins Gilman proposed to professionalize child care at the turn of the century, she was virtually ignored. Even more revealing is the intensity of the conflict over child care centers that emerged within the federal government during World War II, a time when married women were entering the work force in large numbers and government facilities were a palpable necessity.[34]

While stressing women's peculiar adaptability to medicine, women doctors perpetuated an exaggerated concept of womanhood, rendering their arguments inapplicable to other, less obviously "feminine" pursuits. Dr. Frances Emily White attributed women's great success in medicine compared with other professions to a "peculiar fitness" for the work and the lack elsewhere "of equal opportunities for the exercise of those qualities that have become specialized in women."[35] Pursuits like teaching and nursing fit the pattern well, but law did not. Though women lawyers chose to justify their interests in a similar fashion, it was harder for them to claim that their work was an extension of women's natural sphere, and, indeed, few women preferred law to medicine in the 19th and early 20th centuries. All the reasons for this disparity remain complex, but the "natural sphere" argument did exhibit vexing limitations as women moved out of the home and into the world.[36]

A few perceptive individuals struggled uncomfortably with the implications of such reasoning. The journalist Helen Watterson, for example, denounced the woman movement's emphasis on "woman's qualities." Mary Putnam Jacobi quipped that "recently emancipated people are always bores, until they themselves have forgotten all about their emancipation." And Marie Zakrzewska frowned on women who chose medicine out of female "sympathy." The only motives the profession permitted its votaries, she maintained, were "an inborn taste and talent for medicine, and an earnest desire and love of scientific investigation."[37]

The brilliant Jacobi sensed the psychological disadvantages that hampered women physicians from attaining equal status within the profession. Society was still against them, impairing both their own confidence and that of other women in them. Because society refused to judge medical women by their achievements, women doctors were in danger of setting lower standards for themselves. In the 19th century any woman who ventured beyond the domestic role was considered an anomaly. Jacobi insistently urged her students to measure themselves by the highest standards of professional excellence. Mediocre women doctors, she warned, would doom their cause.

Jacobi, forever impatient with the deficiencies of the women's medical schools, tolerated no compromises in quality because of their disadvantaged position. Her tough-mindedness remained a source of inspiration to those who occasionally lost sight of the larger goal. Still the courage and conviction of the early generations of medical women are beyond reproach. In the face of strenuous opposition they pressed for the right of women to study medicine as part of a redefinition of woman's role in a reformed industrial society. Although their goals remained circumscribed by a particular cultural vision, these pioneers effected real changes in their own lives and in the lives of many women around them. They did so without *radical* ideological innovation. Paving the way for the future by their deeds, they failed to understand that true equality between the sexes could not come if women remained confined to a "sphere," no matter how expansively it was defined. Nineteenth-century women doctors passed on a large legacy of unfinished business to their daughters and granddaughters. They left future generations of women to struggle with the implications of Mary Putnam Jacobi's prophetic warning, "if you cannot learn to act without masters, you evidently will never become the real equals of those who do."[38]

## NOTES

1  The last statistic is taken from a survey done by W. C. Hunt, statistician, of Washington, D.C., reprinted in H. Scott Turner, "History of women in medicine," *Los Angeles J. Eclectic Med.*, 1905, 2: 125. The number of male physicians in the United States in 1900 is in dispute. Census records set the figure at 132,000, the A.M.A. at 119,749. See U.S. Bureau of the Census, *Historical Statistics of the United States: Colonial Times to 1970* (Washington, D.C., 1975), Part 1, pp. 75–76.

2  See William B. Walker, "The health reform movement in the United States, 1830–1870" (Ph.D. dissertation, Johns Hopkins Univ., 1955); John Blake, "Health Reform," in *The Rise of Adventism: Religion*

*and Society in Mid-Nineteenth-Century America,* ed. Edwin S. Gaustad (New York, 1975), pp. 30–49. For health reform and women see Regina Markell Morantz, "Nineteenth century health reform and women: a program of self-help," in *Medicine Without Doctors: Home Health Care in American History,* ed. G. Risse, R. Numbers, and J. Leavitt (New York, 1977), pp. 73–93, and "Making women modern: middle class women and health reform in nineteenth century America," *J. Soc. Hist.,* 1977, *10*: 490–507.

3   W. W. Parker, M.D., "Women's place in the Christian world: superior morally, inferior mentally to man — not qualified for medicine or law — the contrariety and harmony of the sexes," *Tr. Med. Soc. St. Va.,* 1892, pp. 86–107.

4   Paul de Lacy Baker, "Shall women be admitted into the medical profession?" *Tr. Med. Assn. St. Ala.,* 1880, *33*: 191–206. See also Julien Picot, "Shall women practice medicine?" *North Carolina Med. J.,* 1885, *16*: 10–21; N. Williams, "A discussion on female physicians," read before the Clay, Lysander and Schroeppel (N.Y.) Medical Association, *Boston Med. & Surg. J.,* 1850, *43*: 69–75; J. F. Ziegler, "Women's sphere," Presidential address to the Medical Society of Pennsylvania, *Tr. Med. Soc. St. Penn.,* 1882, *14*: 25–38; Joseph Spaeth, "The study of medicine by women," *Richmond & Louisville Med. J.,* 1873, *16*: 40–56; *Men and Women Medical Students and the Woman Movement* (Philadelphia, 1869), *passim.*

5   J. S. Weatherly, "Woman: her rights and her wrongs," *Tr. Med. Assn. St. Ala.,* 1872, *24*: 63–80. For a reversal of the argument, defending female medical education as a step *up* from primitive brutality, see Edwin Fussell, *Valedictory Address to the Students of the Female Medical College of Pennsylvania* (Philadelphia, 1857), pp. 5–6.

6   Reynell Coates, *Introductory Lecture to the Class of the Female Medical College of Pennsylvania* (Philadelphia, 1861), pp. 3–4. See also articles cited in n. 4 and n. 5. "Female physicians," *Boston Med. & Surg. J.,* 1856, *54*: 169–174, and "Female practitioners of medicine," *Boston Med. & Surg. J.,* 1867, *76*: 272–274.

7   Medical women, of course, claimed just the reverse. See Weatherly, "Woman: her rights," p. 76; Sophia Jex-Blake, *Medical Women: Two Essays* (Edinburgh, 1872), p. 36; J. P. Chesney, "Woman as a physician," *Richmond & Louisville Med. J.,* 1871, *11*: 6.

8   Samuel Gregory, who founded the New England Female Medical College, was one of those concerned primarily with the improprieties of male accoucheurs.

9   Weatherly, "Woman: her rights," p. 75.

10  See Martin Kaufman, "The admission of women to 19th-century American medical societies," *Bull.*

*Hist. Med.,* 1976, *50*: 251–260. The assessment I give here of the quality of medical education at the women's medical colleges is based on my own preliminary research. Although the majority of male physicians opposed the medical education of women, female physicians had many prominent male supporters who were loyal and enthusiastic. These included Henry I. Bowditch and James Chadwick in Boston; Steven Smith and Abraham Jacobi in New York; Hiram Corson, Henry Hartshorne, and later Alfred Stillé in Philadelphia; and William Byford and I. N. Danforth in Chicago.

11  *Boston Med. & Surg. J.,* 1884, *111*: 90, 1849, *40*: 505; 1873, *89*: 23. "The practice of midwifery by females — by one of the class," *Boston Med. & Surg. J.,* 1849, *41*: 59–61; Coates, *Introductory Lecture,* pp. 3–4; D. W. Graham, "The demand for medically educated women," *J.A.M.A.,* 1886, *6*: 479.

12  Carroll Smith-Rosenberg, "Puberty to menopause: the cycle of femininity," in *Clio's Consciousness Raised,* ed. M. Hartman and L. Banner (New York, 1974), pp. 1–22. The debate over premenstrual tension and the related effects of woman's cycle on her psyche still goes on in medical circles. See K. J. and R. J. Lennane, "Alleged psychogenic disorders in women — a possible manifestation of sexual prejudice," *New Eng. J. Med.,* Feb. 8, 1973, *290*: 288–292.

13  "Female physicians," p. 169; Horatio Storer, "The fitness of women to practice medicine," *J. Gynec. Soc. Boston,* 1870, *2*: 266–267; "Female practitioners of medicine," pp. 272–274; E. H. Clarke, *Sex In Education: Or a Fair Chance for the Girls* (Boston, 1873); Lawrence Irwell, "The competition of the sexes and its results," read before the American Association for the Advancement of Science, August 1896, *Am. Medico-Surg. Bull.,* 1896, *10*: 316–320.

14  Mary Putnam Jacobi, *The Question of Rest for Women During Menstruation* (New York, 1877), p. 227. See also C. Alice Baker to Mary Putnam Jacobi, Nov. 7, 1874, Jacobi MSS, Schlesinger Library, Radcliffe. For studies by other women doctors see Elizabeth R. Thelberg, physician at Vassar, "College education as a factor in the physical life of women," Alumnae Association of the Woman's Medical College of Pennsylvania, *Transactions,* 1899, pp. 73–87; Elizabeth C. Underhill, resident physician at Mt. Holyoke, "The effect of college life on the health of women students," *Woman's Med. J.,* 1913, *22*: 31–33; Clelia Duel Mosher, "Normal menstruation and some factors modifying it," *Johns Hopkins Hosp. Bull.,* 1901, *12*: 178–179.

15  George Gregory, *Medical Morals* (New York, 1852), pp. 5, 20; Rev. William Hosmer, *Appeal to Husbands and Wives in Favor of Female Physicians* (New York,

1853), pp. 3–24; Thomas Ewell, *Letters to Ladies Detailing Important Information Concerning Themselves and Infants* (Philadelphia, 1817), pp. 23–27.

16 Elizabeth Blackwell, *Address on the Medical Education of Women* (New York, 1856), pp. 8–9.

17 For example, G. Fenning, *Every Mother's Book: or the Child's Best Doctor, Being a Complete Course of Directions for the Medical Management of Mothers and Children* (New York, n.d.), or D. Wark, *The Practical Home Doctor for Women* (New York, 1882).

18 Chesney, "Woman as a physician," p. 4.

19 Emmeline Cleveland, *Introductory Lecture to the Class of the Female Medical College of Pennsylvania* (Philadelphia, 1859), p. 7.

20 Elizabeth Blackwell, "Criticism of Gronlund's Cooperative Commonwealth; Chapter X–Woman," given before the Fellowship of New Life, n.d., pp. 9–10; *The Influence of Women in the Profession of Medicine* (London, 1889), p. 11; "Anatomy," Lecture Notes, n.d., all in Blackwell MSS, Library of Congress.

21 Joseph Longshore, *Introductory Lecture to the Class of the Female Medical College of Pennsylvania* (Philadelphia, 1859), p. 11; Joseph Longshore, *The Practical Importance of Female Medical Education* (Philadelphia, 1853), p. 6; Female Medical College of Pennsylvania, "Appeal to the Corporators," Medical College of Pennsylvania Archives [hereafter cited as M.C.P.]; Ann Preston, *Valedictory Address to the Graduating Class of the Female Medical College of Pennsylvania* (Philadelphia, 1858), pp. 9–10.

22 Elizabeth and Emily Blackwell, *Medicine as a Profession for Women* (New York, 1860), pp. 8–9; Richard C. Cabot, "Women in medicine," *J.A.M.A.,* 1915, *65:* 9–17; Cora B. Lattia, "Public health education among women," *N.Y. St. J. Med.,* 1913, *13:* 12–17; "Appeal to the Corporators."

23 Georgiana Glenn, "Are women as capable of becoming physicians as men," *The Clinic,* 1875, *9:* 243–245; Jacobi, "Inaugural Address," Women's Medical College of the New York Infirmary, *Chicago Med. J. & Exam.,* 1881, *42:* 580.

24 A. Lapthorn Smith, "Higher education of women and race suicide," *Popular Science Monthly,* 1905, *66:* 466–473; A. Lapthorn Smith, "What civilization is doing for the human female," *Tr. Southern Surg. & Gynec. Assn.,* 1889, *2:* 352–360; F. W. Van Dyke, "Higher education as the cause of physical decay in women," *Med. Red.,* 1905, *67:* 296–298; William Goodell, R. Gaillard Thomas, M. Allen Starr, J. J. Putnam, "Symposium on the co-education of the sexes," *Med. News, N.Y.,* 1889, *55:* 667–672; J. T. Clegg, "Some of the ailments of woman due to her higher development in the scale of evolution," *Texas Hlth J.,* 1890–91, *3:* 57–59; A. J. C. Skene, *Educa-*

tion and Culture as Related to the Health and Diseases of Women (Detroit, 1889), p. 39.

25 Elizabeth and Emily Blackwell, *Medicine as a Profession,* p. 4; Henry Hartshorne, *Valedictory Address to the Graduating Class of the Woman's Medical College of Pennsylvania* (Philadelphia, 1872), pp. 13–14; Louise Fiske-Byron, "Woman and nature," *N.Y. Med. J.,* 1887, *66:* 627–628. For Ruffin Coleman's remark see "Woman's relation to higher education and the professions as viewed from physiological and other stand points," *Tr. Med. Assn. St. Ala.,* 1889, *42:* 233–247.

26 Emily Blackwell made this argument even before social Darwinism came into vogue: "Mankind," she confided to her diary, "will never be what they should be until women are nobler." Diary, June 4, 1852, p. 83, Blackwell MSS, Library of Congress. See also *J. Hyg. & Herald Hlth.,* 1894, *44:* 236; J. G. Kiernan, "Mental advance in woman and race suicide," *Alienist and Neurologist,* 1910, *30:* 594–599; Elizabeth Blackwell, *Pioneer Work in Opening the Medical Profession to Women* (New York, 1895), p. 253.

27 Samuel Gregory, "Female physicians," *The Living Age,* 1862, *73:* 243–249; Mary Gove Nichols, "Woman the physician," *Water-Cure J.,* 1851, *12:* 3; Thomas Longshore's manuscript is in the M.C.P. Archives, p. 106. See also Marie Zakrzewska to Elizabeth Blackwell, March 21, 1891, Blackwell MSS, Schlesinger Library.

28 Blackwell, *Pioneer Work,* p. 253; Emmeline Cleveland, *Valedictory Address to the Graduating Class of the Woman's Medical College of Pennsylvania* (Philadelphia, 1874), p. 3; Eliza Mosher, "The value of organization—what it has done for women," *Woman's Med. J.,* 1916, *26:* 1–4; James J. Walsh, "Women in the medical world," *N.Y. Med. J.,* 1912, *96:* 1324–1328.

29 Emily Blackwell, "Address at the Thirty-first Annual Commencement of the Women's Medical College of the New York Infirmary," May 25, 1899, printed in *Final Catalogue* (New York, 1899). Also Emily Blackwell, Diary, October 1851, p. 47. Rarely until after 1900 does one come across the argument that medicine is enriching from the standpoint of personal development. It is primarily society which is to benefit; individuals gain *because* they are aiding society.

30 Carroll Smith-Rosenberg, "The female world of love and ritual: women and sexuality in nineteenth century America," *Signs,* Autumn 1975, *1:* 1–29.

31 Margaret Vaupel Clark, "Medical women's contribution to the education of mothers," *Woman's Med. J.,* 1915, *25:* 126–128; Glenn, "Are women as capable," pp. 243–245; "The woman physician and her special obligation and opportunity," *Woman's Med.*

*J.,* 1915, *25*: 74–79. Numerous women doctors gave public health lectures.

32   For the use of the argument see J. Stainbeck Wilson, "Female medical education," *Southern Med. & Surg. J.,* 1854, *10*: 1–17; Emmeline Cleveland, *Valedictory Address to the Graduating Class of the Female Medical College of Pennsylvania* (Philadelphia, 1858), p. 10; Clark, "Medical women's contribution," pp. 126–128; Harriet Williams, "Women in medicine," *Texas Med. News,* 1903, *12*: 613–615.

33   See Jacobi, "Inaugural address," pp. 561–585.

34   Elizabeth Blackwell, for example, opposed public child care. Her belief was that parents as well as children suffered: "Neither can parental responsibility be wisely devolved upon the creche, the nursery, the school and the workshop. . . . No social arrangements must ever be allowed to destroy the essential education which is given to the parent by the children." "Criticism of Gronlund," p. 11. For government ambivalence see William Chafe, *The American Woman* (New York, 1972), pp. 159–172.

35   Frances Emily White, "The American medical woman," *Med. News, N.Y.,* 1895, *67*: 123–128.

36   An interesting example of how conservative this type of argument can be is provided by the situation in India and Pakistan. There "purdah," the seclusion of women, still exists. Yet similar arguments for training a core of professional women to administer to an exclusively female clientele are extremely popular. See Hanna Papenek, "Purdah in Pakistan: seclusion and modern occupations for women," *Journal of Marriage and the Family,* August 1971, pp. 517–530.

37   Helen Watterson, "Woman's excitement over 'Woman'," *Forum,* 1893, *16*: 75–85; Mary Putnam Jacobi, "An address delivered at the Commencement of the Women's Medical College of the New York Infirmary, May 30, 1883," *Arch. Med.,* 1883, *10*: 59–71; Marie Zakrzewska, *Introductory Lecture Before the New England Medical College* (Boston, 1859), pp. 3–26; C. L. Franklin, "Women and medicine," *The Nation,* 1891, *52*: 131.

38   Jacobi, "Commencement address," p. 70.

# 12

## Female Solidarity and Professional Success: The Dilemma of Women Doctors in Late 19th-Century America

### VIRGINIA G. DRACHMAN

In 1886, Edna Dow Cheney, the president of the all-woman's New England Hospital for Women and Children, proudly announced that women's struggle to become doctors was over. "We have no longer to plead woman's right to study medicine," she asserted, "no occasion to ask opportunity for her to practice it."[1] Less than ten years after Cheney made her public declaration of women's progress, Dr. Bertha Van Hoosen, the resident physician at the hospital, wrote to the board of physicians in exasperation, "the interns are unhappy . . . they feel they are losing ground."[2] Together these conflicting statements reflect a paradox of progress which confronted women doctors in the last quarter of the 19th century. On the one hand, they made significant inroads into the medical profession. On the other hand, the progress they made created new problems which often divided women doctors against each other.

Historians have focused on the first part of this story—women's struggle to enter the medical profession. This interpretation might best be understood as the struggle/victory model: male doctors sought to bar women from medicine; in response, female solidarity overcame male opposition, and women entered the medical profession.[3] The vehicles of entry were the medical institutions founded and run by women for women. From this struggle/victory point of view, historians have understood the all-women's medical institutions as the product of female solidarity in the face of male opposition. One historian has aptly described the New England Hospital, for example, as a "feminist show-

place."[4] Indeed, it *was* a triumph to build an all-women's hospital: the New England Hospital and other all-women's medical institutions stood before the public as symbols of the success of feminism.

But, there is a second, more complex chapter to this story which the struggle/victory interpretation masks. As women made inroads into the mainstream of medicine, they struggled more frequently among themselves and acted less and less like a cohesive group with shared values. Many began to question the value of female solidarity. To be sure, some still saw it as crucial to women doctors' professional survival. Yet, others saw female solidarity as an obstacle to their professional progress. This essay focuses on this second chapter in the history of women doctors. It demonstrates that by the late 19th century, women doctors no longer faced only a struggle to break the sexual barriers to the medical profession. Rather, the struggle to become a physician was simply their first battle in the more enduring struggle to *be* one.

The arena for this struggle was often the all-women's medical institutions. Within the walls of their hospitals, colleges, and medical societies women doctors attempted to reconcile their commitment to female solidarity with their desire for professional success. The New England Hospital provides an excellent place to examine 19th-century women doctors as they faced this challenge. While the history of the New England Hospital is important, the more significant story concerns the women doctors who went there to practice medicine and forge their professional lives. It is their story that makes institutions like the New England Hospital important sources for the social history of women and medicine.

Virginia G. Drachman is Associate Professor of History at Tufts University, Medford, Massachusetts.

Reprinted with permission from the *Journal of Social History*, 1982, *15*: 607–619.

Founded in Boston in 1862, the New England Hospital was unique among 19th-century hospitals because its founders were women, its physicians were women, and its patients were women and children. Dr. Marie Zakrzewska, the hospital's founder and central figure until her death in 1902, opened the doors to the New England Hospital with three goals: to provide sick women with medical care from physicians of their own sex, to provide women doctors with clinical training, and to train nurses. To Zakrzewska the central purpose of the hospital was to provide women doctors with equal professional opportunities with male physicians by offering them clinical training. "The most striking feature in its character," Zakrzewska explained of the hospital, "is that it is designed to give to educated women physicians an equal chance of proving their capacity as hospital attendants with their medical brethren, and to admit only female students to its wards, as all other hospitals close their doors to women as medical students."[5] To be sure, clinical training was not readily accessible to the young male doctor-to-be. Since the typical medical school offered lectures exclusively, the would-be doctor seeking practical experience had either to apprentice himself to a physician or work in a hospital.[6] Yet, for the woman doctor seeking clinical experience, the situation was even more difficult: hospitals in New York, Philadelphia, and Boston were closed to women. Zakrzewska sought to duplicate for women at the New England Hospital the clinical advantages and professional opportunities available to men elsewhere. Only in this way, she felt, would women doctors be able to participate as equals with the best of male physicians.

Ironically, embedded within this commitment to professional equality for women and men in medicine were the seeds of new problems and challenges which confronted Zakrzewska in the last quarter of the 19th century. In fact, the closer she saw women doctors come to attaining her goal of professional equality with men, the more she saw her hospital—which had contributed so significantly to women doctors' professional success—lose ground. In her later years, Zakrzewska watched as women doctors increasingly rejected the New England Hospital for other routes to professional success.

When the New England Hospital opened its doors, however, women had few professional alternatives. Only the New England Hospital and the all-women's New York Infirmary provided women doctors with clinical experience and professional opportunities. Faced with few options, a significant number of women who came to the hospital as interns stayed on after their training. During the hospital's first decade, Zakrzewska steadily built up a staff of physicians primarily from interns within the hospital. By 1875, she had eight women doctors working with her, all of whom dedicated their professional lives to the New England Hospital. By 1900, five of the original physicians still worked with Zakrzewska at the hospital. The other three worked there until they became sick or died. With Zakrzewska, these women were the leaders of the hospital. Having come up the ranks within the hospital in its early years, they constituted a distinct group who understood the role of the New England Hospital as Zakrzewska did. As the hospital's board of physicians, this relatively unchanging group of women doctors ran the New England Hospital day in and day out, setting the direction and pace of growth at the hospital throughout the last quarter of the century.

Yet, running the hospital grew steadily more difficult. As the century progressed, the board of physicians frequently encountered dissatisfaction and conflict as they confronted women doctors with different professional experiences, expectations, and options than their own. Over the next few decades, clinical opportunities for women expanded as women opened other hospitals as well as dispensaries in cities around the country. Together with the more than a dozen women's medical colleges which opened in the second half of the century, the New England Hospital became part of a network of women's institutions born out of a need for female solidarity and a desire to provide women with professional opportunities in medicine. Furthermore, the New England Hospital played a significant role in expanding this network. Several women who trained there went on to open other women's medical institutions: Mary Thompson founded the Chicago Hospital for Women and Children and later the Woman's Medical College in Chicago, while Anita Tyng and Mary DeHart opened dispensaries for women in Rhode Island and New Jersey, respectively. Zakrzewska was proud of the contributions her graduates made to expanding this chain of women's medical institutions. "This shows," she boasted publicly in her annual report in 1875, "that the seed sown here has fallen on fertile ground."[7]

In the last decade of the 19th century, women doctors also began to make inroads into the mainstream of medicine. The formerly all-male institutions began to open their doors to women, thereby providing them with access to equal professional training with men, the goal for which Zakrzewska had originally strived when she opened the New England Hospital in 1862. This breakdown of professional barriers was wide-ranging, encompassing medical schools, medical societies, and hospitals. In 1870, for example, the University of Michigan Medical School became coeducational. By 1893, women could attend Tufts University Medical School or Boston University Medical School in Boston. And in the same year, when Johns Hopkins Medical School opened to men and women on an equal basis, women finally gained access to medical training at one of the country's top-level universities. When Cornell followed in 1899, it appeared that women had finally climbed the last rung of the medical school ladder.

While women doctors gained educational advantages, they also found professional colleagueship with male physicians in the formerly male medical societies. By 1882, 17 state societies had a total of 115 female members.[8] And in 1884, the women of Boston took a large step forward when the Massachusetts Medical society voted to accept women as members. Finally in 1915, the American Medical Association opened its membership to female physicians, thereby giving them their ultimate symbol of professional acceptance.

Complementing women's increasing educational and professional opportunities were the expanding clinical opportunities for women at previously all-male hospitals. By the middle of the 1880s, women trained at major hospitals such as Bellevue in New York, Blockley in Philadelphia, Cook County in Chicago, and Boston City in Boston. At the same time, career options for women doctors expanded. Hospitals increasingly placed women on their staffs. By 1890, eight hospitals in New York City alone employed 14 women doctors in their dispensaries. And by 1890, a new area of work opened for women doctors when several states including New York, Ohio, Pennsylvania, and Massachusetts passed legislation requiring the em-

ployment of a woman doctor in every state insane asylum where women were confined.[9] Even private practice proved an increasingly viable option for many women doctors. It took most women doctors only two years to become self-sufficient in their practices, and the average annual income for women doctors by 1881 was $3,000.[10]

Zakrzewska applauded the progress women doctors had made. On the occasion of the New England Hospital's 25th anniversay, she announced with pride that "the women physician is now called for, respected, and welcome in almost every large town."[11] Yet, while Zakrzewska publicly applauded this professional progress, in the privacy of the New England Hospital she confronted new challenges and problems brought on by the very professional advances she wanted for women doctors.[12]

Between 1863 and 1875, while Zakrzewska built up her nucleus of women doctors for the hospital, relative harmony existed between her and the interns she annually trained. Yet, by the end of 1875, the interns began to demonstrate signs of discontent which continued throughout the winter of 1876. After several months of mounting tension, Zakrzewska called the interns together to hear their grievances. Their strongest complaint was that doctors addressed them as "Misses" rather than with the title of "Doctor."[13] In response, Zakrzewska explained that since the hospital did not require interns to have a medical degree, the doctors had always used the title of "Miss" or "Mrs." to minimize differences between interns, some of whom had graduated from medical schools and some of whom had not.[14] Ultimately, the doctors and interns agreed to a compromise. The doctors would continue to address the interns as "Miss" in the hospital but would address them as "Doctor" in the dispensary, the outpatient department of the hospital where the interns had more direct patient contact.

This initial conflict between interns and physicians was resolved relatively simply. Yet, it takes on larger significance because it illuminated two problems which continued to confront Zakrzewska and her board of physicians over the years — namely, the widening gap between the New England Hospital and the medical opportunities for women outside its walls, and the growing conflict between older and younger women doctors over the needs of women in medicine.

From Zakrzewska's point of view, the hospital offered women valuable clinical training which was unavailable to them elsewhere. But, to the interns the opportunity for clinical training at the New England Hospital was not enough. They came to the hospital with expectations of a quality of experience which transcended their appreciation for the opportunity itself. Their heightened expectations were shaped largely by the fact that by 1875 women doctors no longer faced the same professional obstacles that confronted their predecessors a decade before, leading many women doctors to believe that the prejudice against them was fast disappearing. One ex-intern, for example, wrote to Zakrzewska in 1875: "I think whatever prejudice originally existed against women physicians is fast passing away."[15]

The interns who complained to Zakrzewska in 1876 were part of this younger group of medical women whose professional journey was relatively smooth when measured against the rocky path Dr. Zakrzewska and her contemporaries had been forced to blaze. Consequently, they had different expectations and goals from their older colleagues. The meeting in 1876 with the interns illuminated these differences. The interns' request to be referred to as "Drs." rather than as "Misses" revealed their desire for a distinctly professional identity. Zakrzewska, on the other hand, did not seek the same professional identification. "I would prefer never to be called 'Dr.' but rather 'Miss' or 'Madam,'" she explained. "For me," she continued, as well as for many of her contemporaries, "it is far more agreeable to be considered first a woman, and secondarily a doctor."[16] Her preferences for highlighting her gender stood in marked contrast to the interns' preference for emphasizing their professional status. Their differences on this specific issue symbolized a larger difference between them—namely their different evaluations of the importance of female solidarity in their professional lives. Of course, these major differences could not be resolved by a simple compromise over the use of titles. Rather, the tension between the older and younger doctors at the hospital persisted long after that particular group of interns left, and continued to produce conflict throughout the century.

In 1863, for example, the interns refused to cooperate with changes in work assignments brought on by an unusually heavy patient load. Having come to the New England Hospital for a year, expecting to spend three months in the hospital's medical, maternity, and surgical wards, respectively, and three months in its dispensary, they were unwilling to make any adjustments in this pattern of rotation. The situation was indeed untenable, for relations between physicians and interns were so strained that they threatened the orderly management of the hospital.

It is perhaps no accident that the interns' insistence on a particular training experience occurred during the decade of expanding clinical opportunities for women. For Zakrzewska, the opening of previously all-male hospitals to women created a dilemma. On the one hand, she saw it as a major step forward for women doctors, bringing them closer to her original goal of equal opportunity for male and female physicians. On the other hand, she recognized that the increasing clinical options for women at larger, more prestigious hospitals could deter women from choosing the New England Hospital.

This dilemma shaped her response to the interns in 1883. She told them that the hospital offered benefits which transcended the professional opportunities available to them at the previously all-male hospitals and medical schools. "Comparisons are often made between the opportunities offered to medical women now, and twenty-five years ago, but the value of seeing women doing skillful medical work, cannot be over-estimated in its inspiring effect . . . ."[17] From this point of view, Zakrzewska found intolerable the priorities of her interns which placed each individual's professional interests over the needs of the hospital community as a whole. She explained: "All interns ought to work with us in harmony, not for us personally, but for the *cause* of women practitioners in medicine, for whom we older ones broke the path."[18] Yet, the interns were unwilling to give their loyalty unquestioningly. Instead of coming to the New England Hospital with an eagerness to serve the hospital, as Zakrzewska expected, the interns in 1883 brought to the hospital the expectation that the hospital should serve them.

In the last decade of the century, conflict and discontent continued to polarize Zakrzewska and the board of physicians against the younger women at the New England Hospital. In 1893, for example, the older doctors confronted another group of dissatisfied interns. This time, however, the complaints demanded serious attention as well as accommodation by the older doctors. In a letter to the board of physicians, the interns made a series of complaints that amounted to a strong indictment of the New England Hospital. "After having spent three or four years in medical schools of the highest standing, we enter your hospital ready and anxious to do our best. But, we are allowed to *do* absolutely nothing."[19] The interns also expressed discontent with the attitude of the medical staff toward them. "We have no professional standing," they complained, echoing the feelings of the interns in 1876. "We are considered as mere children who come here to be taught."[20] Overall, their complaints stood as a sweeping critique of the training program at the New England Hospital. "Do you think it pays us to spend a year of our time with you and gain so small an amount of practical knowledge?" they charged. "We are not satisfied with what we are getting here!"[21]

To Zakrzewska and the members of the board, an expression of such feelings would have been unthinkable during their years of training. But the situation had changed markedly since their initial struggle to become doctors. The inroads women had made into the medical profession since the 1870s escalated by the mid-1880s. It was in 1886, for example, that the Boston City Hospital agreed to accept women interns. Two years earlier, the medical women of Boston won a major battle when the Massachusetts Medical Society voted to accept women as members. Dr. Emma Call, a physician since 1875, became the Society's first female member.

While Call and two other long-time doctors at the New England Hospital took the exam for admission, the three oldest physicians at the hospital did not seek membership. Zakrzewska, who had unsuccessfully sought admission in 1859 and again in 1864, refused to take the exam and called the Society's offer in her 27th year of practice "condescending." Ironically, her decision foreshadowed the future, for it revealed her choice to allow an important symbol of women doctors' achievements and professionalism to pass her by.

In her response to the interns' letter of complaint, Zakrzewska once again harkened back to the past. Referring to the board of physicians, she

remarked: "All the ladies present have served as interns in this hospital, and all had their grievances, and all had to endure annoyances . . . but just this training," she continued, "which was borne with dignity and silence, has made them superior women, while everyone of the revolting sisterhood have either remained on the lowest step of success or fallen out of the profession entirely."[22] Calling for the unconditional loyalty of all medical women who passed through the New England Hospital, she urged the younger doctors to follow the lead of the older doctors who understood the value of female solidarity. "You are only helpers in one of the greatest historical reforms, which is still in its infancy, and needs a good deal of self-sacrifice yet to arrive at naturally," she told them. "You ought to be willing to assist in such forms and ways as the experienced workers in this cause think safest and wisest to follow."[23]

To Zakrzewska, the interns had taken the New England Hospital for granted. Yet, to the interns, who faced both opportunities for professional training elsewhere as well as pressure to keep up with rising professional standards, the hospital and its older doctors had failed them on both accounts. Both groups of physicians had a legitimate point of view. The New England Hospital no longer afforded women doctors the best training opportunities. In fact, the hospital lacked the financial base ever to catch up with the major hospitals that were now accepting women. For this, Zakrzewska and the older physicians were not totally responsible. The rapidly rising medical standards were difficult for many doctors and medical institutions to maintain. Yet, the older doctors at the New England Hospital did have some responsibility for the problems there. Even as they provided the hospital with continuity and stability, their failure to adjust to the changing medical scene beyond the hospital's walls starved the New England Hospital of fresh ideas. Furthermore, Zakrzewska's stubborn pride in her hospital made it difficult for her to hear or respond objectively to criticism.

Yet, Zakrzewska did recognize that the contents of the interns' complaints deserved serious attention. She had already received similar criticisms from people higher up the hospital hierarchy. Dr. Bertha Van Hoosen, the resident physician in 1891, had made the same criticisms in her statement of resignation. Van Hoosen was a highly respected member of the hospital staff who went on to become an eminent surgeon, professor of obstetrics at Loyola University, and first president of the American Medical Women's Association. Her capabilities and skill were evident to the doctors at the New England Hospital, and her criticisms received serious attention.

Van Hoosen explained that the position of resident physician was "too arduous" and "too disagreeable" for her to continue at the hospital. With despair and frustration she confessed: "I have never felt at the end of any day that I had finished my work in a satisfactory manner." Yet, her problems were small when she compared them to those of the interns whose positions she considered "unendurable." The resident physician, she explained, stood in the way of any practical experience, responsibility, or respect the interns might enjoy.[24]

Van Hoosen proposed a reorganization of hospital staff which included abolishing the position of resident physician. Whereas a similar proposal by the interns had been ignored, within two months of receiving Van Hoosen's letter, the board of physicians drew up a plan for hospital reform which followed the model she proposed.[25] The speed with which such revisions were accepted by the older physicians once Van Hoosen proposed them suggests that by the end of the century the hospital may have needed an influential outsider like her. It needed someone with the objectivity Zakrzewska and the board lacked, who could see that the New England Hospital was becoming out of date. Van Hoosen was more in touch with the growing medical opportunities and pressures for women outside and understood their implications for the New England Hospital. Only a major reorganization of the hospital would help it to maintain its reputation as a valuable training hospital.

But the reforms of 1892 were too little too late. Interns continued to express dissatisfaction in the years immediately following the adoption of Van Hoosen's plan. Lack of clinical experience still prevailed along with an atmosphere of stagnation which made the New England Hospital an increasingly unappealing place for women doctors to train. The tension which had been growing between older and younger physicians since the mid-1870s had by the 1890s set the stage for a crisis of faith in the hospital. As the board of physicians

and younger doctors continued to lock horns, the older doctors watched as the younger ones turned with increasing frequency away from the hospital to seek their opportunities elsewhere.

The experience of one intern—Alice Hamilton—illustrates this trend. Hamilton was accepted as an intern in 1893. On paper, she seemed to be an extremely attractive candidate. She had a glowing recommendation from her professor of chemistry at the University of Michigan Medical School who described her as "a student of superior scholarship and a person of strong intellectual power."[26] With such a positive report, the board of physicians must have felt confident in accepting Hamilton. Similarly, she was delighted to be accepted. "I feel deliciously animated that I shall go to Boston this fall," she wrote her cousin Agnes.[27] Unfortunately, neither Hamilton's expectations of the hospital nor the physicians' expectations of Hamilton were realized. Before her tenure as intern was up, Hamilton requested dismissal from the hospital, and the board readily let her go.

Hamilton encountered the same disappointment and frustration the previous interns endured—inadequate opportunity for clinical training and lack of professional respect. "It is a very strange novelty to me to be in a place where I actually have not enough to do to keep me busy," she complained three weeks after she began work.[28] Less than four weeks later, the situation became intolerable for her. "I feel that I am simply losing a year when I need practical work," she wrote in exasperation. Yet, Hamilton reserved her most scathing comments for the board of physicians. "They are so bland and patronizing and so convinced that there is no hospital like the New England and no advantages like ours. They are narrow women," she continued, "who escape discovering their own inferiority merely by avoiding their superiors."[29] In the spring, Hamilton asked the board of physicians to release her from her contract, and the board, which usually granted such requests only in cases of illness, voted to accept her withdrawal in "the best interests of the hospital."[30]

Hamilton's actions were part of a trend in the 1890s of growing dissatisfaction with and decreasing loyalty to the New England Hospital. This rejection of the hospital took a variety of forms. For example, more and more young women turned down offers of internships at the hospital. Between 1891 and 1895, of the 27 applicants accepted, 7 turned down the offer. Of the four who gave reasons, one took a position at a hospital where she could receive more obstetrical training than the New England Hospital offered, one chose to do "special work" in cystoscopy at Johns Hopkins, one had unspecified "fixed plans," while a fourth received another hospital position.

Once an applicant was on the waiting list, it was even less likely that she would choose to come to the New England Hospital. Of the eight women waitlisted between 1891 and 1895, four rejected eventual offers, while three withdrew their applications. In the interim, all seven made other satisfactory arrangements ranging from finding positions in other hospitals to beginning private practice. Clearly, by the 1890s the New England Hospital was feeling the impact of increased clinical alternatives for young women doctors.

This does not mean that the hospital lacked women seeking to train there. Rather, as the number of women doctors increased throughout the country, so did the number of women seeking internships at the hospital. Whereas 63 women applied between 1891 and 1895, 96 applied between 1900 and 1904. In addition, women were willing to travel farther to come to the hospital. Between 1891 and 1895 more than three-quarters of the applicants were from the Northeast. Between 1900 and 1904, more than one-half were from other parts of the country.[31] Furthermore, individual applicants continued to express a strong desire to come to the New England Hospital. One Mary Findlater, upon graduating from the Woman's Medical College of Pennsylvania, wrote in her application in 1905: "Ever since I started the study of medicine, I have looked forward to my senior year, hoping for an appointment in Boston [at the] New England Hospital, of which I had so often heard."[32] Another candidate expressed her interest somewhat more poetically: "Should you favor my application," she wrote, "I promise I will endeavor to do the work entrusted to me on the principle contained in this little poem which I heard:

> If I were a cobbler, I'd make it my pride,
> the very best cobbler to be.
> If I were a tinker, no other beside
> should mend an old kettle like me.[33]

Nevertheless, despite these signs to the contrary, there was mounting evidence that the hospital was falling to disfavor with growing numbers of women doctors. In 1895, Dr. Mary Hobart, who had been at the hospital for nine years, confronted this dilemma. "It is well known," she stated bluntly at a physicians' meeting, "that the staff of the New England Hospital already has the reputation of being narrow and to repulse bright women who might otherwise be valuable co-workers." Advising the older doctors to be more open to the needs of the young women doctors, she warned, "we must get them and keep them about us. In a few years," she continued, "it will be harder to get women clinicians than now."[34]

Particularly problematic was the fact that the disenchantment with the New England Hospital was no longer limited to interns. Women at all stages of their medical careers displayed their dissatisfaction. One way in which they expressed their discontent was by resigning their positions at the hospital. Between 1862 and 1879, when Zakrzewska built up the New England Hospital, only 6 of the 15 doctors who served on her staff left. But in the "conflict years" between 1880 and 1899, 25 of the 43 staff physicians left. The reasons women gave for leaving were also cause for alarm. In the hospital's early years, death, illness, or retirement were the reasons women doctors left the hospital. In the last decade of the century, however, only 9 of 25 women who gave explanations for leaving left for these same reasons. The remaining 16 resigned because of dissatisfaction with the hospital's facilities, unwillingness to commit so much time to the hospital, opportunities for more lucrative work elsewhere, or a desire to devote more time to private practice.

The irony is inescapable. The closer women came to attaining professional equality with male doctors — the goals for which Zakrzewska founded the New England Hospital — the less they chose the New England Hospital as a route to professional success. This trend revealed a growing difference between the professional route older women doctors had followed in the 1860s and 1870s and the one younger women doctors began to follow in the last decades of the century. Isolated from male medical institutions, the first generation of women doctors relied on the all-women's medical institutions like the New England Hospital. When the male medical institutions began to open to women, a younger generation of women doctors began to turn away from the all-women's institutions in preference for integration into the medical mainstream. To many aspiring women doctors at the end of the century, female solidarity had lost its professional appeal.

Of course, there was not always a sharp division between older women doctors who saw female solidarity as a major priority and younger women doctors who were willing to sacrifice it for their own professional success. There were younger women doctors who continued to share a commitment to women doctors as a group. Gertrude Felker, an intern in 1901, for example, was described as "the kind of girl that will in turn prove helpful to all women."[35] And there were some who stood in both camps. Van Hoosen, for example, went on in later years to found the all-women's American Medical Women's Association.

Nevertheless, by the last decades of the 19th century, there was a clear and growing rejection of the all-women's New England Hospital by younger women doctors. Zakrzewska watched this trend with a mixture of alarm and despair. To be sure, she took the rejection of the hospital personally. But her often inflexible responses to the interns' complaints over the years also revealed her strong convictions about what was best for women doctors. She firmly believed that female solidarity was the only way women would succeed in the medical profession. Even after women attained equal access with men to the best medical institutions, she still maintained that they had to band together if they were to survive. To Zakrzewska, the younger women doctors' rejection of the New England Hospital and the female solidarity upon which it was built represented but the first step in the decline of women in medicine.

While Zakrzewska never gave up these convictions, toward the end of her life she came to understand that the younger women doctors would never fully understand the professional struggles she and her contemporaries had endured. "It is really impossible," she wrote, "to depict the struggles of a pioneer, conditions have so altered, public opinion so changed, that the present generation cannot possibly comprehend the life of fifty years ago."[36]

But, in the years following Zakrzewska's death in 1902, young doctors at the hospital realized they had little understanding of their predecessors. In 1910, the interns recognized that they knew so little about the hospital's early years that they requested a recounting of its history.[37] Their lack of understanding of the older doctors' struggles helps explain young women doctors' discontent and impatience with the New England Hospital, Zakrzewska, and the older doctors. At the same time, their complaints reflected conditions which transcended this generational gap. Rather, from the young doctors' point of view, the rapid advances in medicine beyond the hospital's walls created new professional standards which the New England Hospital did not meet.

In the final analysis, the inroads 19th-century women made into the medical profession created new problems. Female solidarity was initially the best route to professional success for women doctors. But by the end of the century, women doctors had to make difficult decisions about the importance of female solidarity to their professional careers.

But they were not alone, for this dilemma confronted other women toward the end of the century as well. Club women and suffragists, for example, faced similar conflicts in their respective organizations. The general trend in the women's movement was to tread more carefully, and to concentrate more narrowly on reform or professionalism.[38] Thus, younger women doctors chose their individual professional needs over the female solidarity the pioneer women had carefully cultivated. While they believed this was necessary if they were to keep up with male doctors, hindsight suggests that their priorities were somewhat shortsighted. Indeed, the percentage of women doctors declined in the first half of the 20th century.[39] Ironically, Zakrzewska, who was unable to keep up with the new professional standards the younger doctors aspired to, anticipated this trend. In 1883, she had warned the interns: "The cause of women practitioners is by no means to be yet regarded as a permanently established reform, even though many women may be successful in their vocation."[40] Her words were, indeed, prophetic, and carried an important message to all 19th-century women doctors.

## NOTES

Research for this paper was aided by a fellowship from the Rockefeller Foundation and a grant from Tufts University, and was conducted while I was a fellow at the Bunting Institute. An earlier version of this paper was presented at the Conference on Women in the Health Professions, Boston College, November 15, 1980. For their help in the various stages of writing this paper, I would like to thank Steven Fuhrman, Douglas Jones, Ann Lane, Regina Morantz, and the members of the Boston area Medical History Group.

1   *New England Hospital for Women and Children Annual Report* (Boston, 1886), p. 6.

2   Bertha Van Hoosen, Letter of resignation, Sept. 1891, in New England Hospital Collection, Smith College, Northampton.

3   In 1950, Richard Shryock first suggested the importance of feminism to 19th-century women doctors, arguing that the 19th-century women's movement was crucial to women's successful entrance into medicine. Richard Harrison Shryock, "Women in American medicine," *J. Am. Med. Women's Assn.,* Sept. 1950, *5*, reprint. in Richard Harrison Shryock, *Medicine in America: Historical Essays* (Baltimore, 1966), pp. 177–199. John B. Blake examined several of the women who became doctors in the years before the Civil War in "Women and medicine in ante-bellum America," *Bull. Hist. Med.,* 1965, *39*: 99–123. Little else appeared on the topic until Mary Roth Walsh's *"Doctors Wanted: No Women Need Apply": Sexual Barriers in the Medical Profession 1835–1975* (New Haven, 1977). Walsh's book represents the first full-length study of women's entrance into American medicine. Other historians have examined women doctors primarily as professionals and not exclusively within the political sphere. See Regina Markell Morantz and Sue Zschoch, "Professionalism, feminism, and gender roles: a comparative study of nineteenth century medical therapeutics," *J. Am. Hist.,* 1980, *67*: 569–588; Regina Markell Morantz, "The 'Connecting Link': the case for the woman doctor in 19th-century America," in this volume, ch. 11; and Regina Markell Morantz, "The lady and her physician," in *Clio's Consciousness Raised: New Perspectives on the History of Women,* ed. Mary Hartman and Lois W. Banner (New York, 1974), pp. 38–53. See also Virginia G. Drachman, "Gynecological instruments and surgical decisions at a hospital in late nineteenth-century America," *J. Am. Culture,* 1980, *3*: 660–672.

4   Walsh, *"Doctors Wanted: No Women Need Apply,"* Ch. 3.

5   *New England Hospital Annual Report,* 1865, p. 12.

6   For a discussion of 19th-century medical education, see William G. Rothstein, *American Physicians in the 19th-Century: From Sects to Science* (Baltimore, 1972); and Robert P. Hudson, "Abraham Flexner in perspective: American medical education, 1865–1910," in this volume, ch. 10.

7   *New England Hospital Annual Report,* 1875, p. 16.

8   Mary Putnam Jacobi, "Women in medicine," in *Woman's Work in America,* ed. Annie Nathan Meyer (New York, 1891).

9   *Ibid.,* p. 191.

10  *Ibid.,* p. 200.

11  *New England Hospital Annual Report,* 1887, p. 44.

12  The first signs of problems were isolated events brought on by conflicts among the doctors in the hospital. One should not dismiss these conflicts lightly as the expression of normal tension between interns and doctors. Rather, later these specific conflicts began to fit together to reveal a more general pattern of dissatisfaction at the hospital. When taken together, they reveal that larger issues were involved.

13  Marie Zakrzewska, Address to students, Apr. 1, 1876, in New England Hospital Collection, Smith College, Northampton.

14  *Ibid.*

15  *New England Hospital Annual Report,* 1887, p. 17.

16  Zakrzewska, Address to students, Apr. 1, 1876.

17  Marie Zakrzewska, Address to students, Mar. 30, 1883, in New England Hospital Collection, Smith College, Northampton.

18  *Ibid.*

19  Interns' complaints, Oct. 1891, New England Hospital Collection, Smith College, Northampton.

20  *Ibid.*

21  *Ibid.*

22  Marie Zakrzewska, Response to interns, Oct. 30, 1891, in New England Hospital Collection, Smith College, Northampton.

23  *Ibid.*

24  Bertha Van Hoosen, Letter of resignation, Nov. 1891, in New England Hospital Collection, Smith College, Northampton.

25  Revision of hospital management, Oct. 2, 1891, in New England Hospital Collection, Smith College, Northampton.

26  Letter of recommendation from Albert V. Prescott to Dr. Sarah Palmer, Apr. 13, 1893, in New England Hospital Collection, Smith Collection, Northampton.

27  Alice Hamilton to Agnes Hamilton, Aug. 13, 1893, in Schlesinger Library, Radcliffe College, Cambridge, Mass.

28  Alice Hamilton to Agnes Hamilton, Oct. 2, 1893,

in Schlesinger Library, Radcliffe College, Cambridge, Mass.

29   Alice Hamilton to Agnes Hamilton, Oct. 26, 1893, in Schlesinger Library, Radcliffe College, Cambridge, Mass.

30   Minutes of Board of Physicians Meetings, Vol. III, May 4, 1896.

31   All information on interns calculated from applications for internships at the New England Hospital, New England Hospital Collection, Smith College, Northampton.

32   Mary Findlater, Application for internship to New England Hospital, New England Hospital Collection, Smith College, Northampton.

33   Elizabeth McMaster, Application for internship to New England Hospital, New England Hospital Collection, Smith College, Northampton.

34   Mary Hobart to board of physicians, Nov. 1, 1895, in New England Hospital Collection. See also: Francis Kyle to Zakrzewska, Apr. 15, 1890, for alarmed response of a professor at University of Michigan Medical College to practices at New England Hospital; letter from Delia Rice to Zakrzewska, Jan. 6, 1894, expressing concern about applying to the hospital as an intern because of negative rumors about the hospital; both in New England Hospital Collection, Smith College, Northampton.

35   Harriet Lathrop to Emily Pope, May 31, 1900, in New England Hospital Collection, Smith College, Northampton.

36   Marie Zakrzewska to Pauline Pope, Oct. 28, 1901, in New England Hospital Collection, Smith College, Northampton.

37   Interns' request, Dec. 20, 1910, in New England Hospital Collection, Smith College, Northampton.

38   See Karen J. Blair, "The club woman as feminist: the woman's culture club movement in the United States, 1868–1914" (Ph.D. dissertation, SUNY, Buffalo, 1975). Also Mary Jo Buhle, "The nineteenth-century woman's movement: perspectives on woman's labor in industrializing America," presented at the Bunting Institute, Feb. 1979.

39   See Walsh, *Doctors Wanted: No Women Need Apply,* particularly Ch. 6.

40   Marie Zakrzewska, Address to students, Mar. 30, 1883, in New England Hospital Collection, Smith College, Northampton.

# The Health Professions

For well over a century physicians have sought to monopolize, or at least to control, health care in America. Yet despite the acquisition of unparalleled professional power, they have, as Ronald L. Numbers points out, repeatedly been forced to settle for considerably less control than they desired. In addition to the various sectarian healers, whom regular physicians hoped to suppress, there were dentists, midwives, optometrists, podiatrists, pharmacists, and psychologists competing for slices of the health-care pie. The division of labor among these diverse occupational groups seems at times to defy logic. Why, for example, did the treatment of most of the body evolve into medical specialties controlled by physicians, while the care of the teeth and feet fell to practitioners outside the medical profession? History provides some clues.

During the second quarter of the 19th century a handful of physician-dentists sought to turn their field into a medical specialty, like surgery or ophthalmology. But their suggestion that dentistry be included in the medical curriculum met with the response that it was too mechanical. After all, dentists filled and extracted teeth; they did not heal them. Rebuffed by their erstwhile colleagues, these dentists about 1840 founded their own society, started their own journal, and opened their own school, the Baltimore College of Dental Surgery. Within a few decades American dentistry was preeminent in the world, far surpassing American medicine in international repute.

Podiatry, also known as chiropody, developed from a similar quasi-medical background. When doctors specializing in the care and treatment of the feet urged medical schools at the turn of the 20th century to assume responsibility for training in this area, deans turned them away with the comment that corns and bunions were too trivial to warrant such attention. So with the medical profession's blessing, podiatrists, like dentists a half-century earlier, set up their own institutions.

Pharmacists and optometrists trace their roots not primarily to medicine but to the business of drug selling and "spec" peddling. Over the years both professions worked out reasonably harmonious divisions of labor with physicians, distinctions ultimately sanctioned by law. Pharmacists prepared and dispensed drugs, but left the prescribing to physicians. Optometrists tested for corrective lenses, but referred all treatment of the eyes to ophthalmologists.

The female-dominated fields of midwifery and nursing developed along different historical lines. As Frances E. Kobrin demonstrates in her study of the midwife controversy, the medical fraternity did not welcome competition from nonmembers. And it was not as easy for midwives and obstetricians to divide their work as it had been for optometrists and ophthalmologists. Thus some physicians tried to legislate midwives out of business. Nurses, Susan Reverby shows, survived by submitting to the authority of physicians.

On the basis of these few examples, it seems that the medical profession welcomed, or at least tolerated, only those activities that physicians did not want, such as dentistry and podiatry, or that did not encroach substantially on their preserve, such as optometry and pharmacy, or that remained under their direct control, such as nursing.

# 13

## The Fall and Rise
## of the American Medical Profession

### RONALD L. NUMBERS

Midway through the 19th century American medicine lay in a shambles. Addressing the first annual meeting of the American Medical Association in 1848, President Nathaniel Chapman expressed the dejection felt by many physicians. "The profession to which we belong," he lamented, "once venerated on account of its antiquity—its varied and profound science—its elegant literature—its polite accomplishments—its virtues—has become corrupt and degenerate, to the forfeiture of its social position, and with it, of the homage it formerly received spontaneously and universally."[1] The golden age Chapman recalled may have been only an old man's fantasy, but American physicians had unquestionably fallen on hard times. For centuries, at least since the late Middle Ages, Western societies had commonly recognized medicine, along with divinity and law, as one of the prototypical professions, possessing an esoteric body of knowledge, requiring extensive training, and being entitled to exclusive rights protected by law.[2] Although many healers practiced outside the law and failed to acquire professional status, those who earned M.D. degrees or served a protracted apprenticeship formed an occupational elite. By the mid-19th century, however, medicine for many Americans had degenerated into little more than a trade, open to all who wished to try their hand at healing. "Any one, male or female, learned or ignorant, an honest man or a knave, can assume the name of a physician, and 'practice' upon any one, to cure or to kill, as either

RONALD L. NUMBERS is Professor of the History of Medicine and the History of Science at the University of Wisconsin, Madison, Wisconsin.

Courtesy of the University of Notre Dame Press from *The Professions in American History,* forthcoming, edited by Nathan O. Hatch.

may happen, without accountability," wrote one observer in 1850. "'It's a free country!'"[3]

Within a century American physicians and their allies effected a revolution. By 1950, even earlier, medicine had emerged as the strongest and most influential profession in America. Aspiring physicians competed intensely to enter the guild and studied for years to acquire the proper credentials and requisite knowledge. Powerful institutions guarded its interests and regulated its behavior. Laws in every state protected its rights. Indeed, as one lawyer noted enviously, no interest group in the country enjoyed "more freedom from formal control than organized medicine."[4]

### THE FALL

During the early 19th century American physicians viewed their situation with optimism—and rightfully so. Although the country abounded with self-appointed healers and poorly trained doctors, professionally ambitious physicians seemed to be improving their position. With the opening of a medical school at the College of Philadelphia in 1765, Americans could, without going abroad, supplement their apprenticeships with formal lectures and acquire medical degrees. By 1830 the United States boasted 22 such institutions. By this time, also, 13 states had awarded physicians special privileges, usually in the form of laws giving medical societies exclusive rights to license practitioners. Few of these statutes granted licensed practitioners more than the right to sue for unpaid bills; yet they did provide the medical elite with a modicum of social recognition.[5]

In the decades after 1830 several factors converged to undermine the progress physicians seemed to be making: an epidemic of "medical school mania" broke out, the profession fractured into rival sects, and physicians lost the legal standing they had just acquired. Of course, physicians were not the only professionals to suffer a loss of status at this time. As one historian has pointed out, the period from 1830 to 1880 witnessed the general "disestablishment and humbling of the professions" in America.[6] Nevertheless, the particulars of the medical story are unique.

Encouraged by revised state laws that accepted a medical school diploma as the equivalent of a license from an approved medical society, physicians who fancied themselves as professors began flooding the country with low-grade institutions. Already by 1830 the nation's 22 medical schools exceeded by several times the number in European countries of comparable size, and during the next three decades the quantity more than doubled. To make matters worse, most of these institutions, even those nominally affiliated with a college or university, were run for prestige and profit by ill-equipped local practitioners, many of whom could not have matriculated as students in the best European schools. Because of this commercial orientation, requirements for admission—where they existed at all—remained low and graduation often depended more on a student's ability to pay than on his competence. Some medical students could barely read and write, and most had never sat in a college classroom. The best arts students aspired to careers in divinity or law and looked upon medicine as a last resort. "It is very well understood among college boys," wrote one dispirited physician, "that after a man has failed in scholarship, failed in writing, failed in speaking, failed in every purpose for which he entered college; after he has dropped down from class to class; after he has been kicked out of college, there is *one* unfailing city of refuge—the profession of medicine."[7]

Until the last quarter of the century students typically obtained their M.D. degrees by successfully completing eight months of formal training, the last half of which merely duplicated the first. During this brief period they were expected to learn not only the basic sciences like anatomy, physiology, and chemistry, but to acquire clinical skills as well. This became especially true as more and more schools dropped a previous apprenticeship as an entrance requirement. It was no won-

der, commented the medical reformer Nathan Smith Davis in 1845, that 99 out of every 100 American physicians were poorly educated:

> With no *practical* knowledge of chemistry and botany; with but a smattering of anatomy and physiology, hastily caught during a sixteen weeks' attendance on the anatomical theater of a medical college; with still less of real pathology; they enter the profession having mastered just enough of the details of practice to give them the requisite *self-assurance* for commanding the confidence of the public; but without either an adequate fund of knowledge or that degree of mental discipline and habits of patient study which will enable them ever to supply their defects.[8]

Such practitioners, charged another contemporary, tended to pursue "medicine as a trade instead of a profession, [and to] study the science of patient-getting to the neglect of the science of patient-curing."[9]

A second development that undermined the status of medicine was its fragmentation into competing sects, each offering an alternative to the so-called heroic therapy of regular physicians. During the early 19th century practitioners gained considerable notoriety for copius bleeding and the seemingly routine prescribing of calomel, a mercury-based cathartic that often produced harmful and discomforting side effects. Such practices gave rise to a host of critics, among the most vocal and visible of which were the homeopaths and the various botanics, such as the Thomsonians and eclectics.[10]

The pioneer among American sectarians was a New Hampshire farmer, Samuel Thomson, who learned much of his botanic lore from a local female herbalist. Early in his healing career he became convinced that the cause of all disease was cold and that restoring the body's natural heat was the only cure. This he accomplished by steaming, peppering, and puking his patients, relying heavily on lobelia, a botanical emetic long used by American Indians. Not one to ignore the commercial possibilities of his discovery, Thomson in 1806 began selling "Family Rights" to his practice, for which he obtained a patent in 1813. During the 1820s and 1830s his agents fanned out from New England through the southern and western states, urging self-reliant Americans to become their own physicians. By 1840 approximately 100,000 Family Rights had been sold, and Thomson estimated that about 3 million individuals had adopted his system. In states as diverse as Ohio and Mississippi as many as one-half of the citizens reportedly cured themselves the Thomsonian way.

Unlike many sectarians who simply wanted the public to exchange one kind of physician for another, Thomson saw no need for professional healers of any kind. It was high time, he declared, for the common man to throw off the oppressive yoke of priests, lawyers, and physicians and assume his rightful place in a truly democratic society. Contrary to his wishes, his disciples in the 1830s began opening medical schools and competing head-to-head with regular physicians. By the 1840s, however, the Thomsonians were rapidly losing ground to a rival botanical sect, the eclectics, who achieved great popularity in the Midwest, where, in Cincinnati, they operated one of the nation's largest medical schools. Eclectic physicians and surgeons denounced blood-letting and calomel-dosing, but, except for preferring vegetable to mineral remedies, their practice differed little from that of the regulars.

Homeopathy originated in the mind of a regularly educated German physician, Samuel Hahnemann, who during the last decade of the 18th century constructed a novel system of healing based in large part on the healing power of nature and two fundamental principles: the law of similars and the law of infinitesimals. According to the first law, diseases are cured by medicines having the property of producing in healthy persons symptoms similar to those of the disease. An individual suffering from fever, for example, would be treated with a drug known to increase the pulse rate of a person in health. Hahnemann's second law held that medicines are more efficacious the smaller the dose, even down to one-millionth of a gram. Though regular practitioners—or allopaths, as Hahnemann dubbed them—ridiculed this theory, many patients flourished under the mild homeopathic therapy, and they seldom suffered harmful side effects.

Following its appearance in the United States in 1825, homeopathy quickly grew into the nation's largest medical sect, replete with its own medical schools, societies, and journals. Its practitioners, many of whom defected from the regular ranks, were often well educated and well received by the middle and upper classes. By 1860 there were an estimated 2,400 homeopaths nationally, compared with about 60,000 regular physicians, only a third of whom possessed M.D. degrees.[11]

The acrimonious debates between sectarians and regulars—to say nothing of bitter quarrels among the regulars themselves over the efficacy of drug therapy and bleeding—created an atmosphere in which it became fashionable, wrote one editor, "to speak of the Medical Profession as a body of jealous, quarrelsome men, whose chief delight is in the annoyance and ridicule of each other."[12] Although many individual physicians continued to enjoy the respect of their communities, the reputation of the profession as a whole does seem to have declined. Certainly public confidence in medicine was not bolstered when physicians like Harvard's Oliver Wendell Holmes suggested that, with few exceptions, "if the whole materia medica, *as now used*, could be sunk to the bottom of the sea, it would be all the better for mankind—and all the worse for the fishes."[13]

Indicative of the public's low esteem for the medical profession during the 1830s and 1840s was its stripping doctors of their privileged legal status. Although it is difficult to see how early-19th-century licensing laws deterred anyone from practicing medicine, Thomsonians especially felt persecuted and led the fight to repeal the so-called Black Laws. Apparently they were not without popular support, because at one point during the legislative debate in New York Samuel Thomson's son John arrived in the chamber, dramatically pushing a wheelbarrow full of petitions. Swayed by such displays of antimonopolistic sentiment, state legislatures one by one repealed the offending statutes, until by 1850 only two states retained laws in any way restricting the practice of medicine. Society, observed one dejected physician, had thrown the medical profession overboard, "to sink or swim as it can, without even a rope by which to sustain itself."[14]

Unhampered by legal prejudice, healers of every stripe assumed the title "doctor" and hung out their shingles. According to one 1850 survey, of the 201 practitioners in eastern Tennessee, 35 held M.D.'s from regular medical schools, 42 had taken only one course of lectures, 27 identified themselves as botanics, while the rest—nearly half of the total—had picked up their knowledge of medicine from casual reading.[15] With so many marginally qualified practitioners crowding the field, even medical school graduates often found it impossible to live on their medical income alone. It was high time, concluded professional leaders, to launch a counteroffensive — to protect the public health as well as their own pocketbooks.

## EARLY REFORMS

Abandoned to their own devices by the states, medical reformers first explored what they could accomplish through self-regulation. As the editor of the *New York Journal of Medicine* wrote in 1845,

> The profession in almost every state in the union is now left, so far as legal enactments are concerned, to take care of itself; to make its own rules, and adopt its own standard of excellence. For if we cannot make rules or laws which will banish ignorance, stupidity, and empiricism, we can, at least, fix our *own* standard of qualification, and thereby say who *we* will recognize as *our* associates.[16]

To accomplish this end, members of the State Medical Society of New York in 1846 convened a national convention to explore ways of reducing internal discord, isolating sectarians, and, above all, elevating the quality of medical education. Although some medical professors denounced the movement as an "aristocratic" attempt to cripple medical schools, nearly 100 delegates from 16 states showed up.[17] The following year this group launched the American Medical Association, the first national society of regular physicians.

One of the top items on the A.M.A.'s agenda was to draw up a code of ethics, outlining not only the duties of the "professional" physician toward patients and peers, but also the obligations of patients to obey their physicians and avoid quacks. Although the code dealt more with etiquette than ethics, it did establish guidelines governing economic behavior, a source of much contention. In addition to banning advertising, the selling of secret nostrums, and other practices associated with quackery, it recommended the adoption of fee bills in each community to regulate the price of medical services. These schedules of minimum fees were to be binding in all cases except those involving the indigent, brother physicians, and certain public duties. American doctors commonly acknowl-

edged an obligation to put their patients' welfare above personal gain, but they also recognized, as one practitioner explained, that "a physician must train himself to be a professional man when treating patients, and a business man when collecting his bills."[18]

To segregate sectarians and to assist the public in identifying regular physicians, the code stipulated that no A.M.A. member could consult with anyone "whose practice is based on an exclusive dogma." Like the entire code, this provision remained advisory until 1855, when it became mandatory.[19]

No subject attracted greater attention among A.M.A members than medical education, the improvement of which, they hoped, would simultaneously produce better physicians and reduce the number of potential competitors. At its first meeting delegates adopted standards requiring medical schools to offer anatomic dissections and clinical instruction, to extend their terms from four to six months, and to require entering students to possess "a good English education, a knowledge of Natural Philosophy, and the elementary Mathematical Sciences, including Geometry and Algebra, and such an acquaintance, at least, with the Latin and Greek languages as will enable them to appreciate the technical language of medicine, and read and write prescriptions." These standards were so unrealistically high that, in the opinion of one scholar, rigid enforcement "would have closed down practically every medical school in the country, and would have depleted the ranks of formally educated physicians in a few years."[20] Fortunately for medical educators, the A.M.A. represented only a small percentage of American physicians and remained too weak and ineffective throughout the 19th century to reform much of anything.

Medical education did, nevertheless, improve significantly during the latter half of the century. Although the proliferation of substandard schools continued unabated, the best institutions lengthened their curricula to three years, offered a new set of courses each year, required some evidence of preliminary education, and, led by the Harvard Medical College, abandoned proprietary status to become an integral part of a university. The dramatic growth of laboratory-based medical science in the latter half of the century encouraged such reforms, as did the German training of approximately 15,000 American physicians between 1870 and 1914.[21]

No event symbolized the reformation of American medical education more than the opening in 1893 of the Johns Hopkins School of Medicine under the leadership of the German-trained pathologist William H. Welch. At a time when, according to Welch, no American medical school required a preliminary education equal to "that necessary for entrance into the freshman class of a respectable college," the Hopkins faculty, at the insistence of its patron, demanded a bachelor's degree. Modestly following the Hopkins example, more than 20 schools by 1910 raised their entrance requirements to two years of college. This reform, Robert E. Kohler has argued, had far-reaching effects: it "stretched the financial resources of the proprietary school beyond the breaking point. . . . higher entrance requirements disrupted the established market relation with high schools, diminished the pool of qualified applicants, and resulted in a drastic plunge in enrollments. Medical schools could not survive on fees."[22]

A further prod to educational reform came not from within the profession itself, but from the states, every one of which passed some kind of medical licensing act between the mid-1870s and 1900. Although physicians generally led the crusade to restrict the practice of medicine, they were not without external support. As society came to rely on physicians to certify births and deaths, to control infectious diseases, and to commit the insane, it became increasingly apparent that licensing served a public as well as a professional function. In 1888 the Supreme Court in a landmark decision, *Dent v. West Virginia*, upheld the authority of the state medical examining board to deprive a poorly trained eclectic physician of his right to practice. In the opinion of Justice Stephen J. Field, no one had "the right to practice medicine without having the necessary qualifications of learning and skill," and no group had greater competency to judge these qualifications than well-trained physicians.[23] Thus society granted the medical profession one of its most cherished goals: the authority to exclude practitioners deemed unworthy. The fact that other professions won protective legislation at the same time suggests that the physicians' achievement resulted more from a change in so-

cial policy than from a recognition of the improved state of medical science, impressive though it may have been.

The state licensing boards influenced medical education in two ways. First, most of them required candidates to hold a diploma from a reputable medical school, that is, one requiring evidence of preliminary education and, perhaps, offering a three-year course of study, a six-month term, and clinical and laboratory instruction. This forced any school hoping to compete for students to upgrade its curriculum, at least superficially. Second, many states, especially during the late 1880s and 1890s, revised their laws to require all candidates, even those holding medical degrees, to pass an examination. Although some of the weaker schools quickly learned how to coach students to pass these tests, graduates from strong institutions had a much better chance of passing. A shallow medical education no longer paid.[24] The success of the licensing laws convinced professional leaders of the great advantage of legal sanctions over moral suasion in reforming medical education. "It is our opinion," declared the editor of the *Journal of the American Medical Association* in 1895, "that notwithstanding the far-reaching influence of the medical press, and the support of the various medical societies of the country, medical legislation alone caused the healthy reform. It is also apparent that the enforcement of efficient medical legislation in a few States will do more in destroying the dangerous work of the low grade college than all other factors combined."[25]

Medical practice acts not only set standards for licensing physicians, but defined the very practice of medicine. The Nebraska act, for example, stipulated that anyone "who shall operate on, profess to heal, or prescribe for, or otherwise treat any physical or mental ailment of another" was practicing medicine and thus subject to the provisions of the law. For various political reasons, the states often granted exceptions. Many laws specifically exempted dentists, midwives, medical students, and persons who gave emergency aid; and a few states, especially in New England, provided immunity for Christian Scientists and others who engaged in mental healing.[26] However, physicians, whose strategy called for the elimination or subordination of competitors, preferred to define the practice of medicine as broadly as possible. As the sociologist Eliot Freidson has argued, "an essential feature of a useful concept of profession is the possession of something of a monopoly over the exercise of its work."[27] American physicians would have agreed.

Since the appearance of rival sects in the first half of the century, regulars had sought to isolate and discredit them. Nevertheless, well-trained sectarians, especially homeopaths and eclectics, had prospered. During the latter part of the century it became increasingly difficult to distinguish between orthodox and heterodox practice, or to argue that one system was more efficacious than another. In the 1880s, for example, one life insurance company concluded that homeopathy was just as effective as allopathy in saving lives, while a comparative study at Cook County Hospital in Chicago showed the latter to have only a slight edge in mortality rates. Given the training, therapeutic success, and numerical strength of the sectarians, regulars found it impossible to legislate them out of existence; in fact, in at least 20 states they sat on the same licensing boards with homeopaths or eclectics—at a time when the A.M.A. still banned professional intercourse. In only three or four instances did they obtain what they most desired: a single licensing board composed exclusively of regulars.[28]

Although orthodox physicians liked to describe their efforts to suppress sectarians in humanitarian terms, evidence suggests that opposition stemmed as much from fear of competition as from a desire to safeguard the public. After all, as one homeopath perceptively noted, regulars made few attempts to police therapy among themselves:

> If you inform the people that you treat those who come to you according to Similia, so far as drugging goes, you are anathema with the "regular," but if you get inside his fold, you can use any old treatment you please—be it an "electrotherapeutist," a man of "suggestion," or of "serums," calomel, bleeding, anything, and be a "regular physician." Curious, isn't it? Looks as though the real thing at issue was the "recognition of the union" rather than the "welfare of the public."[29]

In addition to battling sectarians, the regular medical profession zealously fought to subordinate and control allied health personnel. As the number of trained nurses increased after the Civil War, physicians expressed concern that these women would attempt to expand their role and presume to act as physicians. Thus doctors attempted to limit the amount of theoretical training nurses received and insisted that nurses strictly obey their orders. As the *Boston Medical and Surgical Journal* explained, the physician's relationship to the nursing staff was to be "like that of the captain to his ship." To win acceptance and approval from the medical profession, nurses themselves went out of their way to reassure the doctors. For example, in her influential *Nursing Ethics* (1900) Isabel Hampton emphasized discipline as the key to success: "The head nurse and her staff should stand to receive the visiting physician, and from the moment of his entrance until his departure, the attending nurses should show themselves alert, attentive, courteous, like soldiers on duty."[30] Such an attitude posed no threat either to pocketbooks or egos.

Physicians experienced much greater difficulty trying to subdue male pharmacists, who not only sold medicines prescribed by doctors but frequently diagnosed minor ailments and suggested remedies. Pharmacists, warned one physician in the early 1880s, had "so industriously and energetically wedged themselves between the 'dear public' and the professional province of the physician" that they threatened to take over the practice of medicine. Incensed doctors denounced this intrusion as dangerous and illegal and sought to revise medical practice acts to ban practices such as over-the-counter prescribing. Their efforts, however, generally failed, and in at least one state (North Dakota) the pharmacists retaliated by securing passage of a law barring physicians from dispensing medicines. "If physicians wish to prevent encroachment on their domain," warned one pharmacist, "they should avoid invading others' property."[31]

Dentistry, which required mechanical skills more than medical knowledge, was one of the few healing activities that physicians attempted neither to crush nor to control. When dentists in the late 1830s tried to win a place for their specialty in the medical school curriculum, one physician quipped "that the author of such a plan, to be consistent, should not fill teeth but treat the constitutional causes of dental caries by bleeding, purging, and leeching his patients."[32] Thus rebuffed, a group of physician-dentists in 1840 established the Baltimore College of Dental Surgery, the first dental school in the country. Although some dentists fretted for decades about their identity—"If we are not medical specialists we are a set of carpenters," said one—the majority, believing that "dentistry was altogether too large to be made the tail end of the kite of medical practice," quietly created a set of institutions paralleling those of the medical profession: societies, schools offering D.D.S. degrees, and separate dental licensing boards. "A professional wall is now being built up," explained one dental leader, "and we hope it will be built so high and strong, that none can scale or break it down, but that all who enter will be compelled to do so through the legitimate and well-guarded gateways." Except for legal loopholes that often allowed physicians to practice dentistry, dentists succeeded by the end of the century in building their professional wall. They failed, however, to win equal standing among physicians, who regarded the filling and pulling of teeth as minor matters. "If dentists are ambitious to be considered medical specialists, they must undergo a general medical education," said one physician condescendingly. "An individual dentist who has taken the medical degree may assuredly be received as a brother practitioner, but a simple D.D.S. never."[33]

In spite of substantial improvements in medical education and the passage of licensing laws, the medical profession at the end of the century still contained, according to one knowledgeable physician, "a vast number of incompetents, large numbers of moral degenerates, and crowds of pure tradesmen." By 1900 there were 151 medical schools, and even the worst institutions sometimes managed to prepare their graduates to pass ineffectual licensing examinations. In one notorious case, the weakest of Chicago's 14 schools—"a school with no entrance requirement, no laboratory teaching, no hospital connections"—outperformed its 13 rivals on the state boards. The medical practice acts, complained one contemporary, allowed all but "the most flagrant quacks and charlatans from carrying on their business unmolested."[34] Thus after a half-century of reform much remained on the medical profession's agenda for elevating its status: the elimination of inferior medical schools, the enactment of stricter licensing laws, and the creation of a powerful national body to represent the interests of physicians.

## THE REFORMATION COMPLETED

The professional leaders of American medicine faced the 20th century determined to complete the reformation they had begun, that is, to reduce the quantity and increase the quality of medical practitioners. Although the ratio of physicians to patients had scarcely changed during the previous 50 years—in fact, it had actually improved from 1:568 in 1850 to 1:576 in 1900—American doctors continued to view the overcrowding of their profession by poorly trained physicians as their greatest problem. Such individuals, argued the reformers, not only provided inadequate and sometimes dangerous care, but also depressed physician income. Well into the 20th century, most American physicians earned less than $2,000 a year. In 1914, for example, less than 60 percent of Wisconsin's approximately 2,800 practitioners earned enough even to pay income taxes; and of those who paid, the average income was only $1,488—well below that of bankers, manufacturers, and lawyers, though more than twice what professors earned.[35]

The profession's first order of business was to create a united front. Since its founding in 1847, the A.M.A. had remained virtually impotent; it had, noted its president sadly in 1901, "exerted relatively little influence on legislation, either state or national." Only about 7 percent of the country's physicians had joined the association, and independent state and county societies often operated at cross purposes to the will of the national body. In response to this situation, an A.M.A. committee in 1901 recommended a complete reorganization: the welding of local, state, and national units into one representative society that would "foster scientific medicine and . . . make the medical profession a power in the social and political life of the republic." Henceforth, membership in a local (generally county) society would automatically carry membership in the state and national organizations. This plan, approved at the 1901 annual session, produced immediate results. Most state societies fell quickly into line, and membership in the A.M.A. multiplied over sevenfold within five years. For the first time American physicians possessed an organization large enough and strong enough to further their interests effectively.[36]

Like its 19th-century parent, the reorganized A.M.A. fought to control access to the profession by tightening the requirements for medical education and licensure. In 1904 it created a Council on Medical Education, which soon began inspecting and grading medical schools. A few years later the council cooperated with the Carnegie Foundation in producing Abraham Flexner's famous report on *Medical Education in the United States and Canada* (1910). This muckraking exposé described conditions — often abysmal — at each of the country's 155 medical schools. The adverse publicity generated by the A.M.A.'s inspections and the Flexner report, together with continuing pressure from licensing bodies and the growing expense of providing laboratory and clinical instruction, forced many institutions to shut down — and finally brought a halt to the overproduction of unqualified physicians. Between 1910 and 1920 the number of medical schools declined from 155 to 85, and it continued falling for the next two decades. By the late 1910s the total number of physicians in the United States was dropping for perhaps the first time in history. The schools that survived this winnowing were, by 1930, generally requiring a bachelor's degree for admission and offering rigorous scientific and clinical training. Unlike the improvements of the 19th century, which had little to do with the A.M.A., these changes often resulted from the A.M.A.'s cozy relationship with the state licensing boards, which delegated to the A.M.A. (sometimes jointly with the American Association of Medical Colleges) the privilege of deciding which schools merited approval for the licensing of their graduates. By this means, and by accrediting hospitals for the training of interns, organized medicine gained considerable control over the education and supply of physicians.[37]

The medical profession enjoyed much less success in its efforts to monopolize the practice of medicine by outlawing rivals and controlling allies. As we have seen, during the last quarter of the 19th century regular physicians often united reluctantly with their old nemeses, the eclectics and homeopaths, to win passage of state licensing laws. In 1903 the A.M.A. took additional steps toward unity by deleting its ethical ban against consulting with irregulars and by welcoming as members eclectics and homeopaths willing to forsake sectarian dogma for scientific truth. This latter act proved to be the kiss of death for eclectic and homeopathic organizations, which, though still

numerically strong, were now struggling to survive. Weakened by internal discord, defecting members, and the lack of state-supported medical schools, they soon ceased to be a factor in American medicine.

The demise of eclectics and homeopaths did not, however, eliminate sectarian competition. During the late 19th century Christian Science, osteopathy, and chiropractic made their appearance, and by the early 20th century these new "cults," as the medical establishment insisted on calling them, began threatening the therapeutic consensus based on scientific medicine as well as the economic goals of physicians. Despite an intensive and protracted campaign by the medical profession to have these sects declared illegal, all three won the legal right to practice their form of healing. The nature of their victory varied from state to state, but their experience in Wisconsin illustrates the various means they used to thwart the medical profession's monopolistic designs.

Like their spiritual leader, Mary Baker Eddy, Christian Science practitioners denied the existence of disease and the need for physicians. Instead of prescribing drugs, they relied on prayer and verbal persuasion to cure individuals who imagined themselves to be ill. Christian Scientists began practicing in Wisconsin in the 1880s, but physicians could do little to stop them before the state passed a medical practice act in 1897. Following enactment of this bill, authorities in Milwaukee arrested two Christian Science practitioners for violating the new law. At their trial the defendants argued that they were not guilty of practicing medicine "because they never administered drugs, never performed surgery, never manipulated the body or even touched their patients." Nevertheless, the court convicted them — only to be overruled by a higher court, which agreed that Christian Science had little in common with medicine. Thereafter, Christian Scientists in Wisconsin faced only the insults of physicians, not the threat of arrest. In some other states, as we have noted, legislators specifically exempted them in defining medical practice.

Osteopathy was founded by a Missouri physician, Andrew Taylor Still, who turned against regular medicine after drug therapy failed to save the lives of his children. Convinced that the human brain functioned as "God's drug store," he attributed all disease to obstructions inhibiting the flow of blood and nervous fluid, which he sought to cure using manual manipulation, particularly of the spine. The first osteopaths arrived in Wisconsin in the 1890s, and by 1900, 19 had located in the state. Charged in that year with illegal practice under the 1897 statute, the osteopaths lost their first court case. Seeking relief, they petitioned the legislature to create a separate licensing board for osteopathy. Regular physicians lobbied instead for the addition of an osteopath to the existing licensing board, believing that the "requirements are so high it is safe to say that but few, if any, osteopaths will ever be able to meet them." The regulars got their wish, but discovered to their chagrin that the underrated osteopaths routinely qualified for licenses to practice. Elsewhere, in over half the states, regulars suffered even greater humiliation, as legislators ignored their pleas and set up separate boards composed only of D.O.'s.

Chiropractic, the brainchild of an Iowa grocer, Daniel David Palmer, explained disease in terms of dislocations of the spine, which allegedly impeded the circulation of nervous fluid. Like osteopaths, with whom they were frequently confused, chiropractors relied therapeutically on adjustments of the spinal column. When the first of them moved to Wisconsin in the early 1900s, they landed in jail for practicing *osteopathy* without a license. Undeterred, they continued to practice illegally until 1915, when the legislature granted them immunity to work as unlicensed practitioners. Ten years later it disregarded the will of the medical profession and, like legislatures in many other states, voted to create a separate chiropractic board of examiners.[38]

In the early 1930s one study of medical care in America reported that "the efforts of the medical profession to prevent legal recognition of the chiropractors have met with almost universal defeat." In fact, by this time nearly a quarter of American healers were Christian Scientists, osteopaths, chiropractors, or irregulars of some stripe. It was clear, concluded the same study, that "in the United States the legislative regulation of the healing art is not accomplishing its acknowledged purpose," that is, creating a monopoly for regular physicians.[39]

Medical doctors encountered equal difficulty keeping assorted other health-care professionals from intruding on what they regarded as their rightful domain. Although they actually assisted podiatrists in achieving their independent status — on the grounds that corn-cutting like tooth-pulling was too trivial to control — they fought continually to limit the activities of such interlopers as optometrists, psychologists, and midwives, who competed directly with physicians specializing in ophthalmology, psychiatry, and obstetrics.[40] The medical profession hoped to restrict the practice of such individuals by defining medicine comprehensively; however, unsympathetic judges and legislators time and again sided with its opponents, as can be seen in the history of relations between physicians and optometrists.

Until the latter part of the 19th century physicians generally left the dispensing of spectacles to itinerant peddlers and other businessmen, who fitted eyeglasses on a trial-and-error basis. But after the 1860s, when a Dutch opthalmologist showed how various visual disorders could be treated by prescribing glasses, physicians became increasingly active in the field — and resentful of opticians who continued to test for lenses. The issue came to a head in 1892, when a couple of New York ophthalmologists warned an optician named Charles F. Prentice that he was violating the state's medical practice act by performing such tests. If he wished to prescribe lenses rather than simply sell them, they argued, "he must first get a degree of M.D. and then a license to practice in this State." Prentice responded to this veiled threat by organizing a state optical society and appealing to the legislature to pass a special practice act for opticians.

During the ensuing debate it became clear that opticians (or optometrists, as they came to be called) sought a status equivalent to dentists, who functioned independently of the medical profession, whereas physicians wanted to relegate optometrists to a position analogous to pharmacists, who simply filled physicians' prescriptions. "The optician must be forbidden to prescribe spectacles," declared one medical journal, "and it should be as illegal for the optician to prescribe glasses as it is for the pharmacist to prescribe morphine or arsenic. Both the optical instrument and the drug are medical agents, and only a physician is fitted to judge of the propriety of their use." Retorted Prentice, "A lens is not a pill."[41]

Despite medical harassment, including occasional arrests for violating medical practice acts, optometrists eventually acquired full legal recognition. During the two decades between 1901 and 1921 they won judicial decisions declaring optometry to be outside the sphere of medical practice, and every state in the Union passed laws setting up examining boards for optometrists. These laws usually barred them from using drugs and, to their great irritation, allowed physicians to refract eyes and prescribe glasses; nevertheless, such statutes represented a clear victory for the optometrists and another humbling defeat for the medical profession, which continued into the 1950s to shun optometrists and to debate whether optometry was a cult or merely a medical sect.[42]

## THE PROFESSION AND THE PUBLIC

A century after the founding of the A.M.A. the American medical profession could look with pride on its various accomplishments. Although its efforts to monopolize the practice of medicine had fallen far short of its goals, it had, through its alliance with the law, eliminated overcrowding in the field, greatly reduced the number of incompetents practicing medicine, and acquired so much prestige and power that medicine became the envy of other professions. By the mid-20th century physicians had become the most admired professionals in the land, and, benefiting especially from the growth of health insurance, had passed bankers and lawyers to become the nation's highest paid workers.[43] Despite mounting criticism of the medical profession during the past couple of decades, physicians have, by and large, retained their elevated position in American society.[44] And despite the increasing intrusion of insurance companies, government agencies, and various allied health professionals into the medical domain, the gains physicians made during the first half of the 20th century have, to a great extent, remained intact.

Medical apologists have long argued that professional advancement brought corresponding gains to the public. "There is nothing for the benefit of medicine unless it is for the benefit of the people," declared one medical society official. "The two interests are identical." In recent years, however, critics of the medical profession have increasingly questioned such assumptions, arguing instead that the reforms we have described "centralized, bureaucratized, modernized and expanded medicine and medical education in the interests of physicians' own professional needs and with little regard for the needs of the public."[45]

The truth, I believe, lies somewhere between these two extremes. On the one hand, there can be little doubt that physicians benefited handsomely from their efforts to regulate and monopolize the practice of medicine. It is equally apparent that the elevation of the profession, in conjunction with other factors, drove up the cost of medical care, created a shortage of American-trained doctors, and damaged the chances for the poor and minorities to pursue careers in medicine.[46] On the other hand, only the most prejudiced observer would argue that the public did not gain as well. Curative medicine may have contributed little to the dramatic reduction in mortality during the past century, but physicians using preventive and ameliorative measures did significantly improve the quality and length of life in America.[47] And although the profession continues to harbor its share of scoundrels, patients today enter doctors' offices with much less cause for fear—and much more hope of being helped—than did their grandparents and great-grandparents. The interests of the profession and the public may not be identical, but neither are they antithetical.

## NOTES

1   N. S. Davis, *History of the American Medical Association* (Philadelphia: Lippincott, Brambo and Co., 1855), p. 56.

2   See, e.g., Vern L. Bullough, *The Development of Medicine as a Profession: The Contribution of the Medieval University to Modern Knowledge* (Basel: S. Karger, 1966).

3   [Lemuel Shattuck], *Report of the Sanitary Commission of Massachusetts* (Boston: Dutton & Wentworth, 1850), p. 58.

4   "The American Medical Association: power, purpose, and politics in organized medicine," *Yale Law J.*, 1954, *63*: 1018.

5   See, e.g., Joseph F. Kett, *The Formation of the American Medical Profession: The Role of Institutions, 1780–1860* (New Haven: Yale Univ. Press, 1968); and

William G. Rothstein, *American Physicians in the Nineteenth Century: From Sects to Science* (Baltimore: Johns Hopkins Univ. Press, 1972).

6 Samuel Haber, "The professions and higher education in America: a historical view," in *Higher Education and the Labor Market*, ed. Margaret S. Gordon (New York: McGraw-Hill Book Co., 1974), p. 251. The "mania" quotation comes from James H. Cassedy, "Why self-help? Americans alone with their diseases, 1800–1850," in *Medicine without Doctors: Home Health Care in American History*, ed. Guenter B. Risse, Ronald L. Numbers, and Judith W. Leavitt (New York: Science History Pubs., 1977), p. 35.

7 "American vs. European medical science again," *Med. Rec.*, 1869, *4*: 183. See also Martin Kaufman, "American medical education," in *The Education of American Physicians: Historical Essays*, ed. Ronald L. Numbers (Berkeley and Los Angeles: Univ. of California Press, 1980), pp. 7–28.

8 Harris L. Coulter, *Divided Legacy: A History of the Schism in Medical Thought*, 3 vols. (Washington, D.C.: McGrath Publishing Co., 1973), III, 143.

9 Worthington Hooker, *Physician and Patient; or, A Practical View of the Mutual Duties, Relations and Interests on the Medical Profession and the Community* (New York: Baker and Scribner, 1849), p. viii.

10 These paragraphs on sectarian medicine are extracted from Ronald L. Numbers, "Do-it-yourself the sectarian way," in *Medicine without Doctors*, pp. 49–72.

11 Kett, *Formation of the American Medical Profession*, p. 186.

12 Richard Harrison Shryock, *Medicine in America: Historical Essays* (Baltimore: Johns Hopkins Press, 1966), p. 151.

13 Rothstein, *American Physicians*, p. 178. For a positive view of medical prestige, see Barbara G. Rosenkrantz, "The search for professional order in 19th century American medicine," *Proc. Int. Cong. Hist. Sci.* 1974, *14* (No. 4): 113–124; see also ch. 16, this book.

14 Kett, *Formation of the American Medical Profession*, pp. 13, 165.

15 Richard Harrison Shryock, *Medical Licensing in America, 1650–1965* (Baltimore: Johns Hopkins Press, 1967), pp. 31–32.

16 Coulter, *Divided Legacy*, p. 182.

17 Davis, *History*, pp. 30–32.

18 J. J. Taylor, *The Physician as a Business Man; or, How to Obtain the Best Financial Results in the Practice of Medicine* (Philadelphia: Medical World, 1981), p. 94; "Code of medical ethics," *Tr. A.M.A.*, 1857, *10*: 607–620.

19 "Code of medical ethics," p. 614.

20 Rothstein, *American Physicians*, p. 120.

21 Robert P. Hudson, "Abraham Flexner in perspective: American medical education, 1865–1910," *Bull. Hist. Med.*, 1972, *56*: 545–561 (ch. 10, this book); Thomas Neville Bonner, *American Doctors and German Universities: A Chapter in International Intellectual Relations, 1870–1914* (Lincoln: Univ. of Nebraska Press, 1963).

22 Simon Flexner and James Thomas Flexner, *William Henry Welch and the Heroic Age of American Medicine* (New York: Viking Press, 1941), pp. 219, 222–223; Robert E. Kohler, "Medical reform and biomedical science: biochemistry—a case study," in *The Therapeutic Revolution: Essays in the Social History of American Medicine*, ed. Morris J. Vogel and Charles Rosenberg (Philadelphia: Univ. of Pennsylvania Press, 1979), p. 32.

23 Haber, "The professions," p. 260.

24 Kaufman, "American medical education," p. 19.

25 Donald E. Konold, *A History of American Medical Ethics, 1847–1912* (Madison: State Historical Society of Wisconsin, 1962), p. 30.

26 Alexander Wilder, *History of Medicine* (New Sharon, Maine: New England Eclectic Publishing Co., 1899), pp. 776–835.

27 Eliot Freidson, *Profession of Medicine: A Study of the Sociology of Applied Knowledge* (New York: Dodd, Mead & Co., 1970), p. 21.

28 John S. Haller, Jr., *American Medicine in Transition, 1840–1910* (Urbana: Univ. of Illinois Press, 1981), pp. 126, 266; Rothstein, *American Physicians*, pp. 308–309.

29 Coulter, *Divided Legacy*, pp. 433–434. For confirmation of this opinion by a regular physician, see Hooker, *Physician and Patient*, p. 255.

30 Philip A. Kalisch and Beatrice J. Kalisch, *The Advance of American Nursing* (Boston: Little, Brown, 1978), pp. 150–153; Mary Roth Walsh, *"Doctors Wanted: No Women Need Apply": Sexual Barriers in the Medical Profession, 1835–1975* (New Haven: Yale Univ. Press, 1977), p. 142; Janet Wilson James, "Isabel Hampton and the professionalization of nursing in the 1890s," in *The Therapeutic Revolution*, p. 221.

31 Haller, *American Medicine in Transition*, pp. 268–272; James G. Burrow, *Organized Medicine in the Progressive Era: The Move toward Monopoly* (Baltimore: Johns Hopkins Univ. Press, 1977), p. 114.

32 L. Laszlo Schwartz, "The historical relations of American dentistry and medicine," *Bull. Hist. Med.*, 1954, *28*: 545.

33 Robert W. McCluggage, *A History of the American Dental Association: A Century of Health Service* (Chicago: American Dental Association, 1959), pp. 155, 169–171. See also William J. Gies, *Dental Education in the United States and Canada* (New York: Carnegie Foundation, 1926), pp. 39–40.

34  Shryock, *Medical Licensing*, p. 60; Abraham Flexner, *Medical Education in the United States and Canada* (New York: Carnegie Foundation, 1910), p. 170; Rothstein, *American Physicians*, p. 310.

35  Ronald L. Numbers, *Almost Persuaded: American Physicians and Compulsory Health Insurance, 1912–1920* (Baltimore: Johns Hopkins Univ. Press, 1978), pp. 4, 9; Committee on Social Insurance, *Statistics Regarding the Medical Profession*, Social Insurance Series Pamphlet No. 7 (Chicago: American Medical Association, [1917]), p. 123.

36  Numbers, *Almost Persuaded*, pp. 27–28.

37  *Ibid.*, pp. 4, 113; Kaufman, "American medical education," p. 20; Shryock, *Medical Licensing*, p. 63; "The American Medical Association," pp. 969–970.

38  Elizabeth Barnaby Keeney, Susan Eyrich Lederer, and Edmond P. Minihan, "Sectarians and scientists: alternatives to orthodox medicine," in *Wisconsin Medicine: Historical Perspectives*, ed. Ronald L. Numbers and Judith Walzer Leavitt (Madison: Univ. of Wisconsin Press, 1981), pp. 59–68; Louis S. Reed, *The Healing Cults: A Study of Sectarian Medical Practice—Its Extent, Causes, and Control* (Chicago: Univ. of Chicago Press, 1932). Regarding osteopathy, see Norman Gevitz, *The D.O.'s: Osteopathic Medicine in America* (Baltimore: Johns Hopkins Univ. Press, 1982); and Erwin A. Blackstone, "The A.M.A. and the osteopaths: a study of the power of organized medicine," *Antitrust Bull.*, 1977, *22*: 405–440.

39  Reed, *The Healing Cults*, pp. 1, 121.

40  See, e.g., Maurice J. Lewi, "Medicine and podiatry in New York State," *N.Y. St. J. Med.*, 1954, *54*: 536–540; John C. Burnham, "The struggle between physicians and paramedical personnel in American psychiatry, 1917–41," *J. Hist. Med.*, 1974, *29*: 93–106; Frances E. Kobrin, "The American midwife controversy: a crisis of professionalization," *Bull. Hist. Med.*, 1966, *40*: 350–363 (ch. 14, this book); and Judy Barrett Litoff, *American Midwives: 1860 to the Present* (Westport, Conn.: Greenwood Press, 1978).

41  Charles F. Prentice, *Legalized Optometry and the Memoirs of Its Founder* (Seattle: Casperin Fletcher Press, 1926), quotations on pp. 27, 55; James R. Gregg, *American Optometric Association: A History* (St. Louis: American Optometric Association, 1972), p. 47.

42  Gregg, *American Optometric Association*, pp. 56–58, 79–80; Louis S. Reed, *Midwives, Chiropodists, and Optometrists: Their Place in Medical Care* (Chicago: University of Chicago Press, 1932), pp. 36–60; *1846–1958 Digest of Official Actions: American Medical Association* (Chicago: American Medical Association, 1959), pp. 536–540.

43  Robert W. Hodge, Paul M. Siegel, and Peter H. Rossi, "Occupational prestige in the United States, 1925–63," *Am. J. Sociol.*, 1964, *70*: 290; Andrea Tyree and Billy G. Smith, "Occupational hierarchy in the United States: 1789–1969," *Social Forces*, 1978, *56*: 887; Ronald L. Numbers, "The third party: health insurance in America," in *The Therapeutic Revolution*, pp. 192–193 (ch. 17, this book).

44  John C. Burnham, "American medicine's golden age: what happened to it?" *Science*, 1982, *215*: 1474–1479 (ch. 18, this book).

45  Ronald L. Numbers, "Public protection and self-interest: medical societies in Wisconsin," in *Wisconsin Medicine*, p. 96; Gerald E. Markowitz and David Karl Rosner, "Doctors in crisis: a study of the use of medical education reform to establish modern professional elitism in medicine," *Am. Quart.*, 1973, *25*: 107.

46  See, e.g., Herbert M. Morais, *The History of the Negro in Medicine* (New York: Publishers Co., 1967); and Walsh, "*Doctors Wanted*," pp. 192–194. Although the percentage of women in medical schools declined during the first half of the 20th century, Walsh argues (p. 237) that they were not driven out of the profession by licensing laws and educational requirements. Rather, she attributes the decline to overt discrimination against women.

47  On the relationship between medicine and mortality in America, see the introduction to this book.

# 14

## The American Midwife Controversy: A Crisis of Professionalization

### FRANCES E. KOBRIN

Although medicine itself has long been an established profession, many of the specialties within medicine have a much shorter history. This diversification is a result not simply of developments within the field itself but has also depended upon the attitude of potential patients — their feeling of a need for such specialization and their ability to take advantage of it. The role of this external factor, however, has varied considerably in the historical development of the several specialties. Surgery became differentiated as soon as the techniques developed enabling it to be practiced safely, whereas other specialties, such as dermatology, plastic surgery, or orthodontics, had to wait until a public attitude evolved which considered ills far less serious than malaria (itself once thought a natural state) as unnatural conditions which require treatment.

Such a specialty was obstetrics, which dealt with what many still consider to be the "natural process" *par excellence*. In the obstetricians' struggle for universal acceptance they faced both medical and nonmedical competition and an almost insuperable economic problem; the level of even the best obstetrical work was almost more of a hindrance than a help. The decade from about 1908 began the contest between the increasingly self-conscious obstetrical specialist and his adversaries, the midwife and her advocates. That such a debate could be carried on with great virulence is itself indicative of the importance of considerations other than the strictly medical. The result, the complete defeat of the United States' variety of midwife and the essential triumph of a "single standard of obstetrics," was not simply a function of the maturity of the obstetric profession.

In the United States in 1910, about 50 percent of all births were reported by midwives,[1] and the percentage for large cities was often higher. At the same time, and continuing well beyond this peak period, the maternal death rate in the United States was the third highest of countries which kept such records.[2] Midwives were employed primarily by Negroes and by the foreign-born and their children, and the midwives themselves usually shared race, nationality, and language with their customers.[3] Because this was a period of unrestricted and heavy immigration (one-third of the population was foreign-born or Negro),[4] the midwife population was swollen considerably.

At this time also, various local medical units in the nation began to assess the situation in their areas, and this resulted in a flood of articles and addresses on "the midwife problem in ——." The big eastern cities, most affected by the heavy immigration, were the most diligent in this regard and produced the bulk of the available data. In 1906, New York commissioned a study which revealed that the New York midwife was essentially medieval, very different from European midwives, for these did not emigrate as rapidly as those who expected such service. According to this report, fully 90 percent were "hopelessly dirty, ignorant, and incompetent."[5] These revelations resulted in the tightening up of existing legislation, and the creation of new, for the licensing and supervision of midwives, and eventually in the establishment of the Bellevue School for Midwives, an institution which lasted for 30 years. Other areas reported similar conditions.

The major failing of the midwife, which this

Frances Kobrin Goldscheider is Associate Professor of Sociology, Brown University, Providence, Rhode Island.

Reprinted with permission from the *Bulletin of the History of Medicine*, 1966, *40*: 350–363.

legislation was to correct, was responsibility for maternal deaths from puerperal sepsis and for neonatal ophthalmia, both preventable with the knowledge available at the time. But it became clear during the controversy that occurred over how to deal with this problem that the midwife was by no means the sole offender in these matters. A survey of professors of obstetrics reached the conclusion that general practitioners were at least as negligent as midwives, as well as being equally responsible for preventable deformities.[6] The overall picture of the obstetrical possibilities open to a prospective patient was not very good. Hospitalization was impossible for all but the very rich or the charity cases in the wards, obstetricians were few, and general practitioners unreliable. Use of a midwife involved many hazards, despite the fact that she was usually a sympathetic woman who would wait and work with the natural labor process (often, of course, for too long) and would also in many cases be in regular attendance for more than a week afterwards, not only caring for mother and infant, but also assuming such duties as were necessary to keep the household functioning normally.

The most obvious cause of this medically unsatisfactory situation was the general opinion that the midwife was an adequate birth attendant. Her success was due to the fact that the rigors of childbirth were still considered normal and risks in the process unavoidable. The general attitude was that nature really controlled the process so that there was little constructive assistance that could be given. This feeling was clearly dominant among the public, although there were signs of change; it was also an important attitude within the medical profession as a whole. One observer, in assessing the lack of interest in obstetrics generally, noted that the word "obstetrics" comes from a Latin word meaning "to stand before" and added, "or as a sneering colleague once said, 'to stand around.'"[7]

The best evidence that this was the judgment of the medical profession was the status of the teaching of obstetrics in United States medical schools. Dr. J. Whitridge Williams, Professor of Obstetrics at Johns Hopkins University, made a comprehensive report on obstetrics as it was studied in United States medical schools in 1912; he found that although medical schools had been improving rapidly, obstetrics was by far the weakest area.[8] He sent a questionnaire to professors of obstetrics in 61 schools rated by the American Medical Association as acceptable (they required entrants to have at least a high school degree) and to 59 nonacceptable schools, receiving 32 and 11 replies respectively. Among his results were the following: Of the 43 professors of obstetrics, only five limited their outside practice to obstetrics, 21 to obstetrics and gynecology, and 17 were in general practice. Only ten had served in lying-in hospitals for more than six months. Only nine had seen more than 1,000 cases of labor as preparation for their post, 13 had seen fewer than 500, five fewer than 100, and one had never seen a woman deliver. Six schools had no connection whatsoever with a lying-in hospital for teaching purposes, and only nine had as many as 500 cases a year for teaching material. The average medical student witnessed but one delivery, and the average for the best 20 medical schools was still only four. Half the schools required a period of service of less than a year in training assistants for their own staff, a level, according to Williams, at which a student is still unable to recognize, much less cope with, a serious emergency. Several of the professors admitted that they themselves were incapable of performing a Caesarean section. Williams concluded that there was only one medical school in the country properly equipped for teaching obstetrics, and he regretted that it was not Johns Hopkins. The result of this neglect of obstetrics, he saw clearly, was that poor schools with poor facilities and poor professors were turning out incompetent products who lost more patients from improper practices than midwives did from infection.[9]

But the obstetricians themselves were fighting this conception of the insignificance of their field. They argued again and again that normal pregnancy and parturition are exceptions and that to consider them to be normal physiologic conditions was a fallacy.[10] It was this view which contributed to much of the unnecessary operative interference that occurred in this period. Amused critics pointed out that women often delivered themselves while their doctors were scrubbing up for a Caesarean,[11] but other results, such as the use of high forceps previous to sufficient dilation, were less fortunate for the health of mother or child.

It was these two fundamentally different approaches to the process of childbirth, based on opposite views of its naturalness, which were responsible for many of the arguments which appeared during this period about the future of the midwife. At one extreme were those who advocated outright abolition of midwives, with legal prosecution of those who continued to practice. This was the official attitude of the state of Massachusetts and also that of most eminent obstetricians.[12] Less adamant was a second group, led by Dr. W. R. Nicholson of the Pennsylvania Bureau of Medical Education and Licensure, which favored eventual abolition, with the existing midwives closely regulated until substitutes could be furnished. A third group was pessimistic about ever abolishing the midwife and thus felt that regulation plus education would elevate the midwife to the relatively safe status she had achieved in England and on the continent. This attitude was reported from Newark, New York State generally, and New York City and Buffalo particularly. Finally, there were those, especially in the South, who felt that if, somehow, midwives could be made to wash their hands and use silver nitrate for the babies' eyes, that would, because of a host of economic and cultural reasons, be the most that could be expected.[13]

Since all but those who held the first position believed that at present there really was no substitute for the midwife, and thus she had at least temporarily to be endured, their views can be conveniently called the public health approach. Their concern was for the immediate future. The first group based its arguments on the necessity of developing obstetrics for the long-term good of American mothers, and so can be identified with the professional approach. An early analyst of this division in medical opinion described it as a conflict between the practical and the ideal,[14] but the actual arguments involved a great deal more than that.

The public health exponents did, in fact, always claim to be realistic, and they accused the professionals of "criminal negligence."[15] The aspects of the situation which they were in a position to consider were certainly important. Since midwives were registering 50 percent of all births, it did not seem likely that the medical profession could expand sufficiently to take care of all. Some public health officials were not even sure that such expansion was desirable. Arguments against it included the record of the medical profession as a whole, the economic problem of supporting the

higher prices charged by doctors, and the attitude of the women themselves. There was also a subterranean problem of status: doctors were often considered less manageable than the more easily supervised midwife.[16]

With regard to the question whether the medical profession ever could absorb all the obstetric cases, Dr. Florence E. Kraker of the Children's Bureau in Washington felt that the midwife problem would actually grow as the preference for hospitals and laboratories among doctors increased, causing them to desert rural areas.[17] Even if sufficient expansion were possible, it would still be necessary, according to New York City Public Health official Dr. S. Josephine Baker, to keep midwives and make them safe, because immigrant women, and particularly their husbands, would allow no male attendants. They expected the simple nursing care and household help that a doctor would not provide, and for this they expected to pay the customary small fee. Providing only doctors for these groups would force them either to pay a higher fee or to use clinics with their implication of charity. Above all, they rejected hospital delivery, which would badly upset the home situation.[18]

What encouraged the proponents of the public health view most was the actual process which had been made through legal recognition, education, and supervision of midwives. England was the chief source of inspiration, since Parliament had, as recently as 1902, established a Central Midwives Board "to secure the better training of midwives and to regulate their practice." Following this change, infant mortality, which had been 151 per 1,000 in 1901, dropped to 106, in 1910, with a commensurate decrease in maternal mortality.[19] A committee of the Russell Sage Foundation, after studying the results, was entirely in favor of the change. In particular, they found that rather than replacing obstetrical practice with trained midwives, it had "increased, improved, and upheld the work of the obstetrician."[20] Germany was also much admired by those of public health persuasion, since the midwife there was a scrupulously regulated institution, trained in government clinics and working in a set district in a defined relationship with a government doctor.[21] The level of obstetric training received by German midwives was recognized as superior to that of most United States doctors.[22]

Major progress had also been made in the United States itself. Newark, after adopting a program of "conference, lectures and personal visits," reported a drop in the three years, 1914–1916, in maternal mortality from 5.3 to 2.2 per 1,000 for the city as a whole, and a level of 1.7 per 1,000 among mothers who "received prenatal supervision from the Child Hygiene Division and were delivered by midwives." This was aggressively compared with the rate of 6.5 for Boston, where midwives were banned. For 1916, again, Newark's infant mortality rate below one month was 8.5 for the special category, as opposed to a city rate of 36.4. The reporting of births was greatly improved, silver nitrate was in universal use, and Board of Health Officer Levy was highly pleased with his results.[23] In Philadelphia a similar program, which emphasized in addition control through registration, gave its director "hope to show statistics unequaled in the history of the world."[24] Midwives, more secure in their licensed status, were calling doctors earlier and oftener, neonatal ophthalmia had vanished, and all at relatively little cost.

Besides pragmatically recognizing the midwife's possibilities, many of her promoters felt a strong sympathy for her and her deficiencies. Ira S. Wile defended her on the grounds that it was "unfair to criticize the lack of an educational standard which has never been established." He felt that abolition was no more the answer than it had been for nurses of the "Sairy Gamp type," 18th-century doctors, or present-day obstetricians, all of whom, by absolute standards, were very bad indeed.[25] Midwives also gained sympathy from their adherents because of the rudeness with which the "arrogant," "unrealistic" obstetricians treated them. Those most in favor of the midwife seemed bent on elevating her to a professional status well above that of a nurse. Recognition was to build self-respect and pride; caste and dignity would bring a more intelligent type of woman into the profession.[26]

It was with these general attitudes that the public health exponents faced the task of elevating the American midwife. The consensus which developed was that midwives should have training for at least six months to a year, including instruction on pregnancy, asepsis, care of labor, and of mother and child after confinement, and, above all, recognition of conditions that indicate when a doctor is needed. These requirements, coupled with legal proscriptions against vaginal examinations, drugs other than laxatives, douches, and the use of instruments, would, they felt, render the midwife a useful member of the community. The further elaboration of linking the midwife to a clinic and to a physician who would make examinations and be available for emergencies was advocated by some, but the problem of maintaining doctors in government employ presented such difficulties that many public health officials were forced to ignore the possibility that a doctor might not be available when needed.[27]

What is important in the plans discussed and occasionally established by public health officials is that in general these men were not simply embracing a distasteful necessity that would otherwise have been avoided. There were some, of course, who felt this way: the official who established the Philadelphia system was well aware of "the incongruity of allowing or actively sanctioning by license, the doing of distinctly medical work by non-medical persons. We cannot adduce a single argument in its favor except . . . *necessity*."[28] But the others were expressing an ideal of obstetric service whereby the ubiquitous process of childbirth could be carried on cheaply and easily, respecting modesty and the integrity of the household, and in a more natural and personal way than if rendered by doctors.

The solution offered by the obstetric profession, on the other hand, was not merely an ideal of obstetric care, but also a very realistic solution for the obstetricians' difficulties. Until this last great wave of immigration, graduating obstetricians had always found sufficient numbers of patients. J. L. Huntington, a Boston obstetrician who was partly responsible for Massachusetts' unique position and was the most vocally concerned of the professionals, observed that the midwife was not — yet — a native product of America. She comes with the immigrant, "but as soon as the immigrant is assimilated, . . . then the midwife is no longer a factor in his home."[29] It was this latest influx of immigrants from southern Europe which had given the midwife problem such dimensions, and, if left alone, her numbers would again dwindle with the slowing of immigration. But if she were given official recognition so that immigrants' sons and grandsons expected such service for their wives, the obstetric profession would, he felt, face grave difficulties.

Huntington believed, therefore, that the greatest danger in recognizing the midwife lay in the effect of such recognition on the general public. If the midwife was sufficient, then calling a G.P. would be the height of caution, and there would be no need felt for obstetricians.[30] He and other obstetricians believed recognition of midwives would set the progress of obstetrics back tremendously. The 50 percent of all cases handled by midwives were useless for advancing obstetrical knowledge. Elevating the midwife and training her would decrease the number of cases in which the stethoscope, pelvimeter, and other newly developed or newly applied techniques could be used to increase obstetrical knowledge. The need for strengthening obstetrics courses in medical schools would diminish, and practicing doctors would think themselves so superior to the strengthened corps of midwives that they would feel no need for improvement.[31] Lowering the standard of adequacy would lower all standards.

Because they believed this situation existed, the obstetricians had very different perspectives from the public health exponents. Some physicians felt the arrangement in Germany was far from ideal, so that even if such a system could be transplanted to the United States the resulting standard of obstetrics would be inadequate. Although German midwives learned obstetrics of high quality in their six-month course, that time was considered insufficient to instill an "aseptic conscience." Further, even in Germany their relationship with the physician was not one of "perfect harmony." According to Huntington's analysis, since it was profitable for a midwife to deliver each case herself, she might postpone calling a physician in time of danger; the physician, as well, might also be insufficiently cautious if he were called in, since the responsibility for complications remained with the midwife. Huntington argued further that in the United States such a plan would be impossible because (stating clearly the issue which so troubled some public health officials) the American medical profession could never be forced by law to respond to the call of the midwife in trouble.[32]

From the professional standpoint, the solution in England was also a bad one. In fact, the more midwives there were, and the more successful they were, the worse the situation would be for the community at large, according to Huntington, because

this would aggravate a "double standard of obstetrics." The 30,000 English midwives had not only taken cases that would have been better cared for by doctors but had also taken enough practice away from physicians to obtain a livelihood.[33] Dr. Charles Ziegler, who was later to become cynical about the whole debate, also complained of the estimated five million dollars collected annually in the United States by midwives "which should be paid to physicians and nurses for doing the work properly."[34] The relationship between the ideal of a "single standard" and the issue of economic competition came up clearly again when obstetricians saw the midwife to be in league with "outside" influences — optometrists, osteopaths, neuropaths, Christian Scientists, and chiropractors — who were all invading the legitimate field of medicine.[35] Massachusetts had just licensed optometrists; "if the midwives are now to be recognized we may fairly ask, where is it going to end?"[36]

The professional ideal, of course, was that all women be delivered by an obstetrician, privately, or, if they could not afford such care, in a hospital-medical school complex. Thus, at a stroke, the midwife would be eliminated and the basis established for enormous advances in obstetrics, since students would then get ample training. In suggesting such a system for New York City, Dr. J. Van D. Young felt that even if it were inaugurated at state expense, "the ultimate good to the profession and to the people would be enormous" and rapidly repaid, and, also, that it would attract serious obstetrical students to New York.[37]

The professionals saw only one way by which their goals could be reached and those of the public health approach thwarted. There had to develop a demand from the public for a higher standard of obstetrics. "We can teach the expectant mother what she deserves, and when she demands it she will get it."[38] They urged accordingly that every mother has a right to such care as shall preserve her and hers in life and health, the care which, they said, the midwife cannot provide since the necessary skills are difficult to teach. Combating the "fallacy" of normal pregnancy and delivery was necessary not only to enhance the value of obstetric skills but also to make the American mother not merely respect, but fear, possible danger and so consider no precaution excessive.

Behind both these perspectives on the midwife

problem was a complicating factor with which neither side dealt adequately. The economic realities of the situation and the costs of the various programs should have been given far more consideration. Since these economic aspects were working against the obstetricians in particular, they were the most guilty in this respect. In general, the public health approach overstated the economic obstacles to the realization of the obstetricians' ideal, whereas the obstetricians tended to ignore such obstacles, with one significant exception. The problem was that the training of an obstetrician was expensive, and his practice had to be sufficiently lucrative to draw able men into the field. In addition, the expansion of hospital and laboratory facilities to train new men and for their use in practice was expensive. Public health officers, who always have many places to spend every appropriation, are not in a position to weigh these facts and their possible consequences; the chief attraction of the midwife for them was that she was cheap. Levy, who established the Newark system, considered as only rhetorical the question whether those who can only afford midwives "should be delivered in finely appointed hospitals at public expense."[39] Others presented the obstetric ideal as a sort of *reductio ad absurdum*. The obstetricians, on the other hand, ignored this difficulty altogether because of their hope of changing what was then a very annoying fact: the same family will pay easily for surgery but expect to pay meagerly for attendance during pregnancy and confinement.[40] All that would be needed was propaganda to solve what they felt was not really an economic problem.

Huntington felt he had another answer to the "economic necessity for the midwife." Boston Lying-In Hospital ran an Out-Patient Department to provide obstetric training for medical students, and the patients, contributing an average of $1.28 each, in 1910 paid "all the expense" of the department, with a surplus of $807.82.[41] But his conclusion that the finest hospital care was itself inexpensive can be seriously questioned. The Boston medical school complex attracted prospective obstetricians from all over the country. Cases used for teaching amounted to nearly 20 percent of the total number of births in Boston in 1913.[42] Huntington thus claims an amazing percentage, and few other areas could hope to rival it, considering the scarcity of obstetricians at that time; yet it still left

80 percent of the births unaccounted for. It can perhaps be safely inferred that the costs of giving the rest similar treatment would rise rapidly, once deliveries had to be accomplished without the help of unpaid medical students. Yet even if the costs were indeed relatively low for caring for everyone on such a basis, the necessary expenditures on facilities to make room for all would be beyond the economic horizon of public officials forced to account closely for their use of public funds.

Only two writers proposed a solution which would make ideal obstetric care possible for all, given all the existing conditions. A. K. Paine, Huntington's only apparent critic in his home state, said that our method of government was not suited to the rigid requirements which the properly regulated midwife demands, but that the "obstetric poor" could be handled on a community basis, if the community would assume the responsibility.[43] Because of the stress Paine gave community responsibility, his argument clearly implied public institutions staffed by government employees and run with tax funds on some level or another.

Charles Ziegler, who earlier had complained of the money wasted on midwives, was a Pittsburgh obstetrician who was concerned with the midwife problem. What happened to him when he attempted to approximate ideal obstetric care for all puts an interesting light on the importance of the "ideal" elements in the original professional argument. Ziegler's experiment also involved inexpensive delivery of the poor and, although he got his funds privately, he had even then the idea that what was essentially obstetric charity should not be borne solely by obstetricians, but should be subsidized by the community.[44] Although he had no access to public funds, he evidently could generate other sources of aid by his enthusiasm for his project. Ziegler wanted to establish a dispensary which could give the best care to those who usually did not get such care, i.e., those not in either of the extreme income categories. The aim was to demonstrate how much mortality statistics could be improved, in the hope, of course, that the result would provide encouragement for others to try to achieve the same result. Six years after opening the dispensary in 1912, $80,000 in contributions had been spent caring for 3,384 confinements on both an in- and an outpatient basis. Fifty-six percent of the cases were foreign-born and 16 percent were Negroes. There were two sets of results. First, maternal mortality was 17 per 10,000 as opposed to a national average of 88.5.[45] This was a remarkable result for the time and clientele. The other result was that the Allegheny County Medical Society found Ziegler guilty of breaches of professional ethics by "solicitation and attendance on cases in families able to pay for a physician [and] . . . solicitation and attendance on cases where a physician had previously been engaged."[46]

Ziegler himself was suspended from the society, and, in 1918, his hospital was commandeered for government service, finishing his experiment.[47] Ziegler concluded after all this that, given the existence of such patients, the cost of caring for them properly (about 20 times Huntington's figure of $1.28), and the strength of the enemies made in the process, the only solution would be municipal, state, and federal aid, not as charity, "but as a matter of wise public policy and of justice to those to whom we look for the perpetuation of our family and national life."[48] He saw the whole obstetric problem as an economic one in which many people could not pay for the services they deserved; an institutional redistribution of such services was therefore necessary.

He believed that his solution would bring opposition from the medical profession, "as they are opposed to any plan which includes municipal or state aid looking toward the solution of the problem on a public-health or public-welfare basis."[49] For although Ziegler's solution ostensibly fulfills the obstetric ideal by granting every American mother her "right," by his method the natural elevation in status of obstetricians which would otherwise have occurred might be jeopardized.

Today the prospective American mother theoretically has access to high quality obstetric care. If she is from a relatively urban environment, this is available through clinics, or through a private obstetrician, for whom a group insurance plan might help pay. If she is from a rural area, a general practitioner graduated from a medical school, whose quality, both overall and in obstetrics, has greatly improved, is likely to be available. Obstetrics, both as a branch of medicine and in professional status, has advanced significantly. Can this result somehow be attributed to the developing superiority of obstetrics as performed by obstetri-

cians, or could the forces arrayed against them have been exaggerated by the obstetricians, making the whole issue just a paper debate?

It appears that despite the potential obstetric superiority of obstetricians over midwives, the triumph of the former was probably due most to the fact that the circumstances debated in this period changed radically. It is certain that the relevant health conditions were not improving in those areas where the midwife was first being superseded. Although in Washington the percentage of births reported by midwives shrank from the 1903 high of 50 percent to 15 percent in 1912, infant mortality in the first day, the first week, and the first month of life had all increased in this period. Also, New York's dwindling corps of midwives achieved significant superiority over New York's doctors in the prevention of both stillbirths and puerperal sepsis.[50] Rather, the obstetricians triumphed because, before the public health programs became firmly established in the public mind, the obstetrician gained tremendous advantages from other sources. Immigration decreased significantly during the war and was afterwards reduced legally to a small fraction of the numbers experienced just before the war. This put time entirely on the side of the physicians, a considerable advantage in itself, while concurrently the economic problem *per se* was greatly reduced. This did not occur simply because of the "prosperity" of the 1920s, which may have had no impact at all; rather, the secular trend towards limitation of family size accelerated to include nearly the entire population. In 1919 in New York City there were 1,700 midwives who were responsible for 40,000 births, or 30 percent of the total. In 1929, though there were still 1,200 midwives, they delivered but 12,000, 12 percent of the total.[51] Not only did the average deliveries per midwife shrink decidedly from 23 to 10 births a year, but also total births decreased by 25 percent. With the limitation of births, it is possible that pregnancy and anticipated delivery seemed sufficiently rare to be generally equated with major operations and worthy of greater expense.

The other secular shift in attitudes from which the obstetricians benefited was a new, general demand for improved obstetrics, the change for which they had been most devoutly hoping. The midwife controversy itself was in some ways a reflection of this change. It was not merely the benevolent concern of public health officials about their vital statistics which was instrumental in effecting all the legislation regulating the midwife. Also responsible was a growing public demand from women, who were becoming increasingly self-conscious about their own welfare, and who were still infected with the reforming zeal of the Progressive Era which was to lead to their enfranchisement. These were, after all, the women who shortly afterward were to deluge their congressmen and senators with pleas for the passage of the Sheppard-Towner Bill. This bill, which Ziegler worked for, provided federal money to the states for the "protection of maternity." With "womanhood" no longer rooted in the domestic, "natural" environment, or perhaps reflecting the struggle for release from such roots, the "natural" way of doing things was losing its appeal for the many emerging American women, and the obstetrician was increasingly there to reap the results of a growing anxiety about childbirth.

In summary, then, the professionalization process was very sensitive to external conditions and attitudes. If conditions had not changed so propitiously, if an economic problem and a conflict of attitudes had continued to exist, the obstetrician might well have found himself in the position of the present-day psychoanalyst with the public realizing that his skills solve but a small part of a complicated problem.

## NOTES

1  Thomas Darlington, "The present status of the midwife," *Am. J. Obst. & Gynec.,* 1911, *63*: 870.
2  E. R. Hardin, "The midwife problem," *Southern Med. J.,* 1925, *18*: 347.
3  See nearly any discussion of the subject at this period, e.g., Darlington, "Present status of the midwife"; J. Clifton Edgar, "The remedy for the midwife problem," *Am. J. Obst. & Gynec.,* 1911, *63*: 882.
4  Darlington, "Present status of the midwife."
5  Edgar, "The remedy for the midwife problem."
6  J. Whitridge Williams, "Medical education and the midwife problem in the United States," *J.A.M.A.,* 1912, *58*: 1–7.
7  C. E. Ziegler, "How can we best solve the midwifery problem," *Am. J. Public Hlth.,* 1922, *12*: 409.
8  Abraham Flexner came to much the same conclusion in his discussion of the clinical years in American medical schools. *Medical Education in the United States and Canada: A Report to the Carnegie Foundation for the Advancement of Teaching.* Bulletin No. 4 (New York, 1910), p. 117.
9  Williams, "Medical education."
10  See, for example, J. F. Moran, "The endowment of motherhood," *J.A.M.A.,* 1915, *64*: 126; J. L. Huntington, "The midwife in Massachusetts: her anomalous position," *Boston Med. & Surg. J.,* 1913, *168*: 419.
11  "Discussion—midwife problem," *N.Y. St. J. Med.,* 1915, *15*: 300.
12  For an impressive list, see Huntington, "The midwife in Massachusetts," p. 420.
13  W. A. Plecker, "The midwife problem in Virginia," *Virginia Medical Semi-Monthly,* 1914–1915, *19*: 457–

458; Helmina Jeidell and Willa M. Fricke, "The midwives of Anne Arundel County, Maryland," *Johns Hopkins Hosp. Bull.,* 1912, *23*: 279–281.
14  A. K. Paine, "The midwife problem," *Boston Med. & Surg. J.,* 1915, *173*: 760.
15  Clara D. Noyes, "The training of midwives in relation to the prevention of infant mortality," *Am. J. Obst. & Gynec.,* 1912, *66*: 1053.
16  "Discussion—midwife problem."
17  Hardin, "The midwife problem," p. 349.
18  Josephine Baker, "The function of the midwife," *Woman's Med. J.,* 1913, *23*: 197.
19  Noyes, "The training of midwives," p. 1054.
20  *Ibid.,* p. 1052.
21  A. B. Emmons and J. L. Huntington, "The midwife: her future in the United States," *Am. J. Obst. & Gynec.,* 1912, *65*: 395–396.
22  Hardin, "The midwife problem," p. 347; Emmons and Huntington, "The midwife," p. 395.
23  Julius Levy, "The maternal and infant mortality in midwifery practice in Newark, N.J.," *Am. J. Obst. & Gynec.,* 1918, *77*: 42.
24  W. R. Nicholson, "The midwife situation . . . ," *Tr. Am. Gynec. Soc.,* 1917, *42*: 632.
25  "Schools for midwives," *Med. Rec.,* 1912, *81*: 517.
26  *Ibid.,* p. 518.
27  See, among others, Hardin, "The midwife problem," p. 349; Plecker, "The midwife problem in Virginia," p. 457; J. A. Foote, "Legislative measures against maternal and infant mortality," *Am. J. Obst. & Gynec.,* 1919, *80*: 550; Edgar, "The remedy for the midwife problem," p. 883.
28  Nicholson, "The midwife situation . . . ," p. 626.

29 Emmons and Huntington, "The midwife," p. 399.
30 Huntington, "The midwife in Massachusetts," p. 419.
31 *Ibid.*
32 Emmons and Huntington, "The midwife," pp. 397–400.
33 *Ibid.*, p. 394.
34 Charles E. Ziegler, "The elimination of the midwife," *J.A.M.A.,* 1913, *60*: 34.
35 "Discussion—midwife problem," p. 299.
36 Huntington, "The midwife in Massachusetts," p. 419.
37 J. Van D. Young, "The midwife problem in the State of New York," *N.Y. St. J. Med.,* 1915, *15*: 295.
38 George C. Marlette, "Discussion," in Hardin, "The midwife problem," p. 350.
39 Levy, "Maternal and infant mortality," p. 41.
40 Paine, "The midwife problem," p. 761.
41 Huntington, "The midwife in Massachusetts," p. 421.
42 Paine, "The midwife problem," p. 762.
43 *Ibid.*, pp. 763–764.
44 Ziegler, "The elimination of the midwife," p. 34.
45 Ziegler, "How can we best solve the midwifery problem," pp. 407–408.
46 *The Weekly Bulletin. Official Journal of the Allegheny County Medical Society, 5*, No. 7 (Feb. 12, 1916), 5.
47 Ziegler, "How can we best solve the midwifery problem," pp. 412–413.
48 *Ibid.*, p. 407.
49 *Ibid.*, p. 413.
50 Baker, "The function of the midwife," p. 196.
51 Hattie Hemschemeyer, "Midwifery in the United States," *Am. J. Nursing,* 1939, *39*: 1182.

# 15

## The Search for the Hospital Yardstick: Nursing and the Rationalization of Hospital Work

### SUSAN REVERBY

Skyrocketing costs and seemingly irrational, un-businesslike procedures have been the major problems ascribed to health care institutions in the 1970s. As concern over these issues has grown, the mantle of service and charity, which for so long has covered hospitals and other health care facilities, has slowly been removed. No longer minor parts of the economy, the hospitals have become business behemoths. They are now expected to run according to capitalist logic as much as any automobile plant or department store.

Because hospitals are labor intensive, much of the concern has focused on ways to curb labor costs and to rationalize the work process.[1] The nurses, because they are the largest group within the hospital work force, have come under particular attention. Attempts to manage and control the nurses are not new, however; only the forms it takes are different. This paper will explore the relationship between hospitals and nursing by examining the managerial reforms for control over the work force and the role that nurses and other direct patient-care workers played in bringing about these changes from the last quarter of the 19th century to the early 1950s. This approach suggests that the labor process in hospitals was shaped by the need of or-ganized nursing to establish its professional status and by the concern of the hospitals to have a loyal work force. I will be examining general tendencies in this process, aware that hospitals are notoriously idiosyncratic facilities where policies can vary between floors, departments, and institutions.

When the editor of the journal *Hospital Management* was searching for an appropriate date for the first annual National Hospital Day in 1921, he settled on May 12 — neither the anniversary of a medical breakthrough, nor the founding date of a great hospital, but the birthday of Florence Nightingale.[2] This symbolic gesture suggests both how closely the histories of hospitals and nursing are tied and how much hospital managements wanted to share in the charitable and saintly image of "the lady with the lamp." But in 1921 hospitals were no longer just charitable institutions, and 75 percent of the "ladies with the lamps" were not working in them.[3]

Hospitals, of course, have always had someone performing some kind of nursing function. Up until the last quarter of the 19th century it was frequently the patients, expected to care for one another when they were ambulatory. There were usually some women employed as nurses, but they were mostly unskilled and provided low level domestic functions. Many were on loan from the adjoining almshouses, although others worked in the hospitals permanently and gained a modicum of skills.[4] An occasional middle- or upper-class "lady" might be trained on the job as head nurse or matron.

The important change in the hospital's nursing work force began in 1873 when the first nurses' training schools were established. Some of the early

SUSAN REVERBY is Director and Assistant Professor of the Women's Studies Program at Wellesley College, Wellesley, Massachusetts.

This paper was originally presented as part of a panel on "Management Reform and Women's Work" at the American Historical Association convention in 1976. It subsequently appeared in *Health Care in America: Essays in Social History*, edited by Susan Reverby and David Rosner (Philadelphia: Temple University Press, 1979), pp. 206–225, and appears here with the permission of the editors.

schools were independent institutions with their own boards, but by the 1880s most schools were organized and controlled by the hospitals, who used the students as a source of nonwage labor. Nursing students were given only small allowances and, along with untrained attendants, became the major employees of most hospitals until the 1930s.

The growth of the hospitals was in part tied to the growth in nursing schools. In 1873, when the first nursing schools were founded, there were 178 hospitals in the United States. By 1923 there were 6,830 hospitals (an increase of over 3,700 percent), and every fourth one included a nursing school. By 1941 the number of hospitals had dropped by 7 percent because of the Depression, but the number of beds had increased by 75 percent.[5]

The two-class health delivery pattern of the late 19th and early 20th centuries meant that upper-class and upper-middle-class patients retained private duty nurses in their homes, or occasionally in hospitals. The poor and working class, especially if they were charity cases, relied on the hospitals and dispensaries. By the 1920s private-duty home care was becoming less common, the hospitals were being used more by all classes, while the two classes of care continued within and between institutions.[6]

The change in the role of hospitals beginning in the Progressive Era was not due to medical science and specialization alone, but also to urbanization, competition for patients between physicians, nurses, and hospitals, and a fiscal crisis within the hospitals resulting in declines in their philanthropic and public charity incomes.[7] Particularly in voluntaries and proprietaries, administrators and trustees had to devise schemes to bring in paying customers as a legitimate way to ease their financial difficulties. They had to convince the general populace that the hospitals were no longer just places where the poor were left to die.[8] In 1908 the superintendent of St. Luke's Hospital in Chicago bluntly declared at an American Hospital Association convention:

> If we can make our hospitals sufficiently attractive to induce patients to remain during convalescence, to come for diagnosis instead of going to hotels and visiting the doctor at his office and to come in for treatment of more or less chronic forms of disease, we will not only increase the number of possible patrons, but the prolonged stay

will mean added work and further, the average profit per patient will be greater.[9]

To the administrators what was being created was both a "workshop for physicians" and a "modern hospital hotel."[10]

Yet the administrators and trustees had an ambivalence about these changes; they shared a sense of hope and a vision of their institutions as scientific centers and efficient businesses, as well as a real uncertainty about giving up their traditions of charity and paternalism.[11] However slowly, hospital care was becoming a commodity, not a charity. Patient payments were becoming the hospitals' most important income source.[12] As health care in the hospitals began to be sold to an increasingly higher class of patients, the administrators and trustees became more and more concerned with their "sales-force." Hospital care may have become a commodity, but it was still one being produced, despite the rhetoric, in a workshop by a largely undifferentiated work force. Unlike commodity producers, however, hospital administrators and trustees did not understand how to determine their own costs, labor or otherwise, lacked any real concept of how to measure productivity, and even questioned if it should be measured at all.

But they were caught up in the early 20th-century rhetoric and concern for efficiency. Many of the businessmen on the boards of trustees, although often aware that the hospital and their own enterprises were quite different, nevertheless felt that an efficient operation, from increasing the number of pay patients to improved nursing service, was part of the hospital's moral obligation to the community. In 1914, appropriately, they invited Frank Gilbreth, one of the fathers of scientific management, to speak at the hospital convention. Gilbreth was highly critical of the hospital's lack of standardization and haphazard organization of work. The commentator on his paper gave lipservice agreement to his ideas. However, the journal *Modern Hospital* reflected the more widespread view when it reprinted his speech, not the commentary, and editorialized that the "dollar yardstick" alone could not be used to measure the hospital's worth.[13]

But the administrators and trustees did believe they needed a new yardstick to measure their employees' worth. As one administrator ruefully commented, "a $15-a-week clerk may have it in her power to alienate a $50,000-a-year endowment," or to drive patients away.[14] Thus, after financing, the most crucial problem, as the administrators perceived it, was the disciplining of their work force.[15]

Nineteenth- and early 20th-century hospital management practices reflected the charity outlook, the unskilled and menial nature of most of the work, and the religious and military origins of hospitals and nursing. Under the rubric that the hospital was a family, the male superintendent (if there was one) or the chief surgeon was regarded as the father, the nursing school superintendent or matron was the mother, and the workers, nursing students, and patients were the children.[16] Both patients and workers were seen as recipients of the institution's charity. Workers were disciplined, like children, through the hospital's control over their daily lives: their food, housing, clothing, sexual activities, even the hours they slept. Rigid lines of authority were reinforced through separate housing entrances and dining facilities.

Women's boards often served as the workers' supervisors, trying to enforce middle-class standards of domestic amenities and measuring work success as if it were domestic service in their homes.[17] Thus appearances, docility, sobriety, cleanliness, and speed, measured by the window shades aligned in a ward or the coverlets on the patients' beds pulled tight by 8:00 A.M., were all signs of proper worker behavior. But hospital managements fully expected their employees, whom they saw as morally flawed, to steal, to cheat the institution at every turn, and to quit with regularity.[18] Despite the paternalism, as Charles Rosenberg has argued, the hospitals frequently had a culture and life of their own over which the administrators, trustees, and visiting committees had very little control.[19]

Nursing students were also subject to this paternalism. Nursing superintendents were responsible for the education of the students, what little of it there was, but mainly for the actual staffing of the hospitals with these students. As would-be employees, students were replaced whenever dropouts occurred. There was little concern for admission standards other than health and strength. Discipline, order, cleanliness, and respectability were all to be the hallmarks of this new creation—the hospital-trained nurse. Character, tact, and obedience, as well as antiseptic and aseptic techniques, were the new nurse's major skills.

Nursing schools ran under a rigid disciplinary model that was supposed to teach "idealism" and "implicit, unquestioning obedience" to a stunted matriarchy in which power only moved downward from the superintendent to the lowliest, newly arrived probationer.[20] Tasks were learned through constant repetition and adherence to each hospital's "one right way," not the "one best way," of performance. A nurse wrote of her training school experience at the turn of the century: "Good care of patients . . . is not made to depend on the individual nurse any more than is absolutely necessary. It is more a matter of a routine being established whose proper working will prevent mistakes on the part of a worker."[21]

Nurses, when they graduated, usually were not employed by hospitals because they were too expensive, too hard to discipline, and too willing to quit. Only those nurses with what was called "executive ability" might expect institutional appointments, and these positions were as nursing superintendents or head nurses, not as general staff nurses.[22] Most graduate nurses therefore became individual entrepreneurs in the uncertain private duty market, where they worked primarily for middle- and upper-class patients in their homes.[23] Those few who accompanied their patients into the hospitals were seen by hospital administrators and nursing matrons as almost dangerous interlopers whose independence might disturb family tranquility.[24]

In private duty the graduates competed for positions with the untrained, with nursing school dropouts, correspondence school, and short-course nurses. By the 1890s nurses in the major cities were complaining about overcrowding, limited training, overwork, and the way in which access to private duty was controlled by the hospitals and physicians running the major nursing registries.[25] The graduate nurse was caught in an ambiguous position. She was a "professional" worker who was expected to perform servant duties; an independent worker who was paid a standard wage and had a busy and slow season like a factory hand; and a skilled worker who was not given any financial incentive, training, or supervision to improve her skills.

When rank-and-file nurses articulated this situation as a severe problem, they were generally blamed by hospitals, physicians, and by many nursing leaders for their lack of character and concern for patients; for their "inability" to choose the proper training school; for their refusal to organize under the leadership of nursing educators whose interests they might see as inimical to their own.[26] Revolt on the part of the nurses was primarily individual: refusing to work for physicians they disliked or distrusted, or to take certain types of difficult cases, gossiping about the hospitals, "floating" from city to city in search of work, or leaving nursing altogether.[27]

By the 1910s the nursing leadership (made up of nursing school superintendents and educators from the larger schools through the National League for Nursing Education and the American Nurses Association), saw that the solution to overcrowding and lack of training in nursing lay in fewer schools, higher admission standards, and less hospital control over the student's education. At the same time, hospital administrators began to realize that their patients were reluctant to accept lower-class workers or untrained students and were bringing more private duty nurses with them into the institutions. Administrators had to agree to some kind of upgrading or training to retain control over their work force. These concerns intensified between 1910 and World War II because of the workers' and nursing students' own response to their conditions.

Nursing leaders complained during the 1920s that women with the "right character" and "proper home training" were not applying to nursing school and that the public saw the school, with its rigidities, as "a sort of respectable reform school where its mental or disciplinary cases can be sent."[28] By the late 1910s and 1920s, as more occupations and white-collar positions were opened for the daughters of the middle-class, nursing was attracting more working-class than middle-class women to its ranks.[29] May Ayres Burgess, the influential author of a 1928 study that was nursing's equivalent to medicine's Flexner Report in 1910, warned both nursing leaders and hospital administrators that the problem was class:

> These undereducated, unprepared women make trouble within the profession. Many of them are drawn from a social group which is not strictly professional in character. They are the ones who are talking trade unionism for nurses. It is natu-

ral that they should. Their fathers, brothers, and sweethearts are ardent members of trade unions. . . . Somehow these undereducated women, of inadequate social and academic background must be kept out of the profession. Fortunately, there is no longer any need for them.[30]

Her fears about unionism were based mainly on future possibilities, although there had been sporadic strikes and union organization among nursing students, nurses, and hospital workers since the 1890s.[31]

On the whole, nurses, nursing students, and other workers in hospitals relied upon subtler forms of revolt. Administrators complained that they refused to answer call buttons, to file reports, to clean up properly, to accept discipline, and would mix medications, complain to patients about the faults of the hospitals, and socialize with each other on hospital time.[32] What they did most visibly was quit. By the 1920s and 1930s hospitals began to realize, as had other industries, that the high turnover rates that they had accepted as inevitable were exceedingly expensive. Improved conditions appeared to be the only solution to the turnover crisis and a way to thwart trade union activity.[33]

The response of hospital administrators and nursing superintendents took several different forms. In general, they made attempts to transform the workers' character rather than to change the actual work process or the inequitable social hierarchy. As in other service industries where the workers' *behavior* is actually part of what is being sold, the administrators concentrated on changing the amenities and refurbishing their 19th-century paternalism in order to obtain a more loyal work force.[34]

Since nurses and workers were often housed in garrets in odd corners of the institutions, administrations began to build fancier nurses' homes, better dining rooms, etc., although the social distinctions between facilities for the different levels of workers were continued.[35] By the Depression the hospitals were moving away from providing full maintenance for all employees with the exception of the nurses. By the 1940s the trend had come full circle and administrators were counseled to "redefine the relationship of employees to the hospital. . . . Non-resident employees should consider the hospital their place of employment and not their home."[36]

Secondly, the appeals for loyalty and greater work effort were made in the language of "joint efficiency" and "mutual cooperation" rather than charitable duties.[37] Since little was done to relieve the drudgery or low pay of the work, in the mid-1920s hospital administrators began to discuss reliance upon a loyal cadre of workers. They later defined this as making it possible to have "the gradual shifting of external authority to internal authority, that is, to an increasing amount of self-control and self-direction."[38] Loyalty was to be obtained by proper training of workers and nursing students to their hierarchical position and to the service ethic of the hospital. The concept of "our hospital" has a more honest ring than when such language becomes "our store" or "our company." Many workers and nurses did feel that way about the hospitals and did have a sense of pride and commitment to caring for patients and sharing the burden of their work. In case the workers did not already have such sentiments, a general service foreman in a San Francisco hospital pointed out "training will imbue them with this essential characteristic."[39] What was new in all of this was that the human relations and industrial psychology techniques of industry were being transplanted to the hospitals. Supervisors, for example, were told to learn about workers' families, to support employee efforts for hard work, and, above all, "to encourage the achievement of personnel stability through the development of personnel loyalty."[40] During the 1920s workers who did not wear uniforms were urged to accept them; administrators hoped this would be a way to promote discipline and instill institutional personalities.[41]

These methods, however, were not employed on a widescale basis, and instead many hospitals came to rely, as did other industries, upon a "flying squadron"—a small core of loyal workers who could be called upon to do a variety of jobs within the hospital.[42] But if the hospital gained this loyal core, it also gained a strong informal network of an "old guard," especially among the nurses. Made up primarily of older single women, these nurses lived together in the hospital residences for nurses and had connections to doctors and the boards of trustees that allowed them to subvert the hospitals' supposed command structures. *Modern Hospital* journal suggested that administrators fire such women when necessary, but such tactics were often unsuccessful when these women had cultivated such high-placed support.[43]

Hospitals were constantly searching for workers who could be relied upon to be loyal, self-motivating within set limits, imbued with the service ethic, willing to accept low wages and their place in a hierarchy, and yet able to transcend normal work loads when emergencies (defined by the administration) or shortages occurred. In the 1920s and 1930s, as medical and nursing practice became more technical and complex, they also began to need nurses who could provide more skilled work. Coupled with organized nursing's desire to upgrade the nurse's position, hospital administrators and nursing leaders together worked out a solution to both their dilemmas: They began to differentiate between the delivery of *nursing care* (which only a trained RN could provide) and the establishment of a *nursing service* (a team of nursing workers on different skill levels).

As early as 1909 the American Hospital Association had suggested the creation of trained subsidiary nursing workers, and physician committees were always suggesting that "subnurses" were really needed.[44] But as long as hospitals and most of the nursing superintendents were convinced that nursing students and untrained attendants were cheaper and more effective, the hospitals were unwilling to begin to think in terms of graded work and a trained assistants' staff. "It was an extraordinary thing," a national nursing report concluded in 1928, "but it seems to be a fact that hospitals regard the suggestion that they pay for their own nursing service as unreasonable . . . the student nurse is seen as an inalienable right."[45] Many nurses also feared that trained nursing assistants would unleash more legitimized lower-priced competition into the already overcrowded private duty market. But if these workers could be given different uniforms, be trained separately, do different work, come from a lower-class or lower-status ethnic group than nurses, as well as stay employed in the hospitals, their threat could be minimized.[46]

Thus, in every generation of nurses there were nursing leaders, many of whom were both nursing educators and hospital administrators, who increasingly saw nursing's future professional status as tied to a rationalized hospital nursing system with a complex division of labor.[47] It was primarily these women who convinced the hospitals both to upgrade the nurse and to subdivide her work because it would be cheaper for hospitals, would give them a disciplined work force through hierarchy and professionalism, and would improve the quality of care. At the turn of the century, they began by questioning the strict ward discipline, citing the fact that the absolute control of the physicians was "short-sighted policy from a business point of view."[48] They argued both that scientific management techniques were applicable to nursing work and that nurses were already unconsciously using them.

It was precisely a concern with detail, systemizing, and proper organization that trained nursing brought to the hospitals. In practice this was usually translated into rigidity and mindless repetition of set patterns. But among nursing's more educated leadership, there was a real willingness to experiment with different forms of work organization and a belief that better training and planning could upgrade the nurse's status and dignity. Anne Goodrich, a nursing educator from Columbia and Yale universities, told the Harvard Medical Club in 1915, "No one is more concerned than a nurse in this standardization of hospitals."[49] Minnie Goodnow, another nursing superintendent and nursing historian, informed the annual hospital convention that nurses were training students "as Mr. Gilbreth does his bricklayers, and as all the efficiency engineers are doing in factories and business offices."[50] M. Adelaide Nutting, the nursing superintendent at Johns Hopkins and later the first full professor of nursing at Columbia, was also interested in the application of scientific management to institutional and home management. A founding member of the American Home Economics Association, she had contacted Lillian Gilbreth, a leading efficiency expert, to enlist her in studying household tasks.[51] The concern with scientific management in both industry and home was therefore transferred by the nurses into the hospitals. By the 1920s the National League for Nursing Education introduced some of the first time-and-motion studies of nursing work.[52]

The major catalyst for change, however, was the Depression, which created another financial crisis for the hospitals. Their income dropped precipitously when demand increased as patients, who could no longer afford either private nursing or physicians, flocked to what they still considered to be charity institutions.[53] Private duty nurses, for whom the Depression had begun in the mid-1920s, found themselves at the point of starvation. By 1932 the American Nurses Association had to send a letter to every hospital in the country urging them to accept graduate nurses on their staffs, to close their nursing schools, and to employ ward assistants.[54] Study after study began to appear in both the nursing and hospital management literature comparing student and graduate labor. The studies were attempts to convince hospitals and reluctant nursing superintendents that graduate nurses were more efficient workers, cheaper because of low wage demands, and easier to discipline both because of their professionalism and because they would be the hospitals' not the patients' employees.[55]

But hospitals were still reluctant to hire graduates as staff nurses. Many institutions did close their nursing schools and the number of schools dropped by 30 percent between 1929 and 1939.[56] But many hospitals substituted a variation on the private duty system called group nursing. The graduate nurse became a hospital employee but was used only with groups of private patients in special rearranged rooms. This allowed the hospital to charge patients extra for this service rather than include it as part of routine hospital care.[57]

The nursing leaders had to convince both hospitals and nurses that the solution to everyone's problems was to have the graduate become a general duty worker in the hospital, not some modified private duty nurse. They faced a reluctant rank and file who saw in hospital work a return to the drudgery, exploitation, and low status they associated with nursing school and institutional employment. Surveys of nursing registries in 1934 and again in 1937 concluded that nurses "are unwilling to accept prevailing conditions of employment for general staff nursing."[58]

The conditions in the hospitals included 12- and 14-hour days on split shifts, excessively strenuous work, rotations from service to service, inadequate pay (often only room and board or a daily salary prorated on a monthly basis), and dismissals when the hospital census dropped. Above all, it meant that once in the hospital the nurse lost her one-to-one relationship with a patient and gained, in the language of the hospital, a "patient load."[59] Overcrowding of patients and understaffing of nurses were chronic dilemmas. For nurses, for whom the very definition of their work was service and comfort to individual patients, the work in hospitals was often an anathema. The nurses reported: "Floor duty in hospitals is too hard and often with not enough help, and one had no time to do the little things for patients that often mean much to add to their comfort and health."[60] But in the hospital the nurse did gain some promise of regular employment when economic conditions were improved. The incorporation of nurses into the hospital became common during the nursing shortages of World War II and in the early 1950s. Time-and-motion studies were used to create a nursing team that divided functions and then assigned them to different level workers, making the RN the foreman of the team. In the words of contemporary critics of current nursing practices, nurses traded control over patient care for some control over other workers.[61]

It should be recalled that in 1914 the hospital administrators and trustees were uncertain about the feasibility of using Frank Gilbreth's yardstick. As late as their 1962 convention, they even showed a film, "Sam Sliderule Surveys the Hospital," which asserted that the efficiency studies of the industrial engineer were not necessarily applicable to the modern hospital.[62] But beginning in the 1920s and growing in the 1950s, nurses provided the hospitals with what they called a "nursing yardstick," by working with industrial engineers, including Lillian Gilbreth, the mother of scientific management, and by sponsoring during the early 1950s over 34 studies on nursing functions in 17 states.[63] The authors of a major hospital engineering textbook in 1966 stated reluctantly: "It is difficult to escape the conclusion that the initiative for the adoption of industrial engineering concepts to hospital activities during the post war years came in large measure from nurses."[64]

But this ultimately proved to be a solution for the hospitals and not for the majority of nurses. As nursing functions were continually spun off, the nurse found herself increasingly task-oriented, tied to paperwork; the nursing station became further and further removed from direct patient care, and the nurse responsible for patients she often never saw or touched. Once incorporated into the administration of the hospital, many nurses quickly gained a stake in its smooth functioning. Advance-

ment in nursing for a few consisted of climbing up the hospital hierarchical ladder, and meant implicit acceptance of the institution's terms. Yet because the hospital's idea of efficiency meant the use of as inexpensive a worker as possible, nurses found themselves (despite legal regulations to the contrary) often doing the same work as aides or licensed practical nurses and trying desperately to define and justify what the differences were between their skills.[65] Chronic understaffing meant nurses were shifted from floor to floor whenever administrators defined the need. As a result, nursing strikes and bargaining issues in the last 30 years have been primarily over staffing patterns and definitions of nursing functions.[66]

As hospitals emerged from their charity base in the 20th century, they grew not so much into full-blown, rationalized, capitalist factories as into capitalist service institutions. As such, their 19th-century paternalism was reformed to meet 20th-century conditions, rather than abandoned. Eric Perkins' view of southern planter-slave relations is equally relevant to hospitals. He points out that "paternalism was never 'pure' in the South because it had to constantly confront the infection of capitalist relations of production and the values associated with it, values measured not by duty or obligation, but by profit and loss."[67] In the hospitals profit and loss were measured less in cash terms and more by numbers of patients, expansion, prestigious research and education; but the same "infection" ran rampant. For the work force, the symptoms were low pay, poor working conditions, high turnover, and constant pressures to accept institutionally defined norms of proper character and service.

Scientific management was therefore more rhetoric than reality in the hospitals in the first half of this century. Nursing leaders, fueled by their need to find nurses a viable work place and to establish their professional role, saw scientific management concepts as meeting their needs and making their work easier. Nursing leadership has continued to see the creation of hierarchy and a caste system as a solution to nursing's professional difficulties. But as nursing leaders struggled to establish the scientific management of nursing work, they were constantly confronted by the objective difficulty of transforming service work into commodity production, the hospitals' unwillingness to use more skilled and expensive labor, and revolts from their own rank and file.

Recent works in nursing history suggest that sexism, male greed, and women's passivity explain nurses' subordination. But nurses must not be seen solely as victims or heroines in a male-dominated system. We must understand both why certain nursing leaders chose the direction they did and how and why their rank and file responded. The American Nurses Association bicentennial history book is entitled *One Strong Voice*, but even a beginning examination of nursing history suggests that there has always been a chorus.

## NOTES

Support from the Milbank Memorial Fund made this research possible. I wish to thank the following for their comments on earlier drafts: Susan Porter Benson, Rosalyn Feldberg, Maurine Greenwald, Diana Long Hall, Lise Vogel, Tim Sieber, David Rosner, Harry Marks, David Montgomery, Sam Bass Warner, Jr., the Work Relations Group.

1 The focus on labor costs has been, in part, because the other costs in the hospitals have been more protected. The use of third-party reimbursements to cover the costs of an additional piece of fancy technology or to pay bank interest charges can be more hidden or justified than wage increases.

2 "First National Hospital Day May 12, organized effort to educate public as to service of institutions begun by HOSPITAL MANAGEMENT, every hospital to benefit," *Hosp. Mgmt.*, Mar. 1921, *11*: 30–33; Malcolm T. MacEachern, "How are you going to celebrate National Hospital Day?" *Hosp. Mgmt.*, Apr. 1931, *31*: 22–26.

3 May Ayres Burgess, *Nurses, Patients and Pocketbooks, Report of A Study of the Economics of Nursing Conducted by the Committee on the Grading of Nursing Schools* (New York, 1928), pp. 248–250.

4 Charles Rosenberg, "And heal the sick: the hospital and the patient in 19th century America," *J. Soc. Hist.*, June 1977, *10*: 428–447.

5 U. S. Bureau of Census, *Historical Statistics of the United States from Colonial Times to 1957* (Washington, D.C., 1959), Series B, pp. 192–194, 235–236; Committee on Hospital Care, *Hospital Care in the United States* (Cambridge, Mass., 1947 and 1957), pp. 52–54.

6 David Rosner, "A once charitable enterprise" (Ph.D. dissertation, Harvard Univ., Dept. of History of Science, 1978); Morris Vogel, "Boston's hospitals, 1880–1930, a social history" (Ph.D. dissertation, Univ. of Chicago, Dept. of History, 1974); Health Policy Advisory Center, *The American Health Empire: Power, Profits and Politics* (New York, 1970).

7 Rosemary Stevens, *American Medicine and the Public Interest* (New Haven, 1971); the analysis is based in part upon my examination of hospital management journals and texts beginning in the 1890s. See also

David Rosner, "Business at the bedside: health care in Brooklyn, 1890–1915," in *Health Care in America: Essays in Social History,* ed. S. Reverby and D. Rosner (Philadelphia, 1979).

8 David Rosner has found that the Brooklyn hospitals began to aggressively advertise their "advantages" during the Progressive Era. In 1923 Somerville Hospital in Somerville, Massachusetts, sent an envelope home with all the school children of the city that informed their parents that: "Your little child might be the next one picked up from underneath a machine and rushed to Somerville Hospital for first aid and his little life saved—THE ONLY HOSPITAL in the city with its doors always open for such cases" (*30th Annual Report,* Somerville Hospital [Somerville, 1923], n.p.).

9 Louis Curtis, "The modern hotel-hospital," *Nat. Hosp. Rec.,* Jan. 15, 1908, *11*: 7.

10 *Ibid.*; George Rosen, "The hospital: historical sociology of a community institution," *From Medical Police to Social Medicine* (New York, 1974), pp. 294–303; Del T. Sutton, "Three years of growth in the hospital field," *Nat. Hosp. Rec.,* Aug. 1900, *3*: 21–26; John A. Hornsby, "The modern hospital—a new entity," *Modern Hosp.,* Oct. 1913, *1*: 112–113; Frederick D. Keppel, "The modern hospital as a health factory," *Modern Hosp.,* Oct. 1916, *7*: 303–306.

11 See, for example, Charlotte Aikens, *Hospital Management* (Philadelphia, 1911); Frank Chapman, *Hospital Organization and Operation* (New York, 1924); Ernest Codman, *A Study in Hospital Efficiency* (Boston, n.d.); John Hornsby and Richard Schmidt, *The Modern Hospital* (Philadelphia, 1913); Albert Ochsner and Meyer Strum, *The Organization, Construction and Management of Hospitals* (Chicago, 1909).

12 C. Rufus Rorem, *The Crisis in Hospital Finance* (Chicago, 1932), pp. 109–115.

13 Frank Gilbreth, "Scientific management in the hospital," *Tr. Am. Hosp. Assn.,* 16th Annual Convention (St. Paul, Minn., 1914), pp. 483–492; Dr. Anker, "Comments on Gilbreth," *ibid.,* pp. 493–494; "The dollar yardstick," *Modern Hosp.,* Nov. 1914, *3*: 318.

14 "Friendliness in the hospital," *Modern Hosp.,* Jan. 1919, *12*: 46.

15  "A symposium on hospital discipline," *Nat. Hosp. Rec.*, June 1905, *7*: 30–35; John Hornsby, "Homes for hospital employees," *Modern Hosp.*, June 1914, *2*: 365–366.

16  See, for example, Nina Dale, "The hospital family—cooperation in domestic management," *Modern Hosp.*, Sept. 1914, *3*: 187–189; Amy Beers, "How nurses may contribute toward a hospital's success," *Modern Hosp.*, Nov. 1914, *3*: 302–304; Asa Bacon, "Nurses and factory labor," *Modern Hosp.*, Apr. 1917, *8*: 299; Charlotte Aikens, "Some opportunities for young women outside the nursing field," *Nat. Hosp. Rec.*, Apr. 1, 1908, *11*: 3–4; George H. M. Rowe, "Observations on hospital organization," *Nat. Hosp. Rec.*, Dec. 1902, *6*: 3–10; this point is more fully developed in JoAnn Ashley, *Hospitals, Paternalism and the Role of the Nurse* (New York, 1976).

17  Janet Wilson James, "Women and the development of health and welfare services in industrial America, 1870–1890," paper presented at the Berkshire Conference on the History of Women, June 1976.

18  "Hospital employees welfare," *Modern Hosp.*, Sept. 1921, *17*: 214; Temple Burling and others, *The Give and Take in Hospitals* (New York, 1956), p. 61; Henry C. Wright, *Report of the Committee of Inquiry into the Departments of Health, Charities, and Bellevue and Allied Hospitals in the City of New York* (New York, 1913), pp. 77–78, 555, 596; Hornsby and Schmidt, *The Modern Hospital*, p. 66; "Discipline," *Trained Nurse & Hosp. Rev.*, Feb. 1913, *50*: 101–102; for the similarity with domestic service, see Lucy M. Salmon, *Domestic Service* (New York, 1897).

19  See note 4 above.

20  Isabel Hampton Robb, *Nursing Ethics* (Cleveland, 1901), p. 46; similarly, see Charlotte Aikens, *Studies in Ethics for Nurses* (Philadelphia, 1916); Lavinia L. Dock, "The relation of training schools to hospitals," *Nursing of the Sick 1893,* reprint of the papers and discussions from the International Congress of Charities, Correction, and Philanthropy, Chicago, 1893 (New York, 1949), p. 20.

21  "With humanity left out" (letter to the editor from a nurse), *Trained Nurse & Hosp. Rev.*, Nov. 1919, *59*: 706.

22  Nancy Tomes, "'Little World of Our Own': the Pennsylvania Hospital Training School for Nurses, 1895–1907," in *Women and Health in America*, ed. Judith Waltzer Leavitt (Madison, 1984), pp. 467–481.

23  Susan Reverby, "'Neither for the Drawing Room nor for the Kitchen,' private duty nursing in Boston, 1873–1920," in *Women and Health in America: Historical Readings*, ed. Judith Walzer Leavitt (Madison: University of Wisconsin Press, 1984), pp. 454–466.

24  "The special nurse" (letter to the editor from "HBJ"), *Trained Nurse & Hosp. Rev.*, Feb. 1915, *54*: 107; Hornsby and Schmidt, *The Modern Hospital, passim*; Janet Geister, "Hearsay and facts in private duty," *Am. J. Nursing*, July 1926, *26*: 80–93.

25  See note 23 above. See also Lavinia L. Dock, "Overcrowding in the nursing profession," *Trained Nurse & Hosp. Rev.*, July 1898, *22*: 8–13; Anita Newcomb McGee, "The growth of the nursing profession in the U.S.," *Trained Nurse & Hosp. Rev.*, June 1900, *24*: 442–445; "Is the profession becoming overcrowded?" *Am. J. Nursing*, Apr. 1903, *3*: 513–515; "An over-supply of nurses," *Pacific Coast Nursing J.*, Jan. 1914, *10*: 3.

26  Between 1897 and 1903 a debate raged in the pages of the *Trained Nurse* on the type of nursing organization that should be formed in New York State, illustrating both the division between rank-and-file graduate nurses and their superintendents and the nature of the attacks on graduate nurses. See "To the graduate nurses of New York State" (letter from superintendents), *Trained Nurse & Hosp. Rev.*, Aug. 1897, *19*: 157–158; "A Jerseyite and a graduate" (letter to the editor), *Trained Nurse & Hosp. Rev.*, Oct. 1897, *19*: 218–219; Lavinia L. Dock, "Trained Nurses Protective Association" (letter to the editor), *Trained Nurse & Hosp. Rev.*, May 1897, *18*: 279–281; Celia R. Heller, "The N.P.A. answers" (letter to the editor), *Trained Nurse & Hosp. Rev.*, June 1897, *18*: 337–340; "New York State legislation," *Trained Nurse & Hosp. Rev.*, Jan. 1900, *24*: 55–56. The debate continued in the *American Journal of Nursing:* Josephine Smetsinger, Letter to the editor, *Am. J. Nursing*, June 1902, *2*: 699–700; "A notice," *Am. J. Nursing*, Mar. 1903, *3*: 495. This debate is discussed by Susan Armeny, "Resistance to professionalization by American trained nurses, 1890–1905," paper presented at the Berkshire Conference on the History of Women, Aug. 25, 1978.

27  "Nurses and state associations," *Trained Nurse & Hosp. Rev.*, Jan. 1911, *46*: 30–31; Letter to the editor, *Pacific Coast Nursing J.*, Mar. 1914, *10*: 130; Ashley, *Hospitals, Paternalism . . . , passim*. Letters in the records of the first nursing registry, the Boston Medical Library Registry of Nurses, also make these points; see Susan Reverby's "Neither for the drawing room . . ."

28  Burgess, *Nurses, Patients and Pocketbooks*, p. 347; see also Charlotte Aikens, "When is a probationer unfit?" *Trained Nurse & Hosp. Rev.*, Feb. 1914, *53*: 103–104; "Personal observation" (letter to the editor from a nurse), *Trained Nurse & Hosp. Rev.*, May 1913, *52*: 306; M. Adelaide Nutting, "Some problems of the training school," *Nat. Hosp. Rec.*, Nov. 1908, *12*: 6–9.

29  The class background of nursing students is currently being studied by several historians. Nancy Tomes (see note 22) and Jane Mottus (NYU Dept. of History) from their work on the Philadelphia and New York hospitals, respectively, suggest that the nursing students, up until World War I, came from middle-class families. My preliminary findings suggest that the smaller schools tended to attract more working-class women and that the shift was, in general, toward working-class women by the 1920s.

30  "Nurses, Patients and Pocketbooks," paper read at the Annual Convention of Nursing Organizations, Louisville, Kentucky, June 7, 1928, *Bull. Am. Hosp. Assn.,* July 1928, *2*: 300–301.

31  "Overworked nurses" (letter to the editor from a graduate), *Trained Nurse & Hosp. Rev.,* Nov. 1890, *5*: 236; "Nurses on strike," *Trained Nurse & Hosp. Rev.,* Feb. 1901, *26*: 95–96; "The profession disgraced," *Am. J. Nursing,* Apr. 1903, *3*: 592; "Nurses' strikes," *Trained Nurse & Hosp. Rev.,* Sept. 1902, *19*: 235–236; "What is the remedy," *Trained Nurse & Hosp. Rev.,* July 1906, *37*: 36–37; "The striking nurse," *Trained Nurse & Hosp. Rev.,* Feb. 1912, *48*: 48; "At the beck of the walking delegate," *The Nurse,* Oct. 1914, *1*: 308–309; "The striking nurse," *Trained Nurse & Hosp. Rev.,* Feb. 1915, *51*: 98; "A trade or a profession," *Trained Nurse & Hosp. Rev.,* June 1920, *56*: 529–530; "Trade unionism and nursing," *Trained Nurse & Hosp. Rev.,* Mar. 1920, *56*: 240.

32  Hornsby and Schmidt, *The Modern Hospital, passim;* Burgess, *Nurses, Patients and Pocketbooks;* Somerville Hospital School of Nursing, Student Records, Somerville, Mass.; Letters in the Boston Medical Library Registry of Nurses, Rare Book Room, Countway Medical Library.

33  "Labor turnover in hospitals," *Modern Hosp.,* Aug. 1923, *21*: 159; Charles Neergaard, "Some causes of labor turnover in hospitals," *Modern Hosp.,* Nov. 1923, *21*: 447–448; Edgar Smith, "Why labor turnover is expensive," *Modern Hosp.,* Mar. 1928, *30*: 58; Jacob Goodfriend, "How can the labor flux be brought to an irreducible minimum?" *Modern Hosp.,* Sept. 1927, *29*: 58; *idem,* "Labor turnover—what will the hospitals do about it?" *Modern Hosp.,* Apr. 1930, *34*: 57; Burgess, *Nurses, Patients and Pocketbooks,* pp. 532–533.

34  For a discussion of this in the department stores, see Susan Porter Benson, "The clerking sisterhood: rationalization and the work culture of saleswomen," *Radical America,* Mar.–Apr. 1978, *12*: 41–55.

35  L. R. Curtis, "Living out versus living in for the hospital employees," *Modern Hosp.,* Apr. 1919, *8*: 253; "Housing the personnel," *Modern Hosp.,* Mar. 1924, *26*: 205.

36  Morris Hinenberg, "Hospital property should not be made PUBLIC," *Modern Hosp.,* Mar. 1943, *60*: 88.

37  "Hospital employees welfare," *Modern Hosp.,* Sept. 1921, *17*: 214; "Welfare work and strikes," *Modern Hosp.,* Sept. 1916, *13*: 263.

38  S. R. Laycock, "A basic need: personnel attributes that satisfy," *Hospitals,* July 1945, *19*: 53–54.

39  John Wylley, "Pathways to better service through proper training of employees," *Modern Hosp.,* June 1924, *22*: 608.

40  Sallie Jeffries, "The personnel problems must be put on a personal basis," *Modern Hosp.,* May 1943, *60*: 55–56; "Discussion—personnel problems," *Tr. Am. Hosp. Assn.,* 38th Annual Conference (Cleveland, 1936), p. 821; Burling and others, *The Give and Take in Hospitals,* pp. 328–333.

41  "Clothes make the man," *Modern Hosp.,* Apr. 1923, *20*: 376–379; John Bresnahan and Harriet Borman, "A uniformed hospital personnel," *Modern Hosp.,* Apr. 1923, *20*: 379.

42  David Montgomery noted that this was particularly common in the rubber and packing industries, but the evidence suggests that the hospitals were not far behind. Discussion with David Montgomery, meeting of the Work Relations Group, Institute for Policy Studies, Washington, D.C., June 6, 1975.

43  "Team work in the hospital," *Modern Hosp.,* Mar. 1915, *4*: 280; "Another source of friction in hospital administration," *Modern Hosp.,* Feb. 1916, *6*: 112. This phenomenon is discussed in the sociological literature; see, in particular, Robert W. Habenstein and Edwin A. Christ, *Professionalizer, Traditionalizer and Utilizer* (Columbia, Mo., 1955); Everett Hughes and others, *20,000 Nurses Tell Their Story* (Philadelphia, 1958); Virginia Walker, *Nursing and Ritualistic Practice* (New York, 1967).

44  Susan Reverby, "Health: women's work," *Prognosis Negative: Crisis in the Health Care System,* ed. David Kotelchuck (New York, 1976), pp. 170–184.

45  Burgess, *Nurses, Patients and Pocketbooks,* p. 434.

46  M, "The attendant, her place and work," *Am. J. Nursing,* Nov. 1919, *20*: 154–155; A. K. Haywood, "The status of the nursing attendant," *Modern Hosp.,* Sept. 1922, *19*: 226–227; A. C. Jensen, "Training nursing attendants," *Modern Hosp.,* Nov. 1938, *51*: 68; Winifred Shepler and others, "Standardized training course for ward aids," *Modern Hosp.,* Dec. 1938, *51*: 68–69; Susan Reverby, "Hospital organizing in the 1950s: an interview with Lillian Roberts," *Signs: Journal of Women in Culture and Society,* Summer 1976, *1*: 1053–1063.

47  I include in this group women whose collective biography has yet to be written: Charlotte Aikens, Mary Riddle, Minnie Goodnow, Anne Goodrich, Shirley Titus, Blanche Pfefferkorn, Eleanor Lambertson.

48  "Why opinions differ," *Trained Nurse & Hosp. Rev.*, Jan. 1908, *40*: 37–38.

49  It is clear from her remarks that Goodrich was concerned with the standardization of nursing duties, not the hospital standardization movement that was beginning at the same time. "Discussion of the Robert Dickinson paper, 'Hospital Organization as Shown by Charts of Personnnel Powers and Functions,'" *Bull. Taylor Soc.*, Oct. 1917, *3*: 8.

50  "Efficiency in the care of the patient," *Tr. Am. Hosp. Assn.*, 16th Annual Conference (St. Paul, 1914), p. 210.

51  Helen E. Marshall, *Mary Adelaide Nutting, Pioneer of Modern Nursing* (Baltimore, 1972), p. 158. My thanks to Delores Hayden for suggesting that I look at the influences of the home economics movement on nursing.

52  Elizabeth Greener, "A study of hospital nursing service," *Modern Hosp.*, Jan. 1921, *16*: 99–102; A. Owens and others, "Some time studies," *Am. J. Nursing*, Feb. 1927, *27*: 99–101; Blanche Pfefferkorn and Marion Rottman, *Clinical Education in Nursing* (New York, 1932); for a review of this literature, see Myrtle Aydelotte, *Nurse Staffing Methodology, A Review and Critique of Selected Literature* (Washington, D.C., 1970).

53  Ronda Kotelchuck, "The Depression and the AMA," *Health PAC Bull.*, Mar.–Apr. 1976 (No. 69): 13–18.

54  "National nursing groups appeal to hospital trustees," *Modern Hosp.*, July 1932, *34*: 108.

55  Malcolm MacEachern, "Which shall we choose — graduate or student service," *Modern Hosp.*, June 1932, *38*: 94–104; Anna Wolf, "Is the use of graduate nurses for floor duty justified?" *Modern Hosp.*, Nov. 1929, *33*: 140–142; "How many students can a graduate nurse replace?" *Modern Hosp.*, Aug. 1933,

*41*: 86; J. C. Geiger, "An important change in policy," *Am. J. Nursing*, Feb. 1932, *32*: 180.

56  U.S. Bureau of Census, Series B, pp. 192–194.

57  Shirley Titus, "Group nursing," *Am. J. Nursing*, July 1930, *30*: 845–850; Shirley Titus, "Graduate nursing, the significance of general duty nursing to our profession," *Am. J. Nursing*, Feb. 1931, *31*: 197–208; Shirley Titus, "Group nursing and how it affects the welfare of the patient," *Modern Hosp.*, Dec. 1930, *35*: 120–128; Subcommittee of the Joint Distribution Committee of the Joint Boards of the Nursing Organizations, "Institutional nursing," *Am. J. Nursing*, June 1931, *31*: 689–692.

58  "What registries did," *Am. J. Nursing*, July 1937, *37*: 736.

59  Carol Taylor, *In Horizontal Orbit, Hospitals and the Cult of Efficiency* (New York, 1973), p. 58.

60  Burgess, *Nurses, Patients and Pocketbooks*, p. 353.

61  Boston Nurses Group, "The false promise: professionalism in nursing," *Science for the People*, May/June 1978, *10*: 20–34.

62  Harold E. Smalley and John R. Freeman, *Hospital Industrial Engineering* (New York, 1966), p. 49.

63  Pfefferkorn and Rottman, *Clinical Education in Nursing*, p. 3; Smalley and Freeman, *Hospital Industrial Engineering*, p. 63; Hughes and others, *20,000 Nurses Tell Their Story*; Aydelotte, *Nurse Staffing Methodology*.

64  Smalley and Freeman, *Hospital Industrial Engineering*, p. 63.

65  Reverby, "Health: women's work."

66  David Gaynor and others, "RN's strike: between the lines," in D. Kotelchuck, *Prognosis Negative*, pp. 229–245.

67  "Roll, Jordan, roll: a Marx for the master class," *Radical Hist. Rev.*, Summer 1976, *3*: 44.

# IMAGE AND INCOME

Despite some slippage in recent years, medicine remains the most trusted and envied of all professions. This was not always so. During the first three hundred years of our country's history the practice of medicine ranked relatively low in professional status. The prestige of physicians reached its nadir in the middle third of the 19th century, with the proliferation of low-quality medical schools, the fragmentation of the profession into quarreling sects, and the repeal of laws regulating the practice of medicine. Even so, as Barbara Gutmann Rosenkrantz points out, American physicians benefited from living in a culture that, lacking an hereditary aristocracy, elevated the professions to a natural aristocracy.

The status of physicians improved during the latter part of the century, as medicine grew more scientific, efficacious, and restrictive. By 1900 most states had enacted licensing laws to exclude incompetents from inflicting themselves on the public. Nevertheless, other occupations, such as law, business, and even the ministry, continued to attract the best and brightest students.

The relatively low income of physicians undoubtedly contributed to medicine's lack of appeal. Although a handful of 19th-century physicians acquired small fortunes, a large percentage of medical-school graduates eventually abandoned medicine to seek greener fields elsewhere. As late as 1913 the American Medical Association estimated that only about 10 percent of physicians in the United States were earning "a comfortable income." The tax records of Wisconsin for the next year lend credence to this statement. Fewer than 60 percent of the state's practitioners earned enough even to be eligible for taxes, and among those required to pay, the average earnings were $1,488 a year, compared to $3,581 for bankers and capitalists, $2,810 for manufacturers, and $2,567 for lawyers.

The financial advantages of medicine did not become apparent until about the time of World War II. As Ronald L. Numbers argues, health insurance—first voluntary, then government-sponsored—played a crucial role in elevating the income of physicians. By the mid-1970s the average American doctor worked approximately 58 hours a week and earned more than $50,000 a year. With increased income came high status, especially in certain specialties, such as thoracic surgery and neurosurgery. Among physicians, general practitioners and physiatrists benefited the least.

Despite frequent complaints about the high costs and low quality of medical care in the United States, characteristic of the end of what John C. Burnham calls the Golden Age of American medicine, most Americans hold their own physicians in high regard. This apparent paradox is illustrated by a survey in the 1970s that found 85 percent of the respondents satisfied with their own doctors, but only 60 percent who thought the quality of medical care in America was good or excellent. Among the young, many of whom fought desperately for a chance to become physicians, no profession held greater promise.

# 16

# The Search for Professional Order
# in 19th-Century American Medicine

## BARBARA GUTMANN ROSENKRANTZ

In the 20th century we insist on the importance of confidence in the medical profession; if all else fails, we expect that the physician's scientific training assures a minimal competence. Few Americans in the mid-19th century could have chosen their doctors with this expectation in mind. So far as medical education was concerned, no agreed-upon body of knowledge about the cause and character of disease justified a systematic theory of pathology. No classification of disease was generally accepted; indeed the names used for identifying diseases and distinguishing among different illnesses defied the creation of order, and since nosologies were not standardized this compounded the difficulty of collecting and interpreting statistics of morbidity and mortality. Nonetheless, despite what we see retrospectively as an unpromising situation, doctors did practice medicine, win their patients' loyalty, and retain plausible confidence in their colleagues' skills.

American doctors were most often trained by a combination of schooling and apprenticeship to more experienced men; the differences among practitioners in different regions of the country were in part a reflection of loyalty to their mentors' schools of thought. They moved about with far greater frequency than most doctors do today, their social origins and intellectual convictions determining where they set up practice. It is difficult to assess the cultural significance of the array of diagnostic and therapeutic options offered by 19th-century prac-

titioners, and today we hold an understandably dim view of the effectiveness of the medical care available to Americans then. We know relatively little about how 19th-century doctors faced their frustrating limitations before the growth of scientific knowledge and effective technology—central to every account of the end of that era—led to the transformation of medical practice in the 20th century. Although medical knowledge and the conquest of many dread diseases have fundamentally altered health and life, historians generally agree that these accomplishments do not fully account for the prestige and power of the medical profession today.[1]

Our own social and ethical dilemmas in the face of evident medical progress make us sensitive, moreover, to an earlier predicament that is both strange and familiar. Between 1870 and 1910 many reputable American doctors advocated more stringent professional standards in order to subdue the disorganization of medical ideas and medical authority, but they also disputed the contribution of science to this end and even called attention to the dangers science posed to accepted medical practice. These physicians' ambivalence toward science undoubtedly had many roots; the psychological, sociological, and economic dimensions of mistrust are indications of what physicians feared for the future as well as evidence of their loyalties to the past. In this paper I draw attention to some of the social meanings of established medical practice and the place convention held in these doctors' memories and experience. I suggest that despite a genuine need and desire for more effective medicine, the status quo represented a reassuring instance of the powerful relationship between security and social authority that conflicted with physicians' efforts to bring about change.[2]

BARBARA GUTMANN ROSENKRANTZ is Professor of the History of Science in the Faculty of Arts and Sciences and the School of Public Health at Harvard University, Cambridge, Massachusetts.

In the first part of the paper I point out that many 19th-century physicians who identified themselves as "regulars," as well as some sectarian practitioners, enjoyed popular recognition that contributed to a favored professional status even though it did not reflect a uniform degree of economic security. We know little about most doctors' incomes, but we do know that public esteem did not eliminate the competition for patients that doctors complained threatened their collection of fees. Doctors bore a portion of the more general antipathy toward special privilege, exemplified by refusal to license qualified physicians and assure their preemptive rights. What bears explanation is how and why positive attitudes toward doctors prevailed in the face of contrary rhetoric, and what practical bonds tied competing medical practitioners together. For despite contesting medical theories, practitioners commonly agreed that knowledge of their patients' personal and social circumstances should guide medical care. Political arguments against privilege and the presumptions that guided medical practice shared a grammar of meaning that was reflected in congruent medical and social rules; in practical terms it appears that commonplace deference and personal hygiene were both best managed by adjustments that essentially fitted the individual to the curve. In the first section of the paper I identify some of the links between culture and explanations of disease that gave respected standing to 19th-century American physicians despite their sometimes blemished personal reputations.

In the second section of the paper I consider some aspects of the intersection of demographic and ideological realities that contribute to "the social construction" of disease. Today we usually identify the causes of disease in the laboratory, and frequently locate symptoms in terms of "objective" data that represent the measurement of biochemical imbalance. We tend to forget that susceptibility to disease is conditioned by social structure, and that exposure to injury as well as the combination of symptoms that are associated in the diagnosis of disease are the products of human culture. Historically, new scientific knowledge has led to discovering one disease where formerly many symptoms were separated and given different names; this was the case when scrofula and consumption were both identified as tuberculosis after the discovery of the tubercle bacillus in 1882. Disease is socially constructed in other ways as well; historians, anthropologists, and sociologists point to those experiences and values that in every age and place give private pain a legitimate, publicly recognized status by validating the links between medical criteria of pathology and social deviance. Sometimes we imagine that because physicians are trained scientific observers their diagnoses and therapies are immunized from the forces that give social meaning to disease.[3] In the second section of this paper I also discuss some of the reasons 19th-century physicians were even less protected from the conceptual and social conflicts associated with the practice of medicine than most doctors practicing in the 20th century. While the social impact of physicians' inner qualms is difficult to calibrate, physicians' disagreements about the underlying causes of susceptibility to disease surely contributed to the heat of arguments over medical training, the exclusion of homeopaths from professional courtesies, and the implications of germ theory for medical practice.

In the last section of this paper I reflect on some of the meanings science held for the medical profession at the close of the 19th century. References to science had long been employed to signal professional integrity and to identify science as the sponsor of medical practice. In this context science associated knowledge and the moral status that assured professional responsibility. By the end of the century references to scientific knowledge among physicians, as well as among lawyers and university-trained men and women, were more refined; that is, science imparted knowledge that was specific to a discipline, and trained the mind. In the third section of the paper I note that this narrower meaning of science made it easier for physicians to defend standards of professional behavior in public, but that it was not necessarily easier to accept the criteria that determined professional responsibility. Although physicians expressed their confidence in science to measure and test their healing arts, many of them found it difficult to adopt a concept of scientific pathology that objectified disease, diminished the patients' contribution to susceptibility, and made the clinician an expert in natural science. That science should be cast as Mephistopheles by its critics is not surprising. But even among physicians who embraced science, the feeling remained powerful that they had compromised a crucial social role. This dilemma had a history that gave meaning to the doctors' doubts.

## I

"Our profession, Gentlemen, is the link that unites Science and Philanthropy," said Alexander Stevens, accepting election to the presidency of the American Medical Association convened in Philadelphia for its first regular meeting in 1847. With rhetoric inspired by the social rather than the sanitary goals of medicine, Dr. Stevens did not explicitly distinguish between the sickroom and the community. The descendent of an old family line, at the age of 58 Stevens represented the most highly trained American physicians; reflecting his own status as an established surgeon and president of the College of Physicians and Surgeons in New York City, Stevens proposed that those gentlemen gathered at the meeting were "one of the strongest ligaments that binds together the elements of society." His assertion that medicine made the rich conscious of their "dependence" and gave the poor "a sense of the innate dignity of their nature" took advantage of commonplace assumptions about personal and public behavior that were as much a part of the 19th-century doctors' armamentarium as the better-known bleeding, cupping, and purging. At a time when disputes over therapy characterized relations among "regulars" (as well as between the orthodox and medical "sects"), Stevens's inaugural message was clearly intended to have a universal appeal.

> In a country, where the population is not crowding on the means of subsistence, and where every individual has the largest opportunity of promoting his own happiness, and of perpetuating it in his posterity, the medical profession, entirely philanthropic in its objects, more intimately connected with the pursuits of science than the other learned professions, and not over shadowed by an hereditary aristocracy, enjoys a pre-eminently high social position, and for all legitimate objects, a commensurate influence.[4]

No doubt Stevens hoped to use this occasion to improve the somewhat tarnished reputation of his profession. Both in this country and abroad physicians were the butt of humor and criticism that often played on allegations of their greed and ignorance. Stevens's lecture suggested that a distinctive New World economy of opportunity for everyone offered a corrective; absent "an hereditary aristocracy" determining who practiced medicine, Americans could enter a profession that welded personal success and public service. Pronouncements of this sort are easy to discount as self-serving rhetoric, and historians have documented less elevated behavior accentuating the entrepreneurial skills and divided doctrinal loyalties of American practitioners — regular and sectarian — as an indication of their "unprofessional" behavior.[5] In any case, doctors in 19th-century America represented a more generous cross section of society than they do today, and contemporary laymen often regarded doctors' manners and education sufficiently heterodox to warrant contempt.

Alexander Stevens's elite audience could, however, have heard his address as an echo of Alexis de Tocqueville's observation that the professions become a natural aristocracy when a nation eschews class distinctions and yet endorses order. Traditional patterns of respect for the learned professions — the Church, medicine, and law — were unclear in this country; although forbidding monopoly of practice to any special group, Americans valued achieved distinction and enhanced the standing of professional men. As fears over corruption and disruption of the social order mounted in the decades before and after the Civil War, physicians increasingly assumed prestigious public roles.[6]

In addition to attracting favorable attention, Stevens intended to elevate the self-image of his audience, reminding them that doing good and doing well were complementary objectives. The multiple opportunities he alluded to were the outcome of conscious strategies as well as historical accident. Few physicians had migrated to the New World colonies, and the practice of medicine continued to be reasonably open to ambitious youth in the 19th century. In those few instances where statute regulated practice or the right to collect fees, state legislatures revoked this privilege from medical societies in the 1820s and 1830s.[7] Without legal distinctions the social differences among doctors became an incentive to advocate competing therapeutic regimens; the appeal of sectarians was in part based on the proposition that medical management was tailored to the patients' constitutions. Regular and sectarian doctors agreed that individual circumstance could modify any disease, and the opportunity for doctors to capitalize on familiarity with patients' experiences also led patients to commend the differences among doctors as beneficial.

Even without reference to the informal systems of medical advice that flourished (then as now), the variety of practice was substantial. This variability was as much a product of the differences among patients as any other single factor, and differences among patients were a reflection of the region and the community, gender, class, and occupation, influences which in turn affected disease and social organization. These variables independently, and in many combinations, shaped physicians' behavior as well. Substantial conflicts among medical practitioners originated, at least in part, because regional and social class identities were important determinants of a practitioner's diagnostic categories and therapeutic preferences. Both sectarian and orthodox doctors underscored the significance of familiarity with their own patients' symptoms when they chose treatments based on their intimate understanding of a patient's particular circumstance, and criticized other remedies as inappropriately "theoretical."

At the same time, regular and sectarian doctors serving patients whose geographic or social locations were similar practiced in quite similar ways. At mid-century when botanic and homeopathic therapies were the clearest challenge to regular doctors, differences in diagnoses could be insignificant compared to de facto agreement reflected in practice, agreement that was predicated on generally acceptable conceptions of adjustment to climate or social situation.[8] This social and psychological environment provided a foundation for professional consultations that later became the emblem of mutual recognition between "allopaths" and homeopaths.[9] Custom and convenience sustained these consultations, especially among urban medical elites, those with hospital appointments and a better class of patients, while at the same time, defense of specific therapies such as bleeding softened among the best-educated physicians who ascribed modifications in treatment to changes in disease itself or in the characteristics of patients.[10] Despite the florid arguments that

often accompanied doctors' reciprocal denunciations, for most of the century doctors succumbed to the advantages of living at peace with each other. Membership of homeopathic physicians alongside regular physicians in local and state medical societies and conferences at the bedside effectively diminished the impact of therapeutic conflict.

Diagnosis, with its implied mastery of prognosis, was the fulcrum of doctor-patient interaction. Diagnostic acumen was an important source of personal distinction for the individual physician, but more to the point, the diagnostic categories employed flowed through a common conceptual funnel so that the premonitory signs and predisposing factors of disease were universally recognizable. And the signs and symptoms of disease that were the clues to diagnosis also provided an explanatory idiom for social disorder. Susceptibility was understood to be the consequence of the conflation of constitutional, behavioral, and environmental influences. Fever, simultaneously the most ubiquitous symptom and the largest class of disease, was an indication of corruption in the body, just as disorder was a sign of alien taint in an increasingly heterogeneous society. It didn't take a doctor to point out that cholera, imported from abroad, festered in the atmosphere contaminated by the immigrant poor.

Beginning in the antebellum period, in the same decades that the concept of self-limited disease promoted the counsel of therapeutic restraint and a sympathetic consideration of homeopathy, physicians were thrown into frenetic medical activity by a vastly documented increase of contagious disease in the urban environment.[11] Sanitary science was not, however, a competing option to be substituted for medical therapy. Instead hygienic knowledge seemed only to reinforce the link between common sense and scientific evidence that pictured disease as an opportunistic interloper taking over when ignorance or negligence permitted. As Charles Rosenberg has pointed out, medicine was a medium that gave meaning to every experience. "Within the shifting etiological world," he writes, "the physician's theoretical responsibility was far broader than mere diagnosis, prognosis, and treatment."[12] In this context Dr. Stevens's marriage of Philanthropy and Science rallied his contemporaries. In later years physicians' social concerns were more often defended with references to their scientific authority, calling to mind a paternal and hierarchical, rather than a conjugal, relationship between the sources and objects of knowledge. The meaning that medicine imparted to experience in 1848 was, however, one important source of a physician's good reputation and status. Dr. Stevens took the ties between medicine, science, and philanthropy for granted; when he cited the medical profession's special relationship with science, he intended to bolster the position of his orthodox colleagues with the assumption that science was a witness everyone could trust. More important, sectarian doctors also expressed their allegiance to science at mid-century, and claimed science as the guide to their specific diagnoses and therapies, so that their patients were not committed to an antiscientific regimen. The categories of this science were still sufficiently generous to accommodate the social distinctions that might otherwise have divided medical practice decisively.

## II

After the Civil War, images of the reconstruction of a nation were reflected in the myths and the realities of American politics and, inevitably, also in the everyday world of American doctors' practices and aspirations. References to the supposed dangers of "city life" figured in medical literature as evidence of social disorder and disease. Despite their questionable reality, these threats were no less insistent, because they shaped Americans' experience indirectly through the imagination. Although the census reported that the proportion of the total population living in cities grew from 19 to 45 percent between 1860 and 1910, this growth was based on enumerations that classified incorporated places of larger than 2,500 in the urban category. Small increments in population eventually brought massive change, but rapid growth occurred in relatively few places; fears of the impact of urbanization on health and medical practice often preceded any substantial rise in mortality rates. In 1860 twice as many people lived in towns of 5,000 to 10,000 as in larger cities of 50,000 and 100,000, and as the nation's population expanded rapidly between 1860 and 1880, the number of people living in very small towns doubled at roughly the same rate as the number living in

larger communities. Even though regional differences in mortality were less significant at the end of the century, recent demographic studies show that the local environment remained the best predictor of variations in disease and death.[13]

Equally important, from the perspective of physicians who had with each succeeding generation moved to cities in increasing numbers, was the fact that between 1860 and 1880, as the number of cities between 50,000 and 100,000 doubled (from 7 to 15), the number of towns with populations of 5,000 and 10,000 increased from 136 to 249. In some respects the practice of medicine seemed impervious to change; the number of doctors kept a steady pace with the rapid growth of the population as a whole; and differences among locations of practice accentuated contesting points of view on every subject from therapeutics to consultation.[14]

Old conflicts that focused on doctors' identities and competing medical theories were heated up again with derogatory remarks about professional training and associations. Controversies about who should practice dominated debate about revisions in the Code of Ethics at national meetings of the A.M.A. and found their way to the floor of state legislatures; by 1881 half of the states required physicians to have a license to practice.[15] Immediate and practical concerns about the most effective methods of disease control were on the table for discussion at the same time as were more reflective considerations about the criteria of professional authority. The situation did not encourage direct and simple answers. Some asked whether contagion could be contained short of eliminating its domestic sources, while others rehearsed the familiar warning that corruption in the cities could not be confined to politics, because, like neglected sewerage, it would seep over endangering the public health.[16] Earlier controversies over yellow fever and cholera were recalled as variously designated authorities claimed that their expert knowledge implied civic responsibility, and appealed to the public for support.

In the last quarter of the century these claims to authority became intertwined with disagreements over the meaning of established rules of behavior; debates about professional responsibility were recapitulated in the context of sweeping references to scientific standards and public accountability. The A.M.A. had first adopted a formal code or "Principles of Medical Ethics" at the Philadelphia meeting where Alexander Stevens spoke. For some time before, state medical societies had included codes of ethics in their by-laws, focusing on proper intraprofessional behavior. State societies denounced the dangers of quack remedies and uneducated doctors, but did not initially require more specific identification of these threats. Massachusetts and New Jersey medical societies enacted ethical rules for physicians in the 18th century, but elsewhere formal principles of behavior derived almost verbatim from a code written by the English physician Thomas Percival. The exclusion of the improperly trained from the ranks of society membership was stated as a matter of principle, but by 1852, and with regularity thereafter, the criteria of exclusion were less than certain. The A.M.A.'s code determined that "a regular medical education furnishes the only presumptive evidence of professional abilities and acquirement," together with "the aids actually furnished by anatomy, physiology, pathology and organic chemistry" and "accumulated experience." This amounted to a pious denial of the status quo in New York and Massachusetts, where homeopaths could be elected to regular medical society membership. The first section of Article IV, on "the duties of physicians in regard to consultations," opened the door to a liberal interpretation of these requirements with the reminder that, since "the patient is the sole object in view" in deciding upon a consultant's qualifications, the patient's request for a specific individual should not ordinarily be denied. Ambiguous in 1848, within the next decade there was additional room for differences of interpretation over the injunction that "no intelligent regular practitioner, who has a license to practise from some medical board of known and acknowledged responsibility, recognized by this Association, and who is in good moral and professional standing in the place in which he resides, should be fastidiously excluded from fellowship, or his aid refused in consultation." By the late 1870s important factions within many of the state organizations contested implementation of the warning that "no one can be considered as a regular practitioner or a fit associate in consultation whose practice is based on an exclusive dogma," and treated this section of the code as less of a safeguard than a provocation. Accommodations in medical practice that

had been made over time were sanctioned by informal rules covering the customary behavior of many doctors and their patients. Underscoring the working harmony of these arrangements between regulars and homeopaths, the first restrictive state practice laws passed in the 1870s focused on punishing quacks, an enemy common to allopathic and homeopathic doctors.[17]

Local resolution of these controversies took on added significance at annual conventions of the A.M.A. with challenges to delegates from state societies that modified the code or failed to enforce the principle of restricting consultation. There was a shift from lenient disposition of these cases to revoking the state delegation's privileges; charges of encouraging promiscuous consultation in the classroom made against a single Michigan physician and professor of medicine were dismissed in 1878, but four years later the Judicial Council refused to seat the New York delegation because that state's abbreviated code implicitly permitted consultation with homeopathic doctors. State delegations fought vigorously for freedom from national oversight, often inspired directly by allegiances that were formed at home.[18] These disputes over the Code of Ethics were not, however, all window dressing or simply a convenient way of combating local enemies at a national level. The insistent pleas for self-regulation were emblematic of more generally eroding confidence in collegiality based on social criteria; disputes were the more painful because all the parties also shared the habit of trust in traditional standards. In states such as Massachusetts, New Jersey, and New York, where social and professional arrangements had, from the perspective of many leading physicians, effectively reinforced each other, a liberal interpretation of consultation was assumed to be the privilege of gentlemen. Ironically, or so it seems to us today, this led members of the medical societies in two of these states to contest the code itself, rather than advocate mediation. In the larger ideological and social contexts of the late 19th century, the most vigorous critics of the code of ethics questioned professional connections when they were primarily based on traditional fellowship.

These conflicts over the principles of professional behavior had roots and branches reaching into other situations where medical and social values were closely related. In several instances physicians within a state society were divided about the preferred criteria for licensing medical practice, and disputes about who should be considered a colleague were sometimes connected to uneasy defense of competing theories of contagion and their implications for public health. Established sanitary practices of quarantine and protection of waste and water emphasized the collaboration of doctors with a public that was sensitized to vigilance through knowledge of personal hygiene. The control of specific diseases through techniques based in laboratories relied less directly on physicians winning public cooperation.[19]

What might have been a wrangle within the profession about privileges and rights to practice was assured a popular audience. Public occasions lent themselves to statements about medical principles and practices. Dr. Austin Flint, a leading New York physician and nationally recognized medical author, proposed that opponents of the Code of Ethics threatened the best medical tradition. In a *Harper's* series on a century of scientific progress, writing in defense of the A.M.A.'s prohibition of promiscuous consultation, Dr. Flint used the argument that current knowledge of etiology was "defective" in insisting that "there is no other standard for medical orthodoxy than the opinions held by respectable physicians and inculcated in the accredited works." Personal reputation confirmed by elite status remained the touchstone of security. Flint's own successful career, which spanned many years and took him to several distinctly different social and physical climates, made it comfortable for him to subscribe to a liberal interpretation of the code's constraints; "there are no restrictions in the way of professional fellowship" so long as the physician "conforms to the established principles of ethics, and does not place himself in an attitude of antagonism toward the honor and dignity of the profession."[20]

Dr. John S. Billings, director of the Surgeon-General's Library, was another stalwart who found tradition a malleable safeguard rather than an obstacle to progress. Reporting on the state of medical education, he criticized uniformity, because it was folly to expect "that all physicians should possess the same qualifications, and be educated to the same standard. This would be," he continued, "like saying that they all should be six feet high."[21] But Billings saw plenty of opportunity for

diversity within the established system, and like Flint, couched his plea for change in terms of continuity and past tradition and practice.

In another transition from implicit standards to formal regulation, physicians were disinclined to rely solely on examinations as criteria for licensure accreditation. There were memories of times and circumstances when, although irregular practice was unequivocally condemned, it had been possible to set the conditions and criteria of practice locally. Now when examinations were used for gatekeeping, questions that would prejudice the chances of success for qualified graduates of homeopathic and eclectic schools were sometimes replaced with questions that were intended to test the mastery of principles and practices specific to the candidate's training. Repeated exceptions became the rule, with emphasis on flexibility in relation to individuals, and a firm position when it came to the condemned "exclusive practice" of homeopathy. A recent study of licensing laws concludes that these concessions to irregular practitioners were made most frequently in states with the largest number of practitioners and where the most securely established sector of the profession practiced.[22]

The troubling ambiguities of determining qualifications were no doubt complicated by competition for "the market," as has been pointed out in many histories of American medicine. We know too little about why and how much that market changed at the end of the 19th century, but it is unimaginable that doctors played an insignificant role in shaping patients' tastes and expectations. If doctors' contributions to treating contagious disease were limited before the advent of antibiotics, their reputations and authority did not wait for or depend on reduction in the numbers of doctors or on the ratio of doctors to the population as a whole, although this fundamental demography surely affected where doctors practiced and their ability to make a living. Evidence of a "crowded" profession was, of course, the argument put forward by medical reformers in their ultimately successful efforts to eliminate the poorly qualified physician from socially acceptable and legally accredited practice. Nonetheless, the analysis of supply and demand that attributes doctors' professional authority entirely to wringing out the medical economy through reducing the number of poorly trained doctors is a post-Flexnerian myth. It would be a mistake to accept the programmatic ethos of reformers in the early 20th century as a statement about the function of professional roles for the 50 years before.[23] Physicians did not, after all, achieve influence for the first time by virtue of their training in the basic sciences.

A symposium on medical ethics in 1882 provided the opportunity to review the status of medical education in the United States. Abraham Jacobi, the distinguished German-born physician, agreed that it would be desirable to remove the opportunity to practice from the unfit doctor, but he suggested that the matter of qualifications was far from settled. In a paper with the solemn title "Requiescat in Pace," he noted that homeopathic principles (as distinguished from Hahnemann's "preposterous" axioms) were found in some measure everywhere in medicine. Jacobi, the first American pediatric specialist, implied, moreover, that the danger from extravagant therapeutic claims was far less damaging to physicians and their patients than the sapped confidence that occurred in the course of controversy.[24] This was, of course, the outlook of an elder statesman, once again the perception of a prominent consultant who represented professional status that had been secured at a time when membership in a respected scientific society spoke for social origins as well as for scientific training.

In a similar vein, Daniel Webster Cathell's popular and practical guide to professional behavior, which was first published in 1881 and reprinted frequently during the next four decades, dismissed the homeopathic therapy of "similars." Scorning the scientific foundations of treatment that emulated the symptoms of disease, Cathell nonetheless reminded the careful physician, "You are bound by an oath to use your best judgment for everyone who puts himself under your care, but neither the Code of Ethics nor the Code of Honor prevents you from sailing as near to every popular breeze as truth and justice will allow." This was not simply the counsel of expedience. Cathell cautioned, "Not a single department of medicine has yet reached scientific exactness, and possibly never will. We, legitimate physicians, are striving to bring its various branches as *near* to perfection as possible, and are willing to learn medical truth and scientific wisdom wherever they can be found."[25] Cathell's lib-

eral view was reinforced by his confidence in the imminent demise of the unorthodox. And Jacobi and Cathell, no less than Flint and Billings, sensed a potential incompatibility between the social and scientific authorities that had been central to professional stability.

A good deal of tension arose from conflicts that were familiar to older doctors who had learned the rules of professional conduct in the course of their medical training and their early years of practice. But there were significant differences in the content and consequences of these late-century confrontations over the regulation and recognition of physicians. Attempts to formalize these proceedings signaled a new relationship between the individual physician and his profession that the disputants on both sides of specific arguments interpreted ominously. Working relations that had become comfortable over time were no longer serviceable. Eventually the institutional props that could order professional affiliations would fill the empty spaces that occurred when social relations failed; standing in medical school, hospital staff membership, and participation in specialists' societies would replace the outworn armatures of latitudinarian collegiality. Defenders of the A.M.A.'s Code of Ethics warned of a dangerous general tendency that occurred when order based on shared social values was replaced by the rampant freedom that was promoted when a physician had the right "to judge his associates on their merits."[26] Opponents of the code's formal restraints accused the A.M.A. of "unscientific attitudes toward science and medicine," while they, riding under the banner of science, defended the right of consultation and the implication that science was the only essential criterion of reliability.[27]

### III

The turn of the century was a time of hope and anxiety for American physicians. Scientific knowledge dramatically "produced" diagnoses and therapies for diseases such as diphtheria and tetanus, while doctors themselves often seemed oddly out of place and out of sorts. Although almost every visible aspect of medical practice—where it took place, what was in the doctor's bag, the doctor's dress and fee—was different from what it is today, critics and admirers of medicine employed arguments that have retained their resonance. Experience and imagination combined to produce stereotypes of medicine—good and bad, scientific and nonscientific—that accentuated popular interest in doctors and their work.[28] Often it seemed that references to science generated contradictory images; predictions of progress when doctors became more scientific, or at least better instructed by science, vied with denunciations of science as the demanding mistress that warped doctors' concerns for patients and patients' confidence in doctors. Even a protagonist of science like the bacteriologist-turned-journalist Paul De Kruif wrote that doctors relied far too much and thoughtlessly on the "few therapeutic and prophylactic weapons" of the scientific laboratory. While he scoffed at physicians' pretensions and ignorance of science, he also underlined their failure to fill their necessary and proper function of "professional sympathizer." In 1922 he saw no prospect of ridding the profession of "this melange of scientist and priest [that] . . . produced curious contradictions and absurdities."[29]

De Kruif's critique of medicine portrayed physicians' conflicting roles without much sympathy for their plight. Nonetheless, this situation had not arisen because of physicians' inadvertent or deliberate neglect of the implications that the growth of scientific knowledge held for medical practice. At the end of the century many physicians were sensitive to aspects of practice they had once deliberately conflated when doctor-patient relations were more explicitly determined by shared values and physical proximity. As I indicated at the beginning of this paper, the status of American doctors early in the 19th century derived in part from opportunities that were available because of incentives for order in a geographically and ideologically fragmented society; respect for medicine was both stimulated and rewarded by the "fit" of contemporary scientific and social explanations of disease and disorder. Outlining the common foundations of diverse medical practices, I pointed to some reasons for the bonds of understanding among doctors and the loyalty medical care promoted between doctors and their patients. Most physicians drew their scientific ideas about health and disease from a general intellectual consensus; their observations of man and nature led to the construction of protean analogies applicable both to individuals and society.

In the second section of the paper I examined the erosion of confidence in standards of professional behavior that troubled a number of prominent physicians in the last half of the 19th century. In most instances controversy was stilled by local adjustments to fit specific circumstances. Doctors' relations with each other continued to be determined by economic and social conditions, and consequently, formal codes of professional behavior had little influence on doctors' work. When consultation of regular physicians with homeopaths became the focus of conflict, opponents of restriction of consultation saw less room for compromise, even though they also, at first, argued from expedience rather than principle. Here too custom, licensing laws, and ideological differences within the sects combined to diminish the importance of "exclusive" medical systems. In 1882, the *New York Medical Journal* urged national support for the state medical society's revised code eliminating prohibition of consultation; reprinting an item from the Canadian *Lancet*, the editorial asked physicians to endorse licensing of qualified homeopaths. Recognition would be an antidote to the profitable martyrdom homeopaths enjoyed when medical societies attacked homeopathic principles.[30]

Benign neglect was not, however, the course physicians chose between 1882 and 1903, when the code of ethics was revised in conjunction with a major reorganization of the A.M.A. A decade earlier efforts to segregate these matters in the Judicial Council and remove them from the floor of annual meetings of the A.M.A. had been partly successful, and now state and local societies bore the brunt of contention. In those instances where differences over revision of the code of ethics continued to structure pronouncements about professional decorum, a conscious distinction was made between behavior that fell under the general heading of etiquette and professional behavior ruled by physicians' unique moral responsibilities. In a series of six articles titled "Medical Ethics and Etiquette," Austin Flint, at this point president-elect of the A.M.A., separately examined the several points at issue, showing scrupulous concern with each turn of the debate. The sequence reflected his indignation, and that of the majority of his colleagues, with the tactics of physicians who proposed that scientific criteria rather than a code of ethics should regulate consultations. At the time, the New York State Medical Society was split in two by a vote that authorized its members to consult with any doctor qualified by law.[31] Dr. Flint colored his discussion with the charge that only zealots proposed to do away with the principles that had guarded the medical profession from association with the "gloomy prognostications" and excessive claims of homeopathic "dogma." He believed that the reputation of the profession was at risk because of internal disputes that might better be settled by rule.

Flint argued that physicians exposed themselves unwisely to alien interests when public law was cited as justification for consultation with homeopathic doctors. It was "absurd" to "take the ground that, because the Legislature of a State has placed on an equal footing different classes of practitioners, those of one class can not refuse to consult with those of another class." Physicians' responsibilities to their patients, Flint insisted, required retaining the medical society's original restriction on consultations. The public must learn, moreover, that although there were no grounds for professional discipline of a physician's eccentric behavior, the medical society guarded its responsibility for determining legitimate criteria of consultation among physicians, and would not tolerate special arrangements based on appeals to superior authority of any kind. When other physicians had come to the conclusion that the debate over consultation was a matter of "medical politics" now that distinctions between the scientifically qualified and the pretender could be settled empirically, Flint's persistent defense of traditional ethics reflected something more than his attachment to the past. Physicians of Flint's eminence did not question that science was the foundation as well as the symbol of the medical profession's authority. Nonetheless Flint's clinical caution linked the regular physician to a muted deference for science. "A well-educated physician," Flint wrote, "must know that he can rarely assume to have warded off an impending disease. The statement to a patient that he has barely escaped an attack of pneumonia, typhoid fever, or apoplexy . . . is either evidence of ignorance on the part of the physician . . . or it is a gross violation of ethics."[32]

Science's entitlement of medicine was unquestioned, and in the 1880s and 1890s, as techniques of physical diagnosis and immunology profoundly altered physicians' understanding of their patients' diseases, the criteria of assurance that shaped professional relations and public reputations separated. Identification of the typhoid or the tubercle bacillus at first changed doctors' self-perceptions even more profoundly than it changed the lives of patients, for science did establish boundaries that determined standards among doctors. They argued that the objective character of scientific criteria and the assurance these criteria gave to the internal legitimation of professional integrity were assured. In that sense, there was no room for an outsider to challenge the regular physician's authority; the challenge physicians faced at the end of the century was to put their own house in order.

In 1903 the A.M.A. adopted the limited code that had once been rejected. In principle this left the settlement of disputes to local societies, and in fact this arrangement fostered self-regulation by physicians in their relations with patients. Those who practiced without accreditation were unlicensed, and therefore illegally in practice. How science would affect the origins and consequences of professional reputation was less certain. If behavior among professionals need no longer be based on a separate code of ethics, would it be necessary, wise, or possible to establish the conditions of responsibility associated with reputation by the same scientific standards? Physicians who had practiced at a time when status was granted by a reputation squeezed out of wisdom, caution, and collegiality were uneasy about professional responsibility that was harnessed to science and the law. At the end of the century as the intellectual and social bases for autonomy were settled, physicians continued to reckon with the consequences their calling had on their conduct.

A little more than a decade after Flint wrote his essays on ethics and etiquette, another distinguished physician of the same generation and standing talked to his fellow physicians about their professional responsibilities. The Philadelphia neurologist Dr. S. Weir Mitchell had a reputation as a scientist and a writer who had crossed over the barriers that might have separated professional and popular audiences. Speaking to a graduating class of medical students, Mitchell pointed to their future as he listed, in effect, the constraints they would have had to reckon with in the past.

I am fond of saying that in our work we sell what neither we who sell nor those who buy can weigh or measure. We have no public to which we bend with abject submission. . . . no judge or jury listens to us. . . . no press or public look on to applaud or condemn. What we do neither the patient nor his friends can fully understand. One silent auditor makes up our moral accounts. That we live very largely a life of self-isolated judgment, that neither scale nor measure approves the amount and integrity of what we sell—this, I think, should make us doubly careful.[33]

Although this was in some respects an oddly troubled and troubling injunction, it was not surprising that Mitchell voiced these concerns. From his point of view a professional ethos in which accountability to science replaced relations with colleagues and patients was a crack in the wall of tradition that had supported the reputation and authority of medicine in the past. It is likely that there were very few in the audience of young physicians who were as uneasy about their responsibilities as Mitchell, in part because they lacked his experience. Science captured their minds and imaginations, and suggested that the power to diagnose and treat the sick would be a better salve than the consolation they might have provided in the past. One might speculate, also, that few of Mitchell's predecessors would have shared his misgivings, since, although they had no less confidence in science, they placed a good deal more trust in the overriding influence of tradition and established practice.

Although doctors often spoke as though these were dilemmas intrinsic to medicine, by the end of the century the struggles over the origins of responsibility and the sources of authority were part of more general social and ideological, personal as well as professional, confrontations with a new kind of expert; determinations of a new set of tasks that the expert might legitimately assume; and professional roles that the expert could accept without being charged with abandoning moral responsibility. Convinced that science would guarantee a more secure professional identity in medicine, and in law and social science as well, many doctors, lawyers, and economists faced parallel qualms about their fields of work; their sense of accomplishment in turn endowed these professionals with a large measure of confidence in their social positions. Professional tensions released in formulating the science of law transformed the legal profession, first inducing a split between the practice and teaching of law and then in efforts to endow the teaching of law with a new activist tradition. Richard T. Ely, the leader of the self-styled, "ethical economists," proposed that scientific analysis of economic conditions "must be met by corresponding changes in society." But the fears that Ely and his American Economics Association colleagues awakened in traditional *laissez-faire* liberals were closely allied to fears expressed by defenders of the A.M.A.'s code of ethics. These were anxieties lest reforming spirits acting in the name of science undermined the morality of the past and destroyed the stability of society.[34]

The emergence of a new professional identity in medicine at the turn of the century was not simply a transformation of vocation authorized by the growth of scientific knowledge, conveniently relegating sectarian practice outside the law. Relations within the profession were profoundly altered as well; neither scale nor measure—to borrow Dr. Mitchell's phrase—drawn from science transmitted ethical principles in quite the way that had been plausible when ethics and etiquette, rather than ethics and science, were closely allied.

## NOTES

This paper was originally prepared for the 14th International Congress of the History of Science (Tokyo, 1974), and published in the *Proceedings* of the meeting. I am grateful to Thomas S. Kuhn for his comments at that meeting, and for the critical attention of colleagues who read the paper over the past decade. The paper was revised while I was a Fellow at the Center for Advanced Study in the Behavioral Sciences, and I would like to thank the National Endowment for the Humanities and the Andrew Mellon Foundation whose support of the Center made my fellowship year (1983–1984) possible. One of the enduring benefits of that year was daily conversation with Charles Rosenberg, whose influence on my work is beyond ordinary measure.

1   Sociologists have written many of the texts that document and interpret the "social factors" integral to medical practice. Social-historical studies of "the professions" identify medicine as the exemplary case in Western culture; see for instance Magali Sarfatti Larson, *The Rise of Professionalism* (Berkeley, 1977). For the special characteristics of physicians' authority in contemporary society, see especially Eliot Freidson, *Professional Dominance: The Social Structure of Medical Care* (Urbana, Ill., 1970). Most recently in a grand sweep that focuses on the marketplace, Paul Starr has described *The Social Transformation of American Medicine* (New York, 1982). For a historian's comment, see Jan Goldstein, "Foucault among the sociologists: the 'disciplines' and the history of the professions," *Hist. & Theory*, 1984, *23*: 170–192. Physicians have long been prominent among historians of medicine concerned with the social contexts of medical knowledge and practice. George Rosen, a physician, editor, and scholar, wrote several historiographical essays that place recent studies in perspective. See "What is social medicine? A genetic analysis of the concept," *Bull. Hist. Med.*, 1947, *21*: 674–733, and "Approaches to a concept of social medicine. A historical survey," *Milbank Mem. Fund Quart. Bull.*, 1948, *26*: 7–21. See also Barbara Gutmann Rosenkrantz, "George Rosen, historian of the field," *Am. J. Public Hlth.*, Oct. 1979.

2   Autobiographical memoirs of 19th- and early 20th-century physicians are useful sources and are not necessarily more difficult to evaluate for historical studies than eagerly sought manuscript records.

3   In the past 20 years many historians of science and medicine have self-consciously employed a model of relations between experience and ideas and between ideology and social order that stimulated their research and interpretations of the past. Two books are regularly cited by historians: Peter L. Berger and Thomas Luckmann, *The Social Construction of Reality: A Treatise on the Sociology of Knowledge* (London, 1966); and Mary Douglas, *Purity and Danger: An Analysis of the Concepts of Pollution and Taboo* (London, 1966). For more recent studies see: *Natural Order, Historical Studies of Scientific Culture*, ed. Barry Barnes and Steven Shapin (London, 1979); and *The Problem of Medical Knowledge: Examining the Social Construction of Medicine*, ed. Peter Wright and Andrew Treacher (Edinburgh, 1982).

4   Alexander H. Stevens, *Tr. A.M.A.*, 1848, *1*: 30. There were only 195 delegates at the first A.M.A. meeting, an unrepresentative fraction of practicing doctors. Nonetheless, among the A.M.A.'s leadership at its founding were well-known physicians whose geographic and social position lent credence to their claims as spokesmen of the profession's in-

terest. For a discussion of contemporary controversy over therapeutics, see John Harley Warner, "'The Nature-Trusting Heresy': American physicians and the concept of the healing power of nature in the 1850's and 1860's," *Perspect. Am. Hist.*, 1977–78, *11*: 291–324.

5   Richard H. Shryock, *Medicine and Society in America, 1660–1860* (Ithaca, N.Y., 1962). For an account of the medical entitlement of social mobility, see Pauline Maier, "Reason and revolution: the radicalism of Dr. Thomas Young," *Am. Quart.*, 1976, *28*: 229–249.

6   Alexis de Tocqueville, *Democracy in America*, trans. Henry Reeve (New York, 1961); Robert Stevens, "Two cheers for 1870: the American law school," *Perspect. Am. Hist.*, 1971, *5*: 424.

7   Richard H. Shryock, *Medical Licensing in America, 1650–1965* (Baltimore, 1967); Joseph Kett, *The Formation of the American Medical Profession: The Role of Institutions, 1780–1860* (New Haven, 1968).

8   Charles E. Rosenberg, "The practice of medicine in New York a century ago," *Bull. Hist. Med.*, 1967, *41*: 223–253, and *idem*, "The therapeutic revolution: medicine, meaning and social change in nineteenth-century America," *Perspect. Biol. & Med.*, 1977, *20*: 485–506 (ch. 3, this volume); John Harley Warner, "The idea of southern medical distinctiveness: medical knowledge and practice in the Old South," in *Science and Medicine in the Old South*, ed. Ronald L. Numbers and Todd L. Savitt, forthcoming (ch. 4, this volume).

9   See, for instance, Oliver Wendell Holmes, *Homeopathy, and Its Kindred Delusions: Two Lectures Delivered Before the Boston Society for the Diffusion of Useful Knowledge* (Boston, 1842).

10  See Warner, "'The Nature-Trusting Heresy,'" especially pp. 306–307. Michael Duffy ("Homeopathy in Massachusetts, 1855–1875" [Senior honors thesis, Department of the History of Science, Harvard College, 1982]) analyzes demographic and social characteristics of homeopathic doctors and their patients.

11  Lemuel Shattuck, *Report to the . . . City Council . . . Embracing Collateral Facts and Statistical Researches Illustrating the Conditions of the Population, and their Means of Progress and Prosperity* (Boston, 1846); John H. Griscom, *Sanitary Condition of the Laboring Population of New York* (New York, 1845); Jacob Bigelow, *Brief Expositions of Rational Medicine . . .* (Boston, 1858).

12  Rosenberg, "The practice of medicine in New York," p. 233.

13  See *Historical Statistics of the United States* (Washington, D.C., 1975), I, pp. 11, 12, for the breakdown of population by size of place. Daniel Scott Smith ("Differential mortality in the United States before

1900," *J. Interdisc. Hist.*, 1983, *13*: 735–759) documents and interprets fluctuations in mortality and analyzes the association and impact of potential variables including medical prophylaxis and therapy. Robert Higgs, "Cycles and trends of mortality in 18 large American cities, 1871–1900," *Explorations Econ. Hist.*, 1979, *16*: 381–408.

14 The ratio of doctors to the whole population was about 1:570 between 1860 and 1900 and declined steadily thereafter for the next three decades, giving a ratio of about 1:700 in 1930, which reflected both an absolute and a relative decline in the number of physicians; see George Rosen, *The Structure of American Medical Practice 1875–1941* (Philadelphia, 1983), pp. 14–15, 55–58, 66. For the determinants and consequences of uneven distribution, see Raymond Pearl, "Distribution of physicians in the United States," *J.A.M.A.*, 1925, *84*: 1024–1028. Rosen (p. 38) uses the percentage of growth of urban populations to illustrate the effect of immigration on cities. The local impact on the structure of medicine that resulted from growing lower-class and foreign-born populations is, of course, another question; see Rosenberg, "The practice of medicine in New York," *passim*; and for later in the century, Judith Walzer Leavitt, *The Healthiest City: Milwaukee and the Politics of Health Reform* (Princeton, N.J., 1982). According to William G. Rothstein (*American Physicians in the Nineteenth Century: From Sects to Science* [Baltimore, 1972], pp. 344–345) homeopathic and eclectic physicians amounted to about 10 percent of practitioners, but he says nothing about their distribution with reference to other doctors or the population.

15 Samuel L. Baker, "Medical licensing in America: an early liberal reform" (Ph.D. dissertation, Department of Economics, Harvard Univ., 1977); Donald E. Konold, *A History of American Medical Ethics, 1847–1912* (Madison, 1962), pp. 14–31.

16 See the *Report of the Council of Hygiene and Public Health of the Citizen's Association in New York Upon the Sanitary Condition of the City* (New York, 1866), and the account of this report's fortunes in Stephen Smith, *The City That Was* (New York, 1911).

17 Chauncey D. Leake ("Percival's Code: a chapter in the historical code of medical ethics," *J.A.M.A.*, 1921, *81*: 366–371) explains the impetus for regulation before publication of Percival's Code and after publication of the third edition (1803), when American medical societies adopted his formulations. Percival originally prepared his essays for the Manchester Infirmary in 1792. Art. IV, A.M.A. Code of Ethics, "Of the duties of physicians in regard to consultations." See also, Morris Fishbein, *History of The American Medical Association from 1847 to 1947*

(Philadelphia, 1947), pp. 35–38; Konold, *American Medical Ethics,* pp. 1–13; Samuel L. Baker, "Physician licensure laws in the United States, 1865–1915," *J. Hist. Med.*, 1984, *39*: 178.

18 *Tr. A.M.A.*, 1878, *29*: 64. The code stipulated that "it is considered derogatory to the interests of the public and the honor of the profession for any physician or teacher to aid, in any way, the medical teaching or graduation of persons knowing them to be supporters and intended practitioners of some irregular and exclusive system of medicine." The Judicial Council concluded in the Michigan case that punitive action would be "more dangerous to the best interest of the profession than all the ends sought to be remedied in the case under consideration." For an analysis of the hidden agenda of the principles in the Massachusetts debate, see Sandra Joan Kopit, "A clash of perspective: the Boston Gynecological Society's challenge of the Massachusetts Medical Society, May, 1870" (Senior honors thesis, Department of the History of Science, Harvard College, 1974).

19 Barbara Gutmann Rosenkrantz, *Public Health and the State: Massachusetts 1842–1936* (Cambridge, Mass.: 1972), Ch. 3 and 4.

20 Austin Flint, "The first century of the Republic: medical and sanitary progress," *Harper's New Monthly Magazine,* 1876, *53*: 81.

21 John S. Billings, "Literature and institutions," in *A Century of American Medicine 1776–1876*, ed. Edward Clarke (Philadelphia, 1876), p. 365.

22 Baker, "Physician licensure laws," pp. 182–183, 187, 193. Three states used licensure examinations in 1885, and it took two more decades to reach agreement on this standard in 43 others. Baker has constructed a chronology based on his search of state legislation showing that inclusion of homeopaths and eclectics on joint boards of accreditation was the practice, unless a separate board for each group was used. His conclusions are based in part on extrapolation from a case study of Massachusetts; see his "Medical licensing in America," and Konold, *American Medical Ethics*, pp. 28–29. Henry G. Piffard ("The status of the medical profession in the state of New York," *N.Y. Med. J.*, 1883, *37*: 402) was one of many physicians on both sides of the controversy to point out that the code was not intended to exclude homeopaths, and adds the point that the homeopathic society had an identical code of ethics with the exception of the section on consultation.

23 Gerald E. Markowitz and David Karl Rosner, "Doctors in crisis: a study of the use of medical education reform to establish modern professional elitism," *Am. Quart.*, 1973, *25*: 83–107. Starr (*Social Transformation of American Medicine*) weighs the fac-

tors associating winning of the medical market and
professional authority. With respect to licensing he
thinks medical societies (he refers to the A.M.A.,
but makes it clear that state societies were really
the ones with the membership that counted) made
a "gesture of accommodation" (p. 109). Contrary
to my study, Starr implies that this was an inconve-
nient marriage; this follows from his view, with
which I would also differ, that earlier in the century "popular" medicine and sects represented a
"counter culture" in an "open market," which resulted in a "dialectic between professionalism and
the nation's democratic culture"; see especially pp.
47–59.

24   Jacobi's paper was published in *An Ethical Symposium:
     Being a Series of Papers Concerning Medical Ethics and
     Etiquette from the Liberal Standpoint,* ed. Alfred C. Post
     (New York, 1883), pp. 156–175. Jacobi argues in
     part that there was no real contest with homeopaths,
     since their influence was dead.

25   D. W. Cathell, *The Physician Himself and What He
     Should Add to His Scientific Requirements,* 2nd ed. (Bal-
     timore, 1882), pp. 142–146.

26   William S. Ely, "The questionable features of our
     medical codes," in *An Ethical Symposium,* p. 11.

27   H. R. Hopkins, "Is it a profession or a trade?" in
     *An Ethical Symposium* pp. 188–189.

28   Fictional representations of doctors in the early
     20th century differed from the semicomic carica-
     tures of an earlier time, replacing ignorance and
     greed with more knowing and powerful self-interest;
     the wise doctor created from this mold also bene-
     fited from increased learning, but he too was a vic-
     tim of the materialism characteristic of American
     life. The best known and the most intellectually ac-
     cessible cast of doctors is in Sinclair Lewis's *Arrow-
     smith* (1925). See Charles E. Rosenberg, "Martin
     Arrowsmith: the scientist as hero," *Am. Quart.,* 1963,
     *15:* 447–458.

29   "Medicine" in *Civilization in the United States: An In-
     quiry by Thirty Americans,* ed. Harold Stearns (New
     York, 1922), p. 443. The article was unsigned, pre-
     sumably because De Kruif was so critical of the
     medical establishment that he feared professional

reprisals. Scorning medicine and "the religion and
folk-lore of sanitation," De Kruif praised biochem-
ists Van Slyke, Folin, and above all Jacques Loeb,
concluding that if there were reason to be pessimistic about medicine, there could be just pride in
American contributions to "the science of the study
of disease."

30   *N.Y. Med. J.,* 1882, *36:* 333. S. Oakley Vanderpoel
     ("The futility of a forced code of ethics," in *An Ethi-
     cal Symposium,* p. 26) represented another option,
     arguing that an alternative would be "to formulate"
     the characteristics of a "gentleman of science" as a
     standard.

31   For a summary of the controversy in New York,
     see Konold, *American Medical Ethics,* pp. 29–31.

32   Austin Flint, "Medical ethics and etiquette, com-
     mentaries on the national code of ethics," *N.Y. Med.
     J.,* 1883, *37:* 340–373. Flint used this opportunity
     to rebuke regular physicians for adopting the term
     *allopath,* reminding his colleagues that it was coined
     by homeopaths to signify a medical theory oppo-
     site to their own. It is a term of "reproach," he
     pointed out, and furthermore "has no pertinency
     as applied to the medical profession." This series
     of seven articles appeared during March and April
     1883 in opposition to the revised code passed by
     the New York State Medical Society in 1882, and
     was later published as a book titled *Medical Ethics
     and Etiquette: The Code of Ethics Adopted by the Ameri-
     can Medical Association, With Commentaries* (New York,
     1883).

33   S. Weir Mitchell, *Two Lectures on the Conduct of Medi-
     cal Life* (Philadelphia, 1893), p. 9. See also, Ger-
     ald L. Geison, "Physiologists and clinicians in the
     American context," in *The Therapeutic Revolution:
     Essays in the Social History of Medicine,* ed. Morris
     Vogel and Charles E. Rosenberg (Philadelphia,
     1979), pp. 67–90.

34   Jerold S. Auerbach, "Enmity and amity: law teach-
     ers and practitioners, 1900-1922," *Perspect. Am. Hist.,*
     1971, *5:* 551–601; William C. Chase, *The American
     Law School and the Rise of Administrative Government*
     (Madison, 1982), pp. 3–22; John G. Sproat, *The
     Best Men* (New York, 1968), pp. 155–157.

# 17

## The Third Party: Health Insurance in America

### RONALD L. NUMBERS

> No third party must be permitted to come between the patient and his physician in any medical matter.
>
> *American Medical Association, 1934*[1]

American medicine in the 19th century was essentially a two-party system: patients and physicians. Medical practice was relatively simple, and doctors —out of economic necessity more than to preserve an intimate physician-patient relationship— personally collected their bills. Most practitioners billed their patients annually or semi-annually, although those with office practices usually insisted on immediate payment.[2] They were not, however, always free to charge what they pleased. In many communities local medical societies established schedules of minimum fees and instructed members never to undercut their colleagues.[3] There was little objection to providing free care for the poor —or to overcharging the wealthy—but generally the American medical profession preferred fixed fees to the so-called "sliding scale."[4] When hospitals began to mushroom late in the century, they, too, charged patients directly according to fixed prices.

But even in the 19th century a small, but undetermined, number of Americans carried some insurance against sickness through an employer, fraternal order, trade union, or commercial insurance company. Most of these early plans, however, were designed primarily to provide income protection, with perhaps a fixed cash benefit for medical expenses; few provided medical care, and those that did, like the plans sponsored by remotely located lumber and mining companies, generally contracted with physicians at the lowest possible prices. This type of "contract" practice restricted the patient's choice of physician, allegedly commercialized the practice of medicine, sometimes resulted in shoddy medical care—and almost always elicited the opposition of organized medicine.[5] During the latter half of the century the American Medical Association (A.M.A.) repeatedly condemned arrangements that provided unlimited medical service for a fixed yearly sum and urged the profession to maintain "the old relations of perfect freedom between physicians and patients, with separate compensation for each separate service."[6]

Widespread interest in health insurance did not develop in the United States until the 1910s, and then the issue was compulsory, not voluntary, health insurance. During the late 19th and early 20th centuries rising costs and increased demands for medical care had prompted many European nations, beginning with Germany in 1883, to provide industrial workers with compulsory health insurance.[7] Americans, however, paid little attention to these foreign experiments before 1911, when the British parliament passed a National Insurance Act.

Inspired by developments abroad and the spirit of Progressive reform at home, the American Association for Labor Legislation in 1912 created a Committee on Social Insurance to prepare a model bill for introduction in state legislatures.[8] By the fall of 1915 this committee had completed a tentative draft and was laying plans for an extensive

RONALD L. NUMBERS is Professor of the History of Medicine and the History of Science at the University of Wisconsin, Madison, Wisconsin.

This essay was prepared originally for *The Therapeutic Revolution: Essays in the Social History of American Medicine*, edited by Morris J. Vogel and Charles E. Rosenberg (Philadelphia: University of Pennsylvania Press, 1979), pp. 177–200.

legislative campaign. Its bill required the participation of virtually all manual laborers earning $100
a month or less, provided both income protection
and complete medical care, and divided the payment of premiums among the state, the employer,
and the employee.[9]

The medical profession's initial response to this
proposal bordered on enthusiasm. Three progressive physicians—Alexander Lambert, Isaac M.
Rubinow, and S. S. Goldwater—had served on the
drafting committee, and for a brief period after
the turn of the century organized medicine was
in a reform-minded mood. Upon receiving a copy
of the A.A.L.L.'s bill, Frederick R. Green, secretary of the A.M.A.'s Council on Health and Public Instruction, informed the bill's sponsors that
their plan for compulsory health insurance was

> exactly in line with the views that I have held for
> a long time regarding the methods which should
> be followed in securing public health legislation.
> . . . Your plans are so entirely in line with our
> own that I want to be of every possible assistance.

Specifically, Green wanted to give the A.A.L.L. "the
assistance and backing of the American Medical
Association in some official way," and he proposed
setting up an A.M.A. Committee on Social Insurance to cooperate with the A.A.L.L. in working out the medical provisions of the bill.[10] As a
result of his efforts, the A.M.A. Board of Trustees
early in 1916 appointed a three-man committee,
with Lambert as chairman. He, in turn, hired Rubinow as executive secretary and set up committee headquarters in the same building with the
A.A.L.L.

The *Journal of the American Medical Association*
hailed the appearance of the model bill as "the in-
auguration of a great movement which ought to
result in an improvement in the health of the industrial population and improve the conditions
for medical service among the wage earners."[11] In
the editor's opinion, "No other social movement
in modern economic development is so pregnant
with benefit to the public."[12] At the A.M.A.'s annual session in June 1916, President Rupert Blue
called compulsory health insurance "the next step
in social legislation,"[13] and Lambert, as chairman
of the Committee on Social Insurance, presented
a report that stopped just short of endorsing the
measure.[14]

Physician support at the state level was similarly
strong. In 1916 the state medical societies of both
Pennsylvania and Wisconsin formally approved the
principle of compulsory health insurance, and the
Council of the Medical Society of the State of New
York did likewise.[15] Reasons for favoring health insurance varied from physician to physician. According to the *Journal of the American Medical Association*, the most convincing argument was "the
failure of many persons in this country at present
to receive medical care";[16] but the average practitioner, who earned less than $2,000 a year, was
probably more impressed by the prospect of a fixed
income and no outstanding bills.[17] Besides, the
coming of health insurance appeared inevitable,
and most doctors preferred cooperating to fighting. "Whether one likes it or not," wrote the editor
of the *Medical Record*,

> social health insurance is bound to come sooner
> or later, and it behooves the medical profession
> to meet this condition with dignity. . . . Blind con-
> demnation will lead nowhere and may bring about
> a repetition of the humiliating experiences suf-
> fered by the medical profession in some of the
> European countries.[18]

By early 1917, however, medical opinion was beginning to shift, especially in New York, where the
A.A.L.L. was concentrating its efforts. One after another of the county medical societies voted against
compulsory health insurance, until finally the
council of the state society rescinded its earlier endorsement.[19] Both friends and foes of the proposed
legislation agreed on one point: the medical profession's chief objection was monetary in nature. As
the exasperated secretary of the A.A.L.L. saw it,
the "crux of the whole problem" was that physicians
were constantly hearing the lie that the model bill
would limit them to 25¢ a visit or about $1,200
a year.[20] "If you boil this health insurance matter
down, it seems to be a question of the remunera-
tion of the doctor," observed one New York physician, who believed that 99 out of 100 physicians
had taken up the practice of medicine primarily "as
a means of earning a livelihood."[21] Another New
York practitioner, who opposed the A.A.L.L.'s bill,
described all other objections besides payment as
"merely camouflage for this one crucial thought."
Medical opposition would melt away, he predicted,
if adequate compensation were guaranteed.[22]

The medical profession was, of course, not alone in opposing compulsory health insurance. Commercial insurance companies, which would have been excluded from any participation, were especially critical; and some labor leaders, like Samuel Gompers, preferred higher wages to paternalistic social legislation.[23]

America's entry into World World I in April 1917 not only interrupted the campaign for compulsory health insurance, but touched off an epidemic of anti-German hysteria. Patriotic citizens lashed out at anything that smacked of Germany, including health insurance, which was reputed to have been "made in Germany." As the war progressed, Americans in increasing numbers began referring to compulsory health insurance as an "unAmerican" device that would lead to the "Prussianization of America."[24]

Shortly before the close of the war California voters, in the only referendum on compulsory health insurance, soundly defeated the measure by a vote of 358,324 to 133,858 and dampened the hopes of insurance advocates.[25] Their spirits revived briefly in the spring of 1919, when the New York State Senate passed a revised version of the model bill, but the bill subsequently died in the Assembly. By 1920 even the A.A.L.L. was rapidly losing interest in an obviously lost cause.

As the prospects for passage of the model bill declined, the stridency of anti-insurance doctors increased. "*Compulsory Health Insurance,*" declared one Brooklyn physician, "is an UnAmerican, Unsafe, Uneconomic, Unscientific, Unfair and Unscrupulous type of Legislation [supported by] Paid Professional Philanthropists, busybody Social Workers, Misguided Clergymen and Hysterical women."[26] In 1919 he and other critics launched a campaign to have the A.M.A.'s House of Delegates officially condemn compulsory health insurance. They failed on their first attempt, but the following year the delegates overwhelmingly approved a resolution stating

> That the American Medical Association declares its opposition to the institution of any plan embodying the system of compulsory contributory insurance against illness, or any other plan of compulsory insurance which provides for medical service to be rendered contributors or their dependents, provided, controlled, or regulated by any state or the Federal Government.[27]

This repudiation of compulsory health insurance was not, as one writer has suggested, the result of "an abdication of responsibility by the scientific and academic leaders of American medicine."[28] Nor was it primarily the product of a rank-and-file takeover by conservative physicians disgruntled with liberal leaders.[29] The doctors who rejected health insurance in 1920 were by and large the same ones who had welcomed — or at least accepted — it only four years earlier. Frederick Green, the person most responsible for the A.M.A.'s early support of compulsory health insurance, was by 1921 describing it as an "economically, socially and scientifically unsound" proposition favored only by "radicals."[30] And his experience was not atypical.

Many factors no doubt contributed to such changes of heart. Opportunism undoubtedly motivated some, and the political climate surely affected the attitudes of others. But more important, it seems, was the growing conviction that compulsory health insurance would lower the incomes of physicians rather than raise them, as many practitioners had earlier believed. With each legislative defeat of the model bill, the coming of compulsory health insurance seemed less and less inevitable, and the self-confidence of the profession grew correspondingly. "[T]his Health Insurance agitation has been good for us," concluded one prominent New York physician as the debate drew to a close. "If it goes no farther it will have brought us more firmly together than any other thing which has ever come to us."[31]

An additional factor affecting the medical profession's attitude toward compulsory health insurance was its recent experience with workmen's compensation, which was probably the most common form of health insurance in America from the 1910s to the 1940s. Beginning in 1911 many states passed laws making employers legally responsible for on-the-job injuries, but few of the early compensation acts provided comprehensive medical benefits. During the war, however, most states added such provisions or liberalized existing ones, giving American doctors their first taste of social insurance. For many, it was not pleasant. Employers often took out accident insurance with commercial companies, which either contracted with physicians to care for the injured or paid local practitioners according to an arbitrary fee schedule.[32] Neither arrangement pleased the medical profession, which complained that the abuses resulting from such practices "were akin to mayhem and murder."[33] It was evident from this experience, reported the A.M.A., that "pus and politics go together."[34]

In 1925 the New York State Medical Society reported that health insurance "is a dead issue in the United States. . . . It is not conceivable that any serious effort will again be made to subsidize medicine as the hand-maiden of the public."[35] The victorious New York physicians had every reason to be confident, but they failed to reckon with economic disaster. The Great Depression invalidated many assumptions about American society and threatened the financial security of both hospitals and physicians. Between 1929 and 1930 hospital receipts per patient declined from $236.12 to $59.26, and occupancy rates fell from 71.28 percent to 64.12 percent.[36] As the Depression continued, income from endowments and contributions decreased by nearly two-thirds, and the charity load almost quadrupled.[37] Particularly hard hit were the private voluntary hospitals, which had been expanding six times faster than the population.[38] The net income of physicians during the first year of the Depression dropped 17 percent, with general practitioners suffering the biggest losses. In some regions, particularly the cotton-growing states, collections from patients fell 50 percent, and the situation grew worse as the Depression continued.[39]

In response to this disaster, several hospitals began experimenting with insurance. Although not the first, the most influential of these experiments was the Baylor University Hospital plan, often described as the "father" of the Blue Cross movement. In December 1929 Baylor Vice-President Justin F. Kimball, former superintendent of the Dallas public schools, enrolled 1,250 public school teachers, who paid 50¢ a month for a maximum of 21 days of hospital care, an arrangement consciously modeled after the prepayment plans used in the lumber and railroad industries.[40] The success of single-hospital insurance at Baylor and other places soon led to the development of multiple-hospital plans that included all hospitals in a given area. The first of these appeared in Sacramento, California, in 1932, and by 1937, when the American Hospital Association began approving such programs, there were 26 in operation with 608,365 participating members.[41]

The motives behind these early endeavors are difficult to determine. In two recent studies of Blue Cross, for example, Odin W. Anderson stresses the altruistic spirit of the pioneers, while Sylvia Law emphasizes their economic interests.[42] There is, as one might expect, some evidence for both interpretations. Voluntary hospital insurance, said Michael M. Davis in 1931, has "the double aim of furnishing a new and broader base of support for hospitals and of helping small income people to meet their big sickness bills."[43] Economic concerns are, however, easier to document than altruism. It is significant that although financially disinterested civic organizations occasionally contributed funds to establish hospital insurance programs, "In most cases the initiative and main drive for the starting of the various plans came from the hospitals of the community—from hospital administrators and trustees."[44] In his 1932 survey of prepayment plans Pierce Williams concluded that hospitals had promoted insurance primarily "to put their finances on a sound basis."[45]

Physician reaction to these early experiments in hospital insurance was mixed. Those affected the most seemed pleased. A physician associated with a Grinnell, Iowa, plan described the attitude of local practitioners as "very cordial,"[46] and Kimball reported that Dallas doctors appreciated both the increased availability of hospital care for their patients and the fact that insurance got "the patient's hospital bill out of the way of the doctor's personal collections."[47] The A.M.A., however, was openly antagonistic, characterizing prepayment plans "as being economically unsound, unethical and inimical to the public interests."[48] According to the director of the Association's Bureau of Medical Economics, such schemes were largely "a result of 'tactics of desperation,' in which hard-pressed hospitals are seeking 'any port in a storm'"[49] The A.M.A.'s solution to the problem of financing health care was "to save for sickness."[50]

Despite these negative pronouncements, health insurance continued to grow—especially after the publication in 1932 of the final report of the Committee on the Costs of Medical Care. This group of 45 to 50 prominent Americans drawn from the fields of medicine, public health, and the social sciences set out in 1927 to ascertain the medical needs of the American people and the resources available to meet them. Ray Lyman Wilbur, a former president of the A.M.A., served as chairman, and over half of the members were physicians. At the end of five years of exhaustive study, funded by several philanthropic organizations, a majority of the committee, including the chairman, modestly recommended the adoption of group practice and voluntary health insurance as the best means of solving the nation's health care problems.[51]

But even this was too radical for eight of the physicians on the committee, who, with one other member, prepared a minority report denouncing "the thoroughly discredited method of voluntary insurance" as being more objectionable than compulsory health insurance. Health insurance, said the minority, would inevitably lead to the

> solicitation of patients, destructive competition among professional groups, inferior medical service, loss of personal relationship of patient and physician, and demoralization of the profession. It is clear that all such schemes are contrary to sound policy and that the shortest road to the commercialization of the practice of medicine is through the supposedly rosy path of insurance.

The dissenting doctors did, however, favor action to alleviate the financial plight of the medical profession, caused in part by having to provide free care to the poor. Thus they recommended that the government relieve physicians of this unfair "burden" by assuming financial responsibility for the care of the indigent. The results of such a plan, they said, "would be far reaching." In particular, the income of physicians would increase and young doctors would find it easier to begin the practice of medicine.[52]

Although some state medical societies (including those in Alabama and Massachusetts) endorsed the majority report,[53] and although more of the committee's physicians had voted with the majority than with the minority, the A.M.A.'s House of Delegates declared that the minority report represented "the collective opinion of the medical profession." Group practice and health insurance, said the delegates, "would be inimical to the best interests of all concerned."[54] Morris Fishbein, the outspoken editor of the association's *Journal*, characteristically reduced the issue to "Americanism versus sovietism for the American people."[55] "The alinement is clear," he wrote,

on the one side the forces representing the great foundations, public health officialdom, social theory—even socialism and communism—inciting to revolution; on the other side, the organized medical profession of this country urging an orderly evolution guided by controlled experimentation.[56]

The alignment may have seemed clear in 1932, but a revival of interest in compulsory health insurance soon blurred it. In 1934, President Franklin D. Roosevelt appointed a Committee on Economic Security to draft legislation for a social security program, which, everyone assumed, would include health insurance. Pressure from organized medicine, however, forced the President to drop health care from the bill he sent to Congress in 1935. Undaunted, progressive members of his administration continued to agitate for compulsory health insurance and in 1938 held a National Health Conference in Washington. This event aroused great popular interest in a government-sponsored health program, resulting the next year in Senator Robert F. Wagner's introduction of a bill to provide medical assistance for the poor, primarily through federal grants to the states.[57]

In view of these developments, the A.M.A. reversed its position on voluntary health insurance, hoping that such action would quiet demands for a compulsory system. In 1937 the House of Delegates approved group hospitalization plans that confined "their benefits strictly to the facilities ordinarily provided by hospitals; viz., hospital room, bed, board, nursing, routine drugs."[58] A short time later the association began taking credit for promoting the growth of hospitalization insurance, which it had so bitterly opposed only a few years before.[59]

At the same time it was giving its blessing to hospitalization insurance, the A.M.A. was working out a physician-controlled plan to provide medical care insurance. In 1934 the House of Delegates took a tentative step in that direction by agreeing on ten principles to govern "the conduct of any social experiments." These included complete physician control of medical services, free choice of physician, the inclusion of all qualified practitioners, and the exclusion of persons living above the "comfort level." The delegates stopped short of endorsing health insurance and made a point of emphasizing the traditional view that medical costs "should be borne by the patient if able to pay at the time the service is rendered."[60]

In February 1935, shortly after the Committee on Economic Security reported to the President, the House of Delegates met in special session — the first since World War I — to reaffirm its opposition to "all forms of compulsory sickness insurance." Recognizing the need to offer an alternative to government-sponsored insurance, the delegates encouraged "local medical organizations to establish plans for the provision of adequate medical service for all of the people . . . by voluntary budgeting to meet the costs of illness."[61] The language was vague, but the intention was clearly to foster the creation of society-controlled medical insurance plans.

In the aftermath of the National Health Conference of 1938 the A.M.A. called a second special session on insurance. This time the House of Delegates approved the development of "cash indemnity insurance plans" for low-income groups, controlled by local medical societies.[62] By offering cash benefits instead of service benefits, physicians hoped to retain their freedom to charge fees higher than the insurance benefits whenever it seemed appropriate.[63] In 1942, to meet competition from commercial insurance companies, the A.M.A. took the final step of approving medical service plans.[64]

By the late 1930s a number of local medical societies, particularly in the Northwest, had already organized "medical service bureaus" offering medical care for a fixed amount per year.[65] In 1939 the California Medical Association, in an effort to stave off compulsory health insurance, established the first statewide medical service plan.[66] Seven years later, when the A.M.A. created Associated Medical Care Plans, the precursor of Blue Shield, there were 43 medical society plans with a combined enrollment of three million members.[67] In most places coverage was limited to low-income families, who would otherwise have been among the least able to pay physicians' fees.

The threat of "socialized medicine" was no doubt the most compelling reason why organized medicine decided to embrace health insurance. As the demand for compulsory health insurance grew, more and more physicians came to see voluntary plans as their "only telling answer to federalization and regimentation."[68] "[I]t is better to inaugurate a voluntary payment plan," advised the secretary of the State Medical Society of Wisconsin, "rather than wait for a state controlled compulsory plan."[69]

But fear of compulsory health insurance was not the only reason why the medical profession changed its mind. By the late 1930s many physicians were also discerning potential benefits in health insurance.[70] A 1938 Gallup poll showed that nearly three-fourths of American doctors favored voluntary medical insurance, and over half were confident that it would increase their incomes.[71] Health insurance, predicted one Milwaukee physician, "would do away with the uncollectible accounts. . . . It would offer to the physician an opportunity of earning a living commensurate with the value of the service that he performs."[72] Furthermore, by paying for expensive services like x-rays and laboratory tests, it would enable doctors to practice a better quality of medicine.[73]

Once the profession recognized these possible benefits, it sought absolute control over medical service plans. In many states physicians won the right to monopolize medical care insurance through special enabling acts, which critics ironically regarded as "un-American."[74] In other places organized medicine tried to discourage physicians from participating in nonsociety plans by threatening expulsion and the denial of hospital privileges. In 1938 such heavy-handed tactics brought the A.M.A. an indictment (and eventual conviction) for violation of antitrust laws.[75]

Despite a genuine concern for the welfare of their patients, doctors did not embrace health insurance primarily to assist the public in obtaining better medical care. In fact, throughout the 1930s spokesmen for organized medicine repeatedly denied that health care in America was inadequate and attributed the good health of Americans to "the present system of medical practice," that is, to the traditional two-party system.[76] The physicians of Massachusetts may, as they claimed, have supported a medical service plan in recognition of "a problem in the distribution of the cost of decent medical care." But even in that progressive state competition from consumer cooperatives was just as important.[77]

Proudly displaying the medical profession's stamp of approval, health insurance entered a period of unprecedented growth (see Fig. 1). By 1952 over half of all Americans had purchased some

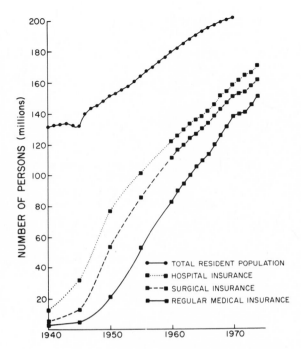

Fig. 1: Growth of health insurance in the United States. Sources: *Source Book of Health Insurance Data, 1975–76* (New York: Health Insurance Institute, 1976), p. 22; U.S. Bureau of the Census, *Historical Statistics of the United States: Colonial Times to 1970* (Washington, D.C.: Government Printing Office, 1975), Part 1, p. 8.

health insurance, and prepayment plans were being described as "the medical success story of the past 15 years."[78] Behind this growth was consumer demand, especially from labor unions, which after the war began bargaining for health insurance to meet rapidly rising medical costs that were making the prospect of sickness the "principal worry" of industrial workers. Following a 1948 Supreme Court ruling that health insurance benefits could be included in collective bargaining, "the engine of the voluntary health insurance movement," to use Raymond Munts's metaphor, moved out under a full head of steam. Within a period of three months the steel industry alone signed 236 contracts for group health insurance, and auto workers were not far behind.[79]

Growth statistics, however, do not tell the whole story. Although most Americans did have some health insurance by mid-century, coverage remained spotty. In 1952 insurance benefits paid only

15 percent of all private expenditures for health care (see Fig. 2). Besides, the persons most likely to be insured were employed workers living in urban, industrial areas, while the unemployed, the poor, the rural, the aged, and the chronically ill — those who needed it the most — went uninsured.[80]

With voluntary plans failing to protect so many Americans, the perennial debate over compulsory health insurance flared up again. Encouraged by organized labor, the Social Security Board in 1943 drafted a bill — named after its congressional sponsors, Senators Robert Wagner and James Murray and Representative John Dingell — providing health insurance to all persons paying social security taxes, as well as to their families. The time, however, was inauspicious. World War II was diverting the nation's attention to other issues, and without the President's active support the bill died quietly in committee.[81]

Two years later, with the war over and Harry S. Truman in the White House, prospects for passage appeared much brighter. Since his days as a county judge in Missouri, Truman had been concerned about the health needs of the poor, and within a few weeks of assuming the presidency he decided to lend his support to the health insurance campaign. Following a strategy session with the President, Wagner, Murray, and Dingell reintroduced their bill, this time adding dental and nursing care to the proposed benefits.[82]

These developments terrified the A.M.A., which viewed the Wagner-Murray-Dingell bill as the first step toward a totalitarian state, where American doctors would become "clock watchers and slaves of a system."[83] To head off passage of such legislation, the A.M.A. in 1946 began backing a substitute bill, sponsored by Senator Robert A. Taft, which authorized federal grants to the states to subsidize private health insurance for the indigent.[84]

The basic problem, as the Association's spokesman Morris Fishbein defined it, was one of "public relations." The medical profession had "to convince the American people that a voluntary sickness insurance system . . . is better for the American people than a federally controlled compulsory sickness insurance system."[85] Actually, most Americans needed little convincing. A 1946 Gallup poll showed that only 12 percent of the public favored extending social security to include health insurance, and more individuals thought the Wagner-

Murray-Dingell proposal would have a negative effect on health care than believed that it would be beneficial.[86]

Truman's surprise victory in 1948, at the close of a campaign that featured health insurance as a major issue, convinced the A.M.A. that it was time to declare all-out war. Shortly after the election returns were in, the House of Delegates voted to assess each member $25 to raise a war chest for combatting socialized medicine, which was defined as "a system of medical administration by which the government promises or attempts to provide for the medical needs of the entire population or a large part thereof."[87] Within a year $2,250,000 had been raised, and the public relations firm of Whitaker and Baxter was putting it to effective use in an effort to "educate" the American people.[88] The showdown came in 1950 when organized medicine won a stunning victory in the off-year elections, forcing many candidates to renounce their earlier support of compulsory health insurance and defeating "nearly 90 percent" of those who refused to back down.[89]

Throughout this controversy representatives of organized medicine insisted that the country did not need compulsory health insurance, just as they had insisted in the early 1930s that voluntary insurance was unnecessary. "There is no health emer-

gency in this country," said a complacent A.M.A. president in 1952. "The health of the American people has never been better."[90] If some individuals could not afford proper medical care, it was probably the result of self-indulgence rather than genuine need:

> Since one out of every four persons in the United States has a motor car, one out of two a radio, and since our people find funds available for such substances as liquors and tobacco in amounts almost as great as the total bill for medical care, one cannot but refer to the priorities and to the lack of suitable education which makes people choose to spend their money for such items rather than for the securing of medical care.[91]

What Americans needed, said the doctors, was more voluntary insurance, which had worked out so well that most physicians by the early 1950s no longer thought coverage should be restricted to low-income groups.[92] The financial and political benefits of health insurance were so great, the medical profession jealously protected it. When rumors began circulating that some surgeons were doubling their fees to insured patients, the A.M.A. called for an immediate crackdown. "Voluntary prepayment plans are the medical profession's greatest bulwark against the socialization of medi-

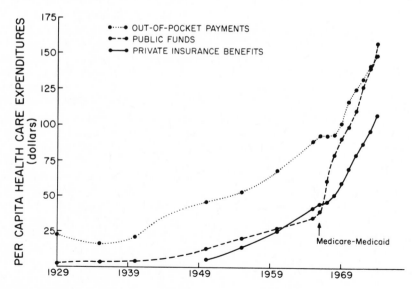

Fig. 2: Sources of health-care expenditures in the United States. Source: Nancy L. Worthington, "National health expenditures, 1929–74," *Social Security Bulletin*, February 1975, *38*: 16.

cine," said one official. "This program must not be jeopardized by avaricious physicians."[93]

The election of a Republican administration in 1952 effectively ended the debate over compulsory health insurance, and organized medicine breathed a sigh of relief. "As far as the medical profession is concerned," wrote the A.M.A. president, "there is general agreement that we are in less danger of socialization than for a number of years. . . . We have been given the opportunity to solve the problems of health in a truly American way."[94] The "American way," it went without saying, was the way of voluntary health insurance.

The Eisenhower years indeed proved to be tranquil ones for the medical profession. Encouraged by their physicians and by the constantly rising costs of medical care, an increasing number of Americans purchased health insurance, until by the early 1960s nearly three-fourths of all American families had some coverage (see Fig. 1). Still, this paid for only 27 percent of their medical bills, and many citizens, especially the poor and the elderly, had no protection at all.[95]

This problem led Representative Aime Forand in the late 1960s to reopen the debate over compulsory health insurance with a proposal limiting coverage to social security beneficiaries. In 1960 Senator John F. Kennedy introduced a similar measure in the Senate.[96] To organized medicine, even such restricted coverage amounted to "creeping socialism,"[97] and the A.M.A. would have none of it. The association's "strongest objection" continued to be that "it is unnecessary and would lower the quality of care rendered," the same argument it had been using since the 1910s. Its only concession was to approve a government plan providing assistance to "the indigent or near indigent," which would benefit physicians as much as the poor.[98] Thus in 1960 Congress, with A.M.A. approval, passed the Kerr-Mills amendment to the Social Security Act, granting federal assistance to the states to meet the health needs of the indigent and the elderly who qualified as "medically indigent."

If the medical profession hoped to forestall the coming of compulsory health insurance by this small compromise, Senator Kennedy's election to the presidency that fall soon convinced them otherwise. Upon occupying the White House, he immediately began laying plans to extend health insurance protection to all persons on social security, whether "medically indigent" or not. The A.M.A. denounced his plans as a "cruel hoax" that would disrupt the doctor-patient relationship, interfere with the free choice of physician, impose centralized control, and — worst of all — undermine the financial incentive to practice medicine. They would not only endanger the quality of medical care, but would discourage the best young people from entering the field.[99] Despite these ominous predictions, Congress in 1965 voted to include health insurance as a social security benefit (Medicare) and to provide for the indigent through grants to the states (Medicaid). Thus, after 50 years of debate, compulsory health insurance finally came to America.

In 1967, just two years after the passage of Medicare, third parties for the first time paid more than half of the nation's medical bills.[100] Many Americans continued to be without health insurance coverage, but seldom by choice.[101] Although critics frequently attacked the insurance business, no one advocated returning to a two-party system. In the opinion of one observer, the acceptance of health insurance was a phenomenon "without parallel in contemporary American life."[102] Prepayment plans benefitted both providers and consumers of medical care, but especially the providers.

Hospitals, the pioneers of voluntary health insurance, profited from the start. In 1947 Louis Reed reported that hospital administrators agreed unanimously that insurance plans had reduced their volume of free care and increased revenues.[103] In the years between 1939 and 1951 the amount of charity care provided by Philadelphia hospitals, for example, fell from 60 percent to 24 percent.[104] Later, in the 1960s and 1970s, the windfall from Medicare and Medicaid enabled many hospitals to improve — or at least to expand — their facilities.

Health insurance also proved advantageous to physicians, especially financially. In the period following the development of medical service plans, their incomes climbed dramatically (see Fig. 3); and, according to some analysts, the "most significant factor" contributing to this increase was third-party payments, which rose from 15.5 percent to nearly 50 percent of physicians' incomes in the two decades between 1950 and 1969.[105] Proving a cause-and-effect relationship is difficult, but the testimony of physicians themselves supports this

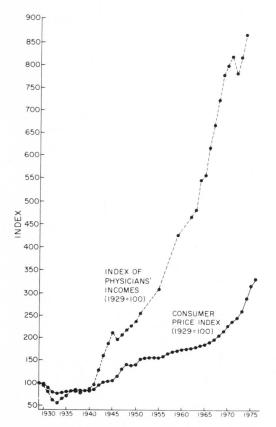

Fig. 3: The income of American physicians, 1929–1975.
Sources: U.S. Bureau of the Census, *Historical Statistics of the United States: Colonial Times to 1970* (Washington, D.C.: Government Printing Office, 1975), Part 1, pp. 175–176, 210–211; U.S. Bureau of the Census, *Statistical Abstract of the United States, 1975* (Washington, D.C.: Government Printing Office, 1975), p. 77; *Medical Economics,* Oct. 24, 1960, *37*: 40, and Nov. 10, 1975, *52*: 184; U.S. Bureau of Labor Statistics, *Consumer Price Index, 1971–76.* Graph prepared by Lawrence D. Lynch.

view. In 1957, for example, over half of the doctors in Michigan reported increased incomes as a result of prepaid medical care, with smalltown physicians and general practitioners registering the greatest gains. The most frequently cited explanations were better bill collecting and more patients.[106]

Certainly there can be little doubt that Medicare and Medicaid benefitted the medical profession handsomely. In fact, Robert and Rosemary Stevens concluded that "it seemed to be the physicians who gained the most."[107] After complaining for years that compulsory health insurance would beggar the profession and reduce the financial incentive to practice medicine, physicians discovered the results to be just the opposite. In the first year under Medicare the rate of increase in physician fees more than doubled (from 3.8 percent to 7.8 percent), while the rate of increase of the Consumer Price Index only rose from 2.0 percent to 3.3. percent.[108] A 1970 Senate Finance Committee investigation turned up at least 4,300 individual physicians who had received $25,000 or more from Medicare in 1968, and 68 of these had gotten over $100,000 each. Although most of this money was earned fairly, reports of questionable practices abounded. Some physicians allegedly saw patients more often than necessary, billed for care never given, and on occasion even resorted to the notorious "gang visit," charging $300 or $400 for one cursory sweep through a hospital ward or nursing home.[109] Such flagrant abuses prompted the president of one local medical society to warn his colleagues "to quit strangling the goose that can lay those golden eggs."[110]

Compared with the relatively tangible benefits of health insurance for hospitals and physicians, those to patients are more difficult to calculate. Prepayment plans undeniably gave Americans greater access to medical care than ever before, eased the financial strain of paying medical bills, and brought peace of mind to millions of policyholders. A grateful public showed its appreciation by buying increasingly comprehensive coverage. But it is not certain that they enjoyed better health for it. On the one hand, there are studies showing that "those who were eligible for Medicaid were likely to have better health than similar groups who were not."[111] But other studies indicate that although Medicare apparently encouraged more expensive types of treatment, like surgery rather than radiation for breast cancer, recovery rates remained roughly the same.[112]

Under health insurance from 1941 to 1970, life expectancy at birth in America did increase from 64.8 years to 70.9 years.[113] But again it is hard to determine how much — if any — of this should be credited to improved medical care, much less to the way in which it was financed. By the early 1970s even organized medicine was downplaying the ability of the medical profession to prolong life and preserve health. As Max H. Parrott of the A.M.A. testified in 1971, choice of life-style had become as important as medical care in determining the nation's health: "No matter how drastic a change is made in our medical care system, no matter how massive a program of national health insurance is undertaken, no matter what sort of system evolves, many of the really significant, underlying causes of ill health will remain largely unaffected."[114] In a society in which heart disease, cancer, accidents, and cirrhosis of the liver all ranked among the top ten killers,[115] it was indeed unrealistic to expect health insurance to cure the nation's ills.

## NOTES

1 Minutes of the 85th annual session, June 11–15, 1934, *J.A.M.A.,* 1934, *102*: 2200.

2 D. W. Cathell, *The Physician Himself and What He Should Add to His Scientific Acquirements,* 3rd ed. (Baltimore: Cushings & Bailey, 1883), pp. 16, 175–176; Charles E. Rosenberg, "The practice of medicine in New York a century ago," *Bull. Hist. Med.,* 1967, *41*: 229–230.

3 George Rosen, *Fees and Fee Bills: Some Economic Aspects of Medical Practice in Nineteenth Century America* (Supplement No. 6, *Bull. Hist. Med.*; Baltimore: Johns Hopkins Press, 1946).

4 Jeffrey Lionel Berlant, *Profession and Monopoly: A Study of Medicine in the United States and Great Britain* (Berkeley: Univ. of California Press, 1975), pp. 101–102.

5 Pierce Williams, *The Purchase of Medical Care through Fixed Periodic Payment* (New York: National Bureau of Economic Research, 1932); Jerome L. Schwartz, "Early history of prepaid medical care plans," *Bull. Hist. Med.,* 1965, *39*: 450–475.

6 *1846–1958 Digest of Official Actions: American Medical Association* (Chicago: A.M.A., 1959), pp. 121–122.

7 For a summary of the European experience, see Richard Harrison Shryock, *The Development of Modern Medicine* (New York: Hafner Publishing Co., 1969), pp. 381–402.

8 This account of the first American debate over compulsory health insurance is based on Ronald L. Numbers, *Almost Persuaded: American Physicians and Compulsory Health Insurance, 1912–1920* (Baltimore: Johns Hopkins Univ. Press, 1978).

9 *Health Insurance: Standards and Tentative Draft of an Act* (New York: American Association for Labor Legislation, 1916).

10 F. R. Green to J. B. Andrews, Nov. 11, 1915, A.A.L.L. Papers, Cornell University.

11 "Industrial insurance," *J.A.M.A.,* 1916, *66*: 433.

12 "Cooperation in social insurance investigation," *ibid.,* pp. 1469–1470.

13 Rupert Blue, "Some of the larger problems of the medical profession," *ibid.,* p. 1901.

14 Report of the Committee on Social Insurance, *ibid.,* 1951–1985.

15 Proceedings of the Medical Society of the State of Pennsylvania, Sept. 18–21, 1916, *Penn. Med. J.,* 1916, *20*: 135, 143; Proceedings of the House of Delegates, State Medical Society of Wisconsin, Oct. 5, 1916, *Wis. Med. J.,* 1916, *15*: 288; Minutes of the Council, Medical Society of the State of New York, Dec. 9, 1916, *N.Y. St. J. Med.,* 1917, *17*: 47–48.

16 "Social insurance in California," *J.A.M.A.,* 1915, *65*: 1560.

17 Income statistics are scarce for this period, but a 1915 survey of physicians and surgeons in Richmond, Virginia, showed that "the very large proportion of physicians were earning less than $2,000," and income tax records for Wisconsin in 1914 indicate that the average income of taxed physicians was $1,488. Committee on Social Insurance, *Statistics Regarding the Medical Profession* (Social Insurance Series Pamphlet No. 7; Chicago: A.M.A., n.d.), pp. 81, 87.

18 "Opposition to the Health Insurance Bill," *Med. Rec.,* 1916, *89*: 424.

19 Report of the Committee on Legislation, *N.Y. St. J. Med.,* 1917, *17*: 234.

20 J. B. Andrews to New York Members of the A.A.L.L., Nov. 3, 1919, A.A.L.L. Papers.

21 "A Symposium on compulsory health insurance presented before the Medical Society of the County of Kings, Oct. 21, 1919," *Long Island Med. J.,* 1919, *13*: 434. George W. Kosmak made the statement.

22 M. Schulman to J. B. Andrews, Feb. 22, 1919, A.A.L.L. Papers.

23 See Gompers' testimony before the *Commission to Study Social Insurance and Unemployment: Hearings before the Committee on Labor, House of Representatives, 64th Congress, First Session, on H. J. Res. 159, April 6 and 11, 1916* (Washington, D.C.: Government Printing Office, 1918), p. 129.

24 See Roy Lubove, *The Struggle for Social Security, 1900–1935* (Cambridge, Mass.: Harvard Univ. Press, 1968), pp. 66–90.

25 On the California debate, see Arthur J. Viseltear, "Compulsory health insurance in California, 1915–18," *J. Hist. Med.,* 1969, *24*: 151–182.

26  "A Symposium on compulsory health insurance," p. 445. John J. A. O'Reilly made the statement.

27  Minutes of the House of Delegates, *J.A.M.A.*, 1920, *74*: 1319.

28  John Gordon Freymann, "Leadership in American medicine: a matter of personal responsibility," *New Eng. J. Med.*, 1964, *270*: 710-715.

29  Elton Rayack, *Professional Power and American Medicine: The Economics of the American Medical Association* (Cleveland: World Publishing Co., 1967), pp. 143-146. For a similar view, see Carleton B. Chapman and John M. Talmadge, "The evolution of the right to health concept in the United States," *Pharos*, 1971, *34*: 39.

30  Frederick R. Green, "The social responsibilities of modern medicine," *Tr. Med. Soc. St. N.C.*, 1921, pp. 401-403.

31  Henry Lyle Winter, "Social insurance," *N.Y. St. J. Med.*, 1920, *20*: 20.

32  On the early history of workmen's compensation in America, see Harry Weiss, "The development of workmen's compensation legislation in the United States" (Ph.D. dissertation, Univ. of Wisconsin, 1933); and Lubove, *The Struggle for Social Security*, pp. 45-65.

33  Bureau of Medical Economics, *An Introduction to Medical Economics* (Chicago: A.M.A., 1935), p. 80.

34  Committee on Social Insurance, *Workmen's Compensation Laws* (Social Insurance Series Pamphlet No. 1; Chicago: A.M.A., [1915]), p. 60.

35  Report of the Committee on Medical Economics, *N.Y. St. J. Med.*, 1925, *25*: 789.

36  Sylvia A. Law, *Blue Cross: What Went Wrong?*, 2nd ed. (New Haven: Yale Univ. Press, 1976), p. 6. According to *J.A.M.A.*, the percentage of occupied beds in nongovernmental hospitals declined from 64.6 percent to 63.2 percent between 1929 and 1930. "Hospital service in the United States," *J.A.M.A.*, 1933, *100*: 892.

37  J. T. Richardson, *The Origin and Development of Group Hospitalization in the United States, 1890-1940* (Univ. of Missouri Studies, Vol. XX, No. 3; Columbia: Univ. of Missouri, 1945), p. 12.

38  "Hospital service in the United States," pp. 892-894.

39  Maurice Leven, *The Incomes of Physicians: An Economic and Statistical Analysis* (Committee on the Costs of Medical Care, Publication No. 24; Chicago: Univ. of Chicago Press, 1932), pp. 76-81. The fraction of California doctors earning less than $6,000 a year rose from approximately one-half in 1929 to three-fourths in 1933. Arthur J. Viseltear, "Compulsory health insurance in California, 1934-1935," *Am. J. Public Hlth.*, 1971, *61*: 2117.

40  J. F. Kimball, "Group hospitalization," *Tr. Am. Hosp. Assn.*, 1931, *33*: 667-668; J. F. Kimball, "Prepay-

ment plan of hospital care,"*American Hospital Association Bulletin*, 1934, *8*: 42-47; Odin W. Anderson, *Blue Cross Since 1929: Accountability and the Public Trust* (Cambridge, Mass.: Ballinger Publishing Co., 1975), pp. 18-19.

41  Louis S. Reed, *Blue Cross and Medical Service Plans* (Washington, D.C.: Government Printing Office, 1947), pp. 10-12.

42  Anderson, *Blue Cross Since 1929*, pp. 29-44; Law, *Blue Cross*, pp. 6-8. Anderson quotes one pioneer, J. Douglas Colman, as saying that "All this notion that it was going to solve the financial problems of hospitals was farthest from their [the Blue Cross founders'] minds." But Colman himself became involved with prepayment plans because hospitals might have to close without them. "An interview with J. Douglas Colman," *Hospitals*, 1965, *39*: 45-46.

43  Michael M. Davis, "Effects of health insurance on hospitals abroad," *Tr. Am. Hosp. Assn.*, 1931, *33*: 585. At the same meeting where Davis read this paper, the president of the A.H.A. called for insurance as a partial answer to the problem of decreasing occupancy rates; *ibid.*, pp. 195-197.

44  Reed, *Blue Cross and Medical Service Plans*, pp. 13-14.

45  Williams, *The Purchase of Medical Care*, p. 219.

46  Letter from E. E. Harris, Dec. 10, 1930, quoted *ibid.*, p. 238.

47  Kimball, "Prepayment plan of hospital care," p. 45.

48  *1846-1958 Digest of Official Actions*, p. 313.

49  R. G. Leland. "Prepayment plans for hospital care," *J.A.M.A.*, 1933, *100*: 871. For similar expressions, see the address of President-Elect Dean Lewis, Minutes of the 84th annual session, June 12-16, 1933, *ibid.*, p. 2021; and the editorial "Hospital insurance and medical care," *ibid.*, p. 973.

50  *1846-1958 Digest of Official Actions*, p. 313.

51  *Medical Care for the American People: The Final Report of the Committee on the Costs of Medical Care* (Committee on the Costs of Medical Care, Publication No. 28; Chicago: Univ. of Chicago Press, 1932), pp. v-viii, 120.

52  *Ibid.*, pp. 164-65, 171-72. The committee's study of the incomes of physicians revealed that "the average volume of free work furnished by physicians throughout the country is only 5 percent of the total." Leven, *The Incomes of Physicians*, p. 66.

53  Oliver Garceau, *The Political Life of the American Medical Association* (Hamden, Conn.: Archon Books, 1961), p. 138.

54  Minutes of the 84th annual session, June 12-16, 1933, p. 48.

55  "The Report of the Committee on the Costs of Medical Care," *J.A.M.A.*, 1932, *99*: 2035.

56  *Ibid.*, p. 1952.

57  The fullest account of this second debate over com-

pulsory health insurance is Daniel S. Hirshfield, *The Lost Reform: The Campaign for Compulsory Health Insurance in the United States from 1932 to 1943* (Cambridge, Mass.: Harvard Univ. Press, 1970). But see also Roy Lubove, "The New Deal and national health," *Current History,* August, 1963, *45:* 77–86, 117; Edwin E. Witte, *The Development of the Social Security Act* (Madison: Univ. of Wisconsin Press, 1962); Arthur J. Altmeyer, *The Formative Years of Social Security* (Madison: Univ. of Wisconsin Press, 1966); and James G. Burrow, *AMA: Voice of American Medicine* (Baltimore: Johns Hopkins Press, 1963), pp. 185–252.

58  Minutes of the 88th annual session, June 7–11, 1937, *J.A.M.A.,* 1937, *108:* 2219.

59  Minutes of the special session, Sept. 16–17, 1938, *ibid.,* 1938, *111:* 1193.

60  Minutes of the 85th annual session, June 11–15, 1934, *ibid.,* 1934, *102:* 2199–2201.

61  Minutes of the special session, Feb. 15–16, 1935, *ibid.,* 1935, *104:* 751.

62  Minutes of the special session, Sept. 16–17, 1938, *ibid.,* 1938, *111:* 1216; *1846–1958 Digest of Official Actions,* pp. 321–322. At this session black physicians representing the National Medical Association pledged to join the struggle against compulsory health insurance, even though it might not be in the best interest of their race. *J.A.M.A.,* 1938, *111:* 1211–1212.

63  Nathan Sinai, Odin W. Anderson, and Melvin L. Dollar, *Health Insurance in the United States* (New York: Commonwealth Fund, 1946), pp. 64–65.

64  Minutes of the 93rd annual session, June 8–12, 1942, *J.A.M.A.,* 1942, *119:* 728.

65  Reed, *Blue Cross and Medical Service Plans,* pp. 136–146.

66  Viseltear, "Compulsory health insurance in California, 1934–1935," pp. 2115–2126; Arthur J. Viseltear, "The California Medical-Economic Survey: Paul A. Dodd versus the California Medical Association," *Bull. Hist. Med.,* 1970, *44:* 151. Although the second debate over compulsory health insurance took place primarily on the national level, many compulsory health insurance bills were also introduced in state legislatures. See Carl W. Strow and Gerhard Hirschfeld, "Health insurance," *J.A.M.A.,* 1945, *128:* 871.

67  Anderson, *Blue Cross Since 1929,* p. 54.

68  R. L. Novy, "In retrospect: changing attitude of the medical profession," *J. Mich. St. Med. Soc.,* 1950, *49:* 708. See also George Farrell, "Development of voluntary nonprofit medical care insurance plans," *N.Y. St. J. Med.,* 1957, *57:* 560–564.

69  J. G. Crownhart, "The economic status of medicine," *Wis. Med. J.,* 1934, *33:* 230. I wish to thank Jennifer Latham for her assistance in locating this and other documents relating to health insurance in Wisconsin.

70  E. Minihan and T. Levi develop this point in their unpublished paper, "The political economy of health care financing: the foundation for medical care in Wisconsin" (April 1975), pp. 22–23.

71  George H. Gallup, *The Gallup Poll: Public Opinion, 1935–1971* (New York: Random House, 1972), I, 107.

72  James C. Sargent, "Shall medicine be socialized?" *Wis. Med. J.,* 1933, *32:* 562. See also Donald K. Freedman and Elinor B. Harvey, "Development of voluntary health insurance in the United States," *N.Y. St. J. Med.,* 1940, *40:* 1704.

73  Reed, *Blue Cross and Medical Service Plans,* p. 230.

74  "Wisconsin Cooperative Association assails State Medical Society," *Wis. Med. J.,* 1946, *45:* 3.

75  *The United States of America, Appellants, vs. The American Medical Association . . . Appellees* (Chicago: A.M.A., 1941).

76  Minutes of the 90th annual session, May 15–19, 1939, *J.A.M.A.,* 1939, *112:* 2295–2296. See also the comments of President-Elect J. H. J. Upham, Minutes of the 88th annual session, June 7–11, 1937, *ibid.,* 1937, *108:* 2132.

77  James C. McCann, "Medical service plans," *ibid.,* 1942, *120:* 1318.

78  President's Commission on the Health Needs of the Nation, *Building America's Health* (Washington, D.C.: Government Printing Office, [1952]), I, 43; II, 257.

79  Raymond Munts, *Bargaining for Health: Labor Unions, Health Insurance, and Medical Care* (Madison: Univ. of Wisconsin Press, 1967), pp. 10–12, 49, 250. See also Frank G. Dickinson, "The trend toward labor health and welfare programs," *J.A.M.A.,* 1947, *133:* 1285–1286.

80  President's Commission on the Health Needs of the Nation, *Building America's Health,* I, 43; II, 253–254; Reed, *Blue Cross and Medical Service Plans,* pp. 28, 119; Sinai, Anderson, and Dollar, *Health Insurance in the United States,* pp. 57–58, 73; Odin W. Anderson and Jacob J. Feldman, *Family Medical Costs and Voluntary Health Insurance: A Nationwide Survey* (New York: McGraw-Hill Book Co., 1956), pp. 14–20.

81  Altmeyer, *The Formative Years of Social Security,* p. 146; Peter A. Corning, *The Evolution of Medicare: From Idea to Law* (Washington, D.C.: Government Printing Office, 1969), pp. 53–55.

82  Monte Mac Poen, "The Truman administration and national health insurance" (Ph.D. dissertation, Univ. of Missouri, 1967), pp. 54–63.

83  "The President's national health program and the

new Wagner bill," *J.A.M.A.*, 1945, *129*: 950–953. See also "Senator Wagner's comments," *ibid.*, 1945, *128*: 667–668.

84 Burrow, *AMA*, p. 347.

85 Morris Fishbein, "The public relations of American medicine," *J.A.M.A.*, 1946, *130*: 511.

86 Gallup, *The Gallup Poll*, I, 578. See also *ibid.*, II, 801–804, 862–863, 886.

87 *1846–1958 Digest of Official Actions*, p. 331; Minutes of the interim session, Nov. 30–Dec. 1, 1948, *J.A.M.A.*, 1948, *138*: 1241; "A call to action against nationalization of medicine," *ibid.*, pp. 1098–1099; "Reply by officers and trustees," *ibid.*, 1949, *139*: 532. A.M.A. officers later referred to this action as "American Medicine's Declaration of Independence"; Report of Co-ordinating Committee, *ibid.*, 1951, *147*: 1692.

88 Burrow, *AMA*, pp. 361–364.

89 R. Cragin Lewis, "New power at the polls," *Medical Economics*, January 1951, *28*: 76.

90 John W. Cline, "The president's page: a special message," *J.A.M.A.*, 1952, *148*: 208.

91 "A call to action against nationalization of medicine," *ibid.*, 1948, *138*: 1098. This comment was made in response to the Federal Security Administrator's statement that millions of Americans could not afford proper medical care. See Oscar R. Ewing, *The Nation's Health: A Report to the President* (September, 1948).

92 Odin W. Anderson, *The Uneasy Equilibrium: Private and Public Financing of Health Services in the United States, 1875–1965* (New Haven: College & Univ. Press, 1968), p. 140.

93 Cline, "The president's page: a special message," p. 1036.

94 Louis H. Bauer, "The president's page," *J.A.M.A.*, 1952, *150*: 1675.

95 Ronald Andersen and Odin W. Anderson, *A Decade of Health Services: Social Survey Trends in Use and Expenditure* (Chicago: Univ. of Chicago Press, 1967), pp. 75, 109, 153. See also Ethel Shanas, *The Health of Older People: A Social Survey* (Cambridge, Mass.: Harvard Univ. Press, 1962).

96 On the events leading up to Medicare, see Max J. Skidmore, *Medicine and the American Rhetoric of Reconciliation* (University: Univ. of Alabama Press, 1970), pp. 75–95.

97 J. H. Houghton, "President's message to the House of Delegates," *Wis. Med. J.*, 1965, *64*: 208.

98 "New drive for compulsory health insurance," *J.A.M.A.*, 1960, *172*: 344–345. See also Edward R. Annis, "House of Delegates report," *ibid.*, 1963, *185*: 202.

99 Donovan F. Ward, "Are 200,000 doctors wrong?" *ibid.*, 1965, *191*: 661–663; *The Case against the King-*

*Anderson Bill* (*H.R. 3820*) (Chicago: A.M.A., 1963), pp. 17, 118–119.

100 Nancy L. Worthington, "National health expenditures, 1929–74," *Social Security Bull.*, February 1975, *38*: 13–14.

101 Estimates of the number of uninsured in the early 1970s varied between 17 and 41 million; see Marjorie Smith Mueller, "Private health insurance in 1973: a review of coverage, enrollment, and financial experience," *ibid.*, p. 21. The likelihood of having health insurance corresponded directly with income. Over 90 percent of families earning above $10,000 in 1970 carried hospital insurance, for example, while less than 40 percent of families with incomes under $3,000 had it. Cambridge Research Institute, *Trends Affecting the U.S. Health Care System* (DHEW Publication No. HRA 76-14503; Washington, D.C.: Government Printing Office, 1976), p. 188.

102 President's Commission on the Health Needs of the Nation, *Building America's Health*, IV, 43.

103 Reed, *Blue Cross and Medical Service Plans*, p. 230.

104 President's Commission on the Health Needs of the Nation, *Building America's Health*, V, 390–391.

105 John Krizay and Andrew Wilson, *The Patient as Consumer: Health Care Financing in the United States* (Lexington, Mass.: Lexington Books, 1974), p. 111. During the 1960s physicians' incomes increased faster than those of other professionals, including chief accountants, attorneys, chemists, and engineers. *Ibid.*, p. 109.

106 *An Opinion Study of Prepaid Medical Care Coverage in Michigan* (Michigan State Med. Soc., 1957), p. 140.

107 Robert Stevens and Rosemary Stevens, *Welfare Medicine in America: A Case Study of Medicaid* (New York: The Free Press, 1974), p. 191. "One unforeseen result of Medicare and Medicaid," say the Stevenses, "was that in formalizing the system of doctors' charges by developing profiles of the 'usual and customary' fees prevailing in each area, some physicians became aware of what others were charging. Quite clearly, there was some 'standardizing-up'. . . ." *Ibid.*, p. 194.

108 Theodore R. Marmor, *The Politics of Medicare* (London: Routledge & Kegan Paul, 1970), p. 89.

109 *Medicare and Medicaid: Problems, Issues, and Alternatives*, Report of the Staff to the Committee on Finance, U.S. Senate (Washington, D.C.: Government Printing Office, 1970), pp. 9–10, 13.

110 Quoted in Stevens and Stevens, *Welfare Medicine in America*, p. 197.

111 *Ibid.*, p. 202.

112 Victor R. Fuchs, *Who Shall Live? Health, Economics, and Social Change* (New York: Basic Books, 1974), pp. 94–95.

113  U.S. Bureau of the Census, *Historical Statistics of the United States: Colonial Times to 1970* (Washington, D.C.: Government Printing Office, 1975), Part 1, p. 55. The great gains came before the 1960s; between 1961 and 1970 life expectancy only increased from 70.2 to 70.9, and actually decreased slightly for black males.

114  *National Health Insurance Proposals: Hearings before the Committee on Ways and Means, House of Representatives, Ninety-Second Congress, First Session on the Subject of National Health Insurance Proposals, Oct.–Nov., 1971* (Washington, D.C.: Government Printing Office, 1972), p. 1950.

115  Monroe Lerner and Odin W. Anderson, *Health Progress in the United States, 1900–1960* (Chicago: Univ. of Chicago Press, 1963), p. 16.

# 18

## American Medicine's Golden Age: What Happened to It?

JOHN C. BURNHAM

During the first half of the 20th century, up until the late 1950s, American physicians enjoyed social esteem and prestige along with an admiration for their work that was unprecedented in any age. Medicine was the model profession, and public opinion polls from the 1930s to the 1950s consistently confirmed that physicians were among the most highly admired individuals, comparable to or better than Supreme Court justices.[1] Highbrow and mass media commentators alike associated medical practice with the "miracles" of science and made few adverse comments on the profession.[2] By the 1970s, however, statesmen of medicine were writing unhappily about being "deprofessionalized" in the wake of attacks by articulate and knowledgeable critics, attacks that by 1981 were reflected specifically in substantial mistrust of the profession among the public at large.[3] One can conduct a historical postmortem of this unexpected turn of events by examining changes in direct public depreciations of the medical profession, using the different kinds and levels of criticism of M.D.'s as indicators of what happened.

The attitudes of leaders and shapers of opinion and of the public toward physicians did not translate directly into the behavior of patients. For economic and social reasons, amounts of money spent by Americans on medicine continued to increase dramatically even when attitudes changed. But, as was revealed both by polls and by a resurgence of alternatives to conventional medical practice, over time the critics not only affected doctors' sensibilities but also demonstrably damaged the social credi-

bility of the profession as a whole.[4] Since public acceptance is necessary for a profession to function, the criticism had tangible effects.

A long and honorable tradition of denigrating doctors was known to Aristophanes and Molière and continued to flourish in 19th-century America.[5] As late as 1908 a set of satirical "Medical Maxims" in this tradition included, for example:

> Diagnose for the rich neurasthenia, brainstorm, gout and appendicitis; for the poor insanity, delirium tremens, rheumatism and gall-stones . . . fatten the thin, thin the fat; stimulate the depressed, depress the stimulated; cure the sick, sicken the cured; but above all, keep them alive or you won't get your money.[6]

But in those same early years of the 20th century, the tradition of doctor baiting tended to die out as the golden age of medicine dawned. Whereas the post-1950s resurgence of criticism that culminated in Ivan Illich's *Medical Nemesis*[7] recalled traditional themes such as physician greed, pretension, and imposition, the later critics were also responding to new and untraditional characteristics of both medical practice and American society.[8] Moreover, the few particular criticisms that survived in the golden age helped shape and define the new deluge.

## EVOLUTION OF THE MEDICAL IMAGE

During the 19th century, physicians seeking to professionalize their calling were fair game for hostile comment, with quacks and sectarians on one side and the practitioners' actual therapeutic impotence on the other. Some aristocrats of medicine and the medical ideal they represented did enjoy high prestige, but most (often deservedly) did not. Occa-

JOHN C. BURNHAM is Professor of History and Lecturer in Psychiatry at Ohio State University, Columbus, Ohio.

Reprinted with permission from *Science,* March 19, 1982, *215*: 1474–1479.

sionally, antimedical diatribes based on these earlier struggles persisted after the 1890s, along with other anachronisms like attacks on the germ theory of disease. But by and large, in the wake of medical, and particularly surgical, successes, publicity about the profession was favorable, and leaders of the American medical profession succeeded by the early 20th century in their campaign to persuade the public to want and expect uniformly well-trained, well-paid physicians who themselves set standards of practice.[9]

So effective was favorable publicity about both science and doctors that Americans in general began to view extensive medical care as a life necessity. Expansion of hospital care at the beginning of the century was an important indication of the change.

After some years, publications of the Committee on the Costs of Medical Care (1928–1933) and other surveys generated much criticism of the medical profession — not for members' inferior technical performance or misbehavior but for their failing to make physician services of any kind available to more people through economic and organizational means.[10] By the late 1930s the modern campaign for "socialized medicine" or compulsory health insurance had begun, and for many decades organized medical groups opposed any change in the structuring and financing of health care delivery.[11] All parties to the controversy, however, continued to agree that medical care was highly desirable.

While many public figures attacked the American Medical Association (A.M.A.) and state and local medical groups for their political activities, the public image of scientific medicine improved constantly.[12] By the 1940s virtually everyone had heard of miracle drugs and many people knew that they owed their lives to them. As writer Evelyn Barkins observed in 1952, "Most patients are as completely under the supposedly scientific yoke of modern medicine as any primitive savage is under the superstitious serfdom of the tribal witch doctor."[13]

Ultimately, however, the socialized medicine debates undermined public confidence in medicine as a profession. The heavily financed publicity campaigns undertaken in the name of the A.M.A. generated political statements that few people could take seriously and raised questions about the claims of members of the profession acting in scientific and clinical roles.[14] Even before World War II the evident social insensitivity of physician groups such as the A.M.A. tended to tarnish the doctor as a public figure, and many people began to associate the physician with another familiar stereotype, the small businessman, who was presumably not only grasping but slightly dishonest.[15] As one writer of the early 1940s observed of organized medicine, its "social outlook turns out to be . . . scarcely distinguishable from that of a plumber's union."[16] Indeed, the actions of physician groups caused the Supreme Court in 1943 officially to refuse to recognize doctors' professional claims and instead to find physician groups, including the A.M.A., guilty of restraint of "trade."[17]

Beginning in the 1940s, a number of reformers within the medical profession worked to expose inferior medical practice and upgrade medicine to a level appropriate for the age of penicillin and high technology. Some of the self-criticism revealed through these efforts was repeated by the general press. The combination of internal criticism and external distrust eventually had a negative effect, just as the social environment for all professions turned from favorable to unfavorable.

## THE END OF THE GOLDEN AGE

The rare public doubters of the medical profession in the late 1940s and early 1950s gradually increased in number. By 1954, Herrymon Maurer, writing in *Fortune*, could cite a series of sensational articles in mass media magazines attacking not only money-making but incompetence in medical practice. Maurer's article was entitled "The M.D.'s Are Off Their Pedestal."[18] A few more years had to pass, however, before the number of recriminations reached the threshold that marked the end of an era.

Despite the ineptitude of the campaigns against socialized medicine, the public image of the physician *per se* was very favorable in the proscientific post-World War II period. This image was reflected, for example, in the activities of Dr. Kildare (a stereotype later known as Marcus Welby, M.D.) who moved from the novel and motion picture to the television screen. Physicians showed up in over half of 800 Hollywood films surveyed in 1949 and 1950. But in only 25 instances was the doctor portrayed as a bad person, and when he was bad there were often extenuating circumstances. He was almost never a humorous character, either.[19]

Around 1950 many physician organizations across the country began systematic campaigns to reduce the number of legitimate complaints of the public against physicians. Leaders in the profession had concluded that actual experiences of everyday Americans with medical care were the source of much of the antipathy directed toward the profession. An early and exemplary effort was that of the California Medical Association, which conducted a double program. First, California M.D.'s made medical care available (but on their own terms) to answer complaints about access to it. Second, and more important, they carried out a campaign to protect the public by hearing complaints against four types of abuses: (i) malpractice; (ii) "unnecessary or incompetent procedures"; (iii) excessive fees; and (iv) unethical acts of physicians. All over the United States grievance committees of local medical societies tried to adjust physician-patient disputes and effect some of the professional self-policing so notoriously absent theretofore.[20]

Grievance committees were, in fact, but one facet of a major attempt of reformer physicians to get each practitioner to emphasize and upgrade his or her personal relationships with patients. The doctors set out to fight bad public relations as one did syphilis, one case at a time but with a cumulative effect.[21] California M.D.'s in 1951 employed the psychologist Ernest Dichter to suggest how each practitioner should manage his or her patients. Every encounter between a physician and patient is, of course, an intensely and unabashedly narcissistic experience for the patient and therefore eminently suitable for psychological manipulation. A patient's gripes about high fees, for example, may mask a real grievance related to some personal slight inflicted by the doctor. Psychological studies and systematic research on patients, analogous to consumer surveys, both gave specificity to concerns about the individual doctor-patient relationship and helped inspire and shape programs to improve such relationships.[22] As an osteopath concluded in 1955, the trust of every patient had to be gained in order to overcome the belief

that medicine was emphasizing business and quantity rather than service or quality.[23] The popular press also soon reflected the medical campaigns, elements of which were familiar from earlier A.M.A. publicity favoring the old family doctor as opposed to the cold, impersonal specialist. By 1959 an article in *Life* was popularizing this idea, portraying physicians favorably but still strongly emphasizing how much they needed to add sympathy to their science.[24]

At the same time that physicians were working on their public relations in the 1950s, overt popular indictments were pushing the profession off the "pedestal." Exactly where and when the final shove came is not certain. In the third quarter of the 20th century there were no fewer than 20 investigations of the New York City health system, and in 1966, after it was clear that the medical profession was in trouble, journalist Martin Gross[25] traced the new criticism to the first of these investigations in the cultural center of the country.[26] In 1965 an anonymous writer in *Consumer Reports*[27] dated modern criticism from the publication of a study conducted in 1956 in which investigators actually rated physician performance. Perhaps the most important date was 1958, when Richard Carter's *The Doctor Business*,[28] the first of a number of muckraking books, appeared. Carter's exposé and others that followed it drew heavily on both public investigations and exposés that members of the profession had written for internal professional purposes. Whatever the source, clearly adverse criticism had entered a novel phase by the end of the 1950s, reflecting and also creating new social circumstances within which physicians practiced.

Indignant lay writers and reformer M.D.'s shared an elevated opinion about what physicians ought to be. They were, wrote a journalist in 1954, supposed to be part of a double picture: "on the one hand, a group of dedicated and white-coated scientists, bending over test tubes and producing marvelous cures for various ailments, and, on the other, equally dedicated practitioners of medicine and surgery, devoting themselves to easing pain and prolonging human life, without thought of personal gain and at considerable self-sacrifice." Both the public and the profession, he noted, were beginning to notice substantial deviations from this widely held ideal and to become filled with "disillusionment . . . tinged with a bitterness which breeds public hostility."[29] Other observers traced the rising level of adverse comment to unrealistic hopes. As the 1950s ended, columnist Dorothy Thompson summarized for readers of the *Ladies' Home Journal* this growing public criticism of American physicians. There was bad hospital care, there were bad doctors, and there were excessive medical costs. But she went on to note the cause:

> In a rather profound sense the current attacks on the medical profession compliment it. People, it seems, *expect* more of physicians than they do of other professional men with the possible exception of the clergy. The medical profession has invited that expectation, and in the opinion of this writer, and with exceptions that only prove the rule, has deserved it.[30]

In later decades, as Americans came to expect the medical profession to furnish comfort, happiness, and well-behaved children as well as health, the disillusionment grew.

## ADAPTING TO CHANGE

Since ancient times, critics—and the public at large—have usually discriminated sharply between their own personal physicians, who command professional trust, and the medical profession as a whole, which does not and which is susceptible to harsh judgments.[31] In the mid-20th century, however, doubts about medicine in general or "the doctor" intensified so much that even personal professional trust was often impaired, especially when a patient could not get the attention that he or she wanted. Critics at all levels who started by blaming the system, particularly the clinic and hospital, inadvertently raised questions about the M.D.'s who collaborated in the faulty operation of the institutions.

As professionals, physicians always functioned in part on the social level. When, in the 20th century, major changes occurred in the immediate social context within which medicine operated, the profession did not adapt quickly in either the formalities of practice or the self image it produced. One of the major new forces was the startling increase of chronic (as opposed to acute) diseases as the dominant concern in practice. A second new force was the growth of huge bureaucratic institutions, particularly hospitals, in the regular health care system. A third force was the greatly increased sophistication of consumers. And a fourth was the rise of psychological explanations for illness, leaving the physician dealing with the uncertainties of psychosomatics. All of these changes were well under way before the 1950s, and each helps to explain what happened to the golden age of medicine.

Critics and reformers outside the profession were also slow to respond to the changed situation. Carter's *The Doctor Business*, for instance, was targeted chiefly on the fee-for-service organization of medicine, and at most only a quarter of the volume was devoted to actual faults in health care. Even in 1960 in perhaps the most crucial of the new critical publications, *The Crisis in American Medicine*, the authors still tended to emphasize the economics of medicine even while recognizing that "millions of people are bitterly dissatisfied with the medical care they are getting."[32]

What eventually transformed the criticism was the addition of another ingredient from society as a whole: widespread anti-institutional sentiment along with a general disillusionment with many aspects of American life.[33] Among the target institutions were the professions, particularly professions based on expertise. In the mid-1950s writers in the highbrow and mass media began to paint negative or at least ambivalent images of many American institutions that in the 1940s had been beyond reproach: the city, the automobile, the large family—and the doctor. In making their unfavorable remarks about doctors, various kinds of public commentators drew from both past and then current concerns to focus on three aspects of the physician's function: the priestly, or sacerdotal, role; the technical role; and the role of the physician as a member of the health care system.

## THE SACERDOTAL ROLE

In the first half of the 20th century, when medical intervention was becoming increasingly effective, such critics as there were tended to concentrate not on the technical role of physicians but on their priestly functioning as they went through medical ceremonies and acted as wise and trusted personages. In this preoccupation, commentators reflected basic popular attitudes. In novels, for example, despite the shift of physician characters from priestly and scholarly roles to scientific, their most important duties still centered on nonphysical problems and relationships.[34] Regardless of the passing of the old-fashioned family doctor, there was a well-understood public demand for a sympathetic personal relationship such as that furnished by the idealized country practitioner. "His successors have much to learn from him," observed an editorial writer in a typical comment as early as 1908. "At all events they must learn to be men, not merely scientists."[35] And even as the socialized medicine debate heated up, the impersonal system rather than individual M.D. performance was the subject of adverse comment.

In all of the criticism during the golden age, the emphasis on priestly personal functions of the physician, as opposed to effectiveness or even competence, is striking. As late as the 1950s, lists of common criticisms to which physicians were sensitive included most prominently "A failure to take a personal interest in the patient and his family," "Inability to get a doctor in cases of emergency," "Waiting time in doctors' offices," and other such items reflecting the continuing demand for personal attention.[36] The only other conspicuous categories of complaint had to do with fees and failure to communicate with the patient. Only in later decades did the demand for competence become very conspicuous.[37]

It is against this background of emphasis on the sacerdotal function of medical personnel that the great constant of criticism, greed, has to be viewed. Greed on the part of a physician violated a sacerdotal stereotype because most Americans expected that under ideal circumstances a physician was a dedicated professional who provided a service because the service was needed, not because it was profitable.[38] Greed showed up earlier as a concern in attacks on quackery, fee-splitting, and then, to a small extent, physician financial interest in laboratory and drug store enterprises.[39] But it was only after physicians had in general substantially increased their incomes that critics fastened on the evident wealth rather than specific fees of M.D.'s as evidence of unseemly grasping. This recent phase had to wait for the development of what David Horrobin has called "the politics of envy" in the late 20th century.[40]

That physician greed was a constant in criticism meant that even in the recent period, when technical as well as priestly performance in medicine was again subject to question, the motive that critics identified in errant physicians was avariciousness. Why else would a rational M.D. commit undesirable acts and reduce the quality of the medical care that he was delivering? And in the continuing socialized medicine controversy, when the physician as entrepreneur was an issue, greed was, again, imputed to medical advocates of *laissez-faire.*[41]

One area in which the public could and did react to physicians in their nontechnical roles was indifference to patients, epitomized in the contrast between house calls and clinic or hospital practice. Personal attention was the theme of the solo practice advocates both inside and outside the profession. It was the chief complaint of detractors of specialization, before and after the late 1950s. It was the object of the local grievance committees set up after World War II. And it was the subject of studies after mid-century by members of a new subspecialty, medical sociologists.

In an era of high technology, when the secrets of medicine became increasingly inaccessible and incomprehensible to the public, responsiveness to the patient remained the one aspect of practice by which most people could judge the M.D. By the 1960s, case histories of patient mistreatment on a social, not technical, level were standard in the growing literature of criticism. But the critics who wanted attention and care from the physician still did not usually specify what the care consisted of until well into the age of malpractice suits.[42]

## THE TECHNICAL ROLE

Although the technical performance of the physician called forth little adverse comment before the 1950s, both the application of medical science and the individual competence of the M.D. in applying it had earlier been traditional and continuing subjects of recrimination. Kept alive for a time in the campaign against obviously incompetent nonphysician quacks, the theme of pretension and ineffective treatment continued to be an issue in occasional attacks on unnecessary surgery. Remarkable, however, was the fact that one type of criticism, that directed toward the laziness, negligence, and incompetence of M.D.'s, remained largely undeveloped for over half a century. There were a few stories about outright malpractice, and there were suggestions (usually made by M.D.'s trying to upgrade the profession) that many physicians were not keeping up with scientific literature.[43] But no rash of damaging exposés appeared until after the 1950s.

One dark side of the physician as technologist was the fear that practitioners would impose too much medicine, not only forcing inoculations and surgery on unwilling persons but, indeed, using patients for experimental purposes. In the 1920s,

Sinclair Lewis's *Arrowsmith* helped keep this traditional fear alive, but the physician as scientist who imposed on patients in the name of technique remained largely a literary figure. For decades, serious critics restricted themselves to the impersonality of the specialist, not his mania for medical intervention and innovation. Lay commentators, in fact, tended to write about fads in medicine in terms of progress and to ignore the discarded fashions. Publicists who did discuss faddism did so gently, like the 1928 humorist in *Collier's* who commented,

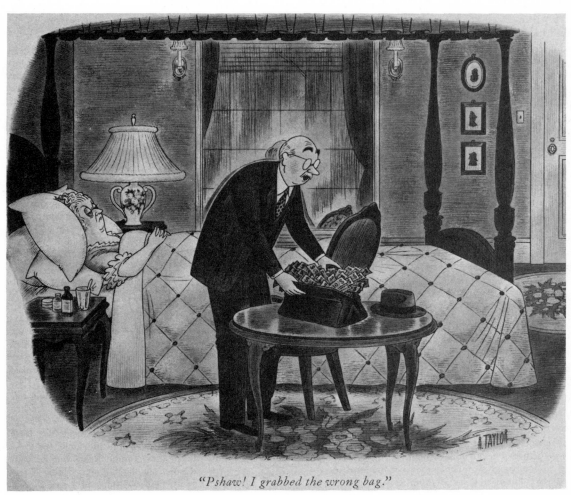

"*Pshaw! I grabbed the wrong bag.*"

Drawing by R. Taylor; © 1959 The New Yorker Magazine, Inc.

An' now it's the gall bladder. Doctors are *mad* over it. The appendix, tonsils, teeth, auto-intoxication, acidosis—all are forgotten; an' the gall bladder is now the undisputed belle of the body. For a medical man it has all the lure an' emotional appeal of a Swinburne poem, a Ziegfeld chorus or a moonlight party in Hollywood.[44]

By the 1960s and 1970s critics were saying that, as one of them put it, medical faddism reflected "the underlying bias of the technological mindset and its activity orientation . . . that newer must be better and that doing more must be better than doing less; hence the possibility of harm is always a second thought. . . ."[45] By this time, then, deliberate risk had been added to lack of knowledge and skill. Moreover, the public ultimately developed a very high level of distrust of what critics had been characterizing as excessive use of drugs and surgery.[46]

## THE SOCIAL ROLE

Beyond the priestly and technical requirements of medical practice, one of the well-understood demands society makes of any professionals in granting them special status has been that their activities be harmless to society (this is one reason that advertising, for example, cannot qualify as a profession). The traditional issue of whether the monopoly granted physicians was or was not antisocial became a crucial one in the 20th century. The reorganizers of American medicine at the turn of the century took pains to show that the newly licensed monopoly, "the medical trust," as early critics characterized it, that outlawed quacks and sectarians and vested licensure in the profession, *was* in the public interest.[47]

Medical leaders succeeded in winning the public's trust and approval.[48] Not even the failure of the self-policing that was a direct (though not essential) concomitant of the monopoly elicited much comment before the 1960s. Only insofar as physicians as a group failed to take positive action to provide medical care for all who wanted it, or as medical groups opposed institutional arrangements designed to improve and extend medical care, did criticism fall on the monopoly. Then, attribution of greed to physicians was one aspect of the accusation, but so also was conservatism, which was

a characteristic of other monopolies that consistently drew criticism in modern America. It was not until the 1960s and 1970s that new, well-educated groups tried to break the monopoly by developing new kinds of "health care deliverers" and by introducing lay control. Such developments grew out of distrust of the intentions and customs of the medical profession.

Attention to the social aspects of medicine was the qualitative characteristic that most clearly differentiated detractors of medicine before and after the 1950s. More recent critics not only decried the monopoly and maldistribution of medical care but also loaded physicians with responsibility for any number of social transgressions: exploiting menials, failing to provide incentives for improving health care delivery, encouraging unnecessary bureaucracies, increasingly setting arbitrary boundaries to illness, ignoring "positive" health, and in general, to use the term of the leading critic, Illich, "medicalizing" the whole society to the detriment of individual dignity and well being.[49]

## THE EROSION OF PROFESSIONAL STATUS

Physicians have always been sensitive to criticism.[50] For half a century they were relatively free from public censure or actual interference in clinical and professional activities, and they enjoyed great public and personal admiration. Few people other than doctors knew about iatrogenic disease or the placebo effect. Criticism—and lack of it—reflected both the impression conveyed in public about the miracles of medicine and the persistence of the sacerdotal role of the physician, demanded by the public at all levels. But the physician as priest was already in some trouble by the 1930s. Attacks on impersonal specialism and on well-meaning social reformers' attempts to spread the technical benefits of medicine through prepayment (that is, insurance) and institutional reorganization laid a basis for doubts about the whole profession. Demand for a priest was still intense, as surveys even in the 1950s showed, but the profession in general was by then set in place to be the object of a more general social attack. This attack portended the end of generous funding for medical research and the end of such extremes of freedom of action as professionals might aspire to.[51]

Commentators with a sense of the tragic, or even just of the ironic, can find in the 20th-century physician ample justification for their views. As sociologist Eliot Freidson pointed out at the beginning of the 1960s, conflict between patient and physician was inevitable because the function of the physician was to apply general knowledge to a particular individual, the patient.[52] Applying knowledge involved trying to control the patient, and the patient in turn was interested in controlling his or her destiny.[53] In attempting to maximize the client-professional trust that would permit patients to yield control, physicians emphasized the validity of their science — and in so doing created a sophisticated public. That public in turn became increasingly competent to expose shortcomings of the profession and to react when physician reformers spoke out about their colleagues' failures.[54] "I wrote about . . . abuses and asked for changes," wrote District of Columbia internist Michael J. Halberstam in the mid-1970s. "And now changes are coming, but alas . . . they will probably be the wrong ones."[55]

One of the major results of the new criticism of the 1960s and 1970s, in which the technical as well as the sacerdotal function of the physician came into question, was therefore a series of demands for greater patient participation in the medical relationship, demands exacerbated by a resurgence of romantic individualism in the culture as a whole.[56] By 1972 one analyst[57] could add to the "engineering" and "priestly" models of health care and delivery two more, the "collegial" and the "contractual." Both of these last models involved patient participation and were flourishing in various settings.[58]

Insofar as the entire society was moving toward social leveling, the high status necessary for professional authority was being eroded throughout most of the century.[59] By the 1960s even the popular image of the physician as portrayed on television reflected a change from a charismatic figure, who used mysterious powers to resolve problems, to a new type of hero, one with only ordinary endowments and who potentially could behave unheroically.[60] But as early as the 1930s the sociologists who surveyed Muncie, Indiana, as "Middletown," had commented that physicians, and lawyers, too, were increasingly less visible as independent community leaders. Older physicians continued to be aware of a change, but few could cite convincing detail as did J. A. Lundy of Worcester, Massachusetts, who in 1952 recalled the time when townspeople customarily tipped their hats to the physician.[61] Another perceived sign of erosion of the physician's place was the fact that patients felt increasingly free to shop around for an M.D. who suited them.[62] The loss was felt not by the technically oriented specialist whose bedside manner might be imperfect, but by the traditional family doctor. By the 1960s and 1970s physicians were complaining not only of lack of deference but of lay interference and assaults on professional privileges. The politics of envy were building in new ways upon traditions of criticism that had been muted in the first half of the 20th century but had not died.

## CONCLUSION

The golden days of the medical profession can be defined by the amount and the content of criticism that the profession received — what little adverse comment there was, was often to the effect that highly desirable professional services were insufficiently available or that physicians had lapsed from their sacerdotal roles. In both cases the critics tended to fasten on the old theme of the doctor whose greed overcame his more professionally disinterested concern. The practice of medicine always involved M.D.'s in ambivalent relationships with both individual patients and society, and high-status professionals who could not or would not respond to patients' personal and selfish concerns of course generated complaints and could even become both personal and social scapegoats.[63] But it was the continuing politics of the socialized medicine debate that first planted the seeds of major and pervasive mistrust. When, after World War II, physicians themselves spoke out to increase the beneficent results of medicine and upgrade the profession in the direction of the professional ideal, they unwittingly opened the door for the latter-day critics who attacked not only priestly pretension but technical performance. The influence of these critics combined with other social forces in movements that in the 1960s and 1970s tended to impair the trust and freedom that had once marked medical practice.[64]

NOTES

A draft on this subject was originally prepared in connection with National Endowment for the Humanities grant FP-0013-79-54 (Seminar for the Professions); the writing was supported in part by a Special Research Assignment from The Ohio State University. For suggestions, thanks are due to members of the NEH seminar and to K. J. Andrien and J. R. Bartholomew.

1  G. H. Gallup, *The Gallup Poll: Public Opinion, 1935–1971* (New York: Random House, 1972), pp. 1152 and 1779–1780.

2  M. J. Halberstam, *Prism*, July–Aug. 1975: 15. Halberstam's is a casual observation: the literature contains no general surveys of the changing fortune of the physician in American organs of information and opinion in the last century, and not even the *Reader's Guide* has been systematically exploited for information about the place of physicians in American society. Sociologists' work on their medical contemporaries dates only from mid-century.

3  F. J. Ingelfinger, *New Eng. J. Med.*, 1976, *294*: 335; American Osteopathic Association, *A Survey of Public Attitudes Toward Medical Care and Medical Professionals* (Chicago: American Osteopathic Association, 1981).

4  American Osteopathic Association, *A Survey of Public Attitudes*; R. W. Hodge, P. M. Siegel, P. H. Rossi, *Am. J. Sociol.*, 1964, *70*: 286; A. Tyree and B. G. Smith, *Soc. Forces*, 1978, *56*: 881.

5  R. H. Shryock, *Ann. Med. Hist.*, 1930, n.s., *2*: 308.

6  Anonymous, *Life*, 1908, *52*: 196.

7  I. Illich, *Medical Nemesis: The Expropriation of Health* (New York: Random House, 1976).

8  The most delightful example is E. Berman, *The Solid Gold Stethoscope* (New York: Macmillan, 1976).

9  J. Duffy, *The Healers: The Rise of the Medical Establishment* (New York: McGraw-Hill, 1976); *J.A.M.A.*, 1967, *200*: 136; M. R. Kaufman, *Mt. Sinai J. Med. N.Y.*, 1976, *43*: 76; G. H. Brieger, *New Physician*, 1970, *19*: 845; B. Rosenkrantz, *Proc. Int. Cong. Hist. Sci.*, 1974, *14*: 113; J. S. Haller, *American Medicine in Transition, 1840–1910* (Urbana: Univ. of Illinois Press, 1981); J. G. Burrow, *Organized Medicine in the Progressive Era: The Move Toward Monopoly* (Baltimore: Johns Hopkins Univ. Press, 1977); *Med. Rev. Rev.*, 1917, *23*: 1; B. Sicherman, in *Nourishing the Humanistic in Medicine*, ed. W. R. Rogers and D. Barnard (Pittsburgh: Univ. of Pittsburgh Press, 1979), p. 95. The famous criticisms in the Flexner Report [A. Flexner, *Medical Education in the United States and Canada* (New York: Carnegie Foundation, 1910)] were aimed at diploma mills, not well-trained M.D.'s; the report spoke for, not against, the profession.

10  F. A. Walker, *Bull. Hist. Med.*, 1979, *53*: 489.

11  The group practice and socialized medicine controversy has been widely researched and is not covered in the present article. Standard sources include S. Kelley, Jr., *Professional Public Relations and Political Power* (Baltimore: Johns Hopkins Press, 1956), pp. 67–106; J. G. Burrow, *AMA: Voice of American Medicine* (Baltimore: Johns Hopkins Press, 1963); E. Rayack, *Professional Power and American Medicine: The Economics of the American Medical Association* (Cleveland: World, 1967); D. S. Hirshfield, *The Lost Reform: The Campaign for Compulsory Health Insurance in the United States from 1932 to 1943* (Cambridge, Mass.: Harvard Univ. Press, 1970); R. Harris, *A Sacred Trust* (New York: New American Library, 1966); R. Numbers, *Almost Persuaded: American Physicians and Compulsory Health Insurance, 1912–1920* (Baltimore: Johns Hopkins Univ. Press, 1978).

12  D. W. Blumhagen, *Ann. Intern. Med.* 1979, *91*: 111.

13  E. Barkins, *Are These Our Doctors?* (New York: Fell, 1952), pp. 171–172. See also a popular work, D. G. Cooley, *The Science Book of Wonder Drugs* (New York: Franklin Watts, 1954).

14  M. J. Gaughan (Thesis, Boston Univ., 1977). For a famous contemporary comment, see B. DeVoto, *Harper's Mag.*, 1951, *202*: 56.

15  A. M. Lee, *Psychiatry*, 1944, *7*: 371.

16  W. Kaempffert, *Am. Mercury*, 1943, *57*: 557.

17  American Medical Association *v.* United States, 317 *U.S. Reports* 519; P. S. Ward, unpublished paper read at American Association for the History of Medicine Meetings, Pittsburgh, May 1978.

18  H. Maurer, *Fortune*, Feb. 1954: 138.

19  R. R. Malmsheimer (Thesis, Univ. of Minnesota, 1978); "Doctors as Hollywood sees them," *Sci. Digest*, Oct. 1953: 60; J. Spears, *Films Rev.*, 1955, *6*: 437; E. H. Vincent, *Quart. Bull. Northwestern Univ. Med. Sch.*, 1950, *24*: 305.

20  J. Hunton, *GP*, 1951, *4*: 110; R. Carter, *The Doctor Business* (New York: Doubleday, 1958), pp. 235–238; G. B. Risse, in *Responsibility in Health Care*, ed. G. J. Agich (Dordrecht: Reidel, 1982).

21  R. W. Elwell, *Ohio State Med. J.*, 1950, *46*: 581.

22  Risse, *Responsibility in Health Care*; R. Waterson and W. Tibbits, *GP*, Oct. 1951, *4*: 93; M. Amrine, *Am. Psychol.*, 1958, *13*: 248. For a summary of the research, see S. Greenberg, *The Troubled Calling: Crisis in the Medical Establishment* (New York: Macmillan, 1965), Ch. 4.

23  *New York Times*, Oct. 16, 1955: 72.

24  *Life*, Oct. 12, 1959: 144; M. Austin, *Look*, Mar. 15, 1949: 34.

25  M. L. Gross, *The Doctors* (New York: Random House, 1966), p. 7.

26  R. R. Alford, *Health Care Politics: Ideological and Interest Group Barriers to Reform* (Chicago: Univ. of Chicago Press, 1975), p. 22. R. Bayer [*Homosexuality and American Psychiatry: The Politics of Diagnosis* (New York: Basic Books, 1981), p. 10] maintains that the public attack on psychiatry prefigured the attacks on medicine as an institution.

27  *Consumer Reports,* Mar. 1965: 146.

28  Previously cited in n. 20.

29  B. McKelway, *Med. Ann. District of Columbia,* 1954, *23:* 457.

30  D. Thompson, *Ladies' Home Journal,* Apr. 1959: 11. Later, television productions greatly intensified unrealistic expectations; G. Gerbner and others, *New Eng. J. Med.,* 1981, *305:* 901.

31  A striking modern survey, showing the generality of the phenomenon in all segments of the population, is Ben Gaffin & Associates, *What Americans Think of the Medical Profession . . . , Report on a Public Opinion Survey* (Chicago: American Medical Association, 1955).

32  M. K. Sanders, ed., *The Crisis in American Medicine* (New York: Harper, 1961), p. vii.

33  R. C. Maulitz, unpublished paper.

34  A. J. Cameron (Thesis, Univ. of Notre Dame, 1973), especially p. 157.

35  *New York Times,* Aug. 21, 1908: 6. An early sociological survey of patients (E. L. Koos, *Am. J. Public Hlth.,* 1955, *45:* 1551) showed that the young modern patients as well as the old who had, for example, actually seen house calls, responded negatively to impersonality in practice. There were probably also changes in the social expectations for the "sick" role; see, for example, E. Kendall, *Harper's Mag.,* 1959, *219:* 29.

36  J. T. T. Hundley, *Va. Med. Mon.,* 1952, *79:* 540; E. Stanton, *J. Maine Med. Assn.,* 1954, *45:* 56.

37  American Osteopathic Association, *A Survey of Public Attitudes.* By 1957 patients were almost evenly divided in wanting most kindly attention or technical skills and results (getting better): G. G. Reader, L. Pratt, M. C. Mudd, *Mod. Hosp.,* 1957, *89:* 88.

38  No attempt is made in this article to deal directly with the issue of professionalization and professional status; there is already a large special literature on the subject.

39  For a particularly good example of the restricted criticism, see an anonymous editorial, "Unprofessional conduct," *J. Med. Soc. N.J.,* 1929, *26:* 326. In the present discussion I treat the explicit content of the criticism and do not utilize the suggestion that complaints about fees were substituted for expressing other grievances.

40  D. F. Horrobin, *Medical Hubris: A Reply to Ivan Illich* (Montreal: Eden, 1977), p. 27. Ironically, high income was one of the factors that contributed to physicians' high prestige (Hodge, Siegel, and Rossi, "Occupational prestige in the United States, 1925–63;" Tyree and Smith, "Hierarchy in the United States: 1789–1969"). P. Starr (*Daedalus,* 1978, *107:* 175) suggests that this type of criticism did not appear conspicuously until after publicity about Medicaid abuses.

41  Stupidity was also an issue, being part of the argument that a reorganized, socialized physician would be better off economically.

42  For example, D. B. Smith and A. D. Kaluzny, *The White Labyrinth: Understanding the Organization of Health Care* (Berkeley: McCutchan, 1975).

43  R. S. Halle, in an article entitled, "Unfit doctors must go" (*Scribner's Mag.,* 1931, *90:* 514), dealt entirely with clear cases of malpractice; and H. M. Robinson (*Am. Mercury,* 1936, *38:* 321) blamed lawyers, patients, and unrealistic expectations for a rash of lawsuits.

44  *Collier's,* Aug. 4, 1928: 27.

45  L. Lander, *Defective Medicine: Risk, Anger, and the Malpractice Crisis* (New York: Farrar, Straus & Giroux, 1978), p. 41.

46  American Osteopathic Association, *A Survey of Public Attitudes.*

47  A. D. Bevan, *Am. Med. Assoc. Bull.,* 1910, *5:* 243.

48  Burrow, *Organized Medicine in the Progressive Era.*

49  See n. 7 above.

50  O. W. Anderson, *Mich. Med.,* 1968, *67:* 455.

51  P. B. Hutt, *Daedalus,* 1978, *107:* 157.

52  E. Freidson, *Patients' Views of Medical Practice — A Study of Subscribers to a Prepaid Medical Plan in the Bronx* (New York: Russell Sage Foundation, 1961), p. 175.

53  Risse, *Responsibility in Health Care.*

54  T. H. Stubbs, *Emory Univ. Quart.,* 1947, *3:* 137.

55  See n. 2 above.

56  D. Nelkin, *Daedalus,* 1978, *107:* 191; E. Dichter (*N.Y. St. J. Med.,* 1954, *54:* 222) is an important example.

57  R. M. Veatch, *Hastings Center Rep.,* June 1972, *2:* 5.

58  *Ibid.*

59  Freidson, *Patients' Views of Medical Practice,* p. 187.

60  B. Myerhoff and W. R. Larson, *Hum. Organ. Clgh. Bull.,* 1964, *24:* 188.

61  J. A. Lundy, *New Eng. J. Med.,* 1952, *246:* 446.

62  R. S. Lynd and H. M. Lynd, *Middletown in Transition: A Study in Cultural Conflicts* (New York: Harcourt, Brace, 1937), p. 427 n; J. Kasteler, R. L. Kane, D. M. Olsen, C. Thetford, *J. Hlth. Soc. Behav.,* 1976, *17:* 328; F. W. Mann, *J. Maine Med. Assn.,* 1925, *16:* 137.

63  N.Y. Hoffman, *J. Am. Med. Assn.,* 1972, *220:* 58.

Another dimension — unchanging pop culture and the dangerous remoteness of the scientist — is not explored in this present article; see G. Basalla, in *Science and Its Public: The Changing Relationship,* ed.

G. Holton and W. H. Blanpied (Dordrecht: Reidel, 1976), p. 261.

64   R. Branson, *Hastings Center Stud.*, 1973, *1*: (No. 2): 17.

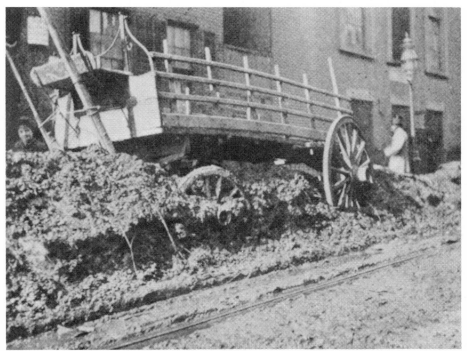

These photographs, taken by the muckraking journalist Jacob Riis, illustrate the transformation brought about by New York City Street Commissioner George Waring after he took office in 1895. Both pictures show the same paved block in front of 212 Sullivan Street. The top photo, taken in March, 1893, depicts a scene typical of American cities in the late 19th century.

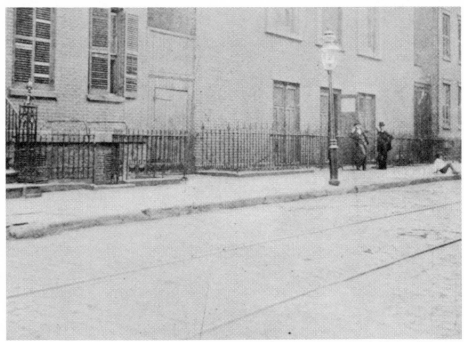

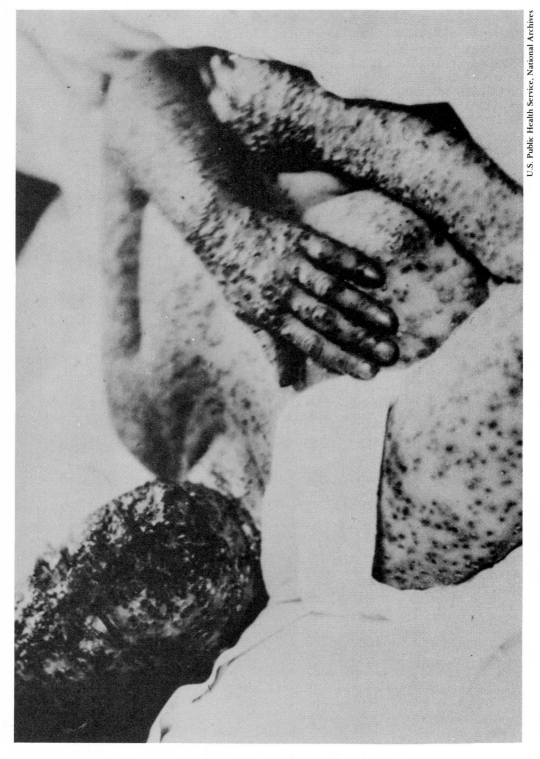

Of all 19th-century threats to health, epidemic diseases aroused the greatest concern. Besides taking many lives, the loathsome smallpox left many of its victims permanently disfigured.

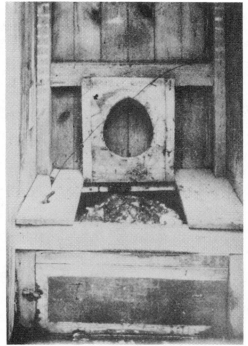

"There Ain't No Law," pamphlet of the National Housing Association (New York, 1913). Courtesy of Clay McShane

Contaminated milk and overflowing privies contributed to the poor health of American city dwellers. The 1858 drawing (below) illustrates one dairy's attempt to obtain the last drop of milk from an obviously sick and dying cow. The 1913 photograph of a privy in Yonkers, New York, graphically portrays the unsanitary condition of one American community in the early 20th century.

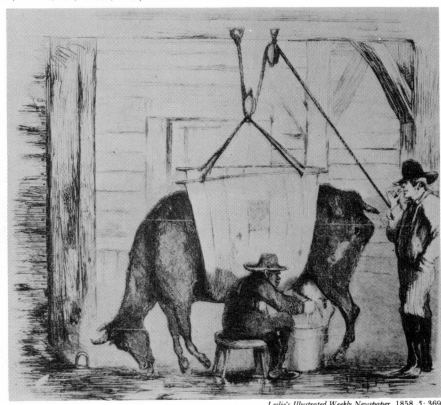

*Leslie's Illustrated Weekly Newspaper*, 1858, 5: 369

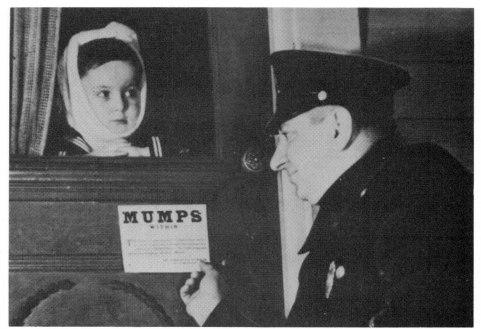

Quarantines and school medical inspections were two of the measures urban health departments employed to reduce sickness among children. These photographs show a Milwaukee health inspector placarding the home of a little boy suffering from mumps and a New York City public health nurse examining the cleanliness of school children.

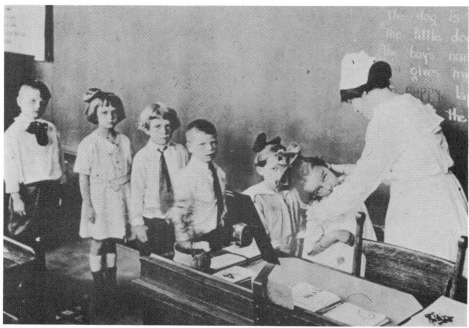

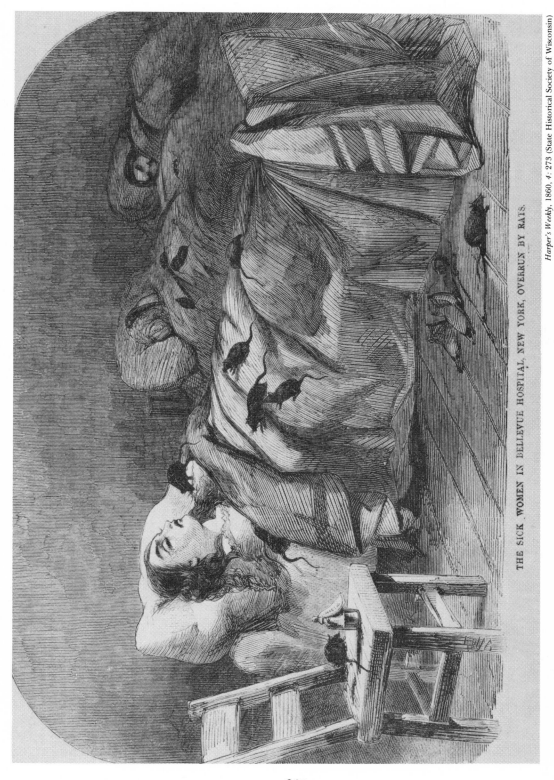

THE SICK WOMEN IN BELLEVUE HOSPITAL, NEW YORK, OVERRUN BY RATS.

*Harper's Weekly*, 1860, 4: 273 (State Historical Society of Wisconsin)

Nineteenth-century hospitals sheltered the suffering poor, but their filthy and understaffed facilities sometimes did more harm than good. In 1860 a woman in New York City's Bellevue Hospital actually lost her newborn baby to the institution's rats.

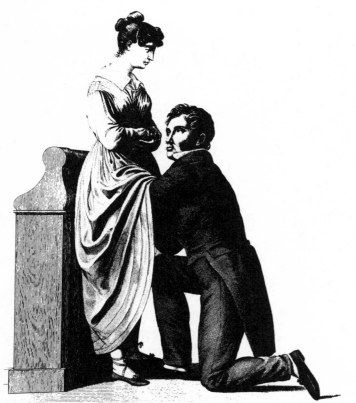

J. P. Maygrier, *Midwifery Illustrated* (New York: Harper Bros., 1834), p. 90

Modesty frequently inhibited women from seeking assistance for sensitive ailments and sometimes affected the treatment they received, as this pelvic examination illustrates. Several health problems resulted from the fashionable 19th-century custom of wearing waist-restricting corsets.

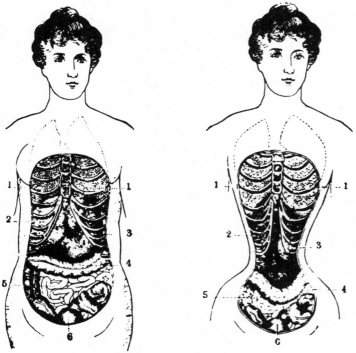

From *The Unfashionable Human Body* by Bernard Rudofsky. Copyright © 1971 by Bernard Rudofsky. Used by permission of Doubleday and Company, Inc.

# FEE-BILL,

## Adopted by the Western Medical Society of the State of Wisconsin, December, 1849.

| | |
|---|---|
| Ordinary office prescription, | $ 0 50 |
| Venesection, or extracting tooth at office. | 50 |
| Opening abscess, | 50 to 5 00 |
| Dresing wound, | 50 " 5 00 |
| Vaccination, | " 1 00 |
| Dividing Fraenum, | 50 " 2 00 |
| Cupping, | 1 00 " 2 00 |
| Introducing Seton or Issue | 1 00 " 2 00 |
| Scarifying Eye, | 1 00 " 5 00 |
| Verbal advice, | 1 00 |
| Written advice, | 2 00 " 5 00 |
| Ordinary visit in Town, | 1 00 |
| Visit after 10 o'clock P. M., | 2 00 |
| Additional patients, same family, (each) | 50 |
| Consultation visit, | 3 00 " 5 00 |
| Malignant Contagious diseases, (first) | 3 00 " 5 00 |
| Subsequent visits, each, | 2 00 |
| Natural Parturition, (ten hours.) | 6 00 " 10 00 |
| Extra Detention, (pr hour.) | 50 |
| Unnecessary Detention, (pr hour.) | 1 00 |
| Twin cases, | 10 00 " 15 00 |
| Instrumental Labor, or Turning, | 15 00 " 25 00 |
| Removing Placenta, | 6 00 " 10 00 |
| Visits after two days, charged as ordinary. | |
| Visit in country under two miles, | 2 00 |
| Do. over two miles, pr mile, | 50 " 1 00 |
| Visit, same neighborhood half price. | |
| Gonorrhœa, (in advance.) | 5 00 " 20 00 |
| Syphilis, (Do.) | 10 00 " 25 00 |
| Introducing Catheter, (first time,) | 2 00 |
| Do. Subsequently, | 1 00 |
| Paracentesis, | 5 00 " 20 00 |
| Excision Tonsils, | 5 00 " 10 00 |
| Operation for Hydrocele, | 5 00 " 25 00 |
| Do. Phimosis, Paraphimosis, | 5 00 " 10 00 |
| Do. Fistula Lachrymalis, | 10 00 " 30 00 |
| Do. " in Ano, | 10 00 " 35 00 |

| | |
|---|---|
| Operation for Imperforate Anus. | $ 5 00 to 25 00 |
| Do. Vagina, | 10 00 " 50 00 |
| Do. Hare-Lip, | 10 00 " 30 00 |
| Do. Hernia, | 25 to 100 00 |
| Do. Cataract, | 50 " 100 00 |
| Do. Strabismus, | 10 " 25 00 |
| Do. Club-Foot, | 25 " 100 00 |
| Do. Stone, | 100 " 200 00 |
| Ligating Arteries, | 10 " 200 00 |
| Extirpating Eye, | 50 " 100 00 |
| Do. Testicle, | 25 " 100 00 |
| Do. Tumors, | 5 " 100 00 |
| Trephining, | 25 " 100 00 |
| Reducing Hernia, | 5 " 15 00 |
| Do. Prolapsus Ani, | 2 " 10 00 |
| Do. Fracture of Thigh, | 25 " 50 00 |
| Do. " Leg, | 10 " 30 00 |
| Do. " Clavicle, | 10 " 25 00 |
| Do. " Arm, Forearm, | 10 " 25 00 |
| Do. " Fingers, Toes, | 3 " 10 00 |
| Dislocation Hip-Joint, | 25 " 100 00 |
| Do. Shoulder-Joint, | 15 " 35 00 |
| Do. Elbow, Wrist, Ankle, | 10 " 25 00 |
| Do. Finger, Toe, | 3 " 10 00 |
| Amputation Thigh, | 50 " 100 00 |
| Do. Leg, Foot, | 25 " 100 00 |
| Do. Finger, Toe, | 5 " 15 00 |
| Do. Arm, Forearm, Wrist, | 25 " 75 00 |
| Do. Hip, or Shoulder Joint, | 100 " 200 00 |
| Do. Breast, | 25 " 100 00 |
| Do. Penis, | 10 " 50 00 |
| Inducing Premature Labor, | 50 " 100 00 |

In all Surgical cases, the charge for subsequent attendance, to be according to time occupied and trouble incurred.

Visits in the country after dark to be considered as night visits, and charged double.

*Resolved*, That the moral, professional and pecuniary interests of this Society, require of its members a uniformity in charges.

*Resolved*, That we, the undersigned, members of the Western Medical Society of the State of Wisconsin, mutually pledge ourselves faithfully to adhere to the foregoing rates of charges.

(SIGNED,)

| | | | |
|---|---|---|---|
| J. W. CLARK, | H. VAN DUSEN, | AZEL P. LADD, | A. SAMPSON, |
| J. S. RUSSELL, | GEO. D. WILBER, | WM. STODDART, | C. A. MILLS, |
| EDWARD CRONIN, | DAVID ROSS, | GEO. W. PHILLIPS, | T. R KIBBE. |

ATTEST, GEO. D. WILBER, *Secretary.*       J. W. CLARK, *President*

History of Medicine Department, University of Wisconsin-Madison

Local medical societies attempted to regulate the costs of medical care and stabilize the income of physicians by publishing schedules of fees like this one for the Western Medical Society of the State of Wisconsin in 1849. Such documents can often tell us as much about the practice of medicine as about medical economics.

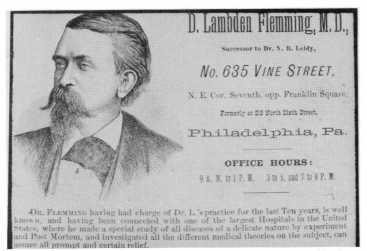

**D. Lambden Flemming, M. D.,**

Successor to Dr. N. B. Leidy,

*No. 635 Vine Street.*

N. E. Cor. Seventh, opp. Franklin Square;

Formerly at 218 North Sixth Street,

Philadelphia, Pa.

**OFFICE HOURS:**

9 A. M. to 1 P. M.    3 to 5, and 7 to 9 P. M.

·DR. FLEMMING having had charge of Dr. L.'s practice for the last Ten years, is well known, and having been connected with one of the largest Hospitals in the United States, where he made a special study of all diseases of a delicate nature by experiment and Post Mortem, and investigated all the different medical theories on the subject, can assure all prompt and certain relief.

Picture Collection, New York Public Library

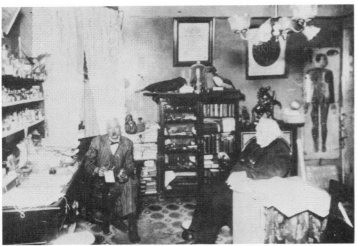

These illustrations suggest changes in the image of the American doctor: the businessman-physician of the 19th century, the family practitioner of the early 20th century, and the striking house staff of a major New York hospital in the 1970s.

State Historical Society of Colorado

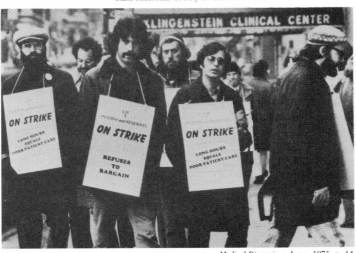

*Medical Dimensions,* June, 1975, p. 14

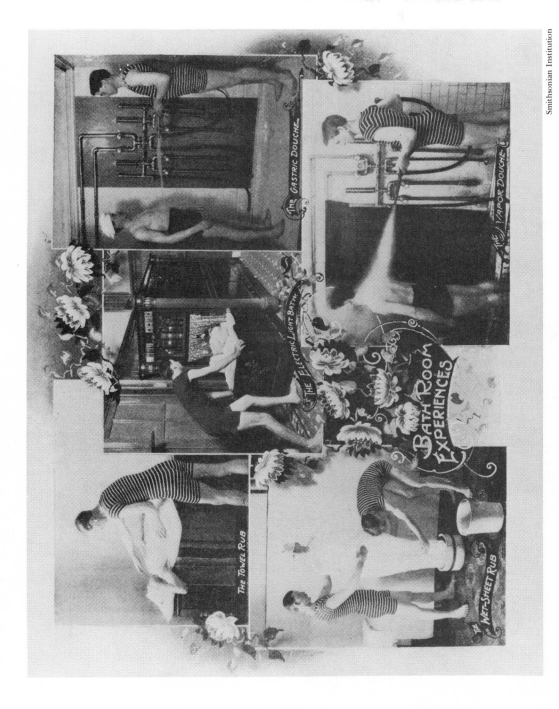

Hydropathy was only one of several medical sects that flourished in 19th-century America. These photographs show the various treatments available at Dr. John Harvey Kellogg's Battle Creek Sanitarium, which prospered well into the 20th century.

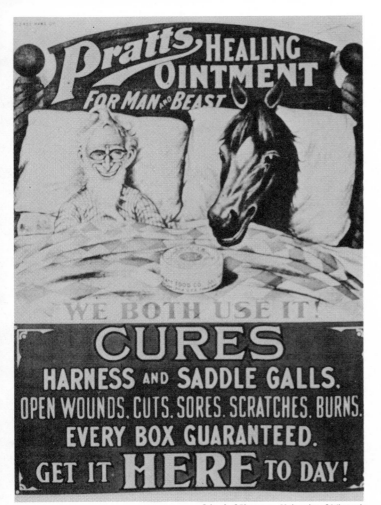

In addition to its regular and sectarian physicians, America offered its sick an almost infinite variety of quacks and cures, from ubiquitous patent remedies like Pratt's Healing Ointment to more elaborate and costly devices like the worthless Electric Couch and Dry Bath.

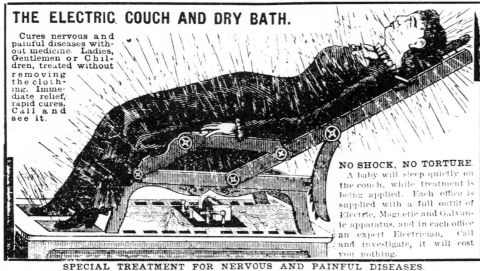

SPECIAL TREATMENT FOR NERVOUS AND PAINFUL DISEASES.

Bellevue Hospital Medical College.
CITY OF NEW YORK.
SESSION 1874-'75.

_Admit_ ............................................................

LECTURES
ON
Physiology and Physiological Anatomy.

_A. Flint jr_— M. D., Professor.

---

Bellevue Hospital Medical College.
CITY OF NEW YORK.
SESSION 1874-'75.

_Admit_ ............................................................

LECTURES
ON
THE PRINCIPLES AND PRACTICE OF MEDICINE.

_Austin Flint_, M. D., Professor.

---

Bellevue Hospital Medical College.
CITY OF NEW YORK.
SESSION 1874-'75.

.................................................... _is entitled_

To all the Privileges of the Department of

PRACTICAL ANATOMY,
Until March 1, 1875.

_A. Flint jr_— M. D., Sec'y of the Faculty.

☞ This Ticket is not an evidence that the holder of it has actually dissected, unless
certified by the Professor of Practical Anatomy. [OVER.]

---

Bellevue Hospital Medical College.
SESSION 1874-'75.

LECTURES ON SURGERY.

_Admit_ ......................

_Frank H Hamilton_ M. D.,
Prof. of Practice of Surgery with Operations.

_Lewis A Sayre_ M. D.,
Prof. of Orthopedic Surgery,

_Alex. B. Mott_ M. D.,
Prof. of Clinical and Operative Surgery,

_Wm. van Buren_ M. D.,
Prof. of the Principles of Surgery with Diseases of the Genito-Urinary System.

---

Until late into the 19th century medical students paid for their tuition by purchasing tickets from each professor whose lectures they wanted to attend.

# INSTITUTIONS

The hospital, so central to health care today, assumed little importance in American medical history until the late 19th century. Except for the almshouses and pesthouses found in large towns along the Atlantic seaboard, there were no hospitals in the British colonies of North America until 1751, when Benjamin Franklin and his Philadelphia friends founded the Pennsylvania Hospital. Modeled after the voluntary hospitals of England, this institution admitted both the mentally and physically ill and accepted those who could pay as well as those who could not.

Because of the nation's predominantly rural population and the social attitudes described by Morris J. Vogel, the idea of hospitals caught on slowly in America. Physicians throughout the 19th century continued to treat most of their patients at home and even to perform surgery there. As late as 1873 there were fewer than 200 hospitals in the United States, about a third of which were for the mentally ill. Yet only 50 years later the number of hospitals was approaching 7,000. This rapid growth resulted as much from the social changes associated with urbanization as from advances in medical technology, such as aseptic surgery and x-rays.

Mental hospitals in America date from 1773, when the colony of Virginia opened an institution in Williamsburg "for persons of insane and disordered minds." It was not until 50 years later, however, with the founding of the Worcester State Lunatic Hospital in Massachusetts, that public-asylum building began in earnest. Thanks in large part to the efforts of Dorothea Dix and other reformers, most states by 1860 had established hospitals to care for the mentally ill. Although founded with the best intentions, these asylums soon found themselves playing a custodial rather than a curative role. As Gerald N. Grob argues, this resulted less from neglect than from a changing patient population.

For the urban poor in the 19th century, the most important medical institution was not the hospital but the dispensary, described by Charles E. Rosenberg. These institutions, which began to appear in the Northeast in the late 18th century, not only dispensed medicines and advice to needy patients but served as an important training ground for medical students and young physicians. With the rise of hospital outpatient departments in the early 20th century and related changes in the values of the medical profession, however, the independent dispensary soon disappeared from the American medical scene.

# 19

## Social Class and Medical Care in 19th-Century America: The Rise and Fall of the Dispensary

### CHARLES E. ROSENBERG

To most mid-20th-century physicians, the term "dispensary" evokes the image of a hectic hospital pharmacy. To his mid-19th-century counterpart, it was both the primary means for providing the urban poor with medical care and a vital link in the prevailing system of medical education. These institutions had an effective life-span of roughly a hundred years. Founded in the closing decades of the 18th century, American dispensaries increased in scale and number throughout the 19th century and remained significant providers of health care well into the 20th century. By the 1920s, however, the dispensaries were on the road to extinction, increasingly submerged in the outpatient departments of urban hospitals. Historians have found the dispensary of little interest; even those contemporary medical activists seeking a usable past for experiments in the delivery of medical care, are hardly aware of their existence.[1] Yet a study of the dispensary illustrates not only an important aspect of medicine and philanthropy in the 19th-century city—but the social logic implicit in their rise and fall underlines permanently significant relationships between general social needs and values and the narrower world of medical men and ideas.

The dispensary was invented in late 18th-century England; it was an autonomous, free-standing institution, created in the hope of providing an alternative to the hospital in providing medical care for the urban poor. Like most such benevolent innovations, it was soon copied by socially conscious

CHARLES E. ROSENBERG is Professor of History and Sociology of Science at the University of Pennsylvania, Philadelphia, Pennsylvania.

Reprinted with permission from the *Journal of the History of Medicine and Allied Sciences,* 1974, *29*: 32–54.

Americans; dispensaries were established in 1786 at Philadelphia, 1791 at New York, 1796 at Boston, and at Baltimore in 1800. Their growth was at first very slow. No additional dispensaries were established until 1816, when the managers of the Philadelphia Dispensary helped establish two new dispensaries, the Northern and Southern, to serve their city's rapidly developing fringes.[2] New Yorkers established the Northern Dispensary in 1827, the Eastern in 1832, the DeMilt in 1851, and North-Western in 1852. By 1874 there were 29 dispensaries in New York, by 1877, 33 in Philadelphia. Their growth was equally impressive in terms of number of patients treated; in New York, for example, the city's dispensaries treated 134,069 patients in 1860, roughly 180,000 in 1866, 213,000 in 1874 and 876,000 in 1900.[3]

The dispensaries shared certain organizational characteristics. Almost all had a central building —with the prominent exception of Boston which had none until the 1850s—and usually employed one full-time employee, an apothecary or house-physician who acted as steward, performed minor surgery, often vaccinated and pulled teeth— as well as prescribed for some patients. (Though most dispensaries limited their aid to prescriptions written by their own staff physicians, a few would fill prescriptions for the indigent patients of any regular physician.)[4] By mid-century the house-physicianship had in the larger dispensaries evolved into two separate positions, resident physician and druggist-apothecary. Most dispensaries also appointed younger physicians who visited patients too ill to attend the dispensary. Such "district visiting" was the principal task of the Philadelphia Dispensary when founded in 1786, remained the sole activity of the Boston Dispensary until 1856 — and was continued by almost all urban dispensaries until the end of the 19th century, though the treatment of ambulatory patients grew proportionately more prominent in all. The dispensaries also appointed attending and consulting staffs from among their community's established practitioners, the attending staff treating patients well enough to visit the dispensary, the consulting staff serving a largely honorary role.

The dispensaries were shoe-string operations. Most, with the exception of those in New York which enjoyed state and city subventions, were supported by private contributions and the often-voluntary services of local physicians.[5] As late as the 1870s and 1880s — when a dispensary might treat over 25,000 patients a year — budgets of four or five thousand dollars were still common and annual reports vied in reporting how little had been spent for prescriptions — an average of under five cents per prescription was common. The Boston Dispensary and Philadelphia Dispensary gradually accumulated some endowment funds, though most others remained financially marginal. All, however, were sensitive to cyclical economic shifts, for contributions declined in periods of depression while patient pressure increased proportionately. As a result of the economy's downturn in 1857, for example, New York's Eastern Dispensary reported an increase of 22 percent in cases over 1858 and 42 percent over 1856.[6] A useful index to the shaky financial condition of many of the dispensaries was their frequent practice of renting a portion of their building to commercial tenants; such income often constituted a substantial portion of the institution's budget and could not be given up even when the dispensary needed room for expansion.[7]

Some of the dispensaries published detailed statistics of the numbers and kinds of ailments treated by their physicians; thus we can begin to reconstruct their everyday responsibilities. Most cases were, of course, relatively minor — for example, bronchitis, colds, or dyspepsia — and rarely were the numbers of deaths equal to more than 2 or 3 percent of the patients treated. Consistently enough, the number of female patients was always greater than that of males, in some instances as much as two to one; working men, that is, had necessarily to tolerate disease symptoms of far greater intensity before feeling able to consult a physician. In those cases serious enough to be treated at home by visiting physicians sex ratios tended to be more nearly equal. (It was not until the end of the century that dispensaries began to consider evening hours for workers.) Although the general level of mortality among all dispensary patients was low, mortality among patients treated in their homes approached the 10 or 11 percent normal for hospitals at the beginning of the century. Such death rates were particularly discouraging, for the district physician never treated many intractable cases. Chronic and degenerative ailments brought incapacity and eventual alms-house incarceration; these cases never found their way into the dispensary's mortality statistics. The dispensaries also performed minor surgery, treating fractures, contusions and lacerations — as well as casual if frequent dentistry, essentially the "indiscriminate extirpation" of offending teeth.[8]

The dispensaries also played an important public health role in providing vaccination for the poor and vaccine matter for the use of private practitioners. From a purely demographic point of view, indeed, vaccination was the most important function performed by the dispensaries. The dispensaries not only made vaccination available without cost, but some mounted door-to-door vaccination programs in their city's tenement districts. In periods of intense demand, most frequently at the outset or threat of a smallpox epidemic, the dispensaries were able to supply large amounts of vaccine matter at short notice. In the opening months of the Civil War for example, the New York Dispensary provided vaccine matter for all the state's recruits.[9]

Despite ventures into surgery, dentistry, and vaccination, dispensary therapeutics were generally synonymous with the writing of prescriptions; dispensaries dispensed. Throughout the first three-quarters of the 19th century, the phrase "prescribing for" was generally synonymous with seeing a patient; busy dispensary physicians could hardly be expected to do more than compose hasty and routine prescriptions. (Dispensary managers tended by mid-century to demand the use of formularies limited in both cost and variety; later in the century some dispensaries were charged with filling prescriptions by number, the dispensing physician being constrained by an abbreviated list of numbered and preformulated prescriptions.)[10] In this routine and exclusive dependence on drug therapy lay the principal difference between the care provided the urban poor and that paid for by the middle class. Physicians in private practice relied consistently in their therapeutics upon adjusting the regimen of their patients, especially in chronic ills; such injunctions were hardly appropriate in dispensary practice. The city poor could not very well vary their diet, take up horse-back riding, visit the seaside, or voyage to the West Indies.

Not surprisingly, the dispensaries tended to develop ties both formal and informal with other urban charities — in New York, for example, with the Commissioners of Emigration, Association for Improving the Condition of the Poor, and Children's Aid Society; in Philadelphia with the Board of Guardians for the Poor.[11] Dispensary physicians were in this sense *de facto* social workers. In New York, for example, a note from the dispensary physician was necessary if the commissioners were to issue a ration of coal; thus a mid-century whimsy referred to "coal fever"—an illness which struck suddenly during cold weather in the city's tenements.[12] In the post-Civil War decades, efforts to provide such physical amenities became somewhat more organized; dispensary physicians continued to work with existing philanthropic agencies and began as well to establish their own auxiliaries in hopes of providing food and nursing in deserving cases. In Philadelphia, the Lying-In and Nurse Charity and the Lying-In Department of the Northern Dispensary had provided some nursing service since the 1830s, while others had paid occasionally for nursing in selected cases since the opening years of the century. In a more contemporary idiom, the Instructive Visiting Nurse Service of the Boston Dispensary began in the 1880s to aid the dispensary's district physicians in their work, not only nursing, but educating the poor in hygiene and diet. In Boston and New York, diet kitchen associations provided nourishing food for patients bearing a dispensary physician's requisition. By 1883, the New York Diet Kitchen Association operated three kitchens in cooperation with the dispensaries and had fed 7,699 patients, filling 53,893 separate requisitions from dispensary physicians during the year.[13]

Another trend marking the 19th-century evolution of the dispensaries, reflecting and paralleling a more general development within the medical profession, was their internal reorganization along specialty lines. As early as 1826, the New York Dispensary reorganized itself, dividing patients treated at the dispensary into "classes" according to the nature of their ailment. Pioneering dispensaries for diseases of the eye and ear had come into being as early as the 1820s. By mid-century, the need for specialty differentiation was unquestioned. When the Brooklyn Dispensary opened in 1847, for example, it announced that patients would be distributed among the following classes: women and children, heart, lungs and throat, skin and vaccination, head and digestive organs, eye and ear, surgery and unclassified diseases. In the second half of the century, specialty designations became increasingly narrow and gradually closer to modern categories; nervous and genito-urinary diseases were, for example, among the most frequently created of such departments in the late 1870s and early 1880s. By 1905, the forward-looking Boston Dispensary boasted these impressively varied out-patient clinics: surgical, general medical, children, skin, nervous system, nose and throat, women, eye and ear, genito-urinary and x-ray.[14] An important related late-19th-century trend was the increasingly frequent establishment of specialized dispensaries, institutions that treated only particular ailments or ailments of particular organs.

These in brief outline were the chief characteristics which marked the growth of the dispensaries between the end of the 18th and last decades of the 19th centuries. Why did the founders and managers of our pioneer dispensaries find them so plausible a response to social need? What factors led to their initial adoption and subsequent growth?

In their appeals for public support, dispensary founders and supporters left abundant records of their conscious motives. Most prominent in the last years of the 18th and opening decades of the 19th centuries was a traditional sense of stewardship. "It is enough for us," as one physician-philanthropist put it, "to be assured that the poor are always with us, and that they are exposed to disease."

> Benevolence [he continued] is not that passive feeling which can be satisfied with doing no injury to our neighbor, or rest contented with mere good wishes for his well-being when he needs our assistance.

The poor, as a prominent New York clergyman explained the need for supporting the dispensary's work, "have feelings as well as we; they are bone of our bone and flesh of our flesh; men of like passions with ourselves."[15] Such sentiments remained deeply felt and were explicitly articulated throughout the first half of the century.

Other, more mundane, motives always coexisted with such humanitarian appeals. One was the familiar mercantilist contention that maintaining the health of the poor would not only save the tax dollars implied by the almshouse or hospital care of chronically ill workers, but would aid the economy more generally by helping maintain the labor force at optimum efficiency. (These appeals assumed, of course, the ability of the dispensary physicians to diagnose ills at a stage when they might still respond to available treatment.) A related argument urged the dispensaries' function as first-line of defense against epidemic disease; though such ills ordinarily began and reached epidemic proportions among the poor, once established they might attack even the comfortable and well-to-do. No household could feel immune when servants and artisans moved easily from the world of their betters to that of tenement-dwelling friends and families.[16] These arguments soon hardened into rhetorical formulae and were ritually intoned throughout the first two-thirds of the century. Thus, for example, a mid-century dispensary spokesman could, in appealing for support, argue that:[17]

> The political economist will find here cheapness and utility combined. The statesman will discover the greatest good of the greatest number combined promoted. The city official will find his sanitary police materially assisted. The heads of families will soon find how much the lives and health of their household are cared for and secured. The tax-payer will see his burdens diminished. The benevolent will have opened to his view in the Dispensary and its kindred and associated charities the widest field for the exercise of good will towards man; and the Christian will find a new proof of the truth that they do not love God less who love mankind more.

Finally, and matter-of-factly, their advocates always contended that dispensaries would serve as much-needed schools of clinical medicine.

But to catalogue the arguments of managers and fund-raisers is not precisely to explain the logic of their commitment. Why did the dispensaries grow so rapidly? Obviously because they worked, worked that is in terms of particular social realities and expectations. At least four such factors help explain the evolution of the dispensary in 19th-century America. First, they were entirely functional in terms of the internal organization of the medical profession. Second, they were entirely consistent with available therapeutic modalities. Third, they were effectively scaled to the needs of a small and comparatively homogeneous community; once established they became indispensable as urban growth dramatically increased their client constituency. Fourth, the dispensaries made sense in terms of their founders' expectations of the roles to be played both by government and private citizens.

Most fundamental was the relationship between the dispensary and the world of medical education and status. Without the initiative and voluntary support of the medical profession dispensaries would not have been created nor could they have survived. Physicians formed the core-group in the formation of almost every American dispensary from the end of the 18th to the beginning of the 20th centuries.[18]

In the first third of the 19th century, when formal clinical training could not be said to exist outside that presumed in the preceptorial relationship, the dispensary helped fill an important pedagogical void. Not only could visiting and attending physicians themselves accumulate experience and reputation while more firmly establishing their private practice — but they could use their dispensary appointment as a means of providing case materials for their apprentices. Thus Benjamin Rush could recommend Drs. Wistar and Griffits as preceptors since both held dispensary positions, "where a young man will see more pratice in a month than with most private physicians in a year." Almost from the first years of the dispensaries, indeed, critics often charged that students and apprentices were allowed to treat the poor. (In Philadelphia, for example, such complaints found their way into newspapers as early as 1791.)[19] In the second quarter of the 19th century, as the preceptorial system grew less significant, the role of the dispensaries in clinical training grew even more prominent; mid-century medical schools vied actively in establishing dispensaries for the benefit of their students.

Most significantly, dispensary physicianships served as a step in the career pattern of elite physicians. Despite the complaints of articulate mid-century critics as to the wretched state of medical education and practice, even a cursory analysis of the profession's structure indicates the existence of a well-defined elite, largely urban, often European-trained, and almost always enjoying the benefits of hospital and dispensary experience. It was just such ambitious young practitioners who served as dispensary visiting and attending physicians while they accumulated experience and gradually made the contacts so important to later success — contacts it should be emphasized, with older established physicians at least as much as with prospective patients.[20] (Prestigious and largely honorary consulting physicianships were normally reserved, in dispensaries as in hospitals, for a community's most influential and respected physicians.) Contemporaries never questioned the dispensary's teaching function. The trustees of the New York Dispensary admitted, for example, in 1854 that their institution served as "a practical school for physicians," but they contended, it was a perfectly defensible policy: "for, by this system, these Physicians must become accomplished practitioners, by the time the growth of their private practice shall oblige them to resign their posts at the Dispensary." With the growing importance of specialization as prerequisite to intellectual status and economic success after mid-century, the increasingly specialized dispensaries served as *de facto* residency programs, allowing ambitious — and often well-connected — young men to accumulate experience and reputation. Though formal statements by medical spokesmen uniformly disowned "exclusive" specialism until long after the Civil War, devotion to a pragmatic specialism was established much earlier in America's cities. In 1839, for example, the editor of the *Boston Medical & Surgical Journal* remarked, in commenting on the specialty organization of New York's Northern Dispensary, that "such is manifestly the tendency in our times, in the great cities, and it is the only way of becoming eminently qualified for rendering the best professional services — to learn to do one thing as well as it can be done."[21]

If the dispensary made excellent sense in terms of the institutional needs of American medicine, it was equally consistent with the technological means available — both at the end of the 18th century, and through the first half of the 19th. Beyond the stethoscope — not routinely applied before mid-century — no special aids to diagnosis were available to any physician, no therapeutics beyond bleeding, cupping, and administration of drugs. Surgery was ordinarily limited, for rich and poor alike, to the treatment of lacerations and fractures, the reduction of occasional dislocations, the lancing of boils and abscesses. Dispensaries seemed, for many decades into the 19th century, fully able to provide both adequate care for the poor and adequate training for their attendants.

The dispensaries seemed equally appropriate to the needs of a small and relatively homogeneous community. The world of the late 18th century assumed — even if it did not necessarily practice — face-to-face interaction between members of different social classes, interactions structured by customary relations of deference and stewardship. This social world-view is concretely illustrated in the acceptance by the dispensaries' founding generation of the contributor recommendation as basis for patient referrals. A certificate of recommendation was necessary, that is, before the dispensary would undertake treatment of a particular patient. This followed English hospital and dispensary practice. As the century progressed, however, the dispensaries which maintained the practice sometimes found it a cause of conflict between medical staff and lay managers. By-laws specified the privileges of recommendation accompanying each contributing membership; a typical arrangement was that which in exchange for a five dollar annual subscription offered the right to recommend two patients at any one time during the year. A 50 dollar subscription typically brought the same privilege for life. Similarly, early dispensary by-laws indicate that members of the boards of managers were expected to play an active and often personal role; the New York Dispensary, for example, created a trustees' committee to accompany visiting physicians on their rounds once a month.[22]

Equally revelatory of the world-view shared by the pious and benevolent Americans who founded the dispensaries was their assumption that a crucial difference separated the dispensary from the hospital patient; the dispensary patients would be drawn from among the worthy poor, hardworking and able to support themselves, except in periods of sickness or general unemployment. Such worthy poor might also include widows, orphans, and the handicapped. The lying-in department of Philadelphia's Northern Dispensary declared in 1835, for example, that it could aid only married women of respectable character, "such as require no aid when in health." Financial support for the dispensary would, the argument followed, keep such honest folk from alms-house residence and morally contaminating contact with those abandoned souls who were its natural inmates. Dispensary spokesmen tirelessly repeated these stylized categories by way of argument even as experience indicated that this neat and comforting ideological distinction failed to reflect reality. In 1830, a physician of the Boston Dispensary could complain indignantly that persons of the "most depraved and abandoned character frequently apply who think they have a right of choice between the Alms-House and the Dispensary." As late as 1869, the Philadelphia Dispensary could still explain that:[23]

> The principal object of this institution is to afford medical relief to the worthy (not the lowest class of) poor, in those cases where removal to a hospital would for any approved reason be ineligible. . . . In a thrifty population like our own, it is the exception . . . where removal to a hospital should be considered eligible.

The dispensaries were founded and grew, finally, because they were entirely consistent with the assumptions of most Americans in regard to the responsibilities of government and appropriate forms and functions of the public institutions which embodied such responsibilities. The prostitute, the drunkard, the lunatic and cripple were the city's responsibility—social subject matter for the alms-house or city physician. The dispensary, on the other hand, represented an appropriate response of humane and thoughtful Americans to the needs of hard-working fellow citizens, a response demanded both by Christian benevolence and community-oriented prudence; it was a form of social intervention limited, conservative and spiritually rewarding. In the second third of the 19th century, as demographic realities shifted inexorably, this traditional view still served to justify the now-expanded work of the dispensaries—

and at the same time to avoid systematic analysis of the changing nature and social condition of the constituency they served. It was only very slowly, and only in the minds of a minority of those associated with dispensary work, that it became clear that many of their city's honest and industrious laboring men were unable to pay for medical care even in times of prosperity.

The dispensary continued to change throughout the second half of the 19th century. We have already referred to their increase in numbers and degree of specialization. Equally significant was expansion of the dispensary form under new kinds of auspices. First, most urban—and even some small town—medical schools anxious to compete for students, established their own dispensaries so as to offer "clinical material" for their embryo physicians. Second, hospitals not only increased in number in the last third of the century, they also began to provide more outpatient care, in some localities duplicating services already offered by dispensaries. In Philadelphia with its flourishing medical schools the rivalry between hospitals and dispensaries emerged as early as 1845.[24] In certain areas outpatient facilities competed for patients, medical school clinics in particular advertising in newspapers and posting handbills. All these events were correlated, of course, with a growing demand within the medical profession for clinical training at every level, for the possession of attending and consulting physicanships, for the accumulation of specialty credentials. At the end of the century, finally, a growing public health movement used the by now familiar dispensary form to shape and deliver medical care and would-be prophylactic measures in slum areas—most conspicuously in the identification and treatment of tuberculosis.

Underlying these developments was a series of parallel changes, first in the scale of the human problems the dispensaries faced, second in the intellectual tools and social organization of the medical profession. First in time came an absolute increase in the numbers and shift in the social origins of those urban Americans calling upon the dispensary. Secondly, in terms of chronology if not significance, were shifts within the world of medicine which made the dispensary increasingly marginal in the priorities of medical men. One need hardly demonstrate the significance to medical practice of increasing specialization, the germ theory and antisepsis, the development of modern surgery, x-ray and clinical laboratory methods, the increasing centrality of the hospital; the way in which demographic and social changes reshaped the dispensaries is perhaps less familiar.

Whatever degree there had been in the original vision of a community bound by common ties of assumption and identity, this unifying vision corresponded less and less to reality as the 19th century progressed. The accustomed social distance between physician and charity patient seemed increasingly unbridgeable. A practical measure of this increasing social distance — and one which correlates with population and immigration statistics — was the growing disquietude of dispensary physicians in contemplating their patients. As early as 1828, New York's Northern Dispensary asked contributors to sympathize with their staff physicians'

> . . . great sacrifices of feeling and comfort, which they must necessarily make, by being forced into daily and hourly association with the miserable and degraded of our species, loathsome from disease, and often still more so by those disgusting habits which go to the utter extinction of decency in all its forms.

The traditional system in which dispensary patients or their messengers called first upon contributors seeking a recommendation and then upon visiting physicians at their regular homes or offices also showed signs of strain. In Boston, where the dispensary's lay managers had long opposed the establishment of a "central office," a major factor helping to overcome this reluctance in the 1850s was the unwillingness of district physicians to have their offices used by so "ignorant and degraded a class." "It is undesirable," as Henry J. Bigelow explained it, "for most physicians to receive at their own apartments the class of applicants who now form the mass of dispensary patients."[25]

The patients who seemed most familiar, closest to the physicians' own experience, were those most capable of evoking sympathy and understanding; thus the plight of those fallen in fortune, of the genteel widow, of the orphaned child of good parents were those which touched visiting physicians most deeply.

It is not infrequently that we witness much feeling manifested by those who have been able to employ their own physicians and purchase their own medicines, when through reverses of fortune they have for the first time applied for assistance from the Institution; such constitute the most interesting portion of our patients.

Other patients were far less interesting.[26]

There were, of course, the venereal and alcoholic; but these had always existed and their existence had always implied a certain conflict between morals and medical care. Far more unsettling by the 1840s were the new immigrants who streamed into America's cities and soon constituted a disproportionate part of the dispensary's clientele. By the early 1850s it was not uncommon for an absolute majority of a particular institution's patients to have been born in Ireland; in the districts of individual visiting physicians over 90 percent of those treated might be foreign born. Not surprisingly, the 1840s and 1850s saw dispensary administrators and trustees pointing again and again to the immigrant as they sought to explain the difficulties of their work and their ever increasing financial need.[27]

It was not only the numbers and the poverty, but the alienness of the immigrants which intensified the differences between them and their would-be medical attendants. It must be recalled that the desirability of dispensary appointments guaranteed their being filled by young physicians of at least middle class background — thus insuring as well a maximum social distance between physician and patient. As early as 1831, for example, Boston Dispensary visiting physicians, dismayed by the conditions they encountered, elected to survey the economic and moral status of their patients. In that age of temperance and pietism, it was only to have been expected that the district physicians found intemperance to be the most important single cause of disease in their patients — and intemperance to be most common among the foreign born. The Irish seemed particularly undesirable, filthy, drunken, generally inhospitable to middle-class standards of behavior. "Upon their habits — their mode of life," a dispensary physician explained in 1850, "depend the frequency and violence of disease. This I am fearful will continue to be the case, since no form of legislation can reach them, or force them to change their habits for those more conducive to cleanliness and health." "Deserving American poor," another Boston Dispensary physician complained, were "often deterred from seeking aid because they shrink from seeming to place themselves on a level with the degraded classes among the Irish."[28] The unfamiliar attitudes and habits of these patients often added to their troublesomeness; they ignored hygienic advice and often defied the physician's simplest requests. The Irish, for example, considered it dangerous to have lymph removed from the lesion of an individual vaccinated for smallpox; thus they refused to return to the dispensary after the required week to have the lesion checked (and to supply the lymph so useful in helping balance the dispensary's budget).[29] Later immigrant groups brought their peculiar beliefs and problems of communication; Jews and Italians replaced the Irish as objects of the dispensary physician's frustration and disdain.

A good many dispensary physicians were, of course, sympathetic to their patients, and in some cases not only sympathetic but convinced that environmental causes contributed to their clients' chronic ill-health. Yet even those individual physicians whose personal convictions made them most sensitive to the deprivation of their city's slum-dwellers, shared the ambivalence and even hostility of their peers. The same mid-century physicians, that is, who denounced basement dwellings, exploitative landlords, rotting meat and adulterated milk — shared a distaste for the intemperance, imprudence, filth, and apparent sexual immorality of those victimized by such conditions. One of the harsher dispensary critics of mid-century tenement conditions could, for example, contend that:

> . . . there is much squalor and other evidences of poverty which might be remedied had the patients more pride in cleanliness and more ambition to be doing well in the world.

As another mid-century physician explained, his patients' degradation and ignorance called "not for pity alone, but for the greatest exercise of patience and forbearance."[30]

A concern with social realities was, moreover, supported by and consistent with mid-19th-century etiological assumptions. Both acute and constitutional ills were seen as related closely to an individual's powers of resistance — itself a product of interaction between constitution and environment.

And the conditions encountered by dispensary physicians were exactly those which seemed to lower resistance and hence increase the incidence and virulence of disease. Thus a dispensary physician could note casually that scarlet fever was particularly virulent one year, since it proved as fatal to the rich as to the poor. Similarly, a pioneer ophthalmologist could urge the need for ophthalmological dispensaries because of the relationship between poverty and diseases of the eye:

> The sickly hue, and the toil worn features of these poor people are but the results of constitutional derangements . . . and as clearly reveal the inseparable union between the health of the body and the health of the eye, as between poverty and disease.

Throughout the century articulate dispensary spokesmen were aware of the need to provide food and clothing for their patients, convinced that medicines could be of only marginal help when patients had to return to work before their complete recovery, while their homes had no adequate heat, their tables only impure and decaying food. "No persons can more readily appreciate than we," as one put it, "the utter uselessness of drugs, if there is no possibility of nourishing and warming the patient."[31]

The attitudes of mid and late 19th-century physicians can best be described in terms not of hostility, but of ambivalence — and perhaps most importantly an ambivalence characterized by a world-view which related disease and morals alike to general social conditions. Both morality and morbidity were seen as resultants of the interactions between environmental circumstance and culpable moral decisions. This mixture of social concern, moralism, meliorism and deep seated antipathy was clearly apparent by mid-century and marked the writings of most dispensary spokesmen until the end of the century; it could not prove the basis of a long-lived commitment to the dispensary and the necessity of its peculiar social function.

Nevertheless, a handful of articulate spokesmen for the dispensary did elaborate a characteristic point of view by the century's end, in which disease was seen not only as related inextricably to environment, but which emphasized the dispensary's capacity to reach out into the homes of the sick poor, so as to deal with problems more fundamental than the symptoms which brought the patient to their attention. The ability of the dispensary to relate to the community surrounding it became in the arguments of such dispensary defenders an indispensable aspect of a socially adequate medical care system. Visiting physicians and nurses could simply not be replaced by a hospital outpatient department. Advocates of this higher dispensary calling argued again and again that one could not simply treat a patient's symptoms and do nothing about an environment which had much to do with causing those very symptoms. Such ideas were implemented perhaps most fully in the tuberculosis dispensaries created so widely in the first decade of the 20th century.[32]

Such would-be rationalizers of American medicine as Edward Corwin, S. S. Goldwater, Richard Cabot, and Michael Davis contended that the dispensary could, in addition to supplying primary treatment for the indigent, supplement the necessarily unfinished work of the general practitioner in those numerous cases where the patient could not afford a specialist's consultation or expensive x-rays and laboratory tests. The dispensary could, that is, serve a vast urban constituency able perhaps to afford the services of a general practitioner but unable to manage the cost of more extended or elaborate medical care. And such occasions increased steadily as the profession's ability to understand and even cure increased. Yet even as they urged such prudent considerations, these advocates of social medicine were well aware of the threat posed to the independence and ultimately to the existence of the dispensary by rapid changes in medical ideas, techniques, and institutional forms.

These arguments were consistent as well with the motivations and social assumptions of the contemporary settlement-house movement and other pioneer social welfare advocates. The settlement houses were often involved in dispensary-like programs themselves. But in a precisely timed irony, the dispensary as a viable independent institution was dying just as its most self-conscious advocates were formulating these brave contentions.

How did this come about? The dispensaries could hardly be said to have lost their social function; we have become quite conscious in recent years that their function is still not being adequately

fulfilled. In retrospect, however, their dissolution was inevitable. By the 1920s, most significantly, the dispensary had become as marginal to the needs of the medical profession as it had been central in the first two-thirds of the 19th century. A century of work in the city's slums, a growing—if always somewhat ambiguous—awareness of the relationship between health and environment, the conscious commitment of a small leadership group to the need for working in that human environment—all proved ultimately of little importance.

As hospital-centered interne and residency programs became a normal part of medical education—following inclusion of clinical training in the undergraduate years—it was inevitable that those elite physicians who would in earlier generations have been anxious to receive a dispensary appointment would now prefer hospital posts. Not only had hospitals increased greatly in number, but they contained beds, laboratory and x-ray facilities, and a cluster of appropriately trained specialists. The hospital's increasingly exclusive claims to practice the best, indeed the only adequate medicine seemed to grow more and more plausible. When, for example, in 1922 the Managers of the Philadelphia Dispensary decided to merge with the Pennsylvania Hospital, they explained that they had "found it practically impossible for an independent dispensary, unassociated with the facilities and specialists of a large modern hospital, to render the public adequate service."[33]

As the intellectual and institutional aspects of medicine changed, economic pressures also pointed toward the centralized and capital-intensive logic of the hospital. Expensive laboratory facilities, x-rays, modern operating rooms all demanded the investment of unprecedently large sums of money. The routine low-budget dosing which characterized the independent 19th-century dispensary seemed no longer a real option; dispensary boards had to face a growing and embarrassing asymmetry between their limited resources and the demands of high quality medical care. The hospital outpatient department seemed to many medical men a substantial and inevitable improvement over its predecessor institution. The growing tendency in the 20th century for medical schools to forge strong hospital ties only increased the centrality of the hospital.

Shorn of its relevance to the career needs of aspiring physicians, the dispensary was left with the clearly residual function of providing public health — charity — medical care, in itself a low-status occupation throughout the 19th century. Dispensary appointments had brought prestige and clinical opportunities in generations during which there were few other badges of status or roads to the acquisition of clinical skills; by the end of the century, there were other, more prestigious options for the ambitious young physician. Positions as municipal "out-door physicians" had a comparatively low status throughout the 19th century. The dominion of fee for service medicine remained essentially unchallenged by the liberal critics of the Progressive generation. Those ambitious young men incapable of remaining content with the mere accumulation of fees were — as the 20th century advanced — ordinarily attracted not by social medicine but increasingly by the "higher" and certainly less ambiguous demands of research; and even clinical investigation seemed in its most demanding forms to have little place in the dispensary.

If the dispensary had lost much of its appeal for the medical elite by the end of the 19th century, it had lost whatever goodwill it had had in the mind of the average practitioner decades earlier. There had always been occasional complaints in regard to the dispensaries intervening unfairly to compete with private physicians for a limited supply of paying patients. From the earliest years of their operation, American dispensaries had warned that their services were only for "such as are really necessitous." None however chose to investigate systematically the means of their patients until after the Civil War. Until the 1870s, criticism was comparatively muted; throughout the last third of the century, however, and into the 20th, the dispensaries were widely attacked as purveyors of ill-considered charity to the unworthy. The more constructive critics sought to find alternatives, the most popular — in addition to simply demanding a small fee — being the provident dispensary, a species of prepaid health plan which had proven workable in some areas in England. In city after city, local practitioners called meetings and commissioned reports predictably concluding that a goodly portion of those using dispensary services were quite capable of paying a private physician's fees.[34] Americans found it difficult to understand the social configuration of the society in which they lived; only abuse

by those in fact capable of paying medical bills could possibly explain the vast numbers who utilized dispensary services. To doubt this was to assume that large numbers of worthy and hard-working Americans were indeed too poor to pay for even minimally adequate medical care.[35]

Physicians were often unwilling to refer their paying patients — even if the payment were only 25 or 50 cents — to the more specialized facilities of neighboring dispensaries. As late as 1914 the director of Pennsylvania's tuberculosis program charged that local practitioners refused to refer patients in the early stages of the disease, unwilling to relinquish treatment until such working-people were too deteriorated to work — and pay. Attacks on the dispensary system were generally supported as well by the charity organization movement which, in city after city, attacked dispensary medicine as an excellent example of that undiscriminating alms-giving which served only to demoralize its recipients. (It should be noted that the majority of empirical studies of dispensary patients completed between the 1870s and World War I indicated that most dispensary patients were not in fact able to pay for medical care.)[36]

By the last quarter of the 19th century the dispensary patient no longer fit into that same vision of an ordered social universe which had guided and inspired the efforts of those benevolent Americans who had founded the first dispensaries a century earlier. Those older views of community and stewardship implied in the contributor-sponsorship system had faded by mid-century, paralleling changes in the environmental reality of America's cities. Similarly, it would have been hardly plausible to argue that New York or Boston tenement-dwellers should be visited in their homes so as to spare them the indignity of hospitalization. The constituency of both hospital and dispensary had changed. By the closing years of the 19th century, the dispensary had very clearly become the provider of charity medicine for a class who — if indeed worthy of such charity — were sharply differentiated from paying patients and who ordinarily lived in a section of the city removed physically from that of contributors, physicians, and private patients. Before mid-century and especially in the first quarter of the 19th century, dispensary managers still sought to enforce requirements that visiting physicians actually reside in the district they served—a natural enough sentiment in the 18th century but impracticable in post-bellum America.[37] The arguments employed by the end of the century to attract contributions had become almost exclusively prudential, appealing little either to explicitly religious convictions or to a feeling of identity with those at risk. Fund-raising circulars emphasized instead the need to avert crime, pauperism and prostitution.

Positive support for the dispensaries was, on the other hand, shaky indeed; aside from the support implicit in the inertia developed by all institutions, only a small group of socially active physicians and proto-social-welfare activists defended the dispensaries as a positive good. Many social workers, as we have indicated, evinced little affection for an institution which seemed to embody so casual and unscientific an approach to philanthropy. Even the oldest dispensaries did not survive as independent institutions past the early 1920s.

Historians have devoted little attention to the dispensary. Yet as our contemporaries begin to concern themselves with the delivery of medical care this neglect may end; for the dispensary provides such would-be reformers with a potentially usable past. The dispensary did at first provide a flexible, informal, and locally oriented framework for the delivery of public medicine. But the analogy to contemporary problems is limited; the flexibility and informality of the dispensary were a result of medicine's still primitive tools, its local orientation a consequence of the contributors being in some sense—or assuming themselves to be—part of the community served by the dispensary. Such conditions ceased to exist well before the end of the 19th century. And even within its own frame of reference, the 19th-century dispensary provided second-class, routine, episodic medicine, was a victim of shabby budgets, and even in its earliest decades marked by unquestioned distance between physician and patient. (A distance *perhaps* made tolerable by traditional attitudes of hierarchy and deference.)

Yet despite these imperfections, the death of the dispensary and the transfer of its functions and client constituency to general hospitals has not been an unqualified success. And though the history of the rise and fall of the dispensary provides no explicit program for contemporary medicine, it does underline a simple moral: any plan for the reordering of medical care must be based on the accommodation of at least three different factors. One is felt social need, felt, that is, by those with power to change social policy. A second factor is general social values and assumptions as they shape the world-view and thus help define the options available to such decision-makers. Third, there are the needs of the medical profession, needs expressed in the career decisions of particular physicians and needs defined by medicine's intellectual tools and institutional forms. Without a strong commitment to government intervention in health matters—a commitment impossible without an appropriate change in general social values—factors internal to the world of medicine have determined most forcefully the specific forms in which medical care has been provided for the American people. Thus the rise and fall of the dispensary; it was doomed neither by policy nor conspiracy but by a steadily shifting configuration of medical perceptions and priorities.

## NOTES

1  The most valuable study of the dispensary is still that by Michael M. Davis, Jr., and Andrew R. Warner, *Dispensaries: Their Management and Development* (New York, 1918). The most useful account of the early years of any single dispensary is [William Lawrence], *A History of the Boston Dispensary* (Boston, 1859). For an example of contemporary interest, see George Rosen, "The first neighborhood health center movement—its rise and fall," *Am. J. Pub. Hlth.*, 1971, *61*: 1620–1637. [See ch. 34 of this book.]

2  Philadelphia Dispensary, Minutebook 18, June 25, 1816, Archives of the Pennsylvania Hospital, Phila-

delphia (Hereafter A.P.H.). Cf. "Brief history of the Southern Dispensary," Southern Dispensary, *81st Annual Report* (Philadelphia, 1898), pp. 6–10.

3  Charles E. Rosenberg, "The practice of medicine in New York a century ago," *Bull. Hist. Med.*, 1967, *41*: 223–253, p. 236; F. B. Kirkbride, *The Dispensary Problem in Philadelphia: A Report made to the Hospital Association of Philadelphia, October 28, 1903* (Philadelphia, 1903). By 1900, Davis and Warner, *Dispensaries,* p. 10, estimated that there were roughly 100 dispensaries in the United States, 75 general and 25 special.

4   As late as 1899, the City of Baltimore still compensated the Baltimore Dispensary when it filled prescriptions for the indigent patients of any legal practitioner. Baltimore General Dispensary, *Character, By-Laws. &c. . . . Revised 1899* (Baltimore, 1899), p. 14.

5   New York's Eastern Dispensary reported in 1857 that the city's donation to the New York Dispensary had been set at $1000 in 1827. As other dispensaries were founded, these too received the same subvention. *23rd Annual Report, 1856* (New York, 1857), p. 19.

6   Eastern Dispensary (New York), *25th Annual Report, 1858* (New York, 1859), pp. 16–17. The panics of 1857, 1873, and 1893, as well as the Civil War years, all represented such periods of stress for the dispensaries. New York's North-Eastern Dispensary, for example, was so pressed by the Panic of 1873 that it could not even publish annual reports in 1874 and 1875. *15th Annual Report, 1876* (New York, 1877), p. 6.

7   As late as 1891, Philadelphia's Northern Dispensary bemoaned the fact that they could still not afford to stop renting their second floor, despite their establishment of five new specialty clinics and consequent need for space. Northern Dispensary, *74th Annual Report, 1891* (Philadelphia, 1892), p. 9. As early as 1803, the Philadelphia Dispensary was happy to rent its basement to a commercial tenant. Minutes, Dec. 12, 1803. The typical pattern was illustrated clearly by the New York Dispensary's decision in 1868 to build a four-story building, the basement, first, third, and fourth levels being rented, only the second used by the dispensary itself. *77th Annual Report, 1868* (New York, 1869), p. 12.

8   Eastern Dispensary (New York), *23rd Annual Report, 1856,* p. 22; S. L. Abbott to G. F. Thayer, April 6, 1844, Chronological File, Boston Dispensary Archives, New England Medical Center, Boston. (Hereinafter B.D.A.) The phrase describing the dispensary's casual dentistry is from New York Dispensary, *81st Annual Report, 1870* (New York, 1871), p. 17.

9   For a convenient summary of early vaccination work by the dispensaries, see DeMilt Dispensary (New York), *25th Annual Report, 1875* (1876), pp. 20–22. For the role of the dispensaries in the Civil War, see New York Dispensary, *72nd Annual Report, 1862* (New York, 1863), pp. 9–10; Eastern Dispensary (New York), *28th Annual Report, 1861* (New York, 1862), pp. 23–25. Though the poor were normally uninterested in vaccination, the threat of epidemics often created a sudden upsurge of interest; in one case, indeed, the New York Dispensary could refer to a "vaccination riot" on their premises. *76th Annual Report, 1865* (New York, 1865) p. 20. Many of the dispensaries were financially dependent on their sale of vaccine matter.

10  George Gould, "Abuse of a great charity," *Med. News, N.Y.,* 1890, *57*: 534–539; Medical College of the Pacific, Faculty Minutes, Jan. 29, 1878, July 22, 1881, Lane Medical Library, Stanford University. New York's Eastern Dispensary was so lacking in funds that its patients were given neither bottles nor printed instructions: "The patients universally bring a bottle or tea-cup to receive and hold the medicine." *28th Annual Report, 1861,* p. 14. There were only occasional conflicts between physicians and lay managers in regard to such cutting of corners. A revealing incident of this kind shook the Boston Dispensary in 1844 when the managers sought to compel their visiting physicians to employ scarification and bleeding instead of the far more expensive leeches. The physicians argued not only that the leeches had a different physiological effect—but that they had well-nigh banished more painful modes of bloodletting from private practice. G. T. Thayer to Visiting Physicians, Feb. 8, 1844; S. L. Abbott et al. to Thayer, April 6, 1844; S. L. Abbott et al. to President and Managers [February 1844], B.D.A.

11  For an example of such ties in a particular dispensary, see DeMilt Dispensary, *2nd Annual Report, 1852–53* (New York, 1853), p. 12; *4th Annual Report, 1855* (New York, 1856), pp. 10–11.

12  Eastern Dispensary (New York), *32nd Annual Report, 1865* (New York, 1866), p. 14.

13  New York Diet Kitchen Association, *11th Annual Report, 1883* (New York, 1884), p. 5. On nursing, see, for example, Philadelphia Dispensary, Minutes, Feb. 15, 1853, Oct. 17, 1854, A.P.H.

14  Brooklyn Dispensary, *Trustee's Report, April, 1847* (New York, 1847), p. 8; Boston Dispensary, *108th Annual Report* (Boston, 1905), pp. 10–12. For the crediting of the New York Dispensary with this particular first, see DeMilt Dispensary, *25th Annual Report, 1875,* p. 19n.

15  John G. Coffin, *An Address delivered before the Contributors of the Boston Dispensary, . . . October 21, 1813* (Boston, 1813), pp. 6, 15; John B. Romeyn, *The Good Samaritan: A Sermon, delivered in the Presbyterian Church, in Cedar-street, New York, . . . for the Benefit of the New York Dispensary* (New York, 1810), p. 16.

16  "Servants," one board of managers argued at midcentury, "who have relations and friends in the lower walks of life, and who are in the habit of visiting them, often in company with the children of their employers, would be subject to more danger than they are now exposed." DeMilt Dispensary, *3rd Annual Report, 1853–54* (New York, 1854), p. 10.

17 DeMilt Dispensary, *5th Annual Report, 1855–56* (New York, 1856), p. 11.

18 For typical examples later in the century, see Central Dispensary and Emergency Hospital of the District of Columbia, *24th Annual Report . . . Including an Historical Sketch of the Institution* (Washington, D.C., 1894), pp. 8–10; Camden City Dispensary, *26th Annual Report, 1892–93* (Camden, N.J., 1893), pp. 6–9.

19 Rush to John Dickinson, Oct. 4, 1791, *Letters of Benjamin Rush*, ed. L. H. Butterfield (Princeton, N.J., 1951), I, 610; Philadelphia *Dunlap's American Daily Advertiser*, Aug. 16, 18, 1791; Minutes, Philadelphia Dispensary, Aug. 26, 1791. Cf. [Lawrence], *History of Boston Dispensary*, pp. 90–91, 98–99. Another dispensary noted at the mid-century that they had "often been accused, as being rather the schools, where the young and inexperienced might find patients to their hands, than benevolent institutions where sufferings might be allayed and diseases cured." DeMilt Dispensary, *2nd Annual Report, 1852–53*, p. 8.

20 Surviving archives of the Boston Dispensary, for example, indicate in letters of recommendation for district physicians the pattern we have suggested: The Bigelows, James Jackson, and Oliver Wendell Holmes recommend and are recommended. Successful candidates had frequently studied in Europe and the Tremont Medical School or served as house physicians at the Massachusetts General Hospital. Cf. James Jackson to Board of Managers, Aug. 3, 1831; O. W. Holmes to William Gray, Sept. 3, 1845, or see letters in 1836 file from John Collins Warren, Jacob Bigelow, and George Hayward recommending O. W. Holmes as a visiting physician. B.D.A.

21 New York Dispensary, *Annual Report, 1854* (New York, 1855), p. 9. A year later, the same dispensary contended that their staff members "in a few years, hope to be the eminent physicians of New York, and it is their right to expect, and of the community to require, that the unequaled advantages, to be found here, should be freely offered them." *Annual Report, 1855* (New York, 1856), p. 10. *Boston Med. & Surg. J.*, 1839, *20*: 351.

22 New York (City) Dispensary, *Charter and By-Laws . . .* (New York, 1814), p. 8. Another indication of the social assumptions of the generation which created the dispensaries was their concern over whether servants and apprentices were appropriate patients. John Bard argued in New York that servants should indeed be treated, but not at their place of work—which would have compelled "gentlemen to visit the servants of families in which they had no acquaintance with the Masters or Mis-

tresses." *A Letter from Dr. John Bard . . . to the Author of Thoughts on the Dispensary . . .* (New York, 1791), p. 20. See the entry for July 17, 1786, in the Minutes of the Philadelphia Dispensary for the question of treating apprentices.

23 Philadelphia Northern Dispensary, Philadelphia Lying-In Hospital, "Rules and Regulations, Adopted November 4, 1835," Historical Collections, College of Physicians of Philadelphia; [?] to Board of Managers, Oct. 1, 1830, B.D.A.; *Rules of the Philadelphia Dispensary with the Annual Report for 1869* (Philadelphia, 1870), p. 10. As late as 1879, the organizers of a specialized New York dispensary contended that they appealed to those patients able to pay a small fee and thus "saved the necessary associations of a public, free dispensary." *Report of the East Side Infirmary for Fistula and other Diseases of the Rectum* (New York, 1879), p. 5. Cf. Pittsburgh Free Dispensary, *3rd Annual Report, 1875* (Pittsburgh, 1876), p. 9.

24 Philadelphia Dispensary, Minutes, Dec. 26, 1845, A.P.H.

25 Northern Dispensary (New York), *1st Annual Report, 1828* (New York, 1828), cont. p. 10; DeMilt Dispensary, *2nd Annual Report, 1853*, p. 12; Bigelow to D. D. Slade, Aug. 22, 1855, B.D.A. Cf. D. D. Slade to My Dear Sir [William Lawrence], Sept. 3, 1855, B.D.A.; [Lawrence,] *History of the Boston Dispensary*, pp. 178–180.

26 Northern Dispensary (Philadelphia), *Annual Report, 1847* (Philadelphia, 1848), p. 10. Such sentiments were familiar ones. A "Contributor" to the Boston Dispensary explained in 1819 that its appropriate clients were those "many persons . . . who have been reduced from a state of competence to one little short of poverty, who while blessed with health, can, by industry, support themselves, but when attacked by sickness, and laid upon a bed of illness, find it impossible to pay the physician and apothecary." *New-England Palladium and Commercial Advertiser*, Jan. 12, 1819. The earliest rules of both Philadelphia and Boston dispensaries emphasized their wish to comfort "those who have seen better days . . . without being humiliated." Boston Dispensary, *Institution of . . . 1817* (Boston, 1817), p. 7.

27 In the New York Dispensary, for example, in 1853, of 7,188 patients treated, 1,582 were born in the United States and 4,886 in Ireland. At the Philadelphia Dispensary in 1857, 1,906 were born in the United States, 3,649 in Ireland. New York Dispensary, *64th Annual Report, 1853* (New York, 1854), p. 12; Philadelphia Dispensary, *Rules . . . with Annual Report for 1857* (Philadelphia, 1858), p. 14. Some dispensaries would not allow venereal cases to be treated, some imposed a special fee, while still others

allowed individual physicians to decide whether they would treat such errant souls.

28 Luther Parks, Jr., to Board of Managers, June 10, 1850, B.D.A. Referring to the Irish, another dispensary physician explained: "Upon their habits, —and mode of life, depend the frequency and violence of disease. This I am fearful will continue to be the case, since no form of legislation can reach them, or force them to change their habits for those more conducive to cleanliness and health." Charles W. Moore to Board of Managers, April 1, 1857, B.D.A. On the temperance question, see, for example, J. B. S. Jackson to Board of Managers, Oct. 8, 1853, B.D.A.

29 New York Dispensary, *64th Annual Report, 1853,* p. 10; New York Dispensary, *72nd Annual Report, 1862,* p. 20. When, in an effort to solve this problem New York's dispensaries initiated a small deposit to be refunded when the patient returned to have the vaccination checked, these intractable—and seemingly ungrateful—patients chose to regard it as a payment absolving them of any responsibility to the institution.

30 J. Trenor, Jr., physician to middle district, Eastern Dispensary (New York), *25th Annual Report, 1858,* p. 32; New York Dispensary, *Annual Report, 1837* (New York, 1838), p. 7.

31 Edward Reynolds, *An Address at the Dedication of the New Building of the Massachusetts Eye and Ear Infirmary, July 3, 1850* (Boston, 1850), p. 15; Mission Hospital and Dispensary for Women and Children, *2nd Annual Report, 1876* (Philadelphia, 1877), p. 10. The scarlet fever reference was by William Bibbins, DeMilt Dispensary, *6th Annual Report, 1856–57* (New York, 1857), p. 17.

32 For useful descriptions of the tuberculosis clinics, see, for example, F. Elisabeth Crowell, *The Work of New York's Tuberculosis Clinics . . .* (New York, 1910); Louis Hamman, "A brief report of the first two years' work in the Phipps Dispensary for tuberculosis of the Johns Hopkins Hospital," *Johns Hopkins Hosp. Bull.,* 1907, *18*: 293–297. For samples of the more positive defense of the dispensary and its appropriate role, see: S. S. Goldwater, "Dispensary ideals: with a plan for dispensary reform . . . ," *Am. J. Med. Sci.,* 1907, n.s. *134*: 313–335; Richard Cabot, "Why should hospitals neglect the care of chronic curable disease in out-patients?" *St. Paul Med. J.,*

1908, *10*: 110–120; Cabot, "Out-patient work: The most important and most neglected part of medical service," *J.A.M.A.,* 1912, *59*: 1688–1689; Good Samaritan Dispensary (New York), *29th Annual Report, 1919* (New York, 1920), p. 8. The most complete statement of a positive dispensary program is to be found in Davis and Warner, *Dispensaries.*

33 Philadelphia Dispensary, Minutes, Jan. 8, 1923, A.P.H. At the end of the 19th century, for example, the Boston Dispensary began a search for beds; it seemed a necessity if bright young men were to be kept on the staff. *Report of the Dinner Given to the Board of Managers of the Boston Dispensary by the Staff of Physicians . . . January 25th, 1909* [Boston, 1909], p. 13. Once allied with a hospital, the dispensary had invariably a lower status. Francis R. Packard charged in 1903 that hospitals would casually spend two or three hundred dollars for new surgical instruments yet balk at ten or fifteen for the dispensary. F. B. Kirkbride, *Dispensary Problem in Philadelphia,* p. 21.

34 Probably most significant is the tone of this debate. It was the ordinary practitioner who generally resented the way in which dispensaries with their elite house staffs attracted cases which might otherwise have remained in the hands of private practitioners. Discussions of "dispensary abuse" also served to express the resentment of many practitioners against the monopolization of hospital and dispensary posts by a minority of well-connected physicians. In its report on charity abuse, for example, the Medical Association of the District of Columbia also urged limited tenure in hospital staff appointments and access to hospital privileges for all "reputable members of the profession." *Report of the Special Committee . . . on the Hospital and Dispensary Abuse in the City of Washington* (Washington, D.C., 1896), pp. 15–16.

35 [William Lawrence], *Medical Relief to the Poor, September, 1877* (Boston, 1877), pp. 3–4; James Keiser, "The abuses in hospital and dispensary practice in Reading," *National Hospital Record,* 1899.

36 Albert P. Francine, "The state tuberculosis dispensaries," *Penn. Med. J.,* 1914, *17*: 940. See Davis and Warner, *Dispensaries,* pp. 42–58, for a brief discussion of patient eligibility.

37 G. F. Thayer to William Gray, April 12, 1838, B.D.A.

# 20

## Patrons, Practitioners, and Patients:
## The Voluntary Hospital in Mid-Victorian Boston

### MORRIS J. VOGEL

The hospital of the immediate post-Civil War period differed little in some respects from its colonial and early 19th-century predecessor. It treated the same socially marginal constituency that American hospitals had always served. Its patients were the poor and those without roots in the community; dependence as much as disease still distinguished them from the public at large. Yet in some other respects the hospital of this era displayed concerns that were typically Victorian—concerns that shaped the transition of the institution into the hospital as we know it.

The general hospital of the 1870s was likely to be a charity, linking the voluntary efforts of doctors and donors in providing free medical care for those without any suitable alternative. For a hospital to exist, doctors had to be willing to provide gratuitous medical service for the sick poor while feeling sufficiently remunerated that they eagerly sought hospital positions. Donors had to be willing to support an institution that they themselves were never likely to use.

Traditionally, Boston's physicians had provided free care for the sick poor who had sought them out. Self-consciously advancing their claim to be professionals rather than businessmen, medical practitioners recognized a responsibility not to refuse advice or treatment to those who could not pay.[1] But in the hospitals and dispensaries organized up to the very end of the 19th century, many

physicians went well beyond their professional obligations and actively made themselves available to patients who could not, and in most instances were forbidden to, pay any fee. Not only did doctors seek duties in such institutions, but often actually founded them, as in the case of inexpensively operated dispensaries, providing only outpatient care. In the case of hospitals, doctors shared leading roles in organizing them with those who provided financial backing.[2]

Hospital and dispensary staff members were part of the city's medical and social elite. They were close in social origins to the donors who supported Boston's voluntary Protestant hospitals, if not directly related to them.[3] This background was part of the reason for their hospital work. The gratuitous treatment they rendered hospital patients was in the same tradition of stewardship as the charitable donations that supported voluntary hospitals.

But free medical treatment was much more than a charitable obligation. As a further consequence of social position, hospital practitioners had professional qualifications and interests that set them apart from their less fortunate medical brethren. In a period when locally available medical training was not advanced, men who later became associated with the city's hospitals were more likely than others to have enjoyed a European medical education after initial training in Boston. Once established in Boston, these upper-class doctors were more likely to assume positions in medical school faculties. And, though conservatives of their own class and background sometimes opposed specialization and even certain imported innovations, young physicians returning from Europe in the second half of the 19th century embraced specialization and the increasing scientific content of

MORRIS J. VOGEL is Professor of History at Temple University, Philadelphia, Pennsylvania.

Reprinted with permission from *Victorian America*, ed. Daniel Walker Howe (Philadelphia: University of Pennsylvania Press, 1976), pp. 121–138. Copyright, 1976, *American Quarterly*, c/o Trustees of the University of Pennsylvania.

medicine more readily than Boston doctors less privileged by birth and social standing.[4]

Hospital positions furnished these upper-class doctors with the clinics that were becoming increasingly necessary for medical school teaching. Teaching brought financial benefits, as former students referred difficult cases to former professors for paying consultations. A hospital position also enabled a medical man to see and treat numbers of special cases, comparatively rare in private practice, and so develop a reputation that would itself be remunerative. Thus, though hospital patients did not pay fees to hospital practitioners, these men received what contemporaries referred to as "certain well-understood advantages."[5]

Hospital physicians earned their livelihoods in the care of well-to-do private patients who paid for the knowledge gained in hospital work. Private practice remained the norm. And because the 19th-century hospital was not the center of the doctor's work world, the few hours he put in there each day during his term of perhaps three months each year did not represent income lost.

Economic motives led nonelite doctors to complain about the abuse of charity they perceived in the medical care offered without fee in hospitals. They saw their natural clientele—the poor and working classes—drained off to the hospitals.[6] When the nature of the hospital patient population changed in the 1890s and in the first decade of the 20th century, complaints about abuse came from a new quarter—from doctors who treated the well-to-do patients beginning to enter hospitals at the turn of the century.[7] These complaints were a significant force in leading the hospital away from its purely charitable organization. But until late in the 19th century, Boston's hospitals, whether municipally or voluntarily supported, were charities.

In part, the wealthy supported these institutions because of their connections with the physicians who staffed them. Amos Lawrence, the mercantile prince, underwrote the entire cost of a children's hospital under the charge of his son, Dr. William R. Lawrence.[8] The staffing of South Boston's Roman Catholic Carney Hospital by Back Bay physicians brought in financial contributions from their friends and families.[9]

In part, too, the wealthy supported these institutions because enlightened selfishness led them to share certain of the physicians' goals. The knowledge and experience doctors gained in treating the poor "raised the standard of medical attainments"; hospital and dispensary practice thus "proved a blessing to rich and poor alike."[10] The Children's Hospital appealed "to all those who have children of their own," reminding them that they had a "double interest" in the institution; "not only on account of the great benefit it will confer on its little inmates, but also because of the advantages it offers for the study of special diseases by which their own offspring may be afflicted."[11] The *Boston Evening Transcript* warned the fortunate that their own well-being depended on the continued well-being of hospitals:

> The aids which society distributes to the hospitals are amply restored by the hospitals to society. . . . Mainly in these institutions the experience and insight, the methods of observation and treatment, the scientific research, are evolved which become employed for the general health of the country. . . . If we could imagine the hospitals abolished, the general death rate in all private practice would be increased.[12]

However, the "double interest" remained a divided interest, for the more fortunate classes did not expect to make direct use of the general hospital in the 1870s. Home care remained the norm. Accident victims, for example, though they might be injured outside the home, were likely to be brought home and cared for there. Speaking in 1864 at the dedication of the Boston City Hospital, its president, Thomas C. Amory, Jr., acknowledged that it was unlikely that hospitalization would replace the ideal of home care. Amory gave an example of what he regarded as a futile attempt to remove the prejudice against hospital care:

> One of our former governors . . . meeting with an accident in the street from which he narrowly escaped with his life, insisted, in order to remove this prejudice, upon being carried to the [Massachusetts General] Hospital. His example may have had its effect. But we doubt if many of our own people, born in Boston, when tolerably comfortable at home, will go, when ill, among strangers to be cured.[13]

When Amory himself was run down by a streetcar in 1886, "a doctor was called and the injured gentleman was removed to his home in carriage."[14]

The pattern of care obtaining at local railroad

accidents is revealing.[15] When a commuter train crashed near Roslindale in 1887, 24 passengers were killed and 14 hospitalized. But most of the nearly 100 victims were taken to their homes.

> The fact that the accident occurred in the midst of a settled suburban district, and that nobody upon the train was more than five miles away from home, made it possible to transport the dead and injured, so far as it was practicable under the circumstances, directly to their homes, and many were so taken.[16]

The severity of their injuries did not separate those hospitalized from those brought home. Only two of the six admitted to the Boston City Hospital were listed as seriously injured, and only one of eight at the Massachusetts General. Of the cases brought to their own homes, a doctor making 55 home visits the day after the wreck reported nine patients in dangerous condition.[17]

The hospital offered patients no medical advantages not available in the home; actually hospital treatment in the 1870s added the risks of sepsis or "hospitalism." The fact that the hospital offered no special medical benefits reinforced a resistance to hospitalization that stemmed from the role of the home as the traditional setting for those undergoing illness and from a negative image of the hospital. That image derived from the actual danger of hospitalism and the traditional identification of the hospital with the pesthole and almshouse. Thus even when home care was unavailable, hospital care was sometimes shunned.

The well-to-do might make use of a hospital in what were labeled peculiar circumstances. This category included individuals away from home because they were from out of town, and old people living alone. For these potential patients, limited separate facilities existed at both the Massachusetts General and Boston City hospitals.[18]

Even the sick poor would avoid the hospital if possible. One of the stated advantages of a dispensary was that outpatient care sidestepped the "dread" which the prospect of hospitalization evoked among many of the poor.[19] The city's two diet kitchens, founded in the 1870s, supplied home meals for dispensary patients too sick or poor to secure their own food.[20] The truly unfortunate shared with that minority of the prosperous classes who used the institution the problem of an inade-

quate or nonexistent home. The Boston Lying-in Hospital received some of its cases from dispensary physicians "who suddenly found themselves called upon to attend some poor woman in quarters utterly unfit for such purposes."[21]

The hospital offered shelter and attention to the sick poor. It replaced comfortless homes "in close courts, narrow alleys, damp cellars or filthy apartments, which the sunshine never enters, nor fresh air purifies." It made up for the absence of "natural protectors" for those without families. It provided relief for "helpless people, who would suffer tenfold more from neglect and ill treatment than they now suffer from disease, were it not for the shelter and care of the hospitals."[22] Indeed the role of hospital was defined in terms of the services it offered the sick and injured victims of a catalog of social ills.

The statistics of hospital use reflected these concerns. An analysis of nativity and occupation shows that patients treated at the Massachusetts General and Boston City Hospital in the 1870s were not a cross-section of the population.

Hospital annual reports listed the occupations admitted; these occupations may be organized according to the socioeconomic classification in Stephan Thernstrom's *The Other Bostonians* and then compared with Thernstrom's observations about the occupational structure of the city.[23] Male patients at the city's two major hospitals were divided into four categories: white-collar, skilled blue-collar, semi-skilled and service, and unskilled and menial. Such an analysis shows occupations with high socioeconomic status were underrepresented among hospital patients in 1870 and 1880, while those with low status were overrepresented.

At the Massachusetts General in 1870, 16.9 percent of the classifiable male patients were in white-collar occupations, while in 1880 that figure was 18.1 percent. In the city population, 32 percent of males were white-collar in 1880. Skilled blue-collar workers accounted for 41.9 percent of Massachusetts General patients in 1870 and 19.4 percent in 1880, while they provided 36 percent of the general male population in 1880. Among patients, 14.2 percent and 11.1 percent were in semi-skilled occupations in 1870 and 1880 respectively, while the city population contained 17 percent in that category in 1880. The unskilled accounted for 26.9 percent (1870) and 51.4 percent (1880) of the patient population and 15 percent of the city population in 1880.[24]

Much the same pattern prevailed at the Boston City Hospital. The largest single occupational category among patients was laborer, consisting of 524 of 1,419 men admitted in 1870/1871 and 792 of 2,696 in 1880/1881. Patients in white-collar occupations totaled 8.2 percent of the hospital's male admissions in 1870/1871 and 10.5 percent in 1880/1881. Skilled blue-collar workers accounted for 36.3 percent of Boston City patients in 1870/1871 and 31.6 percent in 1880/1881. Workers in semi-skilled and service occupations made up 11.8 percent of City Hospital patients in 1870/1871 and 21.7 percent in 1880/1881. As at the Massachusetts General, unskilled (including laborers) and menial workers—43.5 percent and 36.1 percent—were disproportionately over-represented.[25]

Unfortunately, the listing of many women patients as simply wives or widows, and the absence of a satisfactory analysis of the female occupational structure, makes a comparison of female patients with the general female population more difficult. But the fact that nearly half the female patients admitted to both hospitals in the 1870s were identified as domestics reinforces the conclusion based on male employment patterns that hospital patients were drawn disproportionately from among the lower classes.[26]

Though the absolute and relative numbers undergoing hospitalization continued to increase in the 1870s as they had since the city's first hospital opened in 1821, the hospital's constituency remained largely the same, with the greater number of patients coming from an expanded lower class. The continued use of the institution by the stricken and helpless poor served to associate it with the almshouse and reinforced the negative image of the hospital held by society at large. Its image as a refuge for the unfortunate was further heightened by the fact that its patients were not just poor but, after the beginning of large-scale immigration at mid-century, largely foreign born. The Massachusetts General trustees had at first resisted allowing the Irish to enter the hospital as patients, claiming that "the admission of such patients creates in the minds of our citizens a prejudice against the Hospital, making them unwilling to enter it,— and thus tends directly to lower the general standing and character of its inmates." Feeling "the ex-

cess of foreigners among the patients" to be a bane, they had advised the admitting physician to use "the utmost vigilance," but found that "some such admissions must unavoidably take place." Hospital rules directed that all cases of sudden accident were to be admitted, thus bypassing the screening procedure; a very large proportion of accident cases was Irish. In time, the Massachusetts General trustees, "moved by a sense of duty and humanity," opened their wards to the foreign-born.[27]

In 1865, the hospital accepted 628 foreign as against 571 native-born patients. In 1870, the totals showed 718 foreign and 584 Americans, and in 1875 the figures were 1,042 and 799 respectively. The Irish made up the largest segment of the foreign-born population, maintaining at least a majority throughout the 1870s, with those born in the Canadian provinces second.[28] From the opening of the Boston City Hospital in 1864, a majority of its patients was foreign born. In 1865, 647 of its patients were born abroad and 459 in the United States, and in 1870/1871, 1,635 were foreign and 761 native-born. The foreign-born numbered 2,187 and native Americans 993 in 1875/1876. Throughout the period, Irish patients alone outnumbered the native-born.[29]

Just as Irish immigrants tarnished the image of the general hospital, so did the kind of women it cared for taint the image of the lying-in hospital. Maternity care would be among the last reasons causing the comfortable classes to enter hospitals. In the late 19th century women still considered childbirth a natural function, something that could, and should, be performed in the simplest and poorest home.[30] The hospital offered no specialized medical paraphernalia or contrivances, but instead threatened contagion, puerperal fever, and high maternal mortality. Generally, only the most desperate women entered hospitals to have their children. And perhaps the major cause of this desperation was illegitimacy. Small lying-ins, often no more than a few rooms in a tenement or boarding house, kept by midwives or the unscrupulous and untrained, served those seeking "to hide their shame" or having absolutely no alternative. These lying-ins, and the baby farms that sometimes accompanied them, were seen as accessories to vice and degradation, and as adjuncts to brothels. Lying-ins were the first hospitals needing licenses to operate in Massachusetts (1876), but the enforcement problems of the Boston Board of Health suggest that more lying-ins were operated without sanction of law than with it.[31]

Licensed and respectable lying-ins did exist, and did leave records, but their patients, too, were "unfortunate women." Cases included in the first volume of the maternity records of the New England Hospital for Women and Children, covering one-and-one-half years in the early 1870s, list 61 married and 57 unmarried mothers. Over 50 percent of the more than 1,300 mothers delivered in the 1870s at the Boston Lying-in were unmarried. And at St. Mary's Lying-in Hospital, only 20 of 550 patients cared for in the decade from 1874 to 1884 were married.[32] The lying-in hospitals of the period reaffirmed the notion that hospitals were institutions especially for the poor and desperate, and the illegitimacy intimately associated with them added the stigma of immorality.

The hospital was perceived as the kind of place all but the desperate would want to avoid. Yet, although it dealt primarily with the poor, its very nature — the onmipresence of death within its walls — imbued its concerns with a powerful attraction. The community at large was curious as to what went on inside it. This desire to know was heightened by the relative newness of the institution; though its history could be traced back to antiquity, hospitals began to emerge in numbers in Boston and the rest of the nation only after the Civil War. Finally, the curiosity as to what went on within hospitals derived from the fact that even the fortunate individual could not be certain that he would not someday be hospitalized.

Horror was a common response to such a prospect. Joseph Chamberlin, for many years the *Transcript's* "Listener,"[33] reacted strongly after visiting a hospitalized friend:

> If it should fall to the Listener's lot to be called upon to go in sickness to the very best of [hospitals], he would say, "Better a straw cot in an attic at home, with the clumsiest of unprofessional attendance, than the best private room in this place." . . . [T]here is something about the all-pervading presence of Sickness with a large S, this atmosphere of death, either just expected or just escaped, and all of this amiable perfunctoriness of nursing and medical attendance, that is simply horrible. The hospital . . . gives one sickness to think about morning, noon and night.[34]

A visitor might be acutely discomforted by the unnatural concentration of disease and death. But for the patient the environment was threatening:

> The doctors visit you incessantly, and, in spite of their courtesy, you feel as if you were not exactly an ailing human being, but merely a "case" that was being read as one reads a novel which is interesting enough, no doubt, but which is expected to develop a much more interesting phase, to wit, the catastrophe, at almost any moment. And then the grim disquieting presence of all these people like you in the ward around you![35]

The hospital reaffirmed the patient's mortality, but denied his humanity.

Chamberlin told the story of a patient hospitalized for an operation. After surgery, she was put to bed. She lived through a night punctuated by the "wailing and crying" of fellow patients, the death "in dreadful agony" of a neighboring patient, and the quiet but quick, and therefore ghostly, movement of attendants. It was terrifying: "Why it was like being dead and conscious of it!" The next day was quiet, but "spent in anticipating the coming of such another night, was almost as terrible." This particular hospital stay was cut short when a physician inquired "whether I had not any friend to whom I could go," found she had and "made immediate arrangements to have me taken away." Clearly, this patient and many of her contemporaries shared Chamberlin's conclusion: "What a matter for infinite sorrow it is that there should be homes in the world so dismal, so unhealthy, so ill attended, that their inmates are better off in the public wards of the hospital, when they are sick, than they are at home."[36]

Because the hospital was a strange and frightening place, the public welcomed reassurance from the informed. This might take the form of a newspaper article giving the generic history of the hospital and thus implying that it was not simply a modern aberration but an old institution that had proved its value in the past.[37] Or it might take the form of a correspondent's story of a hospital visit or a patient's description of his hospital stay.

Chamberlin's story was idiosyncratic: more common in the Boston press were counterphobic presentations that were almost uniformly formulaic. These addressed fears based on ignorance and substituted for them informed chronicles which denied the presence of death, disease, and pain in the hospital. Insanity, for example, was not mentioned in an extensive account of an insane asylum, though beautiful flowers and homelike accommodations in cottages were.[38] The smallpox hospital emerged from another narrative as a delightful place, serving wonderful food and providing comfortable beds, while smallpox itself, it was concluded, much improved the system.[39] For those hospitals which depended on the beneficence of the public to operate, reassurances that all was well within served a double function in that they encouraged contributions as well as disarmed anxieties.

Boston's City Hospital was supported as a municipal service, but the hospital tradition in Boston, as in the rest of the United States, had been set by the voluntary hospitals, with groups of private individuals undertaking the care of the sick poor as a public trust.[40] The Massachusetts General Hospital and Children's Hospital formed part of the complex of Boston's Protestant charities that owed their founding and existence, at least in part, to the religious doctrine of stewardship. Social and economic inequalities were legitimized by the notion that God meant for them to exist. But the elect, whose heavenly salvation was generally already demonstrated by their earthly riches, held their wealth only as God's trustees. With their wealth came the obligation to aid the less fortunate. The poor provided their economic betters the opportunity, the privilege actually, of spending God's wealth in a way that continually reemphasized their own chosen state.

The Children's Hospital was founded in 1869. It was intended for the poor, for "the little waifs who crowd our poorer streets." In its early years the institution stressed its spiritual role. Making their first annual report, the trustees stated that the institution would provide its patients "Christian nurture."[41] Sickness provided an opportunity for spiritual healing; the philosophy of the Children's Hospital reflected that of a local newspaper, which editorially downgraded the function of hospitals in furnishing medical treatment while commending them for giving patients the best gifts of all, "wrought through a ministry of sorrow."[42] The theological language in which all this was expressed was largely a carry-over from an earlier time; religious terminology provided a familiar and con-

venient vocabulary. Soon, society would no longer justify the hospital in traditional religious terms. One can already sense the beginning of a shift in the hospital's mission during Victorian times, from succoring the sick poor as its role in God's order, to denying that man had to accept God's diseases. Within a generation, this would give the hospital a drastically altered justification. But in the 1870s, these religious terms still symbolized real moral and social concerns.

The Children's Hospital defined its role in terms of the "moral benefit" it offered its patients. Socially, these benefits translated into a program of uplift and social control which it was hoped would help cope with the masses of threatening and increasingly alien poor crowding into the city. The trustees had expected that most of their patients would come from the poorest classes of the community. They found that many came "from the very lowest; from abodes of drunkeness, and vice in almost every form, where the most depressing and corrupting influences were acting both on the body and mind."[43] Hospitalization provided an opportunity to separate these children, at a most impressionable time in their lives, from corrupting influences that, if otherwise permitted to proceed unchecked, could perpetuate an impoverished and vicious class, permanently threatening society.

When a child entered, the hospital first decontaminated its new charge. "On their entrance they are immediately placed in a refreshing bath and clothed in the clean robes of the hospital." Uniform red flannel jackets replaced streetclothes.[44] The decontamination process went deeper; new influences were substituted for old in the hope that, in the few weeks it had, the institution could "help the child-soul to lift itself out of the mud in which it had been born, to assert its native purity in spite of unfortunate surroundings."[45]

Since treatment was not purely medical, the hospital did not restrict its practitioners to the medical profession. The entire Christian community was invited to participate in the healing process, to visit patients and encourage them "by word or counsel."[46] The hospital's first nurses were Episcopalian nuns. Their strength lay less in medical training than in the "Christian nurture" they provided patients. Sister Letitia was a model of this style of charity untainted by medical pretension. "Though enfeebled by disease of the lungs, which she knew must soon terminate her life, yet entirely forgetful of self," she continued nursing—all the while, of course, subjecting her charges to tuberculosis—until she died.[47]

The trustees wanted "to bring [their young patients] under the influence of order, purity and kindness." Among the means employed were tender nursing, books, pictures, "little works of art," and "the visits and attentions of the kind and cultivated."[48] Middle- and upper-class children outside the hospital were encouraged to undertake the painting, as wall decorations, of inspirational mottos that would "cultivate the devotional feelings" of the little sufferers inside. The fortunate who supported the hospital were encouraged to visit the children in its wards at any time of the day, to speak with them, provide role models, and in general to furnish that cultivated influence which the children of the poor had missed.[49] At the same time, parents having children in the hospital were severely restricted in the hours they could see their own children. The original parents' visiting hour allowed one relative at a time between eleven and twelve o'clock on weekdays only, raising difficulties for working fathers (or mothers) who wished to visit. Later, parent visiting was further restricted to the hour between eleven and twelve on Monday, Wednesday, and Friday only.[50] The trustees hoped that this regimen would change the children by "quickening their intellects, refining their manners, and encouraging and softening their hearts."[51]

Supporters of the institution hoped that a different child would leave the hospital than had entered it.[52] Children would leave having been "carefully taught cleanliness of habit, purity of thought and word" and with as much attention "paid to their moral training as can be found in any cultivated family," but the benefits of the hospital would not stop there:

> Think what a widespreading influence this becomes when the children return to their homes. . . . Even among the better class of poor people, the children soon notice the discomforts of careless, untidy habits, and are quick to compare such with the "so much better" at the hospital. In the joy of the child's homecoming, the parents are ready to gratify it by trying the new ways, and all unconsciously rise a little in the social scale by so doing.[53]

"In this wise," the hospital's founder wrote, the institution would "commence the education of the poorer classes."[54]

Even if the child did not go home and improve his family, he himself would be changed by the hospital in a way that would benefit society. The affluent and cultivated were told that they could not tell the difference between their own children and those within the hospital, even though the latter might be immigrant children from the North End. One visitor noted that "the faces of the children quickly lost the expression which we commonly meet in our little street Arabs, and become once more human and civilized."[55] Their hearts softened by kindness, mistrust and hostility evaporated from their faces and they no longer appeared as threatening as they had on the streets.

The hospital promised other far-reaching improvements. The health and strength gained during a hospital stay would not only aid the children, by enabling them to grow into "better men and women," but society as a whole—having escaped childhood invalidism, those healthier adults could support themselves. A promotional article mentioned the institution's success in educating its charges, even implying that it taught some how to read.[56] A hospital stay could help prepare a child for a socially desirable role in adult life.

These perceptions were colored, of course, by expectation. No doubt they express more than actually happened in the hospital in the way of having the children of the poor fulfill the fantasies of the rich. Further, these social expectations were less than the full rationale for the institution. The Children's Hospital was founded by physicians, in part for the sorts of professional reasons earlier suggested. At the same time, however, the founding physicians were responsible for much of this socially oriented promotional rhetoric. There is no reason to believe these doctors did not take their own language seriously. They were members of a social class as well as of a professional group, and shared the didactic concerns typical of Victorian culture.

The Massachusetts General Hospital, a secularly oriented Protestant hospital in the same sense as the Children's Hospital, also began with the mission of uplifting its patients. When founded, it had been intended for native American patients, and had offered to tide them over a bad time and send them on their way having meanwhile reinforced their view of a basically good society in which they could lead good lives.[57] But after the hospital had been overwhelmed by unappealing and apparently intractable and unimprovable adult immigrants, it gave up this aspect of its role. By the 1870s, its literature no longer expressed concern for the character of its patients, and the hospital continued to care for the sick poor with a diminished concern about what it was doing for its patients in a non-physical sense. The hospital kept the support of its donors for a variety of reasons, the chief (probably) being an inertia in which benefactions served as a quiet reaffirmation of stewardship. An obligation to keep the hospital going because it served the needs of medical practitioners was recognized. Finally, the fact that the McLean Asylum for the Insane was a branch of Massachusetts General and served the upper classes in a very direct way maintained their interest in the corporation. Since the asylum generally met its operating expenses from patient revenues, the contributions it generated helped support the hospital.

Yet the loss of reforming zeal brought no relaxation of discipline within Massachusetts General; if anything, it reinforced it. The "influence of order" which pervaded the Children's Hospital furthered that institution's resocialization of its young patients. Order was a concern in Massachusetts General, too, but there it was a reflection of social reality, not part of a vision of social change. Many of the hospital's patients were not bedridden, but able to move around the wards and grounds, and expected to be able to leave the institution to walk about the city or enjoy the carriage rides into the countryside furnished by the Young Men's Christian Union. The hospital treated people new to urban life (through the 1870s the percentage of its patients born in Boston never approached 10 percent) and to the demands of institutional living. To help maintain discipline, its grounds were surrounded by a high wall and an always guarded gate through which patients and visitors had to pass.[58] Patients needed signed passes to leave and reenter the hospital, and visitors were carefully screened.[59] This discipline was maintained for internal reasons; rather than reform a patient who misbehaved, the hospital expelled him.[60]

In one sense, Massachusetts General helped keep order in the general community. Like other hospitals, it functioned as a guarantor of social

stability, or as one supporter of the Children's Hospital put it, "There is a practical side to this charity, which may commend it to thoughtful men." Hospitals provided the working classes with evidence that the wealthy were aware of their responsibilities: "the only sure way to reconcile labor to capital is to show the laborer by actual deeds that the rich man regards himself as the steward of the Master."[61] Until workmen's compensation went into effect, corporations, especially railroads and street railways, underwrote free beds at the Massachusetts General to which they sent employees injured on the job. These accident-prone enterprises provided a paternalistic form of insurance, absolved themselves of responsibility to their injured employees, and attempted to defuse issues that might otherwise build up workers' grievances.[62]

Concern for social order was apparent in the community's support of hospitals in general. One observer noted that "the hospitals act as a kind of insurance system for the laboring classes. They take the risks incidental to their position the more cheerfully, because they know that if injured they are assured of a special provision for their need in our hospitals."[63] Similar reasoning was used to elicit support for the Children's Hospital. Were it not there, or were it unable to admit a suffering child, there would be no telling what even the most respectable worker, distraught over his inability to secure aid for his child, might do. "It is under such circumstances the iron enters a man's soul, and he is ready for a 'strike' or any other desperate remedy that promises better times and money with which to provide good nursing and delicacies for his suffering children." A mother, turned down when applying for admission for her sick child, might go "fiercely on her way, ripe for any evil deed. . . ." But assured that the hospital would care for their sick children, the poor would respond with gratitude rather than violence.[64]

Beside acting as a guarantor of social stability, the hospital was perceived by some as contributing to community prosperity, both through the more tractable labor force it ensured and through the fact that the health of the population was directly translatable into material wealth. In encouraging support for the city's voluntary hospitals, the *Transcript* editorially assured "those who look into the matter [that they would] see that our hospitals are among the very bases of national health and prosperity, and the working of these institutions is, therefore, a matter of general interest and public importance."[65] The hospital thus served much the same function as the public school, to which it was sometimes likened by those arguing that the institution served the entire community and those needing it should use it as a guaranteed right with any cost borne by the community. But of course only a minority fully appreciated all the functions of a hospital; Boston's City Registrar complained that too many of those "by mere fortuitous circumstance different situated" had yet to learn that "the material condition of the whole community is involved in this subject."[66]

Though hospital treatment of the poor protected the established order and added to the wealth of the community, the people for whom it was intended were made to feel recipients of charity and reminded repeatedly that they were enjoying a privilege and their gratitude was expected in return. This attitude was embodied in law. In one case, a man treated gratuitously sued the Massachusetts General Hospital, claiming his broken leg was set improperly. The courts held that even if he had been treated incompetently and negligently, he was not entitled to recover because the institution was a charity.[67] In another case, a woman charity patient operated on at the Free Hospital for Women sued, claiming her operation was not successful. During the course of protracted litigation, "A Friend to our Charities" wrote the *Transcript* complaining that such hospital malpractice

suits arose because "there are some patients so wholly devoid of ordinary gratitude for favors to which they had not a shadow of a claim, as to make their benefactors suffer by reason of their very kindness." When a verdict for the hospital was finally returned, the *Transcript's* headline, "A Victory for Charity," translated the jury's decision into a reaffirmation of the status of the hospital, though only meaning to imply that money given hospitals would not be drained by lawsuits.[68]

It is from this background that the modern hospital emerged. Changes in social attitudes and medical practice — products of social change and scientific progress — have reshaped the institution. But the hospital that was transformed by these forces was itself a shaping force, a product of its own past. It has influenced medical organization and the kind of medical care available. The hospital now cares for patients of all classes, but it is not a classless institution. The hospital allows physicians to practice the best medicine available, but its clinical setting sometimes discourages the human component of caring. And while government financing and third party payment have redistributed the burden of hospital support throughout society, the institution has often remained unresponsive to the mass of its patients. Finally, the hospital has not evolved toward any foreordained perfection. It is no more the ideal form of medical organization today than it was of social consideration for the poor in the second half of the 19th century.

## NOTES

1 See, in this regard, the career of George Cheyne Shattuck (1813–1893), Shattuck Papers, Massachusetts Historical Society.

2 Nathaniel I. Bowditch, *A History of the Massachusetts General Hospital*, 2nd ed. (Boston: The Bowditch Fund, 1872), p. 3; "A statement made by four physicians . . ." (Boston: 1869), in "Papers and Clippings" (hereafter P.&C.), a scrapbook kept by Dr. F. H. Brown about the Children's Hospital, 1869–1879, in the Countway Library, Boston; For the Dispensary for Skin Diseases and the Dispensary for Diseases of the Nervous System, *Boston Med. & Surg. J.*, 1872, *86*: 81, 82; 1872, *87*: 58; F. H. Brown, *Medical Register for the Cities of Boston, Cambridge, Charlestown, and Chelsea* (Boston: J. Wilson & Son, 1873), n.p.

3 Morris J. Vogel, "Boston's hospitals, 1870–1930: a social history" (Ph.D. dissertation, Univ. of Chicago, 1974), pp. 147–150.

4 James Clarke White, *Sketches from My Life, 1833–1913* (Cambridge, Mass.: Riverside Press, 1914), pp. 267–271.

5 *Boston Med. & Surg. J.*, 1882, *107*: 455. See also Henry J. Bigelow, "Fees in hospitals," *Boston Med. & Surg. J.*, 1889, *120*: 378. Bigelow noted: "It has been said, with truth, that these hospital offices would command a considerable premium in money from the best class of practitioners were they annually put up at auction." An annual report of the Boston Dispensary discussed why doctors served: "It is not to be supposed that the motives of the attending physicians have been wholly foreign from

considerations of personal advantage. They have doubtless been actuated by the hope of professional improvement and the prospect of building up an honest fame, as well as by the desires of fulfilling the benevolent intentions of this charity." Quoted in *Boston Med. & Surg. J.*, 1882, *106*: 137.

6   *Boston J. Hlth.*, March 1886, *1*: 100.

7   *Boston Med. & Surg. J.*, 1905, *152*: 295–320.

8   Bowditch, *M.G.H. History*, p. 415.

9   Carney Hospital, *Annual Reports*, 1879–1889.

10  Boston Dispensary, *Annual Report*, quoted in *Boston Med. & Surg. J.*, 1882, *106*: 137.

11  Children's Hospital, *Appeal*, 1869, in P.&C.

12  *Boston Evening Transcript*, April 20, 1881.

13  Boston, *Proceedings at the Dedication of the City Hospital* (Boston: J. E. Farwell, 1865), p. 58.

14  *Boston Evening Transcript*, June 10, 1886.

15  Detailed sources exist for who used hospitals, but since there is no reliable census of accident and illness, it is difficult to deduce what proportion of any different category of sickness or injury was hospitalized and what was not. Catastrophes, like train wrecks, can provide a rough idea. The pattern derived, while inconclusive, is reaffirmed by an examination of actual hospital use in the period.

16  *Boston Evening Transcript*, March 14, 1887.

17  *Boston Evening Transcript*, March 14, 17, 1887; *Boston Med. & Surg. J.*, 1887, *116*: 268. Another "frightful disaster" with the same general pattern occurred with the wreck of an excursion train on the Old Colony Railroad, *Transcript*, Oct. 9, 10, 1878. There was a different pattern after a crash on the Eastern Railroad in Revere. A greater proportion of the injured were hospitalized; probably because an express Pullman was involved, many of the survivors were from out of town. *Transcript*, Aug. 28, 1871.

18  M.G.H., *60th Annual Report, 1873* p. 9; George H. M. Rowe (superintendent, B.C.H.) to John Pratt (superintendent, M.G.H.), March 7, 1894, in M.G.H. archives, Phillips House file.

19  *Boston Med. & Surg. J.*, 1872, *86*: 81, 82.

20  North End Diet Kitchen founded 1874; South End Diet Kitchen a short time later. *Boston Evening Transcript*, Oct. 20, 1874; Nov. 9, 1875; Dec. 2, 1878.

21  Boston Lying-in Hospital, *Annual Report for 1881*, quoted in *Boston Med. & Surg. J.*, 1882, *106*: 462.

22  Children's Hospital, *Appeal*, 1869, in P.&C.; *Boston Evening Transcript*, Oct. 28, 1876; April 1, 1881; Nov. 17, 1883.

23  Thernstrom does not classify census data for 1870 into these socioeconomic categories, so hospital figures for both 1870 and 1880 are compared to data for the general population derived from the 1880 census. Since Thernstrom finds very little change in the city's occupational structure from 1880 to

1920, this is not unreasonable. Stephan Thernstrom, *The Other Bostonians: Poverty and Progress in the American Metropolis, 1880–1970* (Cambridge, Mass.: Harvard Univ. Press, 1973), pp. 50, 51, 289–302.

24  The category of skilled workers in both 1870 and 1880 consisted entirely of Massachusetts General patients listed as "mechanics." This is an ambiguous term and appears to have been applied differently in 1870 and 1880: The number of patients in this category fell from 291 in 1870 to 219 in 1880. Over the same years there was a large jump in laborers (the whole of the unskilled category) from 187 to 580. This suggests that mechanics were not all skilled workers in 1870 and that their 41.9 percent of the male population over-represents skilled workers among the hospital's patients. At the same time, the figure of 26.9 percent may undercount the proportion of hospital patients who were unskilled in 1870. The M.G.H. admitted 780 males (85 unclassified, all minors) in 1870 and 1,363 (235 unclassified) in 1880. Computed from M.G.H., *Annual Reports*.

25  Computed from B.C.H., *Annual Reports*.

26  Computed from M.G.H. and B.C.H., *Annual Reports*.

27  M.G.H., "The Report of a [trustees'] Committee on the Financial Condition of the M.G.H., February 16, 1865." The trustees dated their financial difficulties from the change from "the industrious classes of our native population," many of whom had paid something toward their board, to the foreign-born, who dramatically increased the numbers treated free. The trustees' committee recommended carefully restricting the number of nonpaying patients (read foreign-born) and segregating them in a distinct section of the hospital, so that the institution could get back to serving "the classes for whose advantage it was established." The trustees rejected that suggestion, apparently because of the urging of the medical staff which feared that decreasing the numbers of the really poor would hurt medical education. M.G.H. Trustees [printed letter], April 1, 1865, both in Countway Library; Bowditch, *M.G.H. History*, p. 454.

28  Computed from M.G.H., *Annual Reports*. In 1870, the United States Census listed 35.1 percent of Boston's population as foreign born.

29  Computed from B.C.H., *Annual Reports*.

30  Frances E. Kobrin, "The American midwife controversy: a crisis of professionalization," *Bull. Hist. Med.*, 1966, *40*: 350–363. [See ch 14 in this book.]

31  Boston, Board of Health, *Annual Report for 1879*, p. 20.

32  New England Hospital for Women and Children, MSS Maternity Records, Vol. 1, in Countway Li-

brary; Computed from Boston Lying-in Hospital, *Annual Report for 1930*, p. 58; for St. Mary's, *Boston Med. & Surg. J.,* 1884, *110*: 363, 364.

33   Joseph Edgar Chamberlin, *The Boston Transcript: A History of its First Hundred Years* (Boston: Houghton Mifflin Co., 1930), p. 165.

34   *Boston Evening Transcript,* Feb. 24, 1888.

35   *Ibid.*

36   *Ibid.*

37   E.g., a long feature article, "The origin of hospitals," *ibid.,* July 13, 1886.

38   *Ibid.,* July 10, 1885. This account is of the McLean Asylum, a branch of the M.G.H.

39   *Ibid.,* Nov. 29, 1881.

40   Odin Anderson, *The Uneasy Equilibrium: Public and Private Financing of Health Services in the United States, 1875-1965* (New Haven: College and Univ. Press, 1968), p. 29.

41   Children's Hospital, *1st Annual Report, 1869,* p. 10.

42   *Boston Evening Transcript,* April 20, 1881.

43   Children's Hospital, *3rd Annual Report, 1871,* pp. 7, 8.

44   Charlestown *Chronicle,* Nov. 11, 1871; Boston *Post,* March 1, 1872; both in P.&C.

45   "The Children's Hospital: what 'Fireside' thinks about it," *Boston Evening Transcript,* Jan. 22, 1879.

46   Children's Hospital, *1st Annual Report, 1869,* p. 13; *3rd Annual Report, 1871,* pp. 8-10.

47   Children's Hospital, *8th Annual Report, 1876,* p. 8. It is perhaps unfair to draw so sharp a distinction between medicine and charity in this case. Koch's work was yet to come, and there was no hard medical knowledge of the transmission of tuberculosis.

48   Children's Hospital, *Appeal,* 1869, in P.&C.; Children's Hospital, *1st Annual Report, 1869,* p. 13.

49   Children's Hospital, *3rd Annual Report, 1871,* p. 10; *5th Annual Report, 1873,* p. 9. Young readers of the *Christian Register* were invited to come with their mothers to visit "the dear little occupants." *Christian Register,* May 8, 1869, June 5, 1869; in P.&C.

50   Children's Hospital, *1st Annual Report, 1869,* back cover; *15th Annual Report, 1883,* p. 9.

51   Children's Hospital, *1st Annual Report, 1869,* p. 13.

52   Boston *Post,* March 1, 1872, in P.&C.

53   "Fireside" *Boston Evening Transcript,* Jan. 22, 1879.

54   *Boston Med. & Surg. J.,* 1870, *83*: 140, 141, editorial; the hospital's founder doubled as the editor of the *Journal.*

55   Boston *Sunday Times,* Dec. 29, 1872, in P.&C.; letter to the editor, "My visit to the Children's Hospital," by "A Lady," *Boston Evening Transcript,* Feb. 22, 1875.

56   Boston *Post,* March 1, 1872, in P.&C.; Children's Hospital, *7th Annual Report, 1875,* p. 13.

57   Drs. James Jackson and John C. Warren, "Circular letter," [1810], in Bowditch, *M.G.H. History,* pp. 3-9.

58   Grace W. Myers, *History of the Massachusetts General Hospital: June, 1872 to December, 1900* (Boston: Griffith-Stillings Press, 1929), p. 12.

59   Dr. D. B. St. John Roosa described the visitors lining up at the gate for the twice weekly visiting hour at the New York Hospital, and how visitors were searched before entering. *The Old Hospital and Other Papers* 2nd ed. (New York: W. Wood & Co., 1889), p. 12.

60   E.g., M.G.H. Trustees MSS Records, Aug. 3, 1877, in M.G.H. archives.

61   "Fireside," *Boston Evening Transcript,* Jan. 22, 1879.

62   M.G.H., *Annual Reports, 1870-1910.*

63   *Boston Evening Transcript,* April 20, 1881.

64   Children's Hospital, *7th Annual Report, 1875,* p. 7; *Boston Evening Transcript,* Jan. 22, 1879; a letter from a grateful parent, *Transcript,* Feb. 29 [*sic*], 1874.

65   Registrar's Report of the City of Boston, quoted in *Boston Med. & Surg. J.,* 1871, *85*: 83; *Boston Evening Transcript,* April 20, 1881.

66   Letter to the editor, *Boston Evening Transcript,* Feb. 29, 1888; Registrar's Report, in *Boston Med. & Surg. J.,* 1871, *85*: 84.

67   McDonald vs. M.G.H., 120 Mass. 432, in E. B. Callander, "Torts of hospitals," *Am. Law Rev.,* 1881, *15*: 640; *Boston Evening Transcript,* July 12, 1875.

68   Stogdale vs. Baker, reported in *Boston Evening Transcript,* Nov. 21, 1885, Dec. 12, 1887, Jan. 5, 1888.

# 21

## Abuse in American Mental Hospitals
## in Historical Perspective: Myth and Reality

### GERALD N. GROB

In recent decades the place of mental hospitals in our society has dropped to a new low. Critics have not merely attacked the shortcomings of hospitals, the abuse of patients, and the systematic violation of civil liberties, but have questioned the very legitimacy of the institution itself. Thomas S. Szasz has placed the issue in sharp focus. "To maintain that a social institution suffers from certain 'abuses,'" he has written, "is to imply that it has certain other desirable or good uses. This, in my opinion, has been the fatal weakness of the countless exposés — old and recent, literary and professional — of private and public mental hospitals. My thesis is quite different: Simply put, it is that there are, and can be, no abuses *of* Institutional Psychiatry, because Institutional Psychiatry *is*, itself, an abuse."[1] Szasz's position may be extreme, but his attitude toward mental hospitals accurately reflects a consensus of diverse groups who are united only by a hostility toward institutional care.

The critics of mental hospitals come from many disciplines and occupations: social and behavioral scientists, historians, lawyers, judges, psychiatrists, and members of various other health care occupations. Their arguments against institutional care of the mentally ill take many different forms. Some argue that "mental illness" is, in reality, a culturally determined label for a variety of social deviants — thus justifying their incarceration and preserving the hegemony of elites. Some insist that asylums are institutions whose character is defined by inherent repressiveness. Others assert that madness is a creative response to the cruel realities of life.

GERALD N. GROB is Professor of History at Rutgers University, New Brunswick, New Jersey.

Reprinted with permission from the *International Journal of Law and Psychiatry*, 1980, 3: 295–310.

Advocates of "community care" of the mentally ill have based much of their criticism on the alleged shortcomings of institutional care. Finally, in recent years certain members of the legal profession have raised questions about the rights of patients inside hospitals and the quality of care accorded them.[2]

Let us look first at the charge that mental hospitals serve as institutions to confine social deviants and that the systematic abuse of patients is the norm rather than the exception. This view has its counterpart among scholars who have studied the history of institutional care. To David J. Rothman, for example, the establishment of mental hospitals in the United States (and similar confining institutions such as jails, almshouses, and juvenile homes) resulted from the perceived fears of middle-class Americans of the social disorder associated with the decline of the preindustrial community. The creation of confining institutions in the Jacksonian era, therefore, "represented an effort to insure the cohesion of the community in new and changing circumstances." Even when efforts were made in the early 20th century to individualize care and treatment, the custodial function predominated, thus perpetuating pervasive repression. To Andrew Scull, who has written about the mental hospital in 19th-century England, and to Michael Katz, these institutions were the specific creation of a market-oriented capitalist society. Those individuals who were unable to engage in productive labor were confined in special institutions where they would no longer threaten the social order. The "moral therapy" of the early 19th century, Scull noted, simply represented an effort to redefine lunatics according to the image of bourgeois rationality.[3]

Significantly, the theme of abuse of the institutionalized mentally ill has had a real effect on public policy. Influenced by the opponents of institutionalization, a number of state legislatures during the 1960s and 1970s passed laws whose aim (at least in theory) was to discharge as many involuntarily committed patients as possible and thereby to restore their rightful liberties. An unstated objective of some advocates of such legislation was to abolish all public mental hospitals and to substitute in their place a system of "community care." Contributing to the attack on institutional care was the growing activism of both the federal and state judiciary. A series of judicial decisions involving such issues as the right to the least restrictive treatment, compensation for labor performed within hospitals, freedom from cruel and unusual punishment, the right to refuse medication, and the protection of patient rights by due process tended to undermine the legitimacy of institutional care.[4]

## RHETORIC, LOGIC, AND THE NATURE OF CRITICISM

If there are significant differences among the critics of institutional care, all agree that mental hospitals abuse patients and rarely, if ever, fulfill therapeutic functions. Without in any way judging the validity of this charge, I would like to focus on two general issues that are often overlooked in the discussions. The first pertains to the rhetoric and logic employed in the debates about mental hospitals and psychiatry; the second involves the nature of the evidence used (or ignored) to validate assertions about institutional care. Taken together, both issues raise serious questions about the current controversy over the care and treatment of the mentally ill.

Let us turn first to a brief examination of rhetoric and logic. In much of the critical literature, the term *mental hospital* is employed with distressing frequency. There are virtually no efforts to distinguish between different kinds of institutions; all are regarded as *sui generis*. Yet the very number of such institutions should raise doubts about sweeping generalizations. In 1875 there were more than 60 public mental hospitals; by 1904 the number had increased to over 140; in 1940 the total exceeded 250. There had also been a dramatic rise in the

patient population. Between 1890 and 1940 the number of patients in state institutions rose from about 32,000 to 394,000. Just as we would be offended by any single, all-encompassing generalization about the quality of education in the more than 2,000 American colleges and universities, so we must question claims that assume a unitary character among mental hospitals.

The truth of the matter is that mental hospitals varied greatly both within a single state and between different regions of the country. A study published in 1940 using data from the decade of the 1930s demonstrated that there were, indeed, striking regional differences in a variety of categories, including rates and results of hospitalization, as well as in the quality of care within institutions.[5] In 1940 the average per patient per year maintenance of mentally ill persons in state institutions was $301. Averages, especially those based on aggregate data, however, concealed more than they revealed. New England spent $388 per patient, while the East South Central region spent only $172. The statistics for individual states varied even more than the regional differences. Kentucky had the lowest per patient maintenance cost ($147), while Wisconsin had the highest ($501). Not surprisingly, the former had the worst patient-employee ratio (10:1), while the latter had the best (3.5:1). Even if these figures are adjusted to take into account costs of living in various regions, the differences remain striking. The varying levels of funding reflected the great variations in the quality of care, food, staffs, housing, and recreational and occupational opportunities.[6] Quite obviously, we are dealing with strikingly dissimilar institutions in the different states and regions.

Similarly, the term *abuse* is so broad and all-inclusive that it defies careful and logical analysis. Considering the hundreds of thousands of individuals who were in a mental hospital at some time in their lives, it would be surprising not to find cases of patient abuse. Certainly the opportunity for such abuse existed, commencing with the commitment process and continuing through the period of institutionalization. The fact that there were abuses, however, cannot be construed as proof that such cases were widespread. Individual examples are not by themselves evidence of a general pattern of patient abuse. One historian noted for his critical attitude toward mental institutions recently offered the case of Catherine Lake to prove that individual rights are being systematically violated in mental hospitals. Aside from a completely misleading description of the facts of the case, he offered no evidence to substantiate his charge that such abuse was characteristic.[7] Any generalizations regarding the nature of care and treatment of the institutionalized mentally ill must rest on a firmer foundation than a few unconnected individual cases.

The one-sided notion of all mental hospital care as no more than abuse of patients unfortunately precludes consideration of some probable consequences of closing down all mental hospitals. Contemporary critics of institutionalization, precisely because they discuss the issue of involuntary commitment largely in terms of abstract individual rights, often avoid the far more difficult task of evaluating the moral dilemmas that arise if certain individuals are not commited. An absolutist definition of freedom can negate other humanitarian and ethical principles. It is entirely possible to honor the absolute right to liberty of persons in an advanced state of senility by not hospitalizing them. But at the same time does this not deny them their right to care from society when they are helpless and allow them to die from exposure, starvation, or neglect?

## EVALUATIONS OF FORMER PATIENTS

More serious than the imprecise language and logic used by critics of mental hospitals is the quality and quantity of evidence employed to support generalizations about the nature of institutional care. Admittedly, the surviving historical records do not shed direct light on the issue of institutional abuse of patients. Commitment records provide invaluable demographic data, but reveal little about the internal environment of hospitals. Even where such records describe individual behavior and institutional response, the vagueness of terminology and absence of both data and context make it difficult to arrive at any firm conclusions about the nature and quality of patient care. Similarly, institutional records, including manuscript and printed materials, often reflect the perceptions of managerial and administrative officials, and these are often at variance with the patient's own perceptions.

A large body of primary sources, nevertheless, has survived that helps to shed light on the commitment process itself as well as on the subsequent experiences of patients. Shortly after mental hospitals were established in the early 19th century, a new genre of literature began to appear in print — the narratives of former patients. Obviously these accounts must be used with great care and discrimination. Their authors were atypical, if only because an insignificant percentage of the total institutionalized population ever revealed their thoughts in public. It is virtually impossible, moreover, to judge the validity of the recollections of patients. Despite the problems of a limited sample and lack of corroborating evidence, these narratives are by no means useless.

What did former patients think of their experiences within hospitals? Clearly, a significant number held that mental hospitals were no different than jails. Indeed, patients were often at a greater disadvantage than criminals, since the commitment process did not involve a formal indictment or trial. This was essentially the argument of Robert Fuller, who published one of the earliest exposés of asylum life. Fuller had been confined in the McLean Asylum for the Insane, a private institution opened in 1818 as part of the Massachusetts General Hospital. In 1833 he charged that it was easy to have any person, sane or ill, committed to an asylum, where they were subsequently abused and mistreated. In his view there was little difference between McLean and the Spanish Inquisition; both suppressed individual liberty and freedom. At the asylum patients remained in total isolation; the staff practiced "constant deception"; and the amount charged for care and treatment was but a form of extortion. Conceding that some individuals benefited from their confinement in McLean, Fuller concluded that most patients were injured in the course of their treatment and that "a vast majority would obtain relief in half the time, if permitted to stay with their friends." He demanded that the legislature enact, as he put it, "such laws as shall be necessary to protect the citizens, and promote the happiness of the whole people."[8]

During the succeeding century a modest amount of literature of this genre appeared in print. Some individuals chose to write articles for popular magazines; some arranged for the private publication of pamphlets and books; and others submitted their works to commercial publishers. Curiously enough, the overwhelming majority of authors were unalterably opposed to Fuller's suggestion that insanity could be treated more effectively within a home environment. Even those who were critical of both the commitment process and their experiences within institutions never questioned the legitimacy of the asylum. They argued rather that procedural safeguards during the commitment process and checks upon the authority granted to hospital officials were required. This theme was already evident in the recollections of Elizabeth T. Stone of her experiences in McLean—a work that was published nine years after the appearance of Fuller's pamphlet. "There is no dispute," she wrote,

> but what there should be such an institution as an Insane Assylum [sic], but let it come under the jurisdiction of the Legislature, and not have all the power consigned into the hands of a few individuals, over a distressed class of beings, a money-making system, at the expense of happiness, in a great measure. If it was thought best to have all power put into the hands of one individual, then we should have a King in this country, but it is not thought best. . . . Would it not be well to have it a law that no person should be carried into an Insane Hospital without the advice of a council of physicians, and not have it left to the judgment of one person, for it is not an uncommon thing for persons to be put in there who are not insane, and they cannot help themselves.[9]

Although the literature by former patients varied in tone and content, certain themes appeared constantly. A significant number of accounts emphasized the absence of legal and procedural safeguards which led to the commitment of sane persons. The most spectacular attack on legal incarceration came from E. P. W. Packard, who had been committed to the Illinois State Hospital for the Insane upon petition by her husband. Her charges, unlike those of Fuller and Stone, led to a lengthy investigation by the state legislature and the eventual passage of a personal liberty law in 1867 that provided for jury trials in sanity proceedings. Five years later Packard's efforts contributed to the adoption of a law in Iowa that gave patients complete freedom to write to whomever they pleased and which forbade the superintendent or staff to open or to censor the patients' mail.[10]

A majority of former patients also criticized their experiences within hospitals. Their accounts often emphasized themes which appeared subsequently in the social and behavioral science literature of the 1950s and afterwards. Among their accusations were the following: the deleterious effects of lengthy institutionalization upon personality structure; the important role given to untrained and poorly paid attendants who made ward life so repressive; the deadening effects of an unvarying routine; the occasional brutality toward patients and the use of various forms of restraint; the difficulty in gaining release from the institution; and the great distance that separated patient from physician. "*We were treated in the mass,*" noted one individual who provided a balanced account of her experiences, "*disciplined in the mass, taught in the mass, fed in the mass, and physicked in the mass.*"[11]

Yet some patients, on the other hand, recalled their experiences within hospitals in laudatory terms. They emphasized the positive role of nurses and attendants, and the patience and supportiveness manifested by the medical staff. Conceding that mental hospitals were not "ideal places of residence" and that abuses occasionally took place, one called the state hospital a "marvelous institution." It provided "the best of medical care," maintained an "adequate nursing staff," and relieved families of a "financial burden that in most cases would prove unsupportable."[12]

Finally, one must remember that these accounts are not necessarily reliable historical sources. It was not uncommon for individuals to write about their religious experiences; some repeated direct conversations that they claimed to have had with God.[13] Others provided narratives that strain the credibility of the reader, to say the least.[14]

One common thread runs through virtually all of this literature: at some point the family took an active role in commencing the legal process that ended in commitment. Irrespective of the uniqueness of each of these cases, it is incontrovertible that the internal disruption of the family that followed certain forms of behavior ultimately reached a crisis stage. The existence of hospitals provided an alternative, and some families chose to resolve the problem by institutionalizing one of its members. Such actions were probably taken only after considerable soul-searching and anguish. But the decision to commit the patient generally rested on the belief that the welfare of the family as a whole had to take precedence over the needs of an individual member.

What, then, do all of these accounts by former patients reveal? Any answer to this question can only be ambiguous, for they demonstrate that the experiences of an admittedly atypical group were extremely varied. The majority of the writers were unhappy, but not to the degree that led them to question the legitimacy of mental hospitals. Certainly this was true even in Clifford W. Beers' classic *A Mind That Found Itself*. After gaining his release from several mental hospitals, Beers spent the remainder of his life in an effort to create a national movement to upgrade the quality of institutional care.[15] The perceptions of a minority, on the other hand, were very different. Certainly it is impossible to read this literature as evidence that all hospitals abused patients.[16]

Even where abuses existed, the situation was far more complex than is commonly recognized. The history of involuntary sterilization of the mentally ill is a case in point. Interest in sterilization as a means of social uplift grew out of late 19th-century scientific and intellectual currents. By the end of the century eugenicists were seeking to harness the authority of the state to the theory of heredity. Specifically, they urged the passage of legislation that would prevent socially undesirable groups from propagating themselves, thus raising the quality of the nation's genetic pool. After several failures, eugenicists succeeded in persuading the Indiana legislature in 1907 to enact a law providing for the mandatory sterilization of confirmed criminals, idiots, imbeciles, and rapists when recommended by a board of experts. In the succeeding decade, 15 other states enacted some form of comparable legislation. Most of the laws applied to the mentally ill as well as to others deemed to represent a threat to the nation's biological well-being.[17]

Between 1907 and 1940, a total of 18,552 mentally ill persons in state hospitals were surgically sterilized. The number was not equally distributed among the 30 states that at one time or another had laws authorizing this practice. More than half of all sterilizations were performed in California alone, which together with Virginia and Kansas accounted for nearly three-fourths of the total. Clearly, the experience with sterilization was a function of the state in which patients resided and practices within that state. Neither total population of the state, age distribution, nor any other variable explains these differentials.[18]

Equally significant, there was virtually no unanimity within the medical, legal, and scientific professions or among the public at large regarding the wisdom or advisability of involuntary sterilization. Nor was there a central organization directing the drive to secure enactment of such laws. To be sure, the Eugenics Record Office, founded in 1910 as a center for eugenical research and an agency for the dissemination of propaganda, provided some national cohesion, but it could hardly be termed a pressure group on this issue. Indeed, the National Committee for Mental Hygiene, founded in 1911, refused to support sterilization on the grounds that knowledge about heredity was too fragmentary to justify the practice.[19] In states that enacted legislation, the driving force was either an individual or small group associated with public institutions (mental hospitals, institutions for the feebleminded, and prisons), state boards of charity, private welfare organizations, or institutions of higher learning.[20] Among psychiatrists there was a sharp division of opinion, although most never expressed any view on this question.[21]

Given the differences in attitudes and practices, it is impossible to generalize in any meaningful manner about the country as a whole. A generalization applicable to California and Virginia is inapplicable to many other states where resistance to sterilization existed well before the passage of the Nürnberg laws in Nazi Germany in 1935, which helped to bring the practice into public disrepute. What is required is a more detailed and careful analysis that will enable us to understand why sterilization laws could first be passed and then enforced in some states, passed but not enforced in others, and never passed in still others.

It is possible, of course, to continue to offer other kinds of evidence that call into question the broad generalizations about the past that frequently play a role in the current controversy over mental hospitals. There are, for example, innumerable investigations and exposés — private and public — that purport to demonstrate a pattern of institutional rigidity and patient abuse. In the late 1870s a group of New York neurologists, including physicians such as William A. Hammond, E. C. Spitzka, and lay activists such as Dorman B. Eaton, launched a bitter attack on hospital superintendents that led to an investigation in the state legislature. Shortly thereafter they helped to found the short-lived National Association for the Protection of the Insane and the Prevention of Insanity. Similarly, in 1894 S. Weir Mitchell was invited to address the convention of the American Medico-Psychological Association (now the American Psychiatric Association), and stunned his listeners with a denunciation of institutional psychiatry. Although Hammond, Spitzka, Eaton, and Mitchell were often quoted to validate charges about the depressed character of institutional psychiatry, few took the trouble to analyze the context in which their statements were made. Indeed, contextual knowledge reveals that none of these men were necessarily opposed to institutional care *per se*, and that some of their criticisms reflected different perceptions arising out of their particular specialty and the fact that asylum psychiatrists and urban neurologists handled different kinds of clients.[22] Actually, the challenge to the legitimacy of the mental hospital did not become significant until well into the 20th century. By then university medical centers and opportunities in private practice reduced the attractiveness of hospital-based practice. The result was a shift in interest toward the neuroses and personality disorders and a decline in concern with the seemingly intransigent and debilitating conditions associated with psychoses. My main point should be clear by now: many of the so-called facts that have been offered as evidence of abuse or the low quality of institutional care have either been incomplete or viewed without a proper consideration of their context.

## VIEWING MENTAL HOSPITALS THROUGH HISTORY

What links the approaches previously discussed is the understandable but unfortunate tendency to see and to analyze the past through the eyes of the present. This is, of course, the Whig interpretation of history in another context; Herbert Butterfield's classic observations are as appropriate now as they were a half a century ago. "Real historical understanding," he wrote, "is not achieved by the subordination of the past to the present, but rather by our making the past our present and attempting to see life with the eyes of another century than our own."[23]

When we view mental hospitals from the vantage point of history, they assume a somewhat different character, particularly if a functional approach is pursued. This is not to deny that mental hospitals were coercive institutions. Indeed, a large part of their total population was involuntarily confined, and force—potential and actual—was the major means of control to keep patients confined and to maintain internal discipline.[24] Nevertheless, the coercive nature of these institutions must be placed within an appropriate historical context that permits us to understand the characteristics of patient populations, how and why patients came to be institutionalized, and the kinds of experiences they underwent once admitted. Nor should we assume that hospitals were monolithic and static; just as schools, general hospitals, and other kinds of organizations changed radically over time, so too have mental hospitals passed through a variety of stages.

Rather than providing a comprehensive historical analysis of patients and hospitals, let me offer a few examples. The function and character of mental hospitals were often determined by the nature of the client population rather than by psychiatric theory or practice. Who were these patients? What circumstances led to their commitment? What were their experiences within hospitals? These are only a few of the questions that require answers if we are to understand the nature of institutional care.

Even a cursory analysis of individuals institutionalized in the 19th and 20th centuries provides data that alter the current view that fear of social disorder and perceived threats to the safety of the community led to the establishment and proliferation of mental hospitals. If fear were the sole or most important element in judicial proceedings, we might expect public authorities or social elites to take the lead in initiating involuntary commitment. Such, however, was hardly the case; the majority of commitment proceedings originated within the family. In a recent analysis of commitment proceedings in San Francisco during the first three decades of the 20th century, Richard W. Fox found that 57 percent of commitment proceedings were begun by relatives, 21 percent by physicians, and only 8 percent by the police.[25] The clientele did come from lower-class or lower-middle-class backgrounds, but these were precisely the families that lacked the financial resources to pay for private home or institutional care when one of their members became mentally ill.

Historical studies about conditions within the family that led to the commitment of members to mental hospitals are still lacking. But it is quite clear that in many instances families decided on institutionalization as the lesser of two evils, particularly when confronted with either behavior that threatened its internal integrity or situations with which it could not cope. "I reluctantly enclose application filled out for admission of my mother," a bank employee wrote to the superintendent of the Wisconsin Hospital for the Insane in 1875.

> Of late she had grown materially worse, so that we deem it unsafe for the female portion of the family to be left alone with her during the day and especially unsafe for the little 2 year old that is obliged to remain continually there as she has stated several times of late that she or the children must be sacrificed. Should she destroy another us [sic] could never forgive ourselves if the state has a place provided for their comfort and possible need.

Indeed, many families were reluctant to have members discharged from hospitals for fear that interpersonal relationships might again be disrupted or that an intolerable burden would be placed upon household finances.[26]

The characteristics of institutional populations in the late 19th and early 20th centuries shed considerable light upon the actual workings of mental hospitals, and does not sustain the allegation that hospitals were intended as instruments of social control or, for that matter, served primarily therapeutic functions. For example, nearly 18 percent of all first admissions to New York State mental hospitals in 1920 were diagnosed as psychotic either because of senility or arteriosclerosis. By 1940 this category accounted for nearly 31 percent of all first admissions. During this same period the average age at first admission rose from 42.69 years to 48.47. Indeed, the trend toward an older population continued even after World War II. Between 1949 and 1951, 33.3 percent of all first admissions were over 65 years of age even though only 8.6 percent of the state's population fell into this category. Three decades earlier, by way of contrast, the figures were 13.6 percent and 4.7 percent, respec-

tively. New York was not unique in this respect. Between 1916 and 1925, 16.3 percent of all first admissions to Warren State Hospital in Pennsylvania were 65 and older; the comparable figure for 1936–1945 was 23 percent. The statistics for Illinois and Massachusetts reveal a comparable pattern.[27] What these figures indicate is that mental hospitals were to some extent serving as homes for older persons suffering from some sort of physical and mental impairment.

The number of aged persons in state hospitals varied by period and geographical locale. Within a given state, wide variations among institutions were not uncommon. In 1932 the average age of first admissions committed by the courts in Massachusetts was 48.6 years. Individual hospitals, on the other hand, had widely diverging patterns: the highest average age was 54.4 years (Boston State Hospital); the figures for Taunton State Hospital, Grafton State Hospital, and Boston Psychopathic Hospital were 50.1, 41.7, and 39.1, respectively.[28] Despite institutional variations (which were directly related to varying death, discharge, and retention rates), it is clear that the aged constituted a substantial proportion of the total institutionalized population. By the late 19th century age-specific admission rates of older persons began to rise markedly as compared with admission rates for younger persons. In their classic study of rates of institutionalization covering more than a century, Herbert Goldhamer and Andrew W. Marshall found the greatest increase occurred in the 60 year and older category. In 1885, the age-specific first admission rate in Massachusetts for males 60 years and over was 70.4, and for females 65.5 (per 100,000); by the beginning of World War II the corresponding figures were 279.5 and 223.0. A study of Warren State Hospital in Pennsylvania covering 1916–1950 showed much the same pattern.[29]

Why were aged persons committed to mental hospitals? Communities hardly perceived them as a threat. Nor can it be said that the function of institutionalization was to alter the behavior of such persons or to provide restorative therapy. "The question of the care of the aged is one that will confront us always," noted one superintendent who conceded that no effective treatment was available.[30] Mental hospitals were in fact assuming the function of old-age homes, partly for lack of alternatives. The decline in mortality rates among younger elements in the population, in addition, led to a relative and absolute increase in the numbers of the aged, thereby giving rise to the social problems relating to an aging population. Between 1900 and 1940, the number of persons 65 and over increased from about 3 to 9 million (as compared with a population rise from 76 to slightly more than 131 million).[31]

Older persons ended up in mental hospitals for numerous reasons. Some had no family to provide them with care. Families in many instances lacked the means to care for aged members. Other patients were institutionalized because of the inability or unwillingness of relatives to assume responsibility for them. Certain senile patients exhibited forms of behavior that were difficult for families to cope with. For some indigent aged persons, a mental hospital provided the only means of survival.

The growing proportion of aged persons in mental hospitals undoubtedly reflected a transfer of poulation from almshouses—an institution that had been declining in significance and would eventually become extinct. Between 1904 and 1922 admissions to almshouses fell from 81,412 to 63,807 (a decline from 99.5 to 58.4 persons per 100,000). Although admissions were declining, the almshouse was simultaneously becoming a refuge for the indigent aged. In 1880, 33.2 percent of its population were 60 and over; in 1904 and 1923 this group accounted for 53.1 and 66.6 percent of the total, respectively. For reasons that are not clear, the number of aged, mentally ill persons in these institutions declined precipitously. In 1880 there were over 16,000 mentally ill paupers in American almshouses; by 1923 the number had fallen to about 2,000. The decline was more apparent than real, however, given the steadily rising number of aged mentally ill persons committed to asylums. In effect, the mental hospitals assumed the functions once performed by the almshouse. In 1904, 16.3 percent of patients in mental hospitals were 60 and over; by 1923, 20.8 percent fell into this category.[32]

Psychiatrists and some public officials were well aware of the practice of committing older persons to mental hospitals. Although they were unhappy about this practice, they went along with the custom of confining such persons because there

seemed to be no other alternative. Homes for the aged, which we now see about us, did not become common until after World War II. Dr. Charles C. Wagner, superintendent of the Binghamton State Hospital in New York, defined the issue in simple, yet moving terms. "We are receiving every year a large number of old people, some of them very old, who are simply suffering from the mental decay incident to extreme old age," he wrote in 1900:

A little mental confusion, forgetfulness and garrulity are sometimes the only symptoms exhibited, but the patient is duly certified to us as insane and has no one at home capable or possessed of means to care for him. We are unable to refuse these patients without creating ill-feeling in the community where they reside, nor are we able to assert that they are not insane within the meaning of the statute, for many of them, judged by the ordinary standards of sanity, cannot be regarded as entirely sane.[33]

A similar opinion was expressed by the secretary of the Pennsylvania Board of Public Charities a few years later. The practice of institutionalizing aged senile persons, he noted, was related to the refusal by children to accept responsibility for their ailing parents.

Selfishly neglected by those who owe to them everything they are thrust into seclusion in order that they may not be burdens, and too frequently forgotten and neglected by those through whose veins flows the same blood, they must helplessly and hopelessly wait, receiving kindness and care from those who are neither kith nor kin, until the coming of the Great Messenger shall mercifully relieve them and release them. A crime has been committed and yet a legalized crime and this will be repeated again and again until medical examiners shall more wisely discriminate in their certification of insanity.[34]

Such sentiments were not confined to the early part of the 20th century. A study of the Illinois state hospitals in the early 1930s emphasized the degree to which these institutions were serving as homes for the aged. A major problem, the report emphasized,

is the presence of increasingly large numbers of old people—primarily not mental patients—but described in medical parlance as "senile." Social revolutions, radical changes in housing and living problems, the growth of urban life, and countless other factors have tended to force the old man and or men from their homes. . . . The state mental hospital, organized for quite other purposes, has become their only haven. . . . An illustration of the enormity of this difficulty is found in the Chicago State Hospital which today is being converted into a huge infirmary, with nearly seventy percent of its 4,000 patients aged or infirm, suffering from no psychoses which would be beyond the capacity of the old-fashioned detached city cottage or rural home or of a well-managed county home.[35]

Syphilis as well as senility was another major cause for admitting patients whose abnormal behavior was related to underlying physiological processes. Before the widespread use of penicillin and other antibiotics limited the course of venereal disease, insanity resulting from syphilis accounted for substantial numbers of admissions to asylums. Between 1911 and 1920 about 20 percent of all male first admissions to mental hospitals in New York State were cases of general paresis (the comparable rate for women during this same period was about one third that of men). New York State, once again, was not unique in this respect; other states had comparable rates.[36] Statistics on syphilis became more reliable as the Wassermann test began being routinely administered in all mental hospitals after 1906. This test provided a fairly reliable (although not infallible) serological technique for determining whether the *treponema pallidum* (the organism responsible for syphilis) was present in the blood.

To most Americans in the prepenicillin era, syphilis was more than a physical disease; it symbolized, in part, the penalty for moral corruption. We should not conclude, however, that syphilitic patients committed to mental hospitals were being punished for their transgressions. In the tertiary stage of this disease, massive damage to the central nervous system or brain resulted not only in bizarre behavior but in dramatic neurological symptoms, paralysis, and eventually death. For such cases institutional care was a natural necessity; few households were prepared to cope with such problems. Since general hospitals did not have separate facilities to care for patients in the

tertiary stage (who could live from one to five years), responsibility devolved upon the mental hospital.

Overall, at least one-third (and probably more) of all first admissions to state mental hospitals represented cases where behavioral symptoms were probably of somatic origin. In 1922, for example, 52,472 persons were admitted for the first time into state asylums. Of this number, 15,916 were sent there either because of senility, cerebral arteriosclerosis, general paresis, cerebral syphilis, Huntington's chorea, pellagra, brain tumor or other brain disease, and other somatic illnesses. The statistics a decade later showed much the same pattern. Indeed, between 1933 and 1942 the combined first admissions to state hospitals for paresis, cerebral arteriosclerosis, and senility increased from 31.3 percent to 35.8 percent.[37] There were, of course, significant regional differences. Pellagra (a disease caused by a dietary deficiency, often accompanied by behavioral symptoms) was generally confined to the South. Between 1930 and 1932, the State Hospital at Goldsboro, North Carolina (which was limited to blacks), reported that no less than 19 percent of its admissions were due to pellagra. In northern hospitals, the disease was virtually unknown.[38]

Mental hospitals, in other words, cared for a variety of patients. Some individuals were institutionalized because of physical disability. In other cases, hospitals served as asylums for persons, who, for one reason or another, seemed to require a structured environment. Noting that it was often alleged that public mental hospitals cared for persons who could just as easily have been sent home, the Pennsylvania Commission on Lunacy warned of the dangers of generalizing about such issues. The Commission concluded that many patients no doubt could be sent home, "provided that the home existed, or that conditions at home were suitable for the patient's return"; unfortunately, such conditions did not always exist. Frederick H. Wines, one of the most influential figures in late 19th-century public welfare, observed that many mental hospitals were imposed upon in "that patients are sent to them who should not be so sent, because their friends wish to avoid the responsibility of keeping and caring for them at home."[39]

In dealing with such data, we must be careful

not to read the past in terms of the present. To argue that aged and senile groups as well as persons suffering from physical impairments with accompanying behavioral symptoms, did not belong in mental hospitals, or to insist that individual rights were being ignored, is to misunderstand the nature of social change in the 19th and 20th centuries. In point of fact, high rates of geographical mobility, a rapid increase in the size of urban areas, and the inability of traditional means of alleviating distress and dependency by reliance on familial and community traditions and practices led Americans to turn to quasi-public or public institutions for the care of many dependent groups. Under these circumstances, mental hospitals assumed the responsibility, often unwillingly, for providing care for groups, many of whose members were unable to provide for themselves.[40]

The internal character of mental hospitals, furthermore, was in large measure dictated by the nature of their patient populations as well as by their medical staffs and attendant corps. The absence of a therapeutic environment, for example, may have simply reflected the age or physical condition of individuals for whom no known treatment existed. For such persons hospitals could provide but a form of custodial care at best. Nor were better or more effective alternatives necessarily available at that time. It is debatable whether the chronic nursing homes for the aged that came into existence after the Second World War provided better care than their predecessors.[41]

## MORAL ELEMENTS OF CARING FOR THE MENTALLY ILL

The ongoing debate about modes of care and treatment of the mentally ill generally incorporates two basic elements. The first is a moral element that concerns the manner in which American society *ought* to deal with dependent groups such as (but not limited to) the mentally ill. The second involves the care of the mentally ill in the past. Unfortunately, the two have never been separated, and current moral convictions have given rise to an inaccurate portrait of the past.

That historical knowledge conditions (or reflects) attitudes and behavior in the present is obvious. The issue, therefore, is not whether historical knowledge will be employed to influence decision-making and public policies, but what kind of history will be used. It would be a tragedy if a misunderstanding or erroneous knowledge of the past guided our responses (or served as a rationalization) to the problems presented by mental illness in the present or future.

The thrust of my remarks should not be misinterpreted. I am not arguing that the mentally ill were not "abused," nor am I insisting that mental insitutions were necessarily "benevolent" and "humane" in character. I am rather seeking a balanced historical understanding that takes into account changes in their function and nature. In this respect the current debate about the mentally ill falls far short.[42]

## NOTES

I wish to acknowledge that the research for this paper was supported by a grant from the Public Health Service (HSS), National Library of Medicine, No. 2306.

1   Thomas S. Szasz, *The Manufacture of Madness: A Comparative Study of the Inquisition and the Mental Health Movement* (New York, 1970), pp. xxix–xxxv.

2   Thomas S. Szasz, *The Myth of Mental Illness: Foundations of a Theory of Personal Conduct* (New York, 1961); and *idem, Law, Liberty, and Psychiatry: An Inquiry Into the Social Uses of Mental Health Practices* (New York, 1963); R. D. Laing, *The Politics of Experience* (New York, 1968); Robert Perucci, *Circle of Madness: On Being Insane and Institutionalized in America* (Englewood Cliffs, N.J., 1974); Alexander D. Brooks, *Law,*

*Psychiatry and the Mental Health System* (Boston, 1974); Leona Bachrach, *Deinstitutionalization: An Analytic Review and Sociological Pespective* (Washington, D.C., 1976).

3   David J. Rothman, *The Discovery of the Asylum: Social Order and Disorder in the New Republic,* (Boston, 1971), p. xviii, and *idem, Conscience and Convenience: The Asylum and Its Alternative in Progressive America* (Boston, 1980); Michael B. Katz, "Origins of the institutional state," *Marxist Perspectives,* 1978, *1:* 6–22; Andrew T. Scull, *Museums of Madness: The Social Organization of Insanity in Nineteenth-Century England* (New York, 1979).

4   See Rouse *v.* Cameron, 373 F 2d 451 (D.C. Cir. 1966); Wyatt *v.* Stickney, 344 F. Supp. 373 (M.D.

Ala. 1972), modified *sub nom,* Wyatt *v.* Aderholt, 503 F 2d 1305 (5th Cir. 1974).

5   Joseph Zubin and Grace C. Scholtz, *Regional Differences in the Hospitalization and Care of Patients with Mental Diseases* (Washington, D.C., 1940).

6   The data in this paragraph are drawn from U.S. Bureau of the Census, *Patients in Mental Institutions 1940* (Washington, D.C., 1943), pp. 60, 63.

7   Compare David J. Rothman, "The state as parent: social policy in the Progressive Era," in *Doing Good: The Limits of Benevolence,* ed. Willard Gaylin, Ira Glasser, Steven Marcus and David J. Rothman (New York, 1978), pp. 73, 95, with Lake *v.* Cameron, 364 F. 2d 657 (D.C. Cir. 1966), Brooks, *Law, Psychiatry, and the Mental Health System,* pp. 727–732, and David L. Chambers, "Alternatives to civil commitment of the mentally ill: practical guides and constitutional imperatives," *Mich. Law Rev.,* 1972, *70:* 1108, 1121 n. 59, 1140–1141.

8   Robert Fuller, *An Account of the Imprisonments and Sufferings of Robert Fuller, of Cambridge* (Boston, 1833), pp. 24–29.

9   Elizabeth T. Stone, *A Sketch of the Life of Elizabeth T. Stone, and of Her Persecutions, with an Appendix of Her Treatment and Sufferings While in the Charlestown McLean Asylum, Where She Was Confined Under the Pretence of Insanity* (n.p., 1842), pp. 35–36.

10  For a discussion of Packard's crusade (and a listing of relevant source materials), see Gerald N. Grob, *Mental Institutions in America: Social Policy to 1875* (New York, 1973), pp. 265–269.

11  Margaret Wilson, *Borderland Minds* (Boston, 1940), p. 179.

12  Henry Collins Brown, *A Mind Mislaid* (New York, 1937), pp. 60, 63, 219.

13  See also Jimmy Warde, *Jimmy Warde's Experiences as a Lunatic: A True Story* (Little Rock, c. 1902).

14  See for example, Clarissa Caldwell Lathrop, *A Secret Institution* (New York, 1890).

15  Clifford W. Beers, *A Mind That Found Itself: An Autobiography* (New York, 1908). See also Norman Dain, *Clifford W. Beers: Advocate for the Insane* (Pittsburgh, 1980).

16  The generalizations about patient accounts are based on an examination of more than 50 works published up to 1940. For a further discussion of bibliography see Walter C. Alvarez, *Minds That Came Back* (Philadelphia, 1961).

I have deliberately refrained from analyzing these patient accounts within a psychoanalytic or psychological framework (emphasizing, for example, institutional transference). There are methodological pitfalls in interpreting one class of materials without providing a comparative base (such as letters to superintendents from former patients).

Moreover, virtually nothing is known about the personal lives of many of these literate patients, a fact that magnifies the perils of a psychological interpretation.

17  Mark H. Haller, *Eugenics: Hereditarian Attitudes in American Thought* (New Brunswick, N.J., 1963), pp. 50, 133.

18  Figures from "Sterilizations in state institutions under state laws, 1907–1940," mimeographed table in Association for Voluntary Sterilization Papers, Box 6, Folder 56, Social Welfare History Archives, University of Minnesota, Minneapolis.

19  George K. Pratt to C. F. Williams, Jan. 5, 1932, American Foundation for Mental Hygiene Papers, Uncatalogued, Library of the New York Hospital, New York.

20  See Haller, *Eugenics,* pp. 132–141.

21  For two opposing views, see W. D. Partlow to E. S. Gosney, Mar. 26, 1934, Association for Voluntary Sterilization Papers, Box 5, Folder 48, note 18 above; William A. White to Dr. [?] Fisher, n.d., c.1919, White Papers, Records of Saint Elizabeths Hospital, Record Group 418, National Archives, Washington, D.C. The discussion here is based on a comprehensive analysis of all psychiatric periodicals published in the United States between 1875 and 1940. Historical treatments of sterilization can be found in the following: Haller, *Eugenics,* pp. 50, 133; Rudolph J. Vecoli, "Sterilization: a progressive measure?" *Wisconsin Mag. Hist.,* 1960, *43:* 190–202; Donald K. Pickins, *Eugenics and the Progressives* (Nashville, 1968).

22  For examples of their critiques see the following: Dorman B. Eaton, "Despotism in lunatic asylums," *North Am. Rev.,* 1881, *132:* 263–275; E. C. Spitzka, "What has been done by the Asylum Association in the interest of scientific psychiatry," *Chicago Med. Rev.,* 1880, *1:* 273–280; William A. Hammond, "The non-asylum treatment of the insane," *Tr. Med. Soc. St. N.Y.,* 1879: 280–297; and "The construction, organization and equipment of hospitals for the insane," *Neurol. Contributions,* 1880, *1:* 1–25; S. Weir Mitchell, "Address before the Fiftieth Annual Meeting of the American Medico-Psychological Association, held in Philadelphia, May 16th, 1894," *J. Nerv. & Ment. Dis.,* 1894, *21:* 413–427; also reprinted in *Proc. Am. Medico-Psychological Assn.* (1894), *50:* 101–121.

23  Herbert Butterfield, *The Whig Interpretation of History* (New York, 1951), p. 16.

24  Amitai Etzioni, *A Comparative Analysis of Complex Organizations: On Power, Involvement, and Their Correlates* (New York, 1975), pp. 23–29.

25  Richard W. Fox, *So Far Disordered in Mind: Insanity in California, 1870–1930* (Berkeley, 1978), p. 84.

26 Dale W. Robison, "Wisconsin and the Mentally Ill: a History of the 'Wisconsin Plan' of State and County Care 1860–1915" (Ph.D. dissertation, Marquette Univ., 1976), pp. 7ff. Robison's comments about the role of the family in commitment are based upon an examination of the manuscripts (including incoming correspondence) of the Wisconsin State Hospital for the Insane, located at the State Historical Society of Wisconsin, Madison.

27 New York State Department of Mental Hygiene, *Annual Report*, 1939–1940, *52*: 174–175; Benjamin Malzberg, "A statistical analysis of the ages of first admissions to hospitals for mental disease in New York State," *Psychiatric Quart.* 1949, *23*: 346; *idem*, "A comparison of first admissions to the New York State civil hospitals during 1919–1921 and 1949–1951," *Psychiatric Quart.*, 1954, *28*: 314; United States Bureau of the Census, *Fourteenth Census of the United States*, Vol. II, *Population 1920* (Washington, D.C., 1922), p. 248; *idem, Census of Population: 1950*, Vol. II, *Characteristics of the Population*, Part 32 (Washington, D.C., 1952), p. 58; Morton Kramer, Hyman Goldstein, Robert H. Israel, and Nelson A. Johnson, *A Historical Study of the Disposition of First Admissions to a State Hospital: Experiences of the Warren State Hospital During the Period 1916–50* (Washington, D.C., 1955), p. 10; Carney Landis and Jane E. Farwell, "A trend analysis of age at first admission, age at death, and years of residence for state mental hospitals: 1913–1941," *J. Abnormal & Social Psych.*, 1944, *39*: 3–23.

By the 1930s and 1940s there was a growing appreciation of the age distribution of the mentally ill and some of its implications for psychiatry. For selected examples see the following: Benjamin Malzberg, *Social and Biological Aspects of Mental Disease* (Utica, N.Y., 1940), ch. 2; Neil A. Dayton, *New Facts on Mental Disorders: Study of 89,190 Cases* (Springfield, Ill., 1940), Ch. 8; Harold F. Dorn, "The incidence and future expectancy of mental disease," *Public Hlth. Rep.*, 1938, *53*: 1991–2004; William F. Ogburn and Ellen Winston, "The frequency and probability of insanity," *Am. J. Sociol.*, 1929, *34*: 822–831; Nelson A. Johnson, "The growing problem of old-age psychoses: an analysis of the trend in one state hospital from 1910 to 1944," *Mental Hygiene*, 1946, *30*: 431–450. See also Aubrey Lewis, "Aging and senility: a major problem of psychiatry," *J. Mental Sci.*, 1946, *92*: 150–170.

28 Neil A. Dayton, "A new statistical system for the study of mental disease and some of the attained results," *Bull. Mass. Dept. Mental Dis.*, 1934, *18*: 179–180.

29 Herbert Goldhamer and Andrew W. Marshall, *Psychosis and Civilization: Two Studies in the Frequency of Mental Disease* (Glencoe, Ill., 1953), pp. 54, 91; Kramer and others, *Historical Study . . .*, p. 10.

30 Ohio Department of Public Welfare, *Annual Report*, 1936, *15*: 303–304.

31 United States Bureau of the Census, *Historical Statistics of the United States: Colonial Times to 1970*, 2 vols. (Washington, D.C., 1975), p. 15.

32 United States Bureau of the Census, *Paupers in Almshouses 1904* (Washington, D.C., 1906), pp. 182, 184; *idem, Paupers in Almshouses 1910* (Washington, D.C., 1915), pp. 42–43; *idem, Paupers in Almshouses 1923* (Washington, D.C., 1925), pp. 5, 8, 33; *idem, Insane and Feebleminded in Hospitals and Institutions 1904* (Washington, D.C., 1906), p. 29; *idem, Patients in Hospitals for Mental Diseases 1923* (Washington, D.C., 1926).

33 New York State Commission on Lunacy, *Annual Report*, 1900, *12*: 29–30.

34 Pennsylvania Committee on Lunacy, *Annual Report*, 1904, *22*: 8–9. In Pennsylvania Board of Commissioners of Public Charities, *Annual Report*, 1904, *35*.

35 "The care of the mentally disordered in Illinois: the state hospitals," typed manuscript (c. 1931), pp. 7–8, in American Foundation for Mental Hygiene Papers, Box 4, Library of the New York Hospital.

36 New York State Department of Mental Hygiene, *Annual Report*, 1939–1940, *52*: 176. For other examples see the following: Washington (State) Department of Business Control, *Biennial Report*, 1933–1934, *7*: 27; Ohio Department of Public Welfare, *Annual Report*, 1932–1933, *11–12*: 349, 358–360, and *Annual Report*, 1936, *15*: 304; Oregon State Board of Control, *Biennial Report*, 1919–1920, *4*: 47; Illinois Department of Public Welfare, *Annual Report*, 1928–1929, *12*: 310; North Carolina Charitable, Penal, and Correctional Institutions, *Biennial Report*, 1930–1932, 48.

37 United States Bureau of the Census, *Mental Patients in State Hospitals: 1926 and 1927* (Washington, D.C., 1930), p. 9, and *Mental Patients in State Hospitals: 1931 and 1932* (Washington, D.C., 1934), p. 6; American Psychopathological Association, *Trends of Mental Disease* (New York, 1945), p. 31.

38 North Carolina Charitable, Penal, and Correctional Institutions, *Biennial Report*, 1930–1932, 48.

39 Pennsylvania Committee on Lunacy, *Annual Report*, 1898, *16*: 44–45; in Pennsylvania Board of Commissioners of Public Charities, *Annual Report*, 1898, *29*; *Proc. Nat. Conf. Charities & Corrections*, 1890, *17*: 431.

40 Some scholars have argued that economic and technological changes associated with industrialization introduced a distinction between home and work, thereby undermining the integrated nature of the preindustrial family. In the new industrial society,

public and quasi-public institutions took over functions once performed by families (e.g., education of the young, care of the dependent). This thesis, however attractive, is based on the questionable assumption that the structure and functions of families were simply the result of external forces. The preindustrial family, for example, may have cared for mentally ill members because no alternative was readily available and in spite of the human costs incurred. When presented with an institutional alternative, many families opted for its use. Few families, on the other hand, evinced any eagerness to institutionalize members; the general practice was to retain them at home as long as possible. In offering this analysis, I am not suggesting that changes in social structure did not influence family life, but I am arguing that the behavior of families involved some autonomy on the part of their members. Nor should the strains of retaining mentally ill relatives in a home setting be idealized or minimized.

41  It should be noted that part of the decline in the population of mental hospitals during the past two decades has been more apparent than real. The number of elderly persons in such institutions declined sharply, but the number of aged mentally ill persons in nursing and personal care homes rose sharply. See Richard W. Reddick, "Patterns in use of nursing homes by the aged mentally ill," National Institute of Mental Health, *Statistical Note 107,* 1974. Between 1962 and 1975 the number of first admissions to state and county mental hospitals fell from 163.7 per 100,000 to 36.7. Laura Milazzo-Sayre, "Changes in the age and sex composition of first admissions to state and county mental hospitals, United States 1962–1975" National Institute of Mental Health, *Statistical Note 145,* 1978, p. 9.

42  For a general discussion of the historical development of asylums, see Peter L. Tyor and Jamil S. Zainaldin, "Asylum and society: an approach to institutional change," *J. Soc. Hist.* 1979, *13*: 23–48. My own approach to the history of mental hospitals can be gleaned from the following: *Mental Institutions in America: Social Policy to 1875* (New York, 1973); *The State and the Mentally Ill: A History of Worcester State Hospital in Massachusetts, 1830–1920* (Chapel Hill, 1966); "Rediscovering asylums: the unhistorical history of the mental hospital," in *The Therapeutic Revolution: Essays in the Social History of American Medicine,* ed. Morris J. Vogel & Charles E. Rosenberg (Philadelphia, 1979) pp. 135–157; "Doing good and getting worse: the dilemma of social policy," *Mich. Law Rev.,* 1979, *77*: 761–783; and *Mental Illness and American Society, 1875–1940* (Princeton, 1983).

# RACE AND MEDICINE

Are black people medically different from whites? Apologists for slavery answered in the affirmative, arguing that the peculiar constitution of blacks fitted them for a life of bondage and required unique medical care. In an 1850 essay on "The Diseases and Physical Peculiarities of the Negro Race," Dr. Samuel Cartwright of New Orleans described as a popular northern "error" the notion that "the negro is a white man, but, by some accident of climate or locality, painted black, requiring nothing but liberty and equality—social and political—to wash him white." Not surprisingly, critics of slavery have tended to dismiss such claims as mere rationalizations. For example, in 1956 the historian Kenneth Stampp insisted that "innately Negroes *are*, after all, only white men with black skins, nothing more, nothing less."

Recent studies, reports Todd L. Savitt, have shown that despite basic anatomical and physiological similarities between blacks and whites, some medical differences do exist: blacks possess a greater natural resistance to yellow fever and some forms of malaria than whites, they tolerate humid heat better, and they suffer more readily from such genetically related diseases as sickle cell anemia.

The care sick slaves received, however, depended less on theories of racial differences than on the circumstances of their daily lives. Some planters, eager to protect their investment, contracted with local physicians to treat their slaves for a fixed yearly fee. More commonly, the master, mistress, or overseer—sometimes assisted by a black nurse—treated ailing slaves with home remedies, calling in physicians only for the most serious cases.

Slaves themselves often preferred to rely on their own folk remedies or to seek help from a black root doctor or conjurer.

Because of racial prejudice and their enslaved condition, blacks rarely had the opportunity to become trained physicians. In the years immediately preceding the Civil War a few blacks gained admittance to predominantly white medical schools, but opportunities remained scant until after the war, when black medical schools, beginning with the Howard University School of Medicine in 1868 and Meharry Medical College in 1876, first appeared. Of necessity, black physicians also established their own hospitals and medical societies, including the National Medical Association, created in 1895 because of the discriminatory policies of the American Medical Association.

Blacks and other powerless groups in American society have been particularly vulnerable to exploitation by physicians seeking living bodies for experimentation or cadavers for dissection. Although human experimentation often produced little of value, at least three surgical breakthroughs in the first half of the 19th century depended in part on the use of southern black bodies: Ephraim McDowell's removal of ovaries, Crawford Long's co-discovery of surgical anesthesia, and James Marion Sims's repair of vesico-vaginal fistulae. As Allan M. Brandt shows, the use of blacks for experimental purposes did not end with emancipation. The notorious Tuskegee syphilis study, undertaken by the U.S. Public Health Service in 1932 and involving hundreds of black males, continued until 1972, when public indignation brought it to a halt.

311

# 22

## Black Health on the Plantation:
## Masters, Slaves, and Physicians

### TODD L. SAVITT

Sickness and death were constant worries of 19th-century Americans, especially in the disease-ridden antebellum South, where, by 1860, over 4 million blacks, most of them enslaved, composed much of the work force. Their presence created a special situation for two reasons: first, whites, responsible for slave medical care, in large part dictated the living and working conditions that promoted or destroyed blacks' health; second, some white southerners claimed (and many others believed) that blacks were medically different from whites and so in need of special treatment. This paper will look at the three groups of southerners most directly involved in issues of black health and care — masters, physicians, and the slaves themselves — and consider their relationships to the special problem of slavery.[1]

Section I discusses how southern physicians used their own and others' observations of black medical differences to develop both a partial rationale for enslaving blacks in the American South and an approach to medical care and treatment of Negroes. Section II describes the various ways in which a master's treatment of his plantation slaves affected black health. Finally, Section III deals with black medical care provided by masters, physicians, and slaves and with the interactions of the three groups.

TODD L. SAVITT is Associate Professor of Medical Humanities and History at East Carolina University, Greenville, North Carolina.

This paper was originally prepared for publication in *Science and Medicine in the Old South*, edited by Ronald L. Numbers and Todd L. Savitt, forthcoming, and appears here with permission of the editors.

## WERE BLACKS MEDICALLY DIFFERENT FROM WHITES?

"Scarcely any observant medical man, having charge of negro estates, fails to discover, by experience, important modifications in the diseases and appropriate treatment of the white and black race respectively."[2] Thus wrote the editor of a prominent Virginia medical journal in 1856, in an attempt to impress upon the state's physicians the importance of providing adequate health care to slaves. He could very well have been speaking to all southern doctors, many of whom believed that medical differences existed between blacks and whites. The issue was of both practical and political importance: it involved not only the health care of an entire racial group in the South, but also the partial justification for enslaving them.

Physicians who treated slave diseases had a pecuniary and professional concern with the subject. Their recorded opinions in medical, commercial, and agricultural journals, as well as in personal correspondence, attest to the seriousness with which they approached issues of black health. The politically minded physicians (all of whom practiced medicine) were also resolutely committed to explaining the southern position on slavery. They, too, published for the medical, commercial, and lay public. Men like Josiah Clark Nott of Mobile and Samuel A. Cartwright of New Orleans utilized their knowledge of black medicine to rationalize the necessity and usefulness of slavery. These apologists for the peculiar institution, in order to prove that slavery was humane and economically viable in the South, argued that blacks possessed immunity to certain diseases which devastated whites. Slave-

313

owners, they said, did not sacrifice blacks every time they sent them into the rice fields or cane-brakes. Nor could physicians adequately treat blacks without knowledge of their anatomical and physiological peculiarities and disease proclivities. Blacks were medically different and mentally inferior to whites, they asserted.

In certain obvious physical ways Negroes did vary greatly from Caucasians. Old South writers particularly commented on facial features, hair, posture and gait, skin color, and odor. One school of American scientists spent much time and effort investigating cranium and brain size, as well as other characteristics, in part to discover whether blacks were inferior to whites. Physicians, slave-owners, and other interested persons also detected distinctions in the physical reactions of the two races both to diseases and to treatments. Their observations were often accurate, but at times they allowed racial prejudice to cloud their views. These observers remarked particularly about the relative immunity of blacks to southern fevers, especially intermittent fever (malaria) and yellow fever, susceptibility to intestinal and respiratory diseases, and tolerance of heat and intolerance of cold. Black children, they noted, died more frequently of marasmus (wasting away), convulsions, "teething," and suffocation or overlaying than did whites.[3]

One of the most fascinating subjects about which Old South medical authors wrote was black resistance to malaria, the focus of constant comment during the antebellum period because blacks' liability to it appeared to vary from region to region, plantation to plantation, and individual to individual. In dispute was the degree of susceptibility and the virulence of the disease in Negroes: Could slaves acquire some resistance to malaria by living in constant proximity to its supposed source? Were some slaves naturally immune? Did slaves have milder attacks of the disease than whites?

Modern science has answered many of the questions of immunity and prevention of malaria with which doctors and planters struggled in the antebellum period. Several factors contributed to the phenomenon of malarial immunity. As will be discussed below, many blacks did possess an inherited immunity to one or another form of malaria. But for Caucasians and those Negroes without natural resistance to a particular plasmodium (the organism that causes malaria) type, it was possible to acquire malarial immunity or tolerance only under the conditions stated by the author of an article in the *New Orleans Medical News and Hospital Gazette* (1858–1859) — by suffering repeated infections of the disease over a period of several years. For this to occur, one of the four species of plasmodium — falciparum, vivax, malariae, and ovale — had to be present constantly in the endemic region, so that with each attack a person's supply of antibodies was strengthened against further parasitic invasions. Interruption of this process, such as removal to nonendemic areas for the summer (when exposure to the parasite was useful in building immunity) or for several years (during schooling or travel), prohibited the aggregation of sufficient antibodies to resist infection. In truly endemic areas, acquiring immunity this way was a risky affair: unprotected children struggled for their lives, adults suffered from relapses of infections contracted years before, and partially immune adults worked through mild cases. It is no wonder, then, that slaves sold from, say, Virginia, where one form of malaria was prevalent, to a Louisiana bayou or South Carolina rice plantation, where a different species or strain of plasmodium was endemic, had a high incidence of the disease. Even adult slaves from Africa had to go through a "seasoning" period, because the strains of malarial parasites in this country differed from those in their native lands.

Generally speaking, most malaria in the upper South and in inland piedmont areas was of the milder vivax type, while vivax and the more dangerous falciparum malaria coexisted in coastal and swampy inland portions of both the lower and upper South. Rare pockets of the malariae type (quartan fever) were scattered across the South. Ovale malaria appears not to have been present in the United States. Of course, epidemics of one type or another could strike any neighborhood, resulting in sickness and death even to those who had acquired resistance to the endemic variety. *Plasmodium falciparum* usually caused such epidemics, especially in the temperate regions of the South.[4]

The major reason for black immunity to vivax or falciparum malaria relates not to acquired resistance, but to selective genetic factors. At least three hereditary conditions prevalent among blacks in parts of modern Africa appear to confer immunity to malaria upon their bearers. Recent medical research indicates that the red blood cells of persons lacking a specific factor called Duffy antigen are resistant to invasion of *Plasmodium vivax*. Approximately 90 percent of West Africans lack Duffy antigens, as do about 70 percent of Afro-Americans. This inherited, symptomless, hematologic condition is extremely rare in other racial groups. All evidence points to the conclusion that infection by *Plasmodium vivax* requires the presence of Duffy-positive red blood cells. Since most members of the Negro race do not possess this factor, they are immune to vivax malaria. It can be safely assumed that the vast majority of American slaves and free blacks were likewise resistant to this form of the disease.

Some antebellum blacks had additional protection against malaria resulting from two abnormal genetic hemoglobin conditions, sickle cell disease (a form of anemia) and sickle cell trait (the symptomless carrier state of the sickling gene). People with either of these conditions had milder cases of, and decreased risk of mortality from, the most malignant form of malaria, falciparum. Many of those who had sickle cell *disease* died from its consequences before or during adolescence; however, blacks who had sickle cell *trait* lived entirely normal lives and could then transmit the gene for sickling to their offspring. Since people with the trait had one normal gene and one abnormal gene for sickling (in contrast to those with the disease, who had two of the abnormal genes), their offspring could inherit sickle cell anemia only when each parent contributed a gene for sickling. Because the sickle cell condition was not discovered until 1910, physicians in the antebellum South were unaware that this was one reason why some slaves on plantations appeared to be immune to malarial infections. One other genetic condition with a high incidence within the former slave-trading region probably affords some malarial resistance: deficiency of the enzyme glucose-6-phosphate dehydrogenase (G-6-PD deficiency).

It is impossible to provide an exact calculation of sickle cell and G-6-PD deficiency gene prevalence among antebellum southern blacks. However, an estimate might be ventured based on known gene frequencies among present-day Afro-Americans and those Africans residing in former slave-trading areas. One leading medical authority on abnormal hemoglobins has estimated that at least 22 percent of Africans first brought to this country possessed genes for sickling. Other medical scientists have determined that approximately 20 percent of West Africans have genes for G-6-PD deficiency. Overall, then, using conservative figures, approximately 30–40 percent of newly arrived slaves had one or both of these genes. Recent evidence points to a higher-than-expected frequency of the G-6-PD gene in patients with sickle cell disease, which might reduce this estimate by a few percent. Thus a large proportion of Negroes were immune to the severe effects of falciparum malaria and to the less virulent vivax malaria, facts which planters and physicians in the South could not help but notice and discuss openly.

As with malaria, planters and physicians speculated publicly on blacks' intolerance of cold climates but could never adequately prove their contentions. It was the confirmed opinion of many white southerners that blacks could not withstand cold weather to the same degree as whites because of their dark skin and equatorial origins. Their major concern was that blacks seemed to resist and tolerate respiratory infections less well than whites. Since the germ theory of disease was years in the future, these men and others explained their observations with a combination of then-current though not universally accepted medical, anthropological, and scientific logic—and occasionally with unfounded theories. Blacks, natives of a tropical climate, were physiologically ill suited for the cold winter weather and cool spring and fall nights of the temperate zone. They breathed less air, dissipated a greater amount of "animal heat" through the skin, and eliminated larger quantities of carbon via liver and skin than whites. In addition, blacks were exposed to the elements for much of the year, placing a strain on heat production within the body. One medical extremist, Samuel A. Cartwright of New Orleans, even claimed that Negroes' lungs functioned inefficiently, causing "defective atmospherization of the blood." Some noted that slaves often slept with their heads (rather than their feet) next to the fire and entirely covered by a blanket; this was seen as proof that they required warm, moist air to breathe and to survive in this climate. Blacks were, these men concluded, physiologically different from whites.

Even today there is some confusion among medical authorities regarding the susceptibility of Negroes to severe pulmonary infections. Some claim a racial or genetic predisposition, while others deny it. Historically, blacks have shown a higher incidence and more severe manifestations of respiratory illness than have whites. Explanations for this phenomenon are numerous. First, Negroes did not experience bacterial pneumonias until the coming of the Caucasian. The entire newly exposed population was thus exquisitely sensitive to these infections, and developed much more serious cases than whites, who had had frequent contact with the bacteria since childhood. Second, black African laborers who today move from moist tropical to temperate climates (e.g., to the gold mines of South Africa) contract pneumonia at a much higher rate than whites. Though the incidence of disease decreases with time, it always remains at a more elevated level than among Caucasians. The same phenomenon probably operated during slavery. At first the mortality rate from pneumonia among newly arrived slaves was probably inordinately high, but with time the figure decreased somewhat, though it remains higher than in Caucasians. Third, there appears to be a close relationship between resistance to pulmonary infection and exposure to cool, wet weather. Slaves, who worked outdoors in all seasons and often lived in drafty, damp cabins, were therefore more likely to suffer from respiratory diseases than their masters. Fourth, poor diet, a common slave problem, predisposes people to infections like pneumonia and other respiratory problems.[5] Finally, overcrowding and unsanitary living conditions caused an increased incidence of respiratory diseases. Slaves living in small cottages or grouped together in a large community at the quarters, where intimate and frequent visiting was common, stood a greater chance of contracting airborne infections than did the more isolated whites. Undoubtedly, all these factors combined to increase the occurrence of respiratory illness among southern blacks.

The most serious nonfatal manifestation of cold intolerance was frostbite. At least one proslavery apologist claimed that the Negro race was more susceptible than whites to this condition: "Almost every one has seen negroes in Northern cities, who have lost their legs by frost at sea—a thing rarely witnessed among whites, and yet where a single negro has been thus exposed doubtless a thousand of the former have."[6] The condition was a serious one, especially for slaveowners who stood to lose the labor of valuable workers.

Blacks are in fact more susceptible to cold injury than whites. Studies conducted during and after the Korean War indicate that blacks have a poorer adaptive response to cold exposure than do whites in the following ways: their metabolic rates increase more slowly and not as much as whites; their first shivers (one of the body's defensive responses to cold) occur at a lower skin temperature than for whites; and their incidence of frostbite is higher and their cases more severe than those of whites. Even after blacks have acclimated to cold (and they do so in a manner physiologically similar to whites), they are then only slightly less liable to sustain cold injury than they had been previously. Those antebellum observers who warned against overexposure of slaves to cold were essentially correct.

Racial differences in tolerance to heat also exist but may be modified under certain conditions. Again, antebellum observers agreed that blacks, having originated in an area known for its heat and humidity, were ideally suited for labor in the damp, warm South. One northern physician, John H. Van Evrie, explained blacks' resistance to heat in both religious and physiological terms:

> God has adapted him, both in his physical and mental structure, to the tropics. . . . His head is protected from the rays of a vertical sun by a dense mat of woolly hair, wholly impervious to its fiercest heats, while his entire surface, studded with innumerable sebaceous glands, forming a complete excretory system, relieves him from all those climatic influences so fatal, under the same circumstances, to the sensitive and highly organized white man. Instead of seeking to shelter himself from the burning sun of the tropics, he courts it, enjoys it, delights in its fiercest heats.[7]

Modern medical investigators would not agree with Van Evrie's reasoning. But they have discovered that under normal living conditions Negroes in Africa and the United States are better equipped to tolerate humid heat than whites. However, both races possess the same capacity to acclimatize to hot, humid conditions. The physiological mechanisms by which the human body acclimatizes to heat can be readily observed and measured. Increased external temperature causes the body to perspire more, resulting in a greater evaporative heat loss, a decline in skin and rectal temperatures, and a drop in the heart rate from its initially more rapid pace. When whites and blacks are equally active in the same environment over a period of time, there is little difference in heat tolerance.

From this information it can be assumed that in the Old South slaves and free blacks possessed a higher *natural* tolerance to humid heat stress than did whites. In addition, Negroes became quickly acclimatized to performance of their particular tasks under the prevailing climatic conditions of the region. This natural and acquired acclimatization enabled black laborers to withstand the damp heat of summer better than whites, who were unused to physical exertion under such severe conditions. White farm and general laborers, however, also must have adjusted to the heat and fared as well as blacks. One physiological difference between Caucasians and Negroes which might have affected work performance in the hot, humid South was the latter's inherent ability to discharge smaller amounts of sodium chloride and other vital body salts (electrolytes) into sweat and urine. Excessive loss of these salts leads to heat prostration and heatstroke. Thus conservation of needed electrolytes provided slaves with an advantage over laboring whites, whose requirements for replacement of the substances were greater. In the case of heat tolerance, then, white observers were correct in noting a racial difference, but they tended to ignore the fact that many whites did become acclimatized to the hot, humid environment.

Whites detected, or thought they detected, distinctive variances in black susceptibility to several other medical conditions common in the antebellum South. Many believed that slave women developed prolapsed uteri at a higher rate than white women, though modern anatomists have shown that Negroes are actually less prone to this affliction than Caucasians. Observers also noted that slaves were frequent sufferers of typhoid fever, worms, and dysentery, though we now know that the reason for this high prevalence was environmental rather than racial or genetic. Blacks did, however, have a greater resistance to the yellow fever virus than whites.

One disease that drew great attention because of its frequency and virulence was consumption

(pulmonary tuberculosis), a leading cause of death in 19th-century America for members of both races. A particular form of the disease — characterized by extreme difficulty in breathing, unexplained abdominal pain around the navel, and rapidly progressing debility and emaciation, usually resulting in death — struck blacks so commonly that it came to be known as Negro Consumption or *Struma Africana*. In all likelihood most of the cases which white southerners described as Negro Consumption were miliary tuberculosis, the most serious and fatal form of the disease known, in which tubercles are found in many body organs simultaneously, overwhelming what natural defenses exist. The reason that rapidly fatal varieties of the disease (so-called galloping consumption) afflicted Negroes more frequently than Caucasians may be related to the fact that Caucasians (like Mongolians) had suffered from tuberculosis for many hundreds of years and had developed a strong immune response to the infection, whereas Africans (and American Indians and Eskimos) had been exposed to tuberculosis only since the coming of the white man and had not yet built up this same effective resistance. Others have discounted racial immunity as an explanation and have argued that, as a "virgin" population, blacks were highly susceptible to serious first attacks of tuberculosis. Additional factors such as malnourishment, preexisting illness, or general debility also contributed to the apparent black predisposition to tuberculosis.

Neonatal tetanus (also called *trismus nascentium*) was a common cause of death among newborn slaves throughout the South. Slaveowners and physicians, who recognized its origin in the improper handling of the umbilical stump, often discussed it in their writings. It still kills large numbers of children in undeveloped countries. *Clostridium tetani*, the same bacterium which caused tetanus in older children and adults, also infected newborns through the unwashed and frequently touched umbilical stump. In a typical antebellum case, related by Dr. Albert Snead of Richmond to his colleagues at a medical society meeting in 1853, an eight-day-old black child first refused her mother's breast and gave a few convulsive hand jerks. Soon the baby's entire muscular system was rigid, with her head bent back, fists and jaws clenched, and feet tightly flexed, as the bacterial toxin affected central nervous system tissue. In this case death from suffocation owing to respiratory muscle paralysis did not intervene until the 18th day (though it usually occurred within 7 to 10 days).

One cause of death which Virginians did not consider a disease and which seemed to occur almost exclusively among the slave population was "smothering," "overlaying," or "suffocation." Observers assumed that sleeping mothers simply rolled onto or pressed snugly against their infants, cutting off the air supply, or that angry, fearful parents intentionally destroyed their offspring rather than have them raised in slavery. Modern medical evidence strongly indicates that most of these deaths may be ascribed to a condition presently known as Sudden Infant Death Syndrome (SIDS) or "crib death" which, for reasons yet unexplained, affects blacks more frequently than whites.[8]

The diseases and conditions discussed above represent only some of the several which whites noted affected blacks and whites differently. Others are difficult to trace back to slavery times either through direct records or by implication through comparative West African medicine. Among those not mentioned, the most important is hypertension (high blood pressure). Others include polydactyly (six or more fingers per hand), umbilical hernia, cancers of the cervix, stomach, lungs, esophagus, and prostate, and toxemia of pregnancy. At the same time, Negroes are much less susceptible to hookworm disease, cystic fibrosis, and skin cancer than Caucasians.

Though blacks are not the only racial or ethnic group possessing increased immunity and susceptibility to specific diseases, they were the only group whose medical differences mattered to white residents of the Old South. Reports of black medical "peculiarities" appeared regularly in periodicals and pamphlets, presumably to alert southern physicians of problems they might encounter in practice. Agricultural and medical journal articles and medical student dissertations also discussed racial differences in responses to medical treatments. Most writers agreed that blacks withstood the heroic, depletive therapies of the day (bleeding, purging, vomiting, blistering) less well than whites.

Despite many writings on the subject of black diseases and treatments, no comprehensive discussion existed in any standard textbook for student doctors or practitioners. Some articles on the subject of treatment provided vague information, such

as: "The Caucasian seems to yield more readily to remedies . . . than the African," or, "It is much more difficult to form a just diagnosis or prognosis with the latter [African] than the former [white], consequently the treatment is often more dubious."[9] In 1855 an editor of the *Virginia Medical and Surgical Journal* suggested that a Virginian write a book on "the modifications of disease in the Negro constitution." The subject, he proclaimed, stood "invitingly open"; no medical student, "fresh from Watson or Wood [textbooks of the day], with his new lancet and his armory of antiphlogistics," had been properly trained to treat many of the diseases to which the black man was subject: "Has he been taught that the African constitution sinks before the heavy blows of the 'heroic school' and runs down under the action of purgatives; that when the books say blood letting and calomel, the black man needs nourishment and opium?"[10] Many other southern medical writers put forth urgent pleas for medical school courses and books on black medicine.

John Stainbach Wilson, a Columbus, Georgia, physician who had spent years practicing medicine in southern Alabama, came closest to actually producing a textbook on black health. Its advertised title indicated the wide scope of the proposed contents: *The Plantation and Family Physician; A Work for Families Generally and for Southern Slaveowners Especially; Embracing the Peculiarities and Diseases, the Medical and Hygienic Management of Negroes, Together with the Causes, Symptoms, and Treatment of the Principal Diseases to Whites and Blacks*. But apparently the outbreak of hostilities in 1861 interrupted Wilson's plans. It was not until more than 100 years later, in 1975, that the first *Textbook of Black-Related Diseases* was finally published, written this time by black physicians.

For southern whites, black medical problems and health care had political as well as medical ramifications. Men like Cartwright, Nott, and Wilson were writing for an audience who wished to hear that blacks were distinct from whites. This was, after all, a part of the proslavery argument. Medical theory and practice were still in such a state of flux in the late 18th and early 19th centuries that there was little risk of any true scientific challenge to a medical system based on racial differences. Observers were correct in noting that blacks showed differing susceptibility and immunity to a few specific diseases and conditions. They capitalized on these conditions to illustrate the inferiority of blacks to whites, to rationalize the use of this "less fit" racial group as slaves, to justify subjecting Negro slaves to harsh working conditions in extreme dampness and heat in the malarious regions of the South, and to prove to their critics that they recognized the special medical weaknesses of blacks and took these failings into account when providing for their human chattel. But in terms of an overall theory of medical care predicated on racial inferiority, the issue was a false one. It is instructive to note here, for example, that no writer ventured beyond vague and cautious statements about bleeding or purging blacks less than whites. None presented an account of the amount of blood loss or the dose of medicine which was optimal for blacks. Remarks on the subject were always couched in terms which placed whites in a position of medical and physical superiority over Negroes, perfect for polemics and useless to the practitioner.

## LIVING AND WORKING CONDITIONS

The state of slave health depended not only on disease immunities and susceptibilities but also on living and working conditions. How masters provided for sanitation, housing, food, clothing, and children's and women's special needs, and how they worked and disciplined their human chattel, had a great effect on the health of the black work force.[11] (See Table 1.)

Most bondsmen lived on plantations or farms in a well-defined area known as the quarters. Here was an ideal setting for the spread of disease, similar to the situation which existed in antebellum urban areas. What might have been considered a personal illness in the isolated, white, rural family dwelling became in a three- or ten- or thirty-home slave community a matter of public health and group concern.

At the slave quarters sneezing, coughing, or contact with improperly washed eating utensils and personal belongings promoted transmission of disease-causing microorganisms among family members. Poor ventilation, lack of sufficient windows for sunshine, and damp earthen floors merely added to the problem by aiding the growth of fungus and bacteria on food, clothing, floors, and

utensils, and the development of worm and insect larvae. Improper personal hygiene (infrequent baths, hairbrushings, and haircuts, unwashed clothes, unclean beds) led to such nuisances as bedbugs, body lice (which also carried typhus germs), ringworm of skin and scalp, and pinworms. In a household cramped for space, these diseases became family, not individual, problems. And when two or more families shared homes and facilities, the problem of contagion became further aggravated.

Contacts outside the home also facilitated the dissemination of disease. Children who played together all day under the supervision of a few older women, and then returned to their cabins in the evening, spread their day's accumulation of germs to other family members. Even mere Sunday and evening socializing in an ill neighbor's cabin was enough to "seed" the unsuspecting with disease. Contaminated water, unwashed or poorly cooked food, worm-larvae-infested soil, and disease-carrying farm animals and rodents also contributed their share to the unhealthfulness of the quarters.

The two major types of seasonal diseases which afflicted Old Dominion blacks—respiratory and intestinal—reflected living conditions within most slave communities. Respiratory illnesses prevailed during the cold months, when slaves were forced to spend much time indoors in intimate contact with their families and friends. Several important contagious diseases were spread through contact with respiratory system secretions: tuberculosis, diphtheria, colds and upper respiratory infections, influenza, pneumonia, and streptococcal infections (including sore throats and scarlet fever). The community life of the slave quarters also provided excellent surroundings for dissemination of several year-round diseases contracted through respiratory secretions. People today tend to regard these illnesses—whooping cough, measles, chicken pox, and mumps—as limited to the younger population, but adult slaves who had never experienced an outbreak of, say, measles, in Africa or the United States were quite susceptible to infection and even death. Measles and whooping cough are still important causes of fatality in developing countries, as they were in antebellum Virginia.

As warm weather arrived and workers spent more time outdoors, intestinal diseases caused by

Table 1
Leading Known Causes of Death in Virginia, 1850[a], by Race[b]

| White (N = 8,014)[c] | Percent | Slave (N = 6,284)[c] | Percent | Free Black (N = 558)[c] | Percent |
|---|---|---|---|---|---|
| 1. Tuberculosis[d] | 13.8 | 1. Respiratory diseases[e] | 16.1 | 1. Cholera[j] | 17.2 |
| 2. Respiratory diseases[e] | 9.2 | 2. Tuberculosis[d] | 10.7 | 2. Tuberculosis[d] | 13.8 |
| 3. Nervous system diseases[f] | 8.6 | 3. Nervous system diseases[f] | 7.9 | 3. Respiratory diseases[e] | 10.0 |
| 4. Diarrhea[g] | 8.5 | 4. Old age | 7.3 | 4. Old age | 7.9 |
| 5. Scarlet fever[h] | 6.9 | 5. Dropsy[i] | 6.0 | 5. Dropsy[i] | 7.5 |
| 6. Dropsy[i] | 5.5 | 6. Typhoid[k] | 5.7 | 6. Nervous system diseases[f] | 6.5 |
| 7. Cholera[j] | 4.9 | 7. Diarrhea[g] | 5.5 | 7. Diarrhea[g] | 5.9 |
| 8. Typhoid[k] | 4.7 | 8. Cholera[j] | 5.5 | 8. Accidents[n] | 5.8 |
| 9. Old age | 4.5 | 9. Accidents[n] | 4.5 | 9. Typhoid[k] | 2.9 |
| 10. Digestive system diseases[l] | 4.5 | 10. Digestive system diseases[l] | 3.2 | 10. Digestive system diseases[l] | 2.5 |
| 11. Diphtheria[m] | 3.5 | 11. Diphtheria[m] | 2.3 | 11. Whooping cough | 2.5 |
| 12. Accidents[n] | 3.4 | 12. Suffocation[q] | 2.2 | 12. Maternity[o] | 2.0 |
| 13. Maternity[o] | 2.1 | 13. Scarlet fever[h] | 2.0 | 13. Worms | 2.0 |
| 14. Measles | 1.5 | 14. Worms | 1.8 | 14. Teething | 1.3 |
| 15. Whooping cough | 1.4 | 15. Maternity[o] | 1.8 | 15. Diphtheria[m] | 1.1 |
| 16. Neoplasms[p] | 1.2 | 16. Measles | 1.6 | 16. Intemperance | 1.1 |
| 17. Heart disease | 0.8 | 17. Teething | 1.5 | 17. Malaria[r] | 0.7 |
| 18. Teething | 0.8 | 18. Whooping cough | 1.5 | 18. Scarlet fever[h] | 0.7 |
| 19. Worms | 0.8 | 19. Homicide | 0.9 | 19. Measles | 0.5 |
| 20. Erysipelas | 0.7 | 20. Heart disease | 0.6 | 20. Homicide | 0.5 |
| Fevers (unclassifiable)[s] | 6.5 | Fevers (unclassifiable)[s] | 5.5 | Fevers (unclassifiable)[s] | 4.6 |

[a]Includes figures from the entire state. Compiled from *Mortality Statistics of the Seventh Census of the United States, 1850* (Washington, D.C., 1855), pp. 291–295.

[b]All figures are percentages of the total number of deaths for that race during the designated time period. Causes listed as "unknown" were excluded from the computations.

[c]The numbers in parentheses reflect the total number of deaths from all known causes for that race. Only leading causes are listed for each race.

[d]Consumption, scrofula

[e]Asthma, bronchitis, catarrh, catarrhal fever, influenza, disease of lungs, pleurisy, pneumonia

[f]Apoplexy, disease of brain, chorea, congestion of brain, convulsions, epilepsy, brain fever, inflammation of brain, insanity, neuralgia, paralysis, disease of spine

[g]Cholera infantum, diarrhea, dysentery, summer complaint

[h]Scarlet fever, disease of throat, quinsy

[i]Dropsy, hydrothorax, ascites

[j]Cholera epidemics struck Virgina during the period covered by this census.

[k]Typhoid fever was referred to as typhus fever in the list of causes of death in the 1850 census.

[l]Disease of bowels, colic, cramp, dyspepsia, hernia, inflammation of bowels, inflammation of stomach, jaundice, disease of liver, piles, disease of stomach

[m]Croup

[n]Burns, drownings, scaldings, explosions, shootings, railroad, unspecified

[o]Childbirth, puerperal fever

[p]Cancer, tumor

[q]Many of these deaths are probably attributable to what is known now as crib death or Sudden Infant Death Syndrome (SIDS).

[r]Intermittent fever, remittent fever

[s]Bilious fever, congestive fever, inflammatory fever, fever not specified

poor outdoor sanitation and close contact with the earth became common. Respiratory diseases decreased in frequency and insects became important culprits in the spread of disease — particularly maladies of the digestive tract and various "fevers." What more could a mosquito or housefly wish than a large concentration of human beings, decaying leftover food scraps, scattered human feces, or a compost heap? Mosquitoes discharged yellow fever or malarial parasites while obtaining fresh blood from their victims. Flies transported bacteria such as *Vibrio* (cholera), *Salmonella* (food poisoning and typhoid), and *Shigella* (bacillary dysentery), the virus which causes infectious hepatitis, and the protozoan *Entameba histolytica* (amebic dysentery) from feces to food. Trichina worms, embedded in the muscles of hogs inhabiting yards often shared with bondsmen, were released into a slave's body when the meat was not completely cooked. Finally, there were the large parasitic worms, a concomitant of primitive sanitation.

Intestinal disorders were at least as common among antebellum Virginia's blacks as were respiratory diseases. The human alimentary tract is distinguished among all other body systems in that it receives daily large amounts of foreign material, usually in the form of food, which it must sort and assimilate into a usable form. In the Old South, where living conditions were generally unhygienic, seemingly good food and drink often concealed pathogenic organisms ranging from viruses to worm larvae. Hands entering mouths sometimes contained the germs that others had cast off in feces, urine, or contaminated food. It is not surprising to find that dysentery, typhoid fever, food poisoning, and worm diseases afflicted large numbers of southerners, especially those living in the poorest, most crowded circumstances, without sanitary facilities or time to prepare food properly. Slaves often fit into this category.

Syphilis and its bacteriologically unrelated associate, gonorrhea, are not transmitted through filth or unsanitary living conditions, but they were public health problems in the antebellum South nonetheless. Though morbidity figures for whites and blacks do not exist, the frequency with which these two diseases appeared in physicians' casebooks points to a rate which may be, as one historian has stated, "startling." Masters knew that venereal disease was disseminated by intimate sexual contact, but they also knew how difficult it was to prevent contagion by recognition and isolation of infected individuals.

Old South physicians' records tell only part of the story of gonorrhea and syphilis. For each case that was recorded, many were not, because people treated the disease themselves or waited until it disappeared. They did not realize the potential hazards of concealment to personal and public health. Venereal diseases probably occurred with a frequency which could be considered epidemic. Each newly reported case arose from a person already harboring the microorganisms; that person, in turn, probably had spread the germs to several other unsuspecting victims.

Though the major medical problems at the quarters were communicable diseases, in the course of each day bondsmen faced other health problems unrelated to contagion or parasites. Inadequate clothing and food, poor working conditions, harsh physical punishment, pregnancy, and bodily disorders also made slaves sick or uncomfortable, often rendering them useless to their masters and burdensome to their friends and family.

Though adequate clothing was important for slaves, it did not play as crucial a role in the maintenance of health as did housing. Of course clothing covered and protected the body from exposure to wind, sun, rain, snow, cold, and insects. It also limited the severity of many minor falls to cuts, scrapes, and bruises, and of some industrial accidents to burns over small areas. But only a few disorders are spread by contact with infected clothing (smallpox, body lice, impetigo, typhus) or by contact of exposed skin with other objects (tetanus, yaws, hookworm, brucellosis).

Except in cases where slaves were truly underclothed in winter, possibly causing decreased resistance to respiratory ailments, the danger of contracting disease owing to inadequate or dirty wearing apparel was relatively small. Of articles of clothing which masters provided their bondsmen, shoes were probably the most important in terms of health and disease. Not only did they provide warmth in the winter to feet and toes highly susceptible to frostbite, but they also protected slaves against hookworm penetration, scrapes, scratches, burns, and some puncture wounds which would otherwise have caused tetanus.

Did slaves receive a diet adequate to keep them

healthy, laboring, and producing vigorous off-spring? Opinions vary on this question, for diets differed from individual to individual and our understanding of nutritional needs has changed often. Based on current dietary standards, the daily typical ration, one quart of whole ground, dry, bolted cornmeal, prepared from white corn (the South's favorite), and half a pound of cured, medium-fat ham with no bone or skin, could not have provided enough essential nutrients to sustain a moderately active, 22-year-old male or female, much less a hard-working laborer or a pregnant or lactating woman. Fieldhands fed this diet alone (with water) would soon have become emaciated and sickly and would have shown symptoms of several nutrient deficiencies. It is highly unlikely that any slave could have survived very long on a diet consisting solely of pork and cornmeal.

Most Old Dominion masters provided supplements to the basic hogmeat and cornmeal, a practice most urgently recommended by agricultural writers throughout the state. Vegetables topped the list of required additional foods. Planters could, if they planned ahead, have a ready supply of at least one or two varieties throughout the year. These writers also suggested adding, when available, fish, fresh meat, molasses, milk, and buttermilk to slave diets.

Many agricultural authors and slavemasters indicated in their writings that blacks often raised vegetables, poultry, and even pigs on their own plots of land near the quarters. The assumption was that extra food from this source would supplement rations supplied by the master. Surprisingly, however, some of these same writers also pointed out that slaves usually sold what they raised to the master or at the marketplace, thereby defeating the major purpose of the plan. In all likelihood the slaves did not dispose of all their produce, but saved some for future needs. The fact that there were bondsmen who sold rather than kept food indicates that, other than those saving every available penny to purchase their freedom, some slaves received sufficient nutrition from their regular rations, supplemented by homegrown food, to feel quite comfortable relying on their masters for proper nutrition.

Kenneth Kiple and Virginia H. King, in their recent book on the subject, *Another Dimension to the Black Diaspora*, assess the adequacy of a slave diet consisting primarily of pork and cornmeal supplemented occasionally with other foods.[12] Using recently discovered knowledge of human nutritional needs and nutrient actions and interactions in the body, they conclude that slaves received sufficient amounts of carbohydrates and calories but generally lacked some essential amino acids, vitamin C, riboflavin, niacin, thiamine, vitamin D, calcium, and iron. And slave children, who all too often began life with nutritional deficiencies owing to their mothers' poor pre- and postnatal diets, also lacked sufficient magnesium, calories, and protein in their diets. Not surprisingly, Kiple and King assert, slave adults and children suffered higher morbidity and mortality than whites because of lower resistance to infection and disrupted basic metabolic pathways. Among the most common resultant black health problems were respiratory and intestinal diseases, skin and eye afflictions, "teething," tetanus, "fits and seizures," and rickets. Diet, controlled to a large degree by the master, greatly affected slave health.

In addition to providing food, clothing, and housing, slaveowners also directed working conditions, punishments, and care of women and children. Though warm weather helped the crops grow, it did not always have the same effect on the black Virginians who tended them. Planters recording the effects of excessive heat on their fieldhands made it clear that even though Negroes originated in tropical Africa, they were not immune to sunstroke. Hill Carter of Shirley Plantation wrote, for instance, during the 1825 wheat harvest, "Hotest day ever felt—men gave out & some fainted."[13]

Slaveowners also recognized the potential hazards of overexertion and exposure. Some indulged their slaves by easing their tasks; others found this impossible, especially at certain times of the year. Hill Carter and no doubt many others worked their blacks in intense heat when necessary to harvest a crop. Charles Friend of Prince George County, on the other hand, had second thoughts when the ditching operation to which he had assigned many slaves evolved into a messy and unhealthy job: "We have the ditchers knee deep in water and mud. If I had known how bad it was I should not have put them to work at it but hired labor to do it."[14]

Farm accidents also took their toll on slaves. Falls, overturned carts, runaway wagons, drownings, limbs caught in farm machines, kicks from animals, and cuts from axes or scythe blades were the commonest types. Occasionally slaves suffered more remarkable mishaps, as when a 260-pound Culpepper County fieldhand jumped eight feet from a hay loft onto a pile of hay in which a wooden pitchfork lay concealed. The point punctured the man's scrotum and passed into his abdominal cavity, but miraculously pierced no internal organs. Thanks to prompt surgical attention he was doing "light work" around the plantation about three weeks later.

The whip was an integral part of slave life in the Old Dominion and the Old South. Those bondsmen who had not experienced its sting first-hand were acquainted with persons, usually friends or relatives, who had. Whites held out the threat of whipping as a means of maintaining order. When strong discipline was called for, so, very often, was the lash. Even the mildest and most God-fearing of masters permitted application of this painful instrument in extreme cases, though some insisted that the slave's skin not be cut or that there be a responsible witness present when punishment was administered.

From a medical point of view, whipping inflicted cruel and often permanent injuries upon its victims. Laying stripes across the bare back or buttocks caused indescribable pain, especially when each stroke dug deeper into previously opened wounds. During the interval between lashes, victims anticipated the next in anguish, wishing for postponement or for all due speed, though neither alternative brought relief. In addition to multiple lacerations of the skin, whipping caused loss of blood, injury to muscles (and internal organs, if the lash reached that deep), and shock. (Rubbing salt into these wounds, often complained of as a further mode of torture, actually cleansed the injured, exposed tissues and helped ward off infection). The paddle jarred every part of the body by the violence of the blow, and raised blisters from repeated strokes. In addition to the possibility of death (uncommon), there was the danger that muscle damage inflicted by these instruments might permanently incapacitate a slave or deform him for life. An Old Dominion slave who experienced the sting of the paddle recalled years later: "You be jes' as raw as a piece of beef an' hit eats you up. He loose you an' you go to house no work done

dat day."[15] No work done that day or, in many cases, for several days. Ellick, a rebellious member of Charles Friend's White Hill Plantation slave force, was slapped one day "for not being at the stable in time this morning," and "soundly whipped" the next day for running away and for not submitting to a flogging earlier that morning. He spent the next week recovering in bed, only to receive another whipping upon his return to work. This time he ran off for two days before settling back into the plantation routine.

The daily routines of slave women and children were often upset by health conditions peculiar to these groups. Female slaves probably lost more time from work for menstrual pain, discomfort, and disorders than for any other cause. Planters rarely named illnesses in their diaries or daybooks, but the frequency and regularity with which women of childbearing age appeared on sick lists indicates that menstrual conditions were a leading complaint. A Fauquier County physician considered the loss of four to eight weekdays per month not unusual for slave women. Among the menstrual maladies which afflicted bondswomen most often were amenorrhea (lack of menstrual flow), abnormal bleeding between cycles (sometimes caused by benign and malignant tumors), and abnormal discharges (resulting from such conditions as gonorrhea, tumors, and prolapsed uterus).

Some servants took advantage of their masters by complaining falsely of female indispositions. One unnamed Virginian who owned numerous slaves complained to Frederick Law Olmsted about such malingering women:

> The women on a plantation . . . will hardly earn their salt, after they come to the breeding age; they don't come to the field, and you go to the quarters and ask the old nurse what's the matter, and she says, "oh, she's not well, master; she's not fit to work, sir;" and what can you do? You have to take her word for it that something or other is the matter with her, and you dare not set her to work; and so she lays up till she feels like taking the air again, and plays the lady at your expense.[16]

Masters found it difficult to separate the sick from the falsely ill; as a result they often indulged their breeding-aged women rather than risk unknown complications. Thomas Jefferson, for instance, ordered his overseer not to coerce the female workers into exerting themselves, because "women . . . are destroyed by exposure to wet at certain periodical indispositions to which nature has subjected them."[17]

If white Virginians treated women's gynecological complaints with a certain delicacy, they regarded pregnancy as almost holy. In addition to receiving time off from work and avoiding whippings, expectant women were protected from execution in capital offenses until after parturition.[18] At least three cases arose between the Revolution and the Civil War in which slave women obtained execution postponements for this reason, though all were presumably put to death following delivery.

Children, like women, were exposed to certain unique disorders which caused illness or death. Though their labor did not usually account for much, young slaves' serious illnesses did mean time lost from work for mothers watching over them at home or distractedly worrying about them while performing daily tasks. Slave children suffered more frequently from most illnesses than their white counterparts, especially diarrhea, neonatal tetanus, convulsions, "teething" (not really a disease, but considered a cause of sickness and death prior to the 20th century), diphtheria, respiratory diseases, and whooping cough, owing to poorer living conditions and diet.

Worms occurred frequently in black children. The poor sanitary conditions at many antebellum Virginia slave quarters were conducive to the development of these parasites in the soil. Children playing in the dirt inevitably picked up worm larvae as they put fingers in mouths. Failure to use, or lack of, privy facilities only served to spread worm diseases to other residents of the quarters and to visiting slaves, who then carried these parasites to their own plantation quarters.

Some black children had overt sickle cell disease (noted above) with irregular hemolytic crises, severe joint pains, chronic leg ulcers, and abdominal pains. The medical records relating to antebellum Virginia do not provide any clear descriptions of the disease, probably because its symptoms resemble so many other conditions and because the sickness was not known until 1910. These children were often the "sickly" ones, useless for field work or heavy household duties, expensive to maintain because of frequent infections,

and often unable to bear children if they survived puberty. Their lot was a poor and painful one.

Slave children also developed diseases which no one could identify or treat. John Walker's young servants appeared one day with "head ach sweled faces & belly diseases";[19] Colonel John Ambler's evidenced swollen feet and faces, and bones cutting through the skin; and Landon Carter's had "swelling of the almonds of . . . [their] ears which burst inward and choaked . . . [them]."[20] The white tutor at Nomini Hall, Philip Vickers Fithian, noticed that one slave mother on this Westmoreland County estate had lost seven children successively, none of whom had even reached the age of ten: "The Negroes all seem much alarm'd. . . ."[21] Childhood was generally the least healthy period of a slave's life in antebellum Virginia.

## SLAVE MEDICAL CARE

Bondage placed slaves in a difficult position with regard to health care. When taken ill they had a limited range of choices. Masters usually insisted that their slaves, legally an article of property, immediately inform the person in charge of any sickness so the malady might be arrested before it worsened. But some bondsmen, as people, felt reluctant to submit to the often harsh prescriptions and remedies of 18th- and 19th-century white medical practice. They preferred self-treatment or reliance on cures recommended by friends and older relatives. They depended on Negro herb and root doctors, or on influential conjurers among the local black population. This desire to treat oneself, or at least to have the freedom to choose one's mode of care, came into direct conflict with the demands and wishes of white masters, whose trust in black medicine was usually slight and whose main concern was keeping the slave force intact.

To further compound the problem, unannounced illnesses did not entitle bondsmen to time off from work. To treat their own illnesses slaves had to conceal them or pass them off to the master as less serious than they actually were. Masters who complained that blacks tended to report sickness only after the disease had progressed to a serious stage often discovered that slaves had treated illnesses at home first. The blacks' dilemma, then, was whether to delay reporting illnesses and treat those diseases at home, risking white reprisal; or to submit at once to the medicines of white America and, in a sense, surrender their bodies to their masters. The result was a dual system in which some slaves received treatment both from whites and blacks.

When illness afflicted a slave, white Virginians responded in several ways. They almost always applied treatments derived from European experience. Most often the master, mistress, or overseer first attempted to treat the ailment with home remedies. If the patient failed to respond to these home ministrations, the family physician was summoned. Some slaveowners distrusted "regular" doctors and called instead "irregular" practitioners: Thomsonians, homeopaths, hydropaths, empirics, eclectics, etc. Masters who hired out their bondsmen to others for a period of time arranged for medical care when signing the hiring bond. Whatever the situation, Virginians often displayed concern for the health of blacks in bondage. The reasons were threefold: slaves represented a financial investment which required protection; many masters felt a true humanitarian commitment toward their slaves; and whites realized that certain illnesses could easily spread to their own families if not properly treated and contained.

Those responsible for the care of sick slaves made home treatment the first step in the restorative process. White Virginians recognized that physicians, though possessed of great knowledge of the human body and the effects of certain medicines on it, were severely limited in the amount of good they could perform. Because no one understood the etiology of most diseases, no one could effectively cure them. Astute nonmedical observers could make diagnoses as well as doctors, and could even treat patients just as effectively. Physicians played their most crucial roles in executing certain surgical procedures, assisting mothers at childbirth, and instilling confidence in sick patients through an effective bedside manner. At other times their excessive use of drugs, overready cups and leeches, and ever-present lancets produced positive harm in depleting the body of blood and nourishment and exhausting the already weakened patient with frequent purges, vomits, sweats, and diuretics. Laymen often merely followed the same course of treatment that they had observed their physicians using or that they had read about in one of the ubiquitous domestic medical guides. Anyone could practice blood-letting or dosing with a little experience. And a physician's services cost money, even when no treatment or cure resulted from the consultation.

Home care was not an innovation of 18th-century Virginians, but one that stemmed from man's natural instinct to relieve his own or his family's illness as quickly as possible. The unavailability of physicians, the inaccessibility of many farms to main highways, and the lack of good roads and speedy means of transportation reinforced such thinking among rural Virginians. Even when a doctor was summoned, hours or even a day passed before his arrival, during which time something had to be done to ease the patient's discomfort. People learned to tolerate pain and to cope with death, but the mitigation of suffering was still a primary goal. To that end most Virginians stocked their cabinets with favorite remedies (or the ingredients required for their preparation) in order to be well equipped when relief was demanded. On large plantations with many slaves this was a necessity, as Catherine C. Hopley, tutor at Forest Rill near Tappahannock, Essex County, noted: "A capacious medicine chest is an inseparable part of a Southern establishment; and I have seen medicines enough dispensed to furnish good occupation for an assistant, when colds or epidemics have prevailed."[22] Some physicians made a living selling medicine chests and domestic health guides designed specifically for use on southern plantations. Self-sufficiency in medical care was desirable on farms and even in urban households, especially when financial considerations were important.

An additional feature of home medical care for slaves was the plantation hospital or infirmary. Its form varied from farm to farm and existed primarily on the larger slaveholdings. It was quicker and more efficient to place ailing slaves in one building, where care could be tendered with a minimum amount of wasted movement and where all medicines, special equipment, and other necessary stores could be maintained. Of course, infectious diseases could spread quite rapidly through a hospital, subjecting those with noncontagious conditions to further sickness.

Armed with drugs from the plantation or home dispensary, one person, usually white, had the responsibility of dosing and treating ill slaves. The master, mistress, or overseer spent time each day with those claiming bodily disorders and soon developed a certain facility in handling both patients and drugs. The approach was empirical—if a particular medication or combination of drugs succeeded in arresting symptoms, it became the standard treatment for that malady in that household until a better one came along. Overseers and owners inscribed useful medical recipes into their diaries or journals and clipped suggestions from newspapers, almanacs, and books.

An overseer's or owner's incompetence or negligence was the slave's loss. New and inexperienced farm managers, unskilled in the treatment of illness, necessarily used bondsmen as guinea pigs for their "on-the-job" training. As a consequence of living on the wrong plantation at the wrong time, some slaves probably lost their lives or became invalids at the hands of new, poorly trained, or simply inhumane overseers or masters.

Despite many masters' policy of delaying a call to the physician until late in the course of a slave's disease, there were times when owners desperately wished for the doctor's presence. More practitioners should have retained in their files the numerous hastily scrawled notes from frantic slaveowners begging for medical assistance, or kept a record of each verbal summons to a sick slave at a distant farm or village household. For physicians did play important roles, both physiological and psychological, in the treatment of illness. Dr. Charles Brown of Charlottesville, for instance, had a thriving country practice during the early 19th century. He handled many types of problems: James Old wanted him to determine whether his slave woman, then "in a strange way," was pregnant or not; Bezaleel Brown needed his opinion "if I must bleed her [Jane, who had a pain in her side and suppression of urine] either large or small in quantity"; and Jemima Fretwell wished Brown to "cutt of[f] the arm" of a four-month-old slave which had been "so very badly burnt" that "the [elbow] joint appears like it will drap of[f]."[23] Sometimes physicians made daily visits to dress slaves' wounds or to keep track of household epidemics. In emergencies some owners panicked and fretted away many hours after learning of their physician's temporary absence.

Between the remedies of the household and the standard treatments of the physicians stood "ir-

regular" medicine, often as important but only partially accepted in Virginia. The impact of alternative movements on the medical care of blacks in Virginia was greater than historians have recognized. Most slaveowners either treated with conventional medicines or called in regular doctors, rejecting the new cults as quackery; but a sizable minority, difficult to estimate, became enthusiastic proponents of at least one system—Thomsonianism. This movement with practitioners in areas with heavy slave concentrations (64 percent of the Tidewater counties and 66 percent of the Piedmont counties during the 1830s and 1840s) appealed to masters who were fed up with the ineffective and expensive treatments of their regular physicians. One Tidewater resident turned to Thomsonianism after experienced Norfolk physicians had unsuccessfully managed a household scarlet fever outbreak. All 20 cases, the happy slaveowner reported to the editors of a Thomsonian journal, had been cured. Another man, in Goochland County, stated that a local Thomsonian practitioner had cured his slave of a disease which one of the most respected regular physicians of the area had found intractable to the usual blister and salivation treatments. And a Prince Edward County Thomsonian doctor claimed to have cured a ten-year-old slave who had been suffering from rabies (a misdiagnosis, no doubt). With adherents to the sect so widely diffused throughout the state, the services or success stories of practitioners no doubt reached at least a portion of the slaveholding class and influenced its thinking.

Beyond the master's and overseer's eyes, back in the slaves' cabins, some Virginia blacks took medical matters into their own hands. When under the surveillance of whites, slaves usually (but not always) accepted their treatments. Some even administered them in the name of the master. But others developed or retained from an ancient African heritage their own brand of care, complete with special remedies, medical practitioners, and rituals. The result was a dual system of health care, the two parts of which often conflicted with each other.

Masters did not appreciate slaves overusing the plantation infirmary, medicines, or the family doctor, but they preferred this to black self-care for several reasons. Their quarrel with the bondsmen was the same as the physicians' with the masters:

slaves waited too long before seeking medical assistance and often misdiagnosed illnesses. Most owners permitted blacks a small amount of freedom in treating minor ailments at home, but lost their patience when sickness got out of hand. James L. Hubard, in charge of his father's lands during the latter's vacation at Alleghany Springs, reported that Daphny had treated her own son with vermifuges (worm medicines) for several days before realizing that the boy was suffering not from worms but from dysentery. Hubard quickly altered the medication and summoned a doctor, blaming the entire affair on "the stupidity of Daphny."[24] An enraged Landon Carter found a suckling child with measles at the slave quarters. "The mother," he wrote in his diary, "let nobody know of it until it was almost dead."[25]

Whites also accused slaves of negligence or incompetence in the care of their fellow bondsmen. Dr. G. Lane Corbin of Warwick County, for instance, promoted slaves' use of collodion, a syrupy dressing, because it required so little attention once applied: "This I consider of moment in regard to our slave population, whose negligence and inattention to such matters [as the proper dressing of wounds] must have attracted the notice of the most superficial observer."[26] Negroes frequently were charged with irresponsibility, ignorance, slovenliness, and indifference in the management of other blacks' illnesses. "They will never do right, left to themselves,"[27] declared one Franklin County planter.

Furthermore, some whites argued, slaves did not even care for their own personal health properly. Recovery was retarded and even reversed, Dr. W. S. Morton of Cumberland County remarked, "by their [slaves'] own stupid perversity in refusing confinement to bed, and to follow other important directions when in a very dangerous condition."[28] Masters and physicians often confirmed this but were powerless to combat it. It was difficult for whites, unless they were present at all times, to force ailing blacks to take medicines or to remain constantly in bed. A most spectacular instance of death following defiance of medical orders occurred in Portsmouth when a black male patient of Dr. John W. Trugien, confined to bed with a stab wound of the heart, sustained a massive effusion of blood from that organ upon exerting himself by rising from his pallet.[29]

To offset the failures and harshness of white remedies, or the negligence of masters, or, perhaps, to exert some control over their lives, some slaves treated their own diseases and disorders or turned to other trusted blacks for medical assistance, with or without the master's knowledge.[30] Black home remedies circulated secretly through the slave quarters and were passed down privately from generation to generation. Most of these cures were derived from local plants, though some medicines contained ingredients that had magical value only. Occasionally whites would learn of a particularly effective medicine and adopt it, as when Dr. Richard S. Cauthorn announced in the *Monthly Stethoscope* (1857) that an old folk remedy (milk weed or silk weed, *Asclepias syriaca* in the United States Dispensatory) which had been used for years by blacks in the counties north of Richmond worked almost as well as quinine for agues and fevers.[31] Otherwise most whites simply ignored or tolerated the black medical world until something occurred to bring their attention to it—either a great medical discovery or a slave death caused by abuse.

Because blacks practiced medicine in virtually every portion of the Old Dominion and because their methods were based partially on magic, problems occasionally arose. The main source of trouble was usually not the misuse of home remedies, but the "prescriptions" and activities of so-called conjure doctors. These men and women used trickery, violence, persuasion, and medical proficiency to gain their reputations among local black communities. They were viewed as healers of illness that white doctors could not touch with their medicines, and as perpetrators of sicknesses on any person they wished—all through "spells."

Superstition was a powerful force within the slave community, and a difficult one for white nonadherents to understand or overcome. For instance, the older brother of a slave patient of Dr. A. D. Galt of Williamsburg observed to the doctor that his medicines were useless because Gabriel "had been tricked" and "must have a Negro Doctor" to reverse the progress of the illness. Galt soon claimed to have cured the man, though he did admit that Gabriel suffered frequent relapses, "probably from intemperance in drink."[32] In another case, a slave woman took sick and eventually died on a plantation near Petersburg from what her fellow bondsmen believed were the effects of a conjurer. Some slaves speculated that the young man whom she had refused to marry "poisoned or tricked" her, though the overseer attributed her death to consumption.[33] Virginia Hayes Shepherd, a former slave interviewed at age 83 in 1939, described an incident to illustrate how superstitious her stepfather had been: "He believed he had a bunch something like boils. White doctor bathed it. After a few days it burst and live things came out of the boil and crawled on the floor. He thought he was conjured. He said an enemy of his put something on the horse's back and he rode it and got it on his buttocks and broke him out."[34]

Old Dominion whites did permit blacks to fulfill certain medical functions. Some planters assigned "trusted" slaves to the task of rendering medical assistance to all ailing bondsmen on the farm. In most cases, these blacks simply dispensed white remedies and performed venesection and cupping as learned from the master. Though not complete black self-care, this activity did represent a transitional stage in which slaves had the opportunity to apply some of their own knowledge of herbs, etc., gained from elders, in addition to white remedies. These nurses, predominantly women, usually won the respect of both blacks and whites for their curative skills. "Uncle" Bacchus White, an 89-year-old former slave interviewed in Fredericksburg in 1939, attested, "Aunt Judy uster to tend us when we uns were sic' and anything Aunt Judy couldn't do 'hit won't worth doin."[35] A white lady writing at about the same time provided a similarly romantic view of the black plantation nurse: "One of the house-servants, Amy Green—'Aunt Amy' we children called her —was a skilled nurse. My father kept a store of medicine, his scales, etc. so with Aunt Amy's poultices of horseradish and plattain-leaves and her various cuppings and plasters the ailments of the hundred negroes were well taken in hand."[36] Given

such high testimony and devotion from plantation folk, one could hardly dispute the novelist Louise Clarke Pyrnelle's depiction of Aunt Nancy, a fictional antebellum household nurse who claimed, while dosing several young slaves, "Ef'n hit want fur dat furmifuge [vermifuge—worm medicine], den Marster wouldn't hab all dem niggers w'at yer see hyear."[37]

To Negro women often fell another task: prenatal and obstetrical care of whites and blacks, especially in rural areas. At least one slave on most large Virginia plantations learned and practiced the art of midwifery, not only at home but also throughout the neighborhood. Masters preferred to employ these skilled accouchers in uncomplicated cases rather than pay the relatively high fees of trained physicians. Doctors, remarked one member of the medical profession, attended at less than half of all births in the state. He estimated that 9/10 of all deliveries among the black population (another physician set it at 5/6) were conducted by midwives, most of whom were also black. He further asserted that midwives attended half the white women. Physicians often saw obstetrical cases only when problems arose. As a result of this demand for competent nonprofessional obstetrical services, Negro midwives flourished in the countryside.

Blacks did play a significant role in the health care system of the Old Dominion. They assisted whites and blacks in delivering children, letting blood, pulling teeth, administering medicines, and nursing the sick. The techniques and drugs they used were overtly derived from white medical practices. But unknown to masters, overseers, health officers, or physicians, blacks did also resort to their own treatments derived from their own heritage and experience. Occasionally the white and black medical worlds merged or openly clashed, but usually they remained silently separate.

## NOTES

This paper is extracted in large part from Todd L. Savitt, *Medicine and Slavery: The Diseases and Health Care of Blacks in Antebellum Virginia* (Urbana: Univ. of Illinois Press, 1978), pp. 1–184. I acknowledge the helpful suggestions of Paul Escott, Kenneth Kipple, Ronald Numbers, and James Harvey Young.

1  Except in the first section, where a general overview of black-related diseases is presented, the focus is on Virginia from the Revolution to the Civil War. Health conditions in the Old Dominion at that time were, in many respects, typical of those prevailing throughout the antebellum South. Residents

suffered from malaria, parasitic worm diseases, and dysentery just as Mississippians and Georgians did. Yellow fever struck its major ports, though not as severely or as frequently as at Charleston, Mobile, and New Orleans. Virginia's position on the northern fringe of the slave South perhaps lessened the intensity and duration of warm-weather diseases, but not enough to render its diseases significantly different from those in the lower South.

During the time span under consideration the black population and the health picture in Virginia were relatively stable. The slave trade had ended, there was little black immigration into the state, and tropical diseases brought from Africa and unable to survive in the new environment had all but disappeared.

2  Editorial, *Monthly Steth. & Med. Reptr.,* 1856, *1:* 162–163.

3  These and other diseases and conditions are discussed in a recent, important book on black medical differences: Kenneth Kiple and Virginia H. King, *Another Dimension to the Black Diaspora: Diet, Disease and Racism* (Cambridge, England, 1981).

4  For a discussion of the southern disease environment from colonial times to the present, see Albert Cowdrey, *This Land, This South: An Environmental History* (Lexington, Ky., 1983).

5  Kiple and King (*Another Dimension*) emphasize dietary considerations to explain many slave health problems.

6  John H. Van Evrie, *Negroes and Negro "Slavery"* (New York, 1861), p. 25.

7  Van Evrie, pp. 251, 256.

8  Recent historical discussions of SIDS include Kiple and King, *Another Dimension,* pp. 107–110, and Michael P. Johnson, "Smothered slave infants: Were slave mothers at fault?" *J. Southern Hist.,* 1981, *47:* 493–520.

9  E. M. Pendleton, "On the susceptibility of the Caucasian and African races to the different classes of disease," *Southern Med. Rep.,* 1849, *1:* 336–337.

10  Editorial, "The Medical Society of Virginia," *Va. Med. & Surg. J.,* 1855, *4:* 256–258.

11  For examples of typical planters' writings on the management of slaves, see James O. Breeden, ed., *Advice Among Masters: The Ideal in Slave Management in the Old South* (Westport, Conn., 1980).

12  See notes 3 and 5 above.

13  Shirley on the James Farm Journals, June 23, 1825, Manuscript Room, Library of Congress.

14  Quoted in Wyndham B. Blanton, *Medicine in Virginia in the Eighteenth Century* (Richmond, 1931), p. 161.

15  Interview of William Lee, n.d., WPA Folklore File,

16  Frederick Law Olmsted, *A Journey in the Seaboard Slave States, with Remarks on Their Economy* (New York, 1856), p. 190.

17  Thomas Jefferson to Joel Yancy, Jan. 17, 1819, reproduced in *Thomas Jefferson's Farm Book,* ed. Edwin M. Betts (Princeton, N.J., 1953), p. 43.

18  There were, of course, exceptions to these statements. See, for example, Johnson, "Smothered slave infants," pp. 511–520.

19  John Walker Diary, Apr. 23, 1853, Southern Historical Collection, Univ. of North Carolina at Chapel Hill.

20  Jack P. Greene, ed., *The Diary of Colonel Landon Carter of Sabine Hall, 1752–1778* (Charlottesville, Va., 1965), I, p. 377 (Mar. 31, 1770).

21  Hunter Dickinson Farish, ed., *Journal and Letters of Philip Vickers Fithian, 1773–1774: A Plantation Tutor of the Old Dominion* (Williamsburg, Va., 1957), p. 182.

22  [Catherine C. Hopley], *Life in the South: From the Commencement of the War* (London, England, 1863), I, p. 103.

23  For more examples of such notes, see Todd L. Savitt, "Patient letters to an early nineteenth century Virginia physician," *J. Florida Med. Assn.,* Aug. 1982, *69* (No. 8): 688–694.

24  James L. Hubard to Robert T. Hubard, Aug. 4, 1857, Robert T. Hubard Papers, Univ. of Virginia, Manuscript Room, Alderman Library.

25  Greene, ed., *Carter Diary,* II, p. 812 (May 20, 1774).

26  G. Lane Corbin, "Collodion on stumps of amputated limbs," *Steth. & Va. Med. Gaz.,* 1851, *1:* 489.

27  L. G. Cabell to Bowker Preston, Oct. 8, 1834, John Hook Collection, Univ. of Virginia, Manuscript Room, Alderman Library.

28  W. S. Morton, "Causes of mortality amongst Negroes," *Monthly Steth. & Med. Reptr.,* 1856, *1:* 290.

29  John W. H. Trugien, "A case of wound to the left ventricle of the heart.—Patient survived five days; —with remarks," *Am. J. Med. Sci.,* 1850, n.s., *20:* 99–102.

30  See, for more information and references, Lawrence W. Levine, *Black Culture and Black Consciousness: Afro-American Folk Thought from Slavery to Freedom* (New York, 1977), pp. 55–80.

31  Richard S. Cauthorn, "A new anti-periodic and a substitute for quinia," *Monthly Steth. & Med. Reptr.,* 1857, *2:* 7–14.

32  [A. D. Galt], *Practical Medicine: Illustrated by Cases of the Most Important Diseases,* ed. John M. Galt (Philadelphia, 1843), pp. 295–296.

33  [William McKean to James Dunlap], July 17, 1810, Roslin Plantation Records, Virginia State Library.

Univ. of Virginia, Manuscript Room, Alderman Library.

34   Interview of Virginia Hayes Shepherd, 1939, WPA Folklore File, Univ. of Virginia, Manuscript Room, Alderman Library.

35   Interview of Uncle Bacchus White, 1939, WPA Folklore File, Univ. of Virginia, Manuscript Room, Alderman Library.

36   White Hill Plantation Books, Vol. I, p. 8, Southern Historical Collection, Univ. of North Carolina at Chapel Hill.

37   Louise Carter Pyrnelle, *Diddie, Dumps, and Tot; or Plantation Child-Life* (New York, 1882), quoted in Blanton, *Medicine in Virginia,* p. 49.

# 23

## Racism and Research: The Case of the Tuskegee Syphilis Study

### ALLAN M. BRANDT

In 1932 the U.S. Public Health Service (USPHS) initiated an experiment in Macon County, Alabama, to determine the natural course of untreated, latent syphilis in black males. The test comprised 400 syphilitic men, as well as 200 uninfected men who served as controls. The first published report of the study appeared in 1936 with subsequent papers issued every four to six years, through the 1960s. When penicillin became widely available by the early 1950s as the preferred treatment for syphilis, the men did not receive therapy. In fact on several occasions, the USPHS actually sought to prevent treatment. Moreover, a committee at the federally operated Center for Disease Control decided in 1969 that the study should be continued. Only in 1972, when accounts of the study first appeared in the national press, did the Department of Health, Education and Welfare halt the experiment. At that time 74 of the test subjects were still alive; at least 28, but perhaps more than 100, had died directly from advanced syphilitic lesions.[1] In August 1972, HEW appointed an investigatory panel which issued a report the following year. The panel found the study to have been "ethically unjustified," and argued that penicillin should have been provided to the men.[2]

This article attempts to place the Tuskegee Study in a historical context and to assess its ethical implications. Despite the media attention which the study received, the HEW *Final Report*, and the criticism expressed by several professional organizations, the experiment has been largely misunderstood. The most basic questions of *how* the study

ALLAN M. BRANDT is Assistant Professor of the History of Medicine and the History of Science at Harvard University, Cambridge, Massachusetts.

Reprinted with permission from *Hastings Center Report*, 1978, *8* (No. 6): 21–29.

was undertaken in the first place and *why* it continued for 40 years were never addressed by the HEW investigation. Moreover, the panel misconstrued the nature of the experiment, failing to consult important documents available at the National Archives which bear significantly on its ethical assessment. Only by examining the specific ways in which values are engaged in scientific research can the study be understood.

### RACISM AND MEDICAL OPINION

A brief review of the prevailing scientific thought regarding race and heredity in the early 20th century is fundamental for an understanding of the Tuskegee Study. By the turn of the century, Darwinism had provided a new rationale for American racism.[3] Essentially primitive peoples, it was argued, could not be assimilated into a complex, white civilization. Scientists speculated that in the struggle for survival the Negro in America was doomed. Particularly prone to disease, vice, and crime, black Americans could not be helped by education or philanthropy. Social Darwinists analyzed census data to predict the virtual extinction of the Negro in the 20th century, for they believed the Negro race in America was in the throes of a degenerative evolutionary process.[4]

The medical profession supported these findings of late 19th- and early 20th-century anthropologists, ethnologists, and biologists. Physicians studying the effects of emancipation on health concluded almost universally that freedom had caused the mental, moral, and physical deterioration of the black population.[5] They substantiated this argument by citing examples in the comparative anatomy of the black and white races. As Dr. W. T. English wrote: "A careful inspection reveals the body of the negro a mass of minor defects and imperfections from the crown of the head to the soles of the feet. . . ."[6] Cranial structures, wide nasal apertures, receding chins, projecting jaws, all typed the Negro as the lowest species in the Darwinian hierarchy.[7]

Interest in racial differences centered on the sexual nature of blacks. The Negro, doctors explained, possessed an excessive sexual desire, which threatened the very foundations of white society. As one physician noted in the *Journal of the American Medical Association*, "The negro springs from a southern race, and as such his sexual appetite is strong; all of his environments stimulate this appetite, and as a general rule his emotional type of religion certainly does not decrease it."[8] Doctors reported a complete lack of morality on the part of blacks:

> Virtue in the negro race is like angels' visits — few and far between. In a practice of sixteen years I have never examined a virgin negro over fourteen years of age.[9]

A particularly ominous feature of this overzealous sexuality, doctors argued, was the black males' desire for white women. "A perversion from which most races are exempt," wrote Dr. English, "prompts the negro's inclination towards white women, whereas other races incline towards females of their own."[10] Though English estimated the "gray matter of the negro brain" to be at least 1,000 years behind that of the white races, his genital organs were overdeveloped. As Dr. William Lee Howard noted:

> The attacks on defenseless white women are evidences of racial instincts that are about as amenable to ethical culture as is the inherent odor of the race. . . . When education will reduce the size of the negro's penis as well as bring about the sensitiveness of the terminal fibers which exist in the Caucasian, then will it also be able to prevent the African's birthright to sexual madness and excess.[11]

One southern medical journal proposed "Castration Instead of Lynching," as retribution for black sexual crimes. "An impressive trial by a ghost-like kuklux klan [sic] and a 'ghost' physician or surgeon to perform the operation would make it an event the 'patient' would never forget," noted the editorial.[12]

According to these physicians, lust and immorality, unstable families, and reversion to barbaric tendencies made blacks especially prone to venereal diseases. One doctor estimated that over 50 percent of all Negroes over the age of 25 were syphilitic.[13] Virtually free of disease as slaves, they were now overwhelmed by it, according to informed medical opinion. Moreover, doctors believed that treatment for venereal disease among blacks was impossible, particularly because in its latent stage the symptoms of syphilis become quiescent. As Dr. Thomas W. Murrell wrote:

> They come for treatment at the beginning and at the end. When there are visible manifestations or when harried by pain, they readily come, for as a race they are not averse to physic; but tell them not, though they look well and feel well, that they are still diseased. Here ignorance rates science a fool. . . .[14]

Even the best-educated black, according to Murrell, could not be convinced to seek treatment for syphilis.[15] Venereal disease, according to some doctors, threatened the future of the race. The medical profession attributed the low birth rate among blacks to the high prevalence of venereal disease which caused stillbirths and miscarriages. Moreover, the high rates of syphilis were thought to lead to increased insanity and crime. One doctor writing at the turn of the century estimated that the number of insane Negroes had increased 13-fold since the end of the Civil War.[16] Dr. Murrell's conclusion echoed the most informed anthropological and ethnological data:

> So the scourge sweeps among them. Those that are treated are only half cured, and the effort to assimilate a complex civilization driving their diseased minds until the results are criminal records. Perhaps here, in conjunction with tuberculosis, will be the end of the negro problem. Disease will accomplish what man cannot do.[17]

This particular configuration of ideas formed the core of medical opinion concerning blacks, sex, and disease in the early 20th century. Doctors generally discounted socioeconomic explanations of the state of black health, arguing that better medical care could not alter the evolutionary scheme.[18] These assumptions provide the backdrop for examining the Tuskegee Syphilis Study.

## THE ORIGINS OF THE EXPERIMENT

In 1929, under a grant from the Julius Rosenwald Fund, the USPHS conducted studies in the rural South to determine the prevalence of syphilis among blacks and explore the possibilities for mass treatment. The USPHS found Macon County, Alabama, in which the town of Tuskegee is located, to have the highest syphilis rate of the six counties surveyed. The Rosenwald Study concluded that mass treatment could be successfully implemented among rural blacks.[19] Although it is doubtful that the necessary funds would have been allocated even in the best economic conditions, after the economy collapsed in 1929, the findings were ignored. It is, however, ironic that the Tuskegee Study came to be based on findings of the Rosenwald Study that demonstrated the possibilities of mass treatment.

Three years later, in 1932, Dr. Taliaferro Clark, chief of the USPHS Venereal Disease Division and author of the Rosenwald Study report, decided that conditions in Macon County merited renewed attention. Clark believed the high prevalence of syphilis offered an "unusual opportunity" for observation. From its inception, the USPHS regarded the Tuskegee Study as a classic "study in nature,"* rather than an experiment.[20] As long as syphilis was so prevalent in Macon and most of the blacks went untreated throughout life, it seemed only natural to Clark that it would be valuable to observe the consequences. He described it as a "ready-made situation."[21] Surgeon General H. S. Cumming wrote to R. R. Moton, director of the Tuskegee Institute:

> The recent syphilis control demonstration carried out in Macon County, with the financial assistance of the Julius Rosenwald Fund, revealed the

*In 1865, Claude Bernard, the famous French physiologist, outlined the distinction between a "study in nature" and experimentation. A study in nature required simple observation, an essentially passive act, while experimentation demanded intervention which altered the original condition. The Tuskegee Study was thus clearly not a study in nature. The very act of diagnosis altered the original conditions. "It is on this very possibility of acting or not acting on a body," wrote Bernard, "that the distinction will exclusively rest between sciences called sciences of observation and sciences called experimental."

presence of an unusually high rate in this county and, what is more remarkable, the fact that 99 percent of this group was entirely without previous treatment. This combination, together with the expected cooperation of your hospital, offers an unparalleled opportunity for carrying on this piece of scientific research which probably cannot be duplicated anywhere else in the world.[22]

Although no formal protocol appears to have been written, several letters of Clark and Cumming suggest what the USPHS hoped to find. Clark indicated that it would be important to see how disease affected the daily lives of the men:

> The results of these studies of case records suggest the desirability of making a further study of the effect of untreated syphilis on the human economy among people now living and engaged in their daily pursuits.[23]

It also seems that the USPHS believed the experiment might demonstrate that antisyphilitic treatment was unnecessary. As Cumming noted: "It is expected the results of this study may have a marked bearing on the treatment, or conversely the non-necessity of treatment, of cases of latent syphilis."[24]

The immediate source of Cumming's hypothesis appears to have been the famous Oslo Study of untreated syphilis. Between 1890 and 1910, Professor C. Boeck, the chief of the Oslo Venereal Clinic, withheld treatment from almost 2,000 patients infected with syphilis. He was convinced that therapies then available, primarily mercurial ointment, were of no value. When arsenic therapy became widely available by 1910, after Paul Ehrlich's historic discovery of "606," the study was abandoned. E. Bruusgaard, Boeck's successor, conducted a follow-up study of 473 of the untreated patients from 1925 to 1927. He found that 27.9 percent of these patients had undergone a "spontaneous cure," and now manifested no symptoms of the disease. Moreover, he estimated that as many as 70 percent of all syphilitics went through life without inconvenience from the disease.[25] His study, however, clearly acknowledged the dangers of untreated syphilis for the remaining 30 percent.

Thus every major textbook of syphilis at the time of the Tuskegee Study's inception strongly advocated treating syphilis even in its latent stages, which follow the initial inflammatory reaction. In discussing the Oslo Study, Dr. J. E. Moore, one of the nation's leading venereologists wrote, "This summary of Bruusgaard's study is by no means intended to suggest that syphilis be allowed to pass untreated."[26] If a complete cure could not be effected, at least the most devastating effects of the disease could be avoided. Although the standard therapies of the time, arsenical compounds and bismuth injection, involved certain dangers because of their toxicity, the alternatives were much worse. As the Oslo Study had shown, untreated syphilis could lead to cardiovascular disease, insanity, and premature death.[27] Moore wrote in his 1933 textbook:

> Though it imposes a slight though measurable risk of its own, treatment markedly diminishes the risk from syphilis. In latent syphilis, as I shall show, the probability of progression, relapse, or death is reduced from a probable 25–30 percent without treatment to about 5 percent with it; and the gravity of the relapse if it occurs, is markedly diminished.[28]

"Another compelling reason for treatment," noted Moore, "exists in the fact that every patient with latent syphilis may be, and perhaps is, infectious for others."[29] In 1932, the year in which the Tuskegee Study began, the USPHS sponsored and published a paper by Moore and six other syphilis experts that strongly argued for treating latent syphilis.[30]

The Oslo Study, therefore, could not have provided justification for the USPHS to undertake a study that did not entail treatment. Rather, the suppositions that conditions in Tuskegee existed "naturally" and that the men would not be treated anyway provided the experiment's rationale. In turn, these two assumptions rested on the prevailing medical attitudes concerning blacks, sex, and disease. For example, Clark explained the prevalence of venereal disease in Macon County by emphasizing promiscuity among blacks:

> This state of affairs is due to the paucity of doctors, rather low intelligence of the Negro population in this section, depressed economic conditions, and the very common promiscuous sex relations of this population group which not only contribute to the spread of syphilis but also contribute to the prevailing indifference with regard to treatment.[31]

In fact, Moore, who had written so persuasively in favor of treating latent syphilis, suggested that existing knowledge did not apply to Negroes. Although he had called the Oslo Study "a never-to-be-repeated human experiment,"[32] he served as an expert consultant to the Tuskegee Study:

> I think that such a study as you have contemplated would be of immense value. It will be necessary of course in the consideration of the results to evaluate the special factors introduced by a selection of the material from negro males. Syphilis in the negro is in many respects almost a different disease from syphilis in the white.[33]

Dr. O. C. Wenger, chief of the federally operated venereal disease clinic at Hot Springs, Arkansas, praised Moore's judgment, adding, "This study will emphasize those differences."[34] On another occasion he advised Clark, "We must remember we are dealing with a group of people who are illiterate, have no conception of time, and whose personal history is always indefinite."[35]

The doctors who devised and directed the Tuskegee Study accepted the mainstream assumptions regarding blacks and venereal disease. The premise that blacks, promiscuous and lustful, would not seek or continue treatment, shaped the study. A test of untreated syphilis seemed "natural" because the USPHS presumed the men would never be treated; the Tuskegee Study made that a self-fulfilling prophecy.

## SELECTING THE SUBJECTS

Clark sent Dr. Raymond Vonderlehr to Tuskegee in September 1932 to assemble a sample of men with latent syphilis for the experiment. The basic design of the study called for the selection of syphilitic black males between the ages of 25 and 60, a thorough physical examination including x-rays, and finally, a spinal tap to determine the incidence of neuro-syphilis.[36] They had no intention of providing any treatment for the infected men.[37] The USPHS originally scheduled the whole experiment to last six months; it seemed to be both a simple and inexpensive project.

The task of collecting the sample, however, proved to be more difficult than the USPHS had supposed. Vonderlehr canvassed the largely illiterate, poverty-stricken population of sharecroppers and tenant farmers in search of test subjects. If his circulars requested only men over 25 to attend his clinics, none would appear, suspecting he was conducting draft physicals. Therefore, he was forced to test large numbers of women and men who did not fit the experiment's specifications. This involved considerable expense, since the USPHS had promised the Macon County Board of Health that it would treat those who were infected, but not included in the study.[38] Clark wrote to Vonderlehr about the situation: "It never once occured to me that we would be called upon to treat a large part of the county as return for the privilege of making this study. . . . I am anxious to keep the expenditures for treatment down to the lowest possible point because it is the one item of expenditure in connection with the study most difficult to defend despite our knowledge of the need therefor."[39] Vonderlehr responded: "If we could find from 100 to 200 cases . . . we would not have to do another Wassermann on useless individuals. . . ."[40]

Significantly, the attempt to develop the sample contradicted the prediction the USPHS had made initially regarding the prevalence of the disease in Macon County. Overall rates of syphilis fell well below expectations; as opposed to the USPHS projection of 35 percent, 20 percent of those tested were actually diseased.[41] Moreover, those who had sought and received previous treatment far exceeded the expectations of the USPHS. Clark noted in a letter to Vonderlehr:

> I find your report of March 6th quite interesting but regret the necessity for Wassermanning [*sic*] . . . such a large number of individuals in order to uncover this relatively limited number of untreated cases.[42]

Further difficulties arose in enlisting the subjects to participate in the experiment, to be "Wassermanned," and to return for a subsequent series of examinations. Vonderlehr found that only the offer of treatment elicited the cooperation of the men. They were told they were ill and were promised free care. Offered therapy, they became willing subjects.[43] The USPHS did not tell the men that they were participants in an experiment; on the contrary, the subjects believed they were being treated for "bad blood" — the rural South's colloquialism for syphilis. They thought they were participating in a public health demonstration similar to the one

that had been conducted by the Julius Rosenwald Fund in Tuskegee several years earlier. In the end, the men were so eager for medical care that the number of defaulters in the experiment proved to be insignificant.[44]

To preserve the subjects' interest, Vonderlehr gave most of the men mercurial ointment, a noneffective drug, while some of the younger men apparently received inadequate dosages of neoarsphenamine.[45] This required Vonderlehr to write frequently to Clark requesting supplies. He feared the experiment would fail if the men were not offered treatment.

> It is desirable and essential if the study is to be a success to maintain the interest of each of the cases examined by me through to the time when the spinal puncture can be completed. Expenditure of several hundred dollars for drugs for these men would be well worth while if their interest and cooperation would be maintained in so doing. . . . It is my desire to keep the main purpose of the work from the negroes in the county and continue their interest in treatment. That is what the vast majority wants and the examination seems relatively unimportant to them in comparison. It would probably cause the entire experiment to collapse if the clinics were stopped before the work is completed.[46]

On another occasion he explained:

> Dozens of patients have been sent away without treatment during the past two weeks and it would have been impossible to continue without the free distribution of drugs because of the unfavorable impression made on the negro.[47]

The readiness of the test subjects to participate, of course, contradicted the notion that blacks would not seek or continue therapy.

The final procedure of the experiment was to be a spinal tap to test for evidence of neurosyphilis. The USPHS presented this purely diagnostic exam, which often entails considerable pain and complications, to the men as a "special treatment." Clark explained to Moore:

> We have not yet commenced the spinal punctures. This operation will be deferred to the last in order not to unduly disturb our field work by any adverse reports by the patients subjected to spinal puncture because of some disagreeable sensations following this procedure. These negroes are very

ignorant and easily influenced by things that would be of minor significance in a more intelligent group.[48]

The letter to the subjects announcing the spinal tap read:

> Some time ago you were given a thorough examination and since that time we hope you have gotten a great deal of treatment for bad blood. You will now be given your last chance to get a second examination. This examination is a very special one and after it is finished you will be given a special treatment if it is believed you are in a condition to stand it. . . .
> REMEMBER THIS IS YOUR LAST CHANCE FOR SPECIAL FREE TREATMENT. BE SURE TO MEET THE NURSE.[49]

The HEW investigation did not uncover this crucial fact: the men participated in the study under the guise of treatment.

Despite the fact that their assumption regarding prevalence and black attitudes toward treatment had proved wrong, the USPHS decided in the summer of 1933 to continue the study. Once again, it seemed only "natural" to pursue the research since the sample already existed, and with a depressed economy, the cost of treatment appeared prohibitive—although there is no indication it was ever considered. Vonderlehr first suggested extending the study in letters to Clark and Wenger:

> At the end of this project we shall have a considerable number of cases presenting various complications of syphilis, who have received only mercury and may still be considered untreated in the modern sense of therapy. Should these cases be followed over a period of from five to ten years many interesting facts could be learned regarding the course and complications of untreated syphilis.[50]

"As I see it," responded Wenger, "we have no further interest in these patients *until they die.*"[51] Apparently, the physicians engaged in the experiment believed that only autopsies could scientifically confirm the findings of the study. Surgeon General Cumming explained this in a letter to R. R. Moton, requesting the continued cooperation of the Tuskegee Institute Hospital:

> This study which was predominantly clinical in character points to the frequent occurrence of se-

vere complications involving the various vital organs of the body and indicates that syphilis as a disease does a great deal of damage. Since clinical observations are not considered final in the medical world, it is our desire to continue observation on the cases selected for the recent study and if possible to bring a percentage of these cases to autopsy so that pathological confirmation may be made of the disease processes.[52]

Bringing the men to autopsy required the USPHS to devise a further series of deceptions and inducements. Wenger warned Vonderlehr that the men must not realize that they would be autopsied:

> There is one danger in the latter plan and that is if the colored population become aware that accepting free hospital care means a post-mortem, every darkey will leave Macon County and it will hurt [Dr. Eugene] Dibble's hospital.[53]

"Naturally," responded Vonderlehr, "It is not my intention to let it be generally known that the main object of the present activities is the bringing of the men to necropsy."[54] The subjects' trust in the USPHS made the plan viable. The USPHS gave Dr. Dibble, the director of the Tuskegee Institute Hospital, an interim appointment to the Public Health Service. As Wenger noted:

> One thing is certain. The only way we are going to get post-mortems is to have the demise take place in Dibble's hospital and when these colored folks are told that Doctor Dibble is now a Government doctor too they will have more confidence.[55]*

---

*The degree of black cooperation in conducting the study remains unclear and would be impossible to properly assess in an article of this length. It seems certain that some members of the Tuskegee Institute staff such as R. R. Moton and Eugene Dibble understood the nature of the experiment and gave their support to it. There is, however, evidence that some blacks who assisted the USPHS physicians were not aware of the deceptive nature of the experiment. Dr. Joshua Williams, an intern at the John A. Andrew Memorial Hospital (Tuskegee Institute) in 1932, assisted Vonderlehr in taking blood samples of the test subjects. In 1973 he told the HEW panel: "I know we thought it was merely a service group organized to help the people in the area. We didn't know it was a research project at all at the time." (See "Transcript of proceedings," Tuskegee Syphilis Study Ad Hoc Advisory Panel, Feb. 23, 1973, unpublished typescript,

After the USPHS approved the continuation of the experiment in 1933, Vonderlehr decided that it would be necessary to select a group of healthy, uninfected men to serve as controls. Vonderlehr, who had succeeded Clark as chief of the Venereal Disease Division, sent Dr. J. R. Heller to Tuskegee to gather the control group. Heller distributed drugs (noneffective) to these men, which suggests that they also believed they were undergoing treatment.[56] Control subjects who became syphilitic were simply transferred to the test group — a strikingly inept violation of standard research procedure.[57]

The USPHS offered several inducements to maintain contact and to procure the continued cooperation of the men. Eunice Rivers, a black nurse, was hired to follow their health and to secure approval for autopsies. She gave the men noneffective medicines — "spring tonic" and aspirin — as well as transportation and hot meals on the days of their examinations.[58] More important, Nurse Rivers provided continuity to the project over the entire 40-year period. By supplying "medicinals," the USPHS was able to continue to deceive the participants, who believed that they were receiving therapy from the government doctors. Deceit was integral to the study. When the test subjects complained about spinal taps one doctor wrote:

> They simply do not like spinal punctures. A few of those who were tapped are enthusiastic over the results but to most, the suggestion causes violent shaking of the head; others claim they were robbed of their procreative powers (regardless of the fact that I claim it stimulates them).[59]

Letters to the subjects announcing an impending USPHS visit to Tuskegee explained: "[The doctor] wants to make a special examination to find out how you have been feeling and whether the treatment has improved your health."[60] In fact, after the first six months of the study, the USPHS had furnished no treatment whatsoever.

---

National Library of Medicine, Bethesda, Maryland.) It is also apparent that Eunice Rivers, the black nurse who had primary responsibility for maintaining contact with the men over the 40 years, did not fully understand the dangers of the experiment. In any event, black involvement in the study in no way mitigates the racial assumptions of the experiment, but rather, demonstrates their power.

Finally, because it proved difficult to persuade the men to come to the hospital when they became severely ill, the USPHS promised to cover their burial expenses. The Milbank Memorial Fund provided approximately $50 per man for this purpose beginning in 1935. This was a particularly strong inducement as funeral rites constituted an important component of the cultural life of rural blacks.[61] One report of the study concluded, "Without this suasion it would, we believe, have been impossible to secure the cooperation of the group and their families."[62]

Reports of the study's findings, which appeared regularly in the medical press beginning in 1936, consistently cited the ravages of untreated syphilis. The first paper, read at the 1936 American Medical Association annual meeting, found "that syphilis in this period [latency] tends to greatly increase the frequency of manifestations of cardiovascular disease."[63] Only 16 percent of the subjects gave no sign of morbidity as opposed to 61 percent of the controls. Ten years later, a report noted coldly, "The fact that nearly twice as large a proportion of the syphilitic individuals as of the control group has died is a very striking one." Life expectancy, concluded the doctors, is reduced by about 20 percent.[64]

A 1955 article found that slightly more than 30 percent of the test group autopsied had died *directly* from advanced syphilitic lesions of either the cardiovascular or the central nervous system.[65] Another published account stated, "Review of those still living reveals that an appreciable number have late complications of syphilis which probably will result, for some at least, in contributing materially to the ultimate cause of death."[66] In 1950, Dr. Wenger had concluded, "We now know, where we could only surmise before, that we have contributed to their ailments and shortened their lives."[67] As black physician Vernal Cave, a member of the HEW panel, later wrote, "They proved a point, then proved a point, then proved a point."[68]

During the 40 years of the experiment the USPHS had sought on several occasions to ensure that the subjects did not receive treatment from other sources. To this end, Vonderlehr met with groups of local black doctors in 1934, to ask their cooperation in not treating the men. Lists of subjects were distributed to Macon County physicians along with letters requesting them to refer these men back to the USPHS if they sought care.[69] The USPHS warned the Alabama Health Department not to treat the test subjects when they took a mobile VD unit into Tuskegee in the early 1940s.[70] In 1941, the army drafted several subjects and told them to begin antisyphilitic treatment immediately. The USPHS supplied the draft board with a list of 256 names they desired to have excluded from treatment, and the board complied.[71]

In spite of these efforts, by the early 1950s many of the men had secured some treatment on their own. By 1952, almost 30 percent of the test subjects had received some penicillin, although only 7.5 percent had received what could be considered adequate doses.[72] Vonderlehr wrote to one of the participating physicians, "I hope that the availability of antibiotics has not interfered too much with this project."[73] A report published in 1955 considered whether the treatment that some of the men had obtained had "defeated" the study. The article attempted to explain the relatively low exposure to penicillin in an age of antibiotics, suggesting as a reason: "the stoicism of these men as a group; they still regard hospitals and medicines with suspicion and prefer an occasional dose of time-honored herbs or tonics to modern drugs."[74] The authors failed to note that the men believed they already were under the care of the government doctors and thus saw no need to seek treatment elsewhere. Any treatment which the men might have received, concluded the report, had been insufficient to compromise the experiment.

When the USPHS evaluated the status of the study in the 1960s they continued to rationalize the racial aspects of the experiment. For example, the minutes of a 1965 meeting at the Center for Disease Control recorded:

> Racial issue was mentioned briefly. Will not affect the study. Any questions can be handled by saying these people were at the point that therapy would no longer help them. They are getting better medical care than they would under any other circumstances.[75]

A group of physicians met again at the CDC in 1969 to decide whether or not to terminate the study. Although one doctor argued that the study should be stopped and the men treated, the consensus was to continue. Dr. J. Lawton Smith remarked, "You will never have another study like

this; take advantage of it."[76] A memo prepared by Dr. James B. Lucas, assistant chief of the Venereal Disease Branch stated: "Nothing learned will prevent, find, or cure a single case of infectious syphilis or bring us closer to our basic mission of controlling venereal disease in the United States."[77] He concluded, however, that the study should be continued "along its present lines." When the first accounts of the experiment appeared in the national press in July 1972, data were still being collected and autopsies performed.[78]

## THE HEW FINAL REPORT

HEW finally formed the Tuskegee Syphilis Study Ad Hoc Advisory Panel on August 28, 1972, in response to criticism that the press descriptions of the experiment had triggered. The panel, composed of nine members, five of them black, concentrated on two issues. First, was the study justified in 1932 and had the men given their informed consent? Second, should penicillin have been provided when it became available in the early 1950s? The panel was also charged with determining if the study should be terminated and assessing current policies regarding experimentation with human subjects.[79] The group issued their report in June 1973.

By focusing on the issues of penicillin therapy and informed consent, the *Final Report* and the investigation betrayed a basic misunderstanding of the experiment's purposes and design. The HEW report implied that the failure to provide penicillin constituted the study's major ethical misjudgment; implicit was the assumption that no adequate therapy existed prior to penicillin. Nonetheless medical authorities firmly believed in the efficacy of arsenotherapy for treating syphilis at the time of the experiment's inception in 1932. The panel further failed to recognize that the entire study had been predicated on nontreatment. Provision of effective medication would have violated the rationale of the experiment—to study the natural course of the disease until death. On several occasions, in fact, the USPHS had prevented the men from receiving proper treatment. Indeed, there is no evidence that the USPHS ever considered providing penicillin.

The other focus of the *Final Report*—informed consent—also served to obscure the historical facts of the experiment. In light of the deceptions and exploitations which the experiment perpetrated, it is an understatement to declare, as the *Report* did, that the experiment was "ethically unjustified," because it failed to obtain informed consent from the subjects. The *Final Report's* statement, "Submitting voluntarily is not informed consent," indicated that the panel believed that the men had volunteered *for the experiment*.[80] The records in the National Archives make clear that the men did not submit voluntarily to an experiment; they were told and they believed that they were getting free treatment from expert government doctors for a serious disease. The failure of the HEW *Final Report* to expose this critical fact — that the USPHS lied to the subjects — calls into question the thoroughness and credibility of their investigation.

Failure to place the study in a historical context also made it impossible for the investigation to deal with the essentially racist nature of the experiment. The panel treated the study as an aberration, well intentioned but misguided.[81] Moreover, concern that the *Final Report* might be viewed as a critique of human experimentation in general seems to have severely limited the scope of the inquiry. The *Final Report* is quick to remind the reader on two occasions: "The position of the Panel must not be construed to be a general repudiation of scientific research with human subjects."[82] The *Report* assures

us that a better designed experiment could have been justified:

> It is possible that a scientific study in 1932 of untreated syphilis, properly conceived with a clear protocol and conducted with suitable subjects who fully understood the implications of their involvement, might have been justified in the pre-penicillin era. This is especially true when one considers the uncertain nature of the results of treatment of late latent syphilis and the highly toxic nature of therapeutic agents then available.[83]

This statement is questionable in view of the proven dangers of untreated syphilis known in 1932.

Since the publication of the HEW *Final Report*, a defense of the Tuskegee Study has emerged. These arguments, most clearly articulated by Dr. R. H. Kampmeier in the *Southern Medical Journal*, center on the limited knowledge of effective therapy for latent syphilis when the experiment began. Kampmeier argues that by 1950, penicillin would have been of no value for these men.[84] Others have suggested that the men were fortunate to have been spared the highly toxic treatments of the earlier period.[85] Moreover, even these contemporary defenses assume that the men never would have been treated anyway. As Dr. Charles Barnett of Stanford University wrote in 1974, "The lack of treat-

---

**Claude Bernard on Human Experimentation (1865)**
Experiments, then, may be performed on man, but within what limits? It is our duty and our right to perform an experiment on man whenever it can save his life, cure him or gain him some personal benefit. The principle of medical and surgical morality, therefore, consists in never performing on man an experiment which might be harmful to him to any extent, even though the result might be highly advantageous to science, i.e., to the health of others. But performing experiments and operations exclusively from the point of view of the patient's own advantage does not prevent their turning out profitably to science. . . . For we must not deceive ourselves, morals do not forbid making experiments on one's neighbor or on one's self. Christian morals forbid only one thing, doing ill to one's neighbor. So, among the experiments that may be tried on man, those that can only harm are forbidden, those that are innocent are permissible, and those that may do good are obligatory. Claude Bernard, *An Introduction to the Study of Experimental Medicine* (1865). Trans. Henry C. Green (New York: Dover Publications, 1957).

**From the HEW Final Report (1973)**
1. In retrospect, the Public Health Service Study of Untreated Syphilis in the Male Negro in Macon County, Alabama, was ethically unjustified in 1932. This judgment made in 1973 about the conduct of the study in 1932 is made with the advantage of hindsight acutely sharpened over some forty years, concerning an activity in a different age with different social standards. Nevertheless, one fundamental ethical rule is that a person should not be subjected to avoidable risk of death or physical harm unless he freely and intelligently consents. There is no evidence that such consent was obtained from the participants in this study.

2. Because of the paucity of information available today on the manner in which the study was conceived, designed and sustained, a scientific justification for a short term demonstration study cannot be ruled out. However, the conduct of the longitudinal study as initially reported in 1936 and through the years is judged to be scientifically unsound and its results are disproportionately meager compared with known risks to human subjects involved. . . .

ment was not contrived by the USPHS but was an established fact of which they proposed to take advantage."[86] Several doctors who participated in the study continued to justify the experiment. Dr. J. R. Heller, who on one occasion had referred to the test subjects as the "Ethiopian population," told reporters in 1972:

> I don't see why they should be shocked or hor-rified. There was no racial side to this. It just hap-pened to be in a black community. I feel this was a perfectly straightforward study, perfectly ethi-cal, with controls. Part of our mission as physi-cians is to find out what happens to individuals with disease and without disease.[87]

These apologies, as well as the HEW *Final Re-port*, ignore many of the essential ethical issues which the study poses. The Tuskegee Study reveals the persistence of beliefs within the medical pro-fession about the nature of blacks, sex, and disease — beliefs that had tragic repercussions long after their alleged "scientific" bases were known to be incorrect. Most strikingly, the entire health of a community was jeopardized by leaving a commu-nicable disease untreated.[88] There can be little doubt that the Tuskegee researchers regarded their subjects as less than human.[89] As a result, the ethi-cal canons of experimenting on human subjects were completely disregarded.

The study also raises significant questions about professional self-regulation and scientific bureau-cracy. Once the USPHS decided to extend the ex-periment in the summer of 1933, it was unlikely that the test would be halted short of the men's deaths. The experiment was widely reported for 40 years without evoking any significant protest within the medical community. Nor did any bu-reaucratic mechanism exist within the government for the periodic reassessment of the Tuskegee ex-periment's ethics and scientific value. The USPHS sent physicians to Tuskegee every several years to check on the study's progress, but never subjected the morality or usefulness of the experiment to serious scrutiny. Only the press accounts of 1972 finally punctured the continued rationalizations of the USPHS and brought the study to an end. Even the HEW investigation was compromised by fear that it would be considered a threat to future hu-man experimentation.

In retrospect the Tuskegee Study revealed more about the pathology of racism than it did about the pathology of syphilis; more about the nature of scientific inquiry than the nature of the disease process. The injustice committed by the experi-ment went well beyond the facts outlined in the press and the HEW *Final Report*. The degree of deception and damages have been seriously under-estimated. As this history of the study suggests, the notion that science is a value-free discipline must be rejected. The need for greater vigilance in assessing the specific ways in which social val-ues and attitudes affect professional behavior is clearly indicated.[90]

## NOTES

1  The best general accounts of the study are "The 40-year death watch," *Medical World News,* Aug. 18, 1972: 15–17; and Dolores Katz, "Why 430 blacks with syphilis went uncured for 40 years," Detroit *Free Press,* Nov. 5, 1972. The mortality figure is based on a published report of the study which ap-peared in 1955. See Jesse J. Peters, James H. Peers, Sidney Olansky, John C. Cutler, and Geraldine Gleeson, "Untreated syphilis in the male Negro: pathologic findings in syphilitic and nonsyphilitic patients," *J. Chron. Dis.,* Feb. 1955, *1*: 127–148. The article estimated that 30.4 percent of the untreated men would die from syphilitic lesions.

2  *Final Report* of the Tuskegee Syphilis Study Ad Hoc Advisory Panel, Department of Health, Education, and Welfare (Washington, D.C.: Government Print-ing Office, 1973). (Hereafter, HEW *Final Report*).

3  See George M. Fredrickson, *The Black Image in the White Mind* (New York: Harper and Row, 1971), pp. 228–255. Also, John H. Haller, *Outcasts From Evolution* (Urbana: Univ. of Illinois Press, 1971), pp. 40–68.

4  Frederickson, *The Black Image,* pp. 247–249.

5  "Deterioration of the American Negro," *Atlanta J.-Rec. Med.,* July 1903, *5*: 287–288. See also J. A. Rodgers, "The effect of freedom upon the psycho-logical development of the Negro," *Proc. Am. Medico-Psychological Assn.,* 1900, *7*: 88–99. "From the most healthy race in the country forty years ago," con-cluded Dr. Henry McHatton, "he is today the most

diseased." "The sexual status of the Negro—past and present," *Am. J. Dermatology & Genito-Urinary Dis.,* Jan. 1906, *10:* 7–9.

6  W. T. English, "The Negro problem from the physician's point of view," *Atlanta J.-Rec. Med.,* Oct. 1903, *5:* 461. See also, "Racial anatomical peculiarities," *N.Y. Med. J.,* Apr. 1896, *63:* 500–501.

7  "Racial anatomical peculiarities," p. 501. Also, Charles S. Bacon, "The race problem," *Medicine* (Detroit), May 1903, *9:* 338–343.

8  H. H. Hazen, "Syphilis in the American Negro," *J.A.M.A.,* Aug. 8, 1914, *63:* 463. For deeper background into the historical relationship of racism and sexuality, see Winthrop D. Jordan, *White Over Black* (Chapel Hill: Univ. of North Carolina Press, 1968; Pelican Books, 1969), pp. 32–40.

9  Daniel David Quillian, "Racial peculiarities: a cause of the prevalence of syphilis in Negroes," *Am. J. Dermatology & Genito-Urinary Dis.,* July 1906, *10:* 277.

10  English, "The Negro problem . . . ," p. 463.

11  William Lee Howard, "The Negro as a distinct ethnic factor in civilization," *Medicine* (Detroit), June 1903, *9:* 424. See also, Thomas W. Murrell, "Syphilis in the American Negro," *J.A.M.A.,* Mar. 12, 1910, *54:* 848.

12  "Castration instead of lynching," *Atlanta J.-Rec. Med.,* Oct. 1906, *8:* 457. The editorial added: "The badge of disgrace and emasculation might be branded upon the face or forehead, as a warning, in the form of an 'R,' emblematic of the crime for which this punishment was and will be inflicted."

13  Searle Harris, "The future of the Negro from the standpoint of the southern physician," *Alabama Med. J.,* Jan. 1902, *14:* 62. Other articles on the prevalence of venereal disease among blacks are: H. L. McNeil, "Syphilis in the southern Negro," *J.A.M.A.,* Sept. 30, 1916, *67:* 1001–1004; Ernest Philip Boas, "The relative prevalence of syphilis among Negroes and whites," *Social Hygiene,* Sept. 1915, *1:* 610–616. Doctors went to considerable trouble to distinguish the morbidity and mortality of various diseases among blacks and whites. See, for example, Marion M. Torchia, "Tuberculosis among American Negroes: medical research on a racial disease, 1830–1950," *J. Hist. Med.,* July 1977, *32:* 252–279.

14  Thomas W. Murrell, "Syphilis in the Negro: its bearing on the race problem," *Am. J. Dermatology & Genito-Urinary Dis.,* Aug. 1906, *10:* 307.

15  "Even among the educated, only a very few will carry out the most elementary instructions as to personal hygiene. One thing you cannot do, and that is to convince the negro that he has a disease that he cannot see or feel. This is due to lack of concentration rather than lack of faith; even if he does believe, he does not care; a child of fancy, the sensations of the passing hour are his only guides to the future." Murrell, "Syphilis in the American Negro," p. 847.

16  "Deterioration of the American Negro," *Atlanta J.-Rec. Med.,* July 1903, *5:* 288.

17  Murrell, "Syphilis in the Negro; its bearing on the race problem," p. 307.

18  "The anatomical and physiological conditions of the African must be understood, his place in the anthropological scale realized, and his biological basis accepted as being unchangeable by man, before we shall be able to govern his natural uncontrollable sexual passions." See, "As ye sow that shall ye also reap," *Atlanta J.-Rec. Med.,* June 1899, *1:* 266.

19  Taliaferro Clark, *The Control of Syphilis in Southern Rural Areas* (Chicago: Julius Rosenwald Fund, 1932), pp. 53–58. Approximately 35 percent of the inhabitants of Macon County who were examined were found to be syphilitic.

20  See Claude Bernard, *An Introduction to the Study of Experimental Medicine* (New York: Dover, 1865, 1957), pp. 5–26.

21  Taliaferro Clark to M. M. Davis, Oct. 29, 1932. Records of the USPHS Venereal Disease Division, Record Group 90, Box 239, National Archives, Washington National Record Center, Suitland, Maryland. (Hereafter, NA-WNRC). Materials in this collection which relate to the early history of the study were apparently never consulted by the HEW investigation. Included are letters, reports, and memoranda written by the physicians engaged in the study.

22  H. S. Cumming to R. R. Moton, Sept. 20, 1932, NA-WNRC.

23  Clark to Davis, Oct. 29, 1932, NA-WNRC.

24  Cumming to Moton, Sept. 20, 1932, NA-WNRC.

25  Bruusgaard was able to locate 309 living patients, as well as records from 164 who were deceased. His findings were published as "Ueber das Schicksal der nicht specifizch behandelten Luetiken," *Arch. Dermatology & Syphilis,* 1929, *157:* 309–332. The best discussion of the Boeck-Bruusgaard data is E. Gurney Clark and Niels Danbolt, "The Oslo Study of the natural history of untreated syphilis," *J. Chron. Dis.,* Sept. 1955, *2:* 311–344.

26  Joseph Earle Moore, *The Modern Treatment of Syphilis* (Baltimore: Charles C. Thomas, 1933), p. 24.

27  *Ibid.,* pp. 231–247; see also John H. Stokes, *Modern Clinical Syphilology* (Philadelphia: W. B. Saunders, 1928), pp. 231–239.

28  Moore, *Modern Treatment of Syphilis,* p. 237.

29  *Ibid.,* p. 236.

30  J. E. Moore, H. N. Cole, P. A. O'Leary, J. H.

Stokes, U. J. Wile, T. Clark, T. Parran, J. H. Usilton, "Cooperative clinical studies in the treatment of syphilis: latent syphilis," *Venereal Disease Information,* (Sept. 20, 1932), *13*: 351. The authors also concluded that the latently syphilitic were potential carriers of the disease, thus meriting treatment.

31  Clark to Paul A. O'Leary, Sept. 27, 1932, NA-WNRC. O'Leary, of the Mayo Clinic, misunderstood the design of the study, replying: "The investigation which you are planning in Alabama is indeed an intriguing one, particularly because of the opportunity it affords of observing treatment in a previously untreated group. I assure you such a study is of interest to me, and I shall look forward to its report in the future." O'Leary to Clark, Oct. 3, 1932, NA-WNRC.

32  Joseph Earle Moore, "Latent syphilis," unpublished typescript, n.d., p. 7. American Social Hygiene Association Papers, Social Welfare History Archives Center, University of Minnesota, Minneapolis.

33  Moore to Clark, Sept. 28, 1932, NA-WNRC. Moore had written in his textbook, "In late syphilis the negro is particularly prone to the development of bone or cardiovascular lesions." See Moore, *The Modern Treatment of Syphilis,* p. 35.

34  O. C. Wenger to Clark, Oct. 3, 1932, NA-WNRC.

35  *Ibid.,* Sept. 29, 1932.

36  Clark memorandum, Sept. 26, 1932, NA-WNRC. See also, Clark to Davis, Oct. 29, 1932, NA-WNRC.

37  As Clark wrote: "You will observe that our plan has nothing to do with treatment. It is purely a diagnostic procedure carried out to determine what has happened to the syphilitic Negro who has had no treatment." Clark to Paul A. O'Leary, Sept. 27, 1932, NA-WNRC.

38  D. G. Gill to O. C. Wenger, Oct. 10, 1932, NA-WNRC.

39  Clark to Vonderlehr, Jan. 25, 1933, NA-WNRC.

40  Vonderlehr to Clark, Feb. 28, 1933, NA-WNRC.

41  *Ibid.,* Nov. 2, 1932. Also, *ibid.,* Feb. 6, 1933.

42  Clark to Vonderlehr, Mar. 9, 1933, NA-WNRC.

43  Vonderlehr later explained: "The reason treatment was given to many of these men was twofold: First, when the study was started in the fall of 1932, no plans had been made for its continuation and a few of the patients were treated before we fully realized the need for continuing the project on a permanent basis. Second it was difficult to hold the interest of the group of Negroes in Macon County unless some treatment was given." Vonderlehr to Austin V. Diebert, Dec. 5, 1938, Tuskegee Syphilis Study Ad Hoc Advisory Panel Papers, Box 1, National Library of Medicine, Bethesda, Maryland. (Hereafter, TSS-NLM.) This collection contains the materials assembled by the HEW investigation in 1972.

44  Vonderlehr to Clark, Feb. 6, 1933, NA-WNRC.

45  H. S. Cumming to J. N. Baker, Aug. 5, 1933, NA-WNRC.

46  Vonderlehr to Clark, Jan. 22, 1933; Jan. 12, 1933, NA-WNRC.

47  Vonderlehr to Clark, Jan. 28, 1933, NA-WNRC.

48  Clark to Moore, Mar. 25, 1933, NA-WNRC.

49  Macon County Health Department, "Letter to subjects," n.d., NA-WNRC.

50  Vonderlehr to Clark, Apr. 8, 1933, NA-WNRC. See also, Vonderlehr to Wenger, July 18, 1933, NA-WNRC.

51  Wenger to Vonderlehr, July 21, 1933, NA-WNRC. The italics are Wenger's.

52  Cumming to Moton, July 27, 1933, NA-WNRC.

53  Wenger to Vonderlehr, July 21, 1933, NA-WNRC.

54  Vonderlehr to Murray Smith, July 27, 1933, NA-WNRC.

55  Wenger to Vonderlehr, Aug. 5, 1933, NA-WNRC.

56  Vonderlehr to Wenger, Oct. 24, 1933, NA-WNRC. Controls were given salicylates.

57  Austin V. Diebert and Martha C. Bruyere, "Untreated syphilis in the male Negro, III," *Venereal Disease Information,* Dec. 1946, *27*: 301–314.

58  Eunice Rivers, Stanley Schuman, Lloyd Simpson, Sidney Olansky, "Twenty-years of followup experience in a long-range medical study," *Public Hlth. Rep.,* Apr. 1953, *68*: 391–395. In this article Nurse Rivers explains her role in the experiment. She wrote: "Because of the low educational status of the majority of the patients, it was impossible to appeal to them from a purely scientific approach. Therefore, various methods were used to maintain their interest. Free medicines, burial assistance or insurance (the project being referred to as 'Miss Rivers' Lodge'), free hot meals on the days of examination, transportation to and from the hospital, and an opportunity to stop in town on the return trip to shop or visit with their friends on the streets all helped. In spite of these attractions, there were some who refused their examinations because they were not sick and did not see that they were being benefitted" (p. 393).

59  Austin V. Diebert to Raymond Vonderlehr, Mar. 29, 1939, TSS-NLM, Box 1.

60  Murray Smith to subjects, 1938, TSS-NLM, Box 1. See also, Sidney Olansky to John C. Cutler, Nov. 6, 1951, TSS-NLM, Box 2.

61  The USPHS originally requested that the Julius Rosenwald Fund meet this expense. See Cumming to Davis, Oct. 4, 1934, NA-WNRC. This money was usually divided between the undertaker, pathologist, and hospital. Lloyd Isaacs to Raymond Vonderlehr, Apr. 23, 1940, TSS-NLM, Box 1.

62  Stanley H. Schuman, Sidney Olansky, Eunice

Rivers, C. A. Smith, Dorothy S. Rambo, "Untreated syphilis in the male Negro: background and current status of patients in the Tuskegee study," *J. Chron. Dis.,* Nov. 1955, *2*: 555.

63  R. A. Vonderlehr and Taliaferro Clark, "Untreated syphilis in the male Negro," *Venereal Disease Information,* Sept. 1936, *17*: 262.

64  J. R. Heller and P. T. Bruyere, "Untreated syphilis in the male Negro: II. Mortality during 12 years of observation," *Venereal Disease Information,* Feb. 1946, *27*: 34–38.

65  Jesse J. Peters, James H. Peers, Sidney Olansky, John C. Cutler, and Geraldine Gleeson, "Untreated syphilis in the male Negro: pathologic findings in syphilitic and non-syphilitic patients," *J. Chron. Dis.,* Feb. 1955, *1*: 127–148.

66  Sidney Olansky, Stanley H. Schuman, Jesse J. Peters, C. A. Smith, and Dorothy S. Rambo, "Untreated syphilis in the male Negro, X. Twenty years of clinical observation of untreated syphilitic and presumably nonsyphilitic groups," *J. Chron. Dis.,* Aug. 1956, *4*: 184.

67  O. C. Wenger, "Untreated syphilis in male Negro," unpublished typescript, 1950, p. 3. Tuskegee Files, Center for Disease Control, Atlanta, Georgia. (Hereafter TF-CDC).

68  Vernal G. Cave, "Proper uses and abuses of the health care delivery system for minorities with special reference to the Tuskegee syphilis study," *J. Nat. Med. Assn.,* Jan. 1975, *67*: 83.

69  See for example, Vonderlehr to B. W. Booth, Apr. 18, 1934; and Vonderlehr to E. R. Lett, Nov. 20, 1933, NA-WNRC.

70  "Transcript of proceedings—Tuskegee Syphilis Ad Hoc Advisory Panel," Feb. 23, 1973, unpublished typescript, TSS-NLM, Box 1.

71  Raymond Vonderlehr to Murray Smith, Apr. 30, 1942; and Smith to Vonderlehr, June 8, 1942, TSS-NLM, Box 1.

72  Stanley H. Schuman, Sidney Olansky, Eunice Rivers, C. A. Smith, and Dorothy S. Rambo, "Untreated syphilis in the male Negro: background and current status of patients in the Tuskegee study," *J. Chron. Dis.,* Nov. 1955, *2*: 550–553.

73  Raymond Vonderlehr to Stanley H. Schuman, Feb. 5, 1952, TSS-NLM, Box 2.

74  Schuman and others, "Untreated syphilis . . .," p. 550.

75  "Minutes, April 5, 1965" unpublished typescript, TSS-NLM, Box 1.

76  "Tuskegee Ad Hoc Committee meeting—minutes, February 6, 1969," TF-CDC.

77  James B. Lucas to William J. Brown, Sept. 10, 1970, TF-CDC.

78  Elizabeth M. Kennebrew to Arnold C. Schroeter, Feb. 24, 1971, TSS-NLM, Box 1.

79  See *Medical Tribune,* Sept. 13, 1972: 1, 20; and Report on HEW's Tuskegee Report," *Medical World News,* Sept. 14, 1973: 57–58.

80  HEW *Final Report,* p. 7.

81  The notable exception is Jay Katz's eloquent "Reservations about the panel report on Charge 1," HEW *Final Report,* pp. 14–15.

82  HEW *Final Report,* pp. 8, 12.

83  *Ibid.*

84  See R. H. Kampmeier, "The Tuskegee Study of untreated syphilis," *Southern Med. J.,* Oct. 1972, *65*: 1247–1251; and "Final report on the 'Tuskegee Syphilis Study,'" *Southern Med. J.,* Nov. 1974, *67*: 1349–1353.

85  Leonard J. Goldwater, "The Tuskegee Study in historical perspective," unpublished typescript, TSS-NLM; see also "Treponemes and Tuskegee," *Lancet,* June 23, 1973: 1438; and Louis Lasagna, *The VD Epidemic* (Philadelphia: Temple Univ. Press, 1975), pp. 64–66.

86  Quoted in "Debate revives on the PHS study," *Medical World News,* Apr. 19, 1974: 37.

87  Heller to Vonderlehr, Nov. 28, 1933, NA-WNRC; quoted in *Medical Tribune,* Aug. 23, 1972: 14.

88  Although it is now known that syphilis is rarely infectious after its early phase, at the time of the study's inception latent syphilis was thought to be communicable. The fact that members of the control group were placed in the test group when they became syphilitic proves that at least some infectious men were denied treatment.

89  When the subjects are drawn from minority groups, especially those with which the researcher cannot identify, basic human rights may be compromised. Hans Jonas has clearly explicated the problem in his "Philosophical reflections on experimenting with human subjects," *Daedalus,* Spring 1969, *98*: 234–237. As Jonas writes: "If the properties we adduced as the particular qualifications of the members of the scientific fraternity itself are taken as general criteria of selection, then one should look for additional subjects where a maximum of identification, understanding, and spontaneity can be expected—that is, among the most highly motivated, the most highly educated, and the least 'captive' members of the community."

90  Since the original publication of this article, a full-length study of the Tuskegee Experiment has appeared. See James H. Jones, *Bad Blood: The Tuskegee Syphilis Experiment* (New York: Free Press, 1981).

# EPIDEMICS

Although epidemics have seldom taken more lives than endemic diseases, they have always attracted more attention. Sweeping inexorably through town after town, these unpredictable plagues aroused more fear and anxiety than more deadly but common everyday killers like pneumonia and tuberculosis. Cholera visited the United States only four times — in 1832, 1849, 1866, and 1873 — but the mere thought of this viciously dehydrating disease struck fear in the heart of virtually every American throughout the 19th century. Even today the threat of an epidemic that might cost a few thousand lives excites more concern than automobile accidents, for example, which annually take tens of thousands of lives.

Among the most feared of all epidemics were smallpox and yellow fever. Smallpox, a physically repulsive and often disfiguring disease, arrived in the New World with the European settlers, slaying many American Indians and taking the lives of numerous immigrants. When smallpox struck, colonials typically quarantined the affected area and isolated the sick, either at home or in a pesthouse. In 1721 Cotton Mather attempted to introduce another means of stopping this loathsome disease. John B. Blake tells about the controversy in Boston that the introduction of inoculation (or variolation) ignited. Although this preventive measure seemed to lower mortality from smallpox, it was not without its risks, as opponents vigorously pointed out. A second debate over smallpox immunization developed in the 19th century, after Benjamin Waterhouse brought William Jenner's method of vaccination with cowpox virus to America. As Judith Walzer Leavitt relates, even with this safer technique, resistance — political as well as medical — continued until the 20th century. The Milwaukee experience illustrates that some epidemics, instead of encouraging public action to prevent future occurrences, impeded the course of public health reform.

Yellow fever, a distinctive disease characterized by yellowish skin, black vomit, and high death rates, likewise stirred political and medical passions, as Martin S. Pernick shows in his study of the Philadelphia epidemic of 1793. That epidemic served as a terrifying reminder of yellow fever's destructive abilities for the next hundred years. Although yellow fever disappeared from the northern states after the early 19th century, it remained a threat in the South until 1900, when Walter Reed and his associates discovered the role of the mosquito in transmitting the infection.

With the exception of the 1918–19 influenza epidemic, which killed more Americans than World War I, the United States has been remarkably free of major epidemics during the 20th century. But as the swine flu scare of 1976 illustrated, we still live in fear of an attack by a mysterious new killer. The recent example of AIDS (Acquired Immune Deficiency Syndrome), which affected only about 800 Americans before 1983 but almost 4,000 in the single year 1984, serves as a contemporary example of the helplessness and fear engendered by unexplainable disaster.

# 24

## The Inoculation Controversy in Boston, 1721–1722

### JOHN B. BLAKE

Of all the diseases affecting colonial America, none caused more consternation than smallpox. Highly contagious, once it gained a foothold, it spread rapidly and with fearful mortality. Recognizing these facts, the authorities of Massachusetts developed certain techniques designed to keep this scourge under control. They required incoming vessels with smallpox aboard to perform quarantine at Spectacle Island in Boston harbor, and when cases appeared in town, the selectmen removed the patients to a pesthouse or placed guards about the infected dwellings. Although these precautions often proved successful, they were unable entirely to prevent periodic epidemics. During one of these outbreaks, in 1721, inoculation of the smallpox was first tried in the colonies. It enraged the town and called forth a bitter newspaper and pamphlet war, but it was the earliest important experiment in preventive medicine in America.

The practice was not new in 1721. People in certain parts of Africa, India, and China had been using inoculation for centuries. Even in Europe there was some reference to it in a verse production of the School of Salerno in the 10th or 11th century. The first authentic reports were published in Leipzig between 1670 and 1705. In other parts of Europe it was employed as a part of folkmedicine.[1] Late in the 17th century, accounts of the Asiatic practice began arriving in England, and in February 1699/1700, Dr. Clopton Havers called it to the attention of the of the Royal Society. Certainly by this time many Englishmen had heard of the art.[2]

JOHN B. BLAKE, formerly Chief of the History of Medicine Division, National Library of Medicine, Bethesda, Maryland, is now retired.

Reprinted with permission from the *New England Quarterly*, 1952, *25*: 489–506.

In the following two decades, after inoculation had become popular in Turkey, it was more fully studied, reported, and recommended in the western world. During a smallpox epidemic in 1713 it again came up for discussion in the Royal Society. In May 1714, Dr. John Woodward, Professor of Physic at Gresham College, communicated to this scientific organization an enthusiastic endorsement from Dr. Emanuel Timonius of Constantinople.[3] Other correspondents also reported on the practice, and two years later the society published another favorable account by Jacobus Pylarinus.[4] Not until April 1721, however, did the first recorded inoculation take place in England, on the daughter of Lady Mary Wortley Montagu. Another child received the treatment in May. Princess Caroline became interested, and in August six felons offered themselves for experiment. After other trials the two royal daughters were successfully inoculated in April 1722.[5]

In Massachusetts, meanwhile, some of Cotton Mather's parishioners gave him a Negro slave in 1706. No doubt Mather asked him if he had had the smallpox, and received then his first confused intimation of the practice of inoculation as some of the African natives carried it out. Further questioning of several other Negroes and some Guinea slave traders confirmed the tale. Sometime before July 1716, Mather also received a copy of Timonius's communication in the *Philosophical Transactions*. In a letter to Dr. Woodward of July 12, 1716, he corroborated this account with what he had heard and inquired why the practice was not tried in England. "For my own part," he wrote, "if I should live to see the *Small-Pox* again enter into our City, I would immediately procure a Consult of our Physicians, to Introduce a Practice, which may be of so very happy a Tendency."[6] At least five years in advance, therefore, Mather had seriously considered the policy he was later to follow.[7]

On April 22, 1721, among several ships arriving from the West Indies was H.M.S. *Seahorse*, which brought the smallpox. Not until May 8, however, did the selectmen learn that a Negro who came on the naval vessel was in town with the disease. When they heard of another case at Captain Wentworth Paxton's house, they ordered two men to stand guard there and let no one in or out without their permission. A few days later, at the request of the town, the governor and council ordered the *Seahorse* down to Bird Island to prevent further infection from this source, but not until after several other sick members of the company had come ashore. As late as May 20 the selectmen could find no more cases, but two days later the town nevertheless instructed its representatives to seek further legislation to enable the selectmen to prevent the spread of infectious sickness. On the twenty-fourth the selectmen set 26 free Negroes to work cleaning the streets as a preventive measure, but without avail. On May 27 there were eight known cases, and by the middle of June the disease was in so many houses that the selectmen abandoned the system of guards.[8]

By this time Cotton Mather had decided to carry out his previous plan. Considering it his Christian duty—and worrying about his own children—on June 6 he circulated a letter about inoculation among the physicians of Boston, along with an abstract of the accounts by Timonius and Pylarinus. "*Gentlemen,*" he wrote, My *request* is, that you would *meet for a Consultation* upon this Occasion, and to *deliberate* upon it, that whoever first begins this practise, (*if you approve that it should be begun at all*) may have the concurrence of his *worthy Brethren* to fortify him in it."[9] Whatever their reasons, they made no reply. On June 24, after the guards had been taken off the houses, he wrote another letter strongly recommending the technique to Dr. Zabdiel Boylston.[10] This may have convinced the physician, for two days later he inoculated his six-year-old son Thomas and two of his Negroes. After several anxious days the experiment proved successful, and on July 12 he inoculated Joshua Cheever. Two days later John Helyer and another Negro underwent the operation. On the seventeenth Boylston treated his son John, and on the nineteenth three more people, bringing the total to ten.[11]

The populace was quickly aroused. The idea had caused talk soon after Mather brought it up; within four days after Boylston's first experiment it "raised an horrid Clamour. . . ."[12] In an advertisement in the *Boston Gazette* on July 17 the physician justified his action on the grounds of the reports of Timonius and Pylarinus and his own successful experiments, but when he indicated his intention to continue by the announcement that "*in a few Weeks more, I hope to give you some further proof of their just and reasonable Account,*" he no doubt increased the people's wrath. Cotton Mather, convinced of the value of the practice, thought the Devil had "taken a strange Possession of the People," and noted sadly in his diary that not only Boylston but he himself was also "an Object of their Fury; their furious Obloquies and Invectives."[13]

Soon the selectmen felt they must act. On July 21 they and some justices of the peace met with several members of the medical profession. Disregarding Boylston's invitation to see some of his patients,[14] they accepted instead Dr. Lawrence Dalhonde's statement that inoculation in Italy, Spain, and Flanders had led to horrible sequelae, and pronounced that it "has proved the Death of many Persons," that it "Tends to spread and continue the Infection," and that its continuance "is likely to prove of most dangerous consequence."[15] On this basis the selectmen and justices severely reprimanded Boylston and forbade him to continue the practice.[16]

Three days later Dr. William Douglass, who led the professional opposition, tried a new attack in a communication to the *News-Letter*. He credited Mather with "a Pious & Charitable design of doing good," but attacked Boylston for "*His mischievous propagating the Infection* in the most Publick Trading Place of the Town. . . ." He called on the ministers to determine "how the trusting more the extra groundless *Machinations of Men* than to our Preserver in the ordinary course of Nature, may be consistent with that Devotion and Subjection we owe to the *all-wise Providence* of GOD Almighty." Of the lawyers he inquired "how it may be construed a *Propagating of Infection and Criminal.*"[17] On the thirty-first the ministers' reply appeared in the *Gazette*, signed by Increase and Cotton Mather, Benjamin Colman, Thomas Prince, John Webb, and William Cooper. After upholding Boylston's professional skill, they declared that if, as they believed, inoculation could save lives, they accepted it "with all thankfulness and joy as the gracious Discovery of a *Kind Providence* to Mankind. . . ." Use of this operation, they said, like that of any other medical treatment, depended on God's blessing and was fully consistent with "*a humble Trust . . . and a due Subjection*" to the Lord. When James Franklin's new paper, the *New-England Courant*, appeared on August 7, the anti-inoculators had their medium, and a furious newspaper and pamphlet war ensued.

Boylston, meanwhile, backed by the six ministers, disregarded the selectmen's orders and on August 5 resumed inoculating. During that month he performed the operation on 17 people, in September on 31, and the next month on 18. Among the last were three men from Roxbury who, after their recovery, returned to recommend it there. November was his busiest month, with 104 inoculations. Several ministers and other prominent men encouraged the practice by their example. On September 23 the Honorable Thomas Fitch, Esq., tried the new technique. Others included the Reverend Thomas Walter on October 31, and in November, the Reverend Ebenezer Pierpont, Anthony Stoddard, Esq., John White, Esq., the Honorable Judge Quincy's son Edmund, Edward Wigglesworth and William Welsteed, professor and fellow respectively at Harvard, Justice Samuel Sewall's grandson Samuel Hirst, the Honorable Jonathan Belcher's son Andrew, and the Reverend Nehemiah Walter. On December 8, even a doctor, Elijah Danforth of Roxbury, submitted to the test.[18]

Whatever the clergymen and esquires may have thought of inoculation, the people as a whole continued to oppose it violently. They were urged on by most of the local physicians, one of whom went so far as to assert that it would breed in Boston bubonic plague, which was then devastating southern France.[19] One man vented his feelings about three in the morning of November 14 by throwing a lighted grenade into Cotton Mather's house.[20] Ten days previously, shortly after Boylston began receiving patients from Roxbury and Charlestown, the town had expressed its official attitude by voting that anyone who came into Boston to be inoculated should be forthwith sent to the pesthouse unless he returned home, "Least by alowing this practis the Town be made an Hospi-

tal for that which may prove worse then the Smal pox, which has already put So many into mourning. . . ."[21] The selectmen thereupon requested the justices for warrants to remove such persons.[22] When several ministers were accused of encouraging country people to come into Boston to be inoculated despite the town's vote, the selectmen called them to a meeting, but "after some hot Discourse on both sides" they denied it.[23]

Meanwhile the epidemic also raged. Soon after it began, trade was disrupted, and many people fled. One person died in May, 8 in June, 11 in July, and 26 in August.[24] That month the General Court, which was sitting at the George Tavern on the Neck, appointed three men to stand guard at the door of the House of Representatives to prevent anyone from Boston entering without special license.[25] In September, when the deaths jumped to 101, the selectmen severely limited the length of time funeral bells could toll.[26] When the sloopmen who normally supplied the town with wood refused to bring it in, the selectmen made special arrangements to allay their fear and avert a fuel shortage, perhaps on the suggestion of Cotton Mather.[27] When the General Court met again on November 7, in Cambridge, the members were "very solicitous of Returning to their Homes as soon as may be,"[28] for by then the smallpox was in the college town. The session lasted only ten days, most of the time being taken up with the Indian war in Maine and quarrels with the governor. The legislators did find time, however, to tighten up the law against peddlers, who were charged with spreading the disease.[29] More helpful was the thousand pounds voted from the public treasury for the selectmen and overseers of the poor to distribute among the many people "reduced to Very Great Strieghts & Necessitous Circumstances," who could otherwise have supported their families comfortably.[30] Along with the contributions from other towns, it was no doubt gratefully received.[31]

By then the epidemic was beginning to decline. October had been the worse month, with 411 deaths. In November the total dropped to 249, and by mid-December, according to the selectmen, the mortality was not much higher than in time of health.[32] During January and February Boylston inoculated only 12 people, none in Boston.[33] On February 26 the selectmen issued an official statement that there were no more known cases in the town. Altogether, since April, 5,889 people, of whom 844 died, had had the smallpox. This one disease caused more than three-fourths of all the deaths in Boston during the year of the epidemic.[34] During the same period Boylston inoculated 242 persons, with 6 deaths.[35] Except for a few recurrences in April and May the epidemic was over in the capital.[36]

Then, on May 11, 1722, Boylston inoculated Samuel Sewall, a Boston merchant and nephew of the diarist, his wife, three boys in his household, and Joanna Alford, the first he had done since February 24, and the first in Boston since December.[37] The people were incensed. The selectmen quickly removed these new cases to Spectacle Island to keep them from communicating the infection to anyone else,[38] and called Boylston before the town meeting, where he "did solemnly promise to Inoculate no more without the knowledge & approbation of the Authority of the Town."[39] Douglass gloated:

> Last January *Inoculation* made a Sort of *Exit*, like the Infatuation Thirty Years ago, after several had fallen Victims to the mistaken Notions of Dr. *M–r* and other learned Clerks concerning Witchcraft. But finding Inoculation in this Town, like the Serpents in Summer, beginning to crawl abroad again the last Week, it was in time, and effectually crushed in the Bud, by the *Justices, Select-Men,* and the *unanimous Vote* of a general Town-Meeting.[40]

The voters also instructed their representatives to seek legislation regulating inoculation and prohibiting it in any town without the selectmen's permission. Since some question had arisen over the interpretation of the act relating to contagious diseases, the people wanted their officials "Clothed with full power to obtain the great End & Designe of that Law, which is for the Preservation, Health, and Safty, of the Inhabitants."[41]

The House had already passed a "Bill to prevent the Spreading of the Infection of the Small-Pox by the practice of Inoculation" in March 1721/1722, but the council had turned it down.[42] Perhaps for this reason the representatives made no further attempt to pass a general law. Their attitude, however, was unchanged. When the Boston assemblymen brought up the subject of Samuel Sewall and the others sent to Spectacle Island, the

General Court resolved on June 2, 1722, that they should not come to Boston as long as the legislature was in session. As late as July 3 the House denied a petition passed by the council to rescind this order.[43]

An analysis of the whole controversy shows that several factors were involved. One source of opposition to inoculation was the religious scruples of earnest and devout people. Some maintained that it was a sin for a healthy person to bring the sickness upon himself, especially since he might otherwise escape it altogether, and that he should in submission to God's will leave it to Him to determine whether or not he would suffer the disease. Another argument was that since the epidemic was sent by God, the only proper recourse was repentance and reformation; inoculation only increased the guilt because it was a rebellious attempt to take God's work out of His hands and showed distrust in His promises:[44]

> It is impossible that any *Humane Means*, or *preventive Physick* should defend us from, or Over-rule a *Judicial National Sickness*; for were it so, Wicked and Atheistical Men would have the same terms and conditions of *Security* in a *Physical Respect*, with the most Holy and Religious. And *National Judgments* would not have the Designed Ends for which they were sent *National Amendment*.[45]

Some of Boston's leading ministers, however, easily answered these arguments. It was not unlawful to make oneself sick in this manner, they declared; rather it was a duty because it was a protection against a worse sickness. In the same way, they pointed out, other preventive medicines such as purges and vomits were used, and no one considered that sinful. William Cooper provided the most complete rebuttal. It was not faith, he said, but presumption for anyone to think that God would preserve him when walking in an infected atmosphere. One must, of course, rely primarily on the Lord, he said, but this did not preclude the use of the best human help afforded by His providence. Recourse to inoculation did not take God's work from His hands, for both inoculated and natural smallpox were secondary causes and therefore under Him the First Cause. While agreeing that the epidemic was God's judgment for the sins of the community, he believed that the people should be thankful for His mercy in sending the means to escape the extremity of destruction. Inoculation, he said, might be God's chosen instrument to preserve life as long as He had predestined it; no one, he pointed out, relied on predestination to keep himself from starving. Admittedly there was no guarantee that an inoculated person would not die. But after serious consideration of this, the knottiest problem of all, Cooper believed that if a person died under this operation, he died in the use of the most likely means he knew to save his life in time of peril, and, therefore, in the way of duty and so in God's way.[46]

The religious question, though significant, should not be overemphasized. While much of the argument was couched in religious terms, the real dividing point was medical. The Sixth Commandment was frequently mentioned, but whether for or against depended on what the medical results of inoculation were alleged to be. None of the opponents was content to rest his case on the necessity of trusting in God's providence; however they phrased it, they all thought the practice harmful to the health and lives of their fellow-citizens.

In the passion of the fight both sides exaggerated either the ease and safety of the practice on the one hand, or its horrors and dangers on the other. The proponents' fundamental argument, however, was that it gave the patient a mild case of smallpox which protected him from the natural one. They cited the reports of Timonius and Pylarinus, and Boylston published Mather's abstracts.[47] They pointed out that in Africa the Negroes had long carried on this practice to great advantage. They ridiculed the assertions that it would cause plague or debilitate the constitution. In particular they called to witness the results of Boylston's own trials. Old and young, weak and strong, had been inoculated, they said, with success beyond expectation. After making excuses for the sole death at the time he wrote, Increase Mather declared:

> It is then a wonderful Providence of GOD, that all that were *Inoculated* should have their Lives preserved; so that the Safety and Usefulness of this Experiment is confirmed to us by Ocular Demonstration: I confess I am afraid, that the Discouraging of this Practice, may cause many a Life to be lost, which for my own part, I should be loth to have any hand in, *because of the Sixth Commandment.*[48]

When we see how easily it enables people to pass through smallpox, said Benjamin Colman, we should praise the Lord for His mercy in providing it.[49] "*In fine;*" added Cotton Mather, "*Experience has declared, that there never was a more* unfailing Remedy *employed among the Children of Men.*"[50]

Although some objections were fantastic and some picayune, anti-inoculators also had sound arguments. They emphasized the known deaths among the inoculated—which the Mathers tried to explain away—and hinted of others. They said, rightly, that the technique endangered the individual who submitted to it. Their chief contention was that inoculation as performed by Boylston spread the epidemic. John Williams maintained that anyone who voluntarily took the smallpox violated the moral law of God—"Therefore all things whatsoever ye would that Men should do to you, do ye even so to them"—by bringing the disease to his neighbor.[51]

The anonymous author of *A Letter from One in the Country, to His Friend in the City* expressed this viewpoint ably. As he saw it, Boylston introduced the practice without the consent of the other physicians soon after the guards had been removed from stricken houses, when there was still a possibility that the epidemic would not spread. Is it not an offense against the government, he asked, to infect one's own family with the smallpox despite the cries of civil authority, professional brethren, and neighbors? "If a man should wilfully throw a Bomb into a Town . . . ought he not to die? so if a man should wilfully bring Infection from a person sick of a deadly and contagious Disease, into a place of Health; is not the mischief as great?"[52] The author was willing to allow those who favored inoculation to practice it, but only where they would not threaten the rest of the community. He felt sure, and he was right, that the people who urged the new technique never thought of regulating it, "which ought to have been the very first step in a matter of such concernment to a people."[53] He hoped the General Court would act:

> That if they allow it, there may be proper Pest Houses in solitary places, to receive those that have a mind thus voluntarily to infect themselves, with severe penalties on those that shall dare to do otherwise, to the endangering the lives of their honest Neighbours. . . .[54]

This was a sound suggestion. Unfortunately it was not carried out for many years.

Religious and medical divisions were not the only causes of the heat of the controversy. In part they were due to the personalities involved, particularly those of Cotton Mather and William Douglass. The former, pedantic, tactless, egotistical, convinced that those who opposed him were possessed of the Devil, yet rejoicing in the prospect of martyrdom at the hands of Satan's minions (the town), asserted that raving and railing against *"the* Ministers, *and other serious* Christians, *who favour this Practice, is a very crying Iniquity; and to call it a* Work of the Devil . . . *is a shocking* Blasphemy. . . ."[55] He or one of his cohorts accused the anti-inoculation physicians of being another "Hell-Fire Club," a current, notorious group of blasphemers in England.[56] Douglass, on the other hand, accused Mather of credulity, whim, and vanity, of omissions and errors in his abstracts of Timonius and Pylarinus, and of misrepresentation; and he called Boylston an illiterate quack.[57] Douglass, apparently, thought he should be the leader of whatever was happening in local medical affairs and was prone to disparage any who were not his sycophants. Nine years later he declared that Mather had "surreptitiously" set Boylston to work, "that he might have the honour of a New-fangled notion."[58] One suspects that some of his bitterness resulted from his own failure to take the lead. Eventually he came to favor the practice, but he never forgave his two opponents.[59]

The clash between Mather and Douglass stemmed from more than their personalities, for they also stood for two different principles. The minister was in effect maintaining the right of his profession to interfere with and control the life of the community. This is why he and his father — the ordained leaders in all things — became so incensed when others defied them. We say that inoculation is good and lawful, they seemed to assert; therefore all men must believe it. The wise and judicious people of Massachusetts approved it, wrote Increase Mather, referring to the magistrates and ministers, himself and his son. Those who opposed were of a different breed:

> Furthermore, I have made some Enquiry, Whether there are many Persons of a Prophane Life and Conversation, that do Approve and Defend *Inoculation*, and I have been answered, that

they know but of very few such. This is to me a weighty Consideration. But on the other hand, tho' there are some Worthy Persons, that are not clear about it; nevertheless, it cannot be denied, but that the known Children of the Wicked one, are generally fierce Enemies to Inoculation.[60]

To those with a troubled conscience, Mather suggested that they seek guidance from their religious advisers. But as for Douglass, no one could "in rational Charity" think that he had

> the least spark of Grace in his heart . . . ; for in his Pamphlet there are many impudent and malicious Lies, and the whole design of it is to jeer and abuse the faithful Messengers of GOD, which is far from a sign of Piety. 2 Chron. 36. 16.[61]

Douglass, on the other hand, was defending the integrity of the medical profession against the interference of those whom he considered to be credulous laymen. He pointed out that no one should accept all the quaint things published in the *Philosophical Transactions*, that Mather's sources of information — accounts from the Levant and from untutored Negroes — were at best questionable.[62] His principal complaint was that despite the opposition of the town, the selectmen, and the medical profession, *"Six Gentlemen of Piety and Learning, profoundly ignorant of the Matter,"* rashly advocated a new and doubtful procedure in "a Disease one of the most intricate practical Cases in Physick. . . ."[63] By January 1721/1722, Douglas was willing to admit that inoculated smallpox was frequently more favorable than natural and that the practice was at least a temporary, palliative preventive. Though pessimistic, he thought that it might with improvement become a specific smallpox preventive. But, he declared, it must be allowed by an act of the legislature and carried out by "abler hands, than *Greek old Women, Madmen and Fools.*" He wanted a period of cautious experimentation. "For my own Part," he said, *"till after a few Years, I shall pass no positive Judgment of this bold Practice."*[64]

Douglass' attitude toward the clergy brought him allies who opposed them chiefly for political reasons. Among them was John Williams. Much of his stuff was nonsense, some of it mildly amusing, but a large part was devoted to comprehensive attacks on the ministers. Claiming that inoculation was "a Delusion of the Devil," he compared it to "the Time of the Witchcraft at Salem, when so many innocent Persons lost their Lives. . . ."[65] He blasted the ministers for going outside their calling by trying to control such public affairs as inoculation and paper money. "Now the People are afraid," he declared, "the Ministers do affect a Rule over them in Temporals, as the Pope of *Rome* does temporally as well as spiritually, rule and determine things."[66]

James Franklin also seized this opportunity to belabor the clery. "I pray Sir," asked "Layman" in a debate with "Clergyman" printed in Franklin's *Courant*:

> who have been Instruments of Mischief and Trouble both in Church and State, from the Witchcraft to Inoculation? who is it that takes the Liberty to Villify a whole Town, in Words too black to be repeated? Who is it that in common Conversation makes no Bones of calling the Town a MOB? [67]

Another *Friendly Debate* which he published just before the annual meeting for choosing town officers used the controversy to introduce an attack on the ministers, particularly Cotton Mather, for electioneering against the incumbent selectmen, for attempting to run the town, and for scorning the "Leather Apron Men."[68]

Boston's religious leaders were not the sort to turn the other cheek. One of their supporters damned "this Impious and Abominable Courant" as a weekly libel sheet whose "main intention" was to "Vilify and Abuse the best Men we have, and especially the Principal Ministers of Religion in the Country."[69] Increase Mather added his condemnation and his lamentations for the degeneracy of his native land. "I can well remember," he declared, "when the Civil Government could have taken an effectual Course to suppress such a *Cursed Libel*!"[70] The most thorough rebuttal was a pamphlet inspired by Cotton Mather,[71] the *Vindication of the Ministers of Boston*. The anonymous author lauded the clergy as worthy men seeking the best for their people and gave the pro-Mather version of the beginning of the whole controversy. He was chiefly concerned, however, with maintaining the ministers' leadership in all things:

> If this *impious* & Satanic Custom [of attacking the clergy] prevail, we shall involve our selves into a thousand pernicious *Evils*. . . . Our *Reprovers* and *Prophets* being Silenced, *Iniquity* and every *Abomination* will break in among us, and bear down like an irresistible Torrent, all *Virtue*, and *Religion* before it. And what is mostly to be deprecated, all manner of *Spiritual Plagues* will follow this our degeneracy; and the *Town* grow ripe for a *Wrath unto the Uttermost*.[72]

Inoculation had become a bitter party cause.

Reviewing the controversy, we must credit Cotton Mather and Boylston for their courage in experimenting with and continuing what seemed on fairly good evidence to be a means of saving life. But they cannot escape censure for their neglect of the rights of the community by their failure to take any steps to prevent those who were inoculated from transmitting the disease to others. Moreover, though Mather was not as credulous in this case as Douglass thought, it is difficult to escape the conclusion that he and Boylston were lucky that the experiment worked so well. On the other hand, Douglass' cautious approach toward an obviously dangerous medical innovation was a sane one. Unfortunately the vehemence of his opposition and his credulity in accepting Dalhonde's report becloud the positive values of his attitude. Furthermore, despite his expressed preference for cautious experiments, he himself would probably never have undertaken them.

## NOTES

1 Arnold C. Klebs, "The historic evolution of variolation," *Johns Hopkins Hosp. Bull.*, 1913, *24*: 70; Charles G. Cumston, "Historical notes on smallpox and inoculation," *Ann. Med. Hist.*, 1924, 6: 469.

2 Raymond P. Stearns and George Pasti, Jr., "Remarks upon the introduction of inoculation for smallpox in England," *Bull. Hist. Med.*, 1950, *24*: 106–108.

3 Emanuel Timonius, "An account, or history, of the procuring the small pox by incision, or inoculation; as it has for some time been practised at Constantinople," Royal Society of London, *Philosophical Transactions*, No. 339, April-May-June 1714, *29*: 72–82.

4 Jacobus Pylarinus, "Nova & tuta variolas excitandi per transplantationem methodus, nuper inventa & in usum tracta," Royal Society of London, *Philosophical Transactions*, No. 347, January-February-March 1716, *29*: 393–399.

5  Stearns and Pasti, "Introduction of inoculation in England," pp. 109–114; Klebs, "Evolution of variolation," pp. 71–72.

6  George L. Kittredge, "Introduction," Increase Mather, *Several Reasons Proving That Inoculating or Transplanting the Small Pox, Is a Lawful Practice, and That It Has Been Blessed by God for the Saving of Many a Life* (Cleveland, 1921), p. 5.

7  *Ibid.,* pp. 2–6; George L. Kittredge, "Some lost works of Cotton Mather," Massachusetts Historical Society, *Proceedings,* 1911–1912, *65*: 420–427.

8  Boston Record Commissioners, *Report* (Boston, 1876–1898), VIII, 154–155; XIII, 81–83; Massachusetts General Court, *The Acts and Resolves, Public and Private, of the Province of the Massachusetts Bay* (Boston, 1869–1922), X, 105; *Boston News-Letter,* May 22, 29, 1721; William Douglass to Cadwallader Colden, May 1, 1722, New-York Historical Society, *Collections,* 1917, *50*: 141–142.

9  *A Vindication of the Ministers of Boston, from the Abuses & Scandals, Lately Cast upon Them, in Diverse Printed Papers* (Boston, 1722), p. 8; Cotton Mather, *Diary* (Massachusetts Historical Society, *Collections,* 7th series, VII–VIII, 1911–1912), II, 620–622.

10  Reginald H. Fitz, *Zabdiel Boylston, Inoculator, and the Epidemic of Smallpox in Boston in 1721* (n.p., [1911], reprinted from *Johns Hopkins Hosp. Bull.,* 1911, *22*: 315–327), p. 10.

11  Zabdiel Boylston, *An Historical Account of the Small-Pox Inoculated in New England, upon All Sorts of Persons, Whites, Blacks, and of All Ages and Constitutions* . . . 2nd ed. (London, 1726; reprinted at Boston, 1730), pp. 2–7.

12  C. Mather, *Diary,* II, 628.

13  *Ibid.,* p. 632.

14  Boylston, *Historical Account,* pp. 3–4; *Boston Gazette,* July 31, 1721.

15  *News-Letter,* July 24, 1721.

16  [Cotton Mather], *An Account of the Method and Success of Inoculating the Small-Pox, in Boston in New-England* (London, 1722), p. 11; *New-England Courant,* Aug. 7, 1721.

17  *News-Letter,* July 24, 1721. As was his wont, Douglass added several gratuitous insults to Boylston.

18  Boylston, *Historical Account,* pp. 7–31, 50; *News-Letter,* March 5, 1729/30.

19  *Courant,* Aug. 14, 1721.

20  C. Mather, *Diary,* II, 657–658; *News-Letter,* Nov. 20, 1721.

21  Boston Record Commissioners, *Report,* VIII, 159.

22  Boston Record Commissioners, *Report,* XIII, 90–91.

23  *Courant,* Nov. 20, 1721. Yet as late as Jan. 13, 1721/22, Cotton Mather recorded in his *Diary* (II, 670): "Make an offer to a Minister at *Marble-head,* likely to be murdered by an abominable People, that will

not lett him save his Life, from the Small-Pox, in the Way of Inoculation. Offer to receive and cover him."

24  *News-Letter,* Feb. 26, 1721/22.

25  Mass. *Acts and Resolves,* X, 105.

26  Boston Record Commissioners, *Report,* XIII, 87.

27  *Ibid.,* pp. 88–89; *News-Letter,* Sept. 25, 1721; C. Mather, *Diary,* II, 646.

28  Massachusetts General Court, House of Representatives, *Journals* (Boston, 1919–), III, 146.

29  1721–1722, ch. 6, Mass. *Acts and Resolves,* II, 232.

30  Mass. *Acts and Resolves,* X, 123.

31  Boston Record Commissioners, *Report,* VIII, 159; *Courant,* Jan. 1, 1721/22.

32  *News-Letter,* Feb. 26, 1721/22; Boston Record Commissioners, *Report,* XIII, 92.

33  Boylston, *Historical Account,* pp. 32-duplicate 31.

34  *News-Letter,* Feb. 26, Mar. 12, 1721/22.

35  Boylston, *Historical Account,* p. 50; *News-Letter,* March 5, 1729/30.

36  Boston Record Commissioners, *Report,* XIII, 96; *News-Letter,* April 16, 1722; *Gazette,* May 21, 1722.

37  Boylston, *Historical Account,* pp. duplicate 31-duplicate 32; Frederick G. Kilgour, "Thomas Robie (1689–1729), colonial scientist and physician," *Isis,* 1939, *30*: 486–487.

38  Boston Record Commissioners, *Report,* VIII, 165; XIII, 97–98; *Gazette,* May 21, 1722.

39  *Gazette,* May 21, 1722.

40  *Courant,* May 21, 1722.

41  Boston Record Commissioners, *Report,* VIII, 166–167.

42  House *Journals,* III, 178, 181, 184–185; Thomas Hutchinson, *The History of the Colony and Province of Massachusetts-Bay,* ed. Lawrence S. Mayo (Cambridge, Mass., 1936), II, 208.

43  Mass. *Acts and Resolves,* X, 161; House *Journals,* IV, 66.

44  *The Imposition of Inoculation as a Duty Religiously Considered in a Letter to a Gentleman in the Country Inclin'd to Admit It* (Boston, 1721), pp. 4–15; *Courant,* Aug. 28, 1721.

45  *Imposition of Inoculation Religiously Considered,* p. 9.

46  [William Cooper], *A Letter to a Friend in the Country, Attempting a Solution of the Scruples & Objections of a Conscientious or Religious Nature, Commonly Made against the New Way of Receiving the Small-Pox* (Boston, 1721), pp. 3–11.

47  Zabdiel Boylston, publisher, *Some Account of What Is Said of Inoculating or Transplanting the Small Pox* (Boston, 1721).

48  I. Mather, *Several Reasons,* p. 72.

49  Benjamin Colman, *Some Observations on the New Method of Receiving the Small-Pox by Ingrafting or Inoculating* (Boston, 1721), pp. 1–5.

50  Cotton Mather, *Sentiments on the Small Pox Inoculated* (with I. Mather, *Several Reasons,* Cleveland, 1921), p. 76.

51  John Williams, *Several Arguments, Proving that Inoculating the Small Pox Is Not Contained in the Law of Physick, Either Natural or Divine, and Therefore Unlawful,* 2nd ed. (Boston, 1721), pp. 3–4.

52  *A Letter from One in the Country, to His Friend in the City: in Relation to Their Distresses Occasioned by the Doubtful and Prevailing Practice of the Inocculation of the Small-Pox* (Boston, 1721), pp. 3–4.

53  *Ibid.,* p. 7.

54  *Ibid.,* p. 8.

55  C. Mather, *Sentiments on the Small Pox Inoculated,* pp. 78–79; Mather's *Diary* for the period (II, 620–674) is full of such opinions.

56  *News-Letter,* Aug. 28, 1721.

57  [William Douglass], *The Abuses and Scandals of Some Late Pamphlets in Favour of Inoculation of the Small Pox, Modestly Obviated, and Inoculation Further Consider'd in a Letter to A—— S—— M. D. & F. R. S. in London* (Boston, 1722), pp. 6–7; [William Douglass], *Inoculation of the Small Pox as Practised in Boston, Consider'd in a Letter to A—— S—— M. D. & F. R. S.* (Boston, 1722), pp. 1–13; *News-Letter,* July 24, 1721.

58  [William Douglass], *A Dissertation Concerning Inoculation of the Small-Pox* (Boston, 1730), p. 2.

59  William Douglass, *A Summary, Historical and Political, of the First Planting, Progressive Improvements, and Present State of the British Settlements in North-America* (London, 1755), II, 409.

60  I. Mather, *Several Reasons,* p. 73.

61  Increase Mather, *Some Further Account from London, of the Small-Pox Inoculated,* 2nd ed. (Boston, 1721), p. 5.

62  [Douglass], *Inoculation as Practised in Boston,* pp. 1–9; [Douglass], *Abuses and Scandals,* pp. 6–10.

63  *Courant,* Aug. 7, 1721.

64  [Douglass], *Inoculation as Practised in Boston,* p. 20.

65  John Williams, *An Answer to a Late Pamphlet, Intitled, a Letter to a Friend in the Country* (Boston, 1722), p. 4.

66  *Ibid.,* p. 11.

67  *Courant,* Jan. 22, 1721/22.

68  *A Friendly Debate; or, a Dialogue between Rusticus and Academicus about the Late Performance of Cademicus* (Boston, 1722).

69  *Gazette,* Jan. 15, 1721/22.

70  *Gazette,* Jan. 29, 1721/22.

71  Kittredge, "Introduction," I. Mather, *Several Reasons,* pp. 39–41.

72  *Vindication of Ministers,* p. 12.

# 25

## Politics, Parties, and Pestilence: Epidemic Yellow Fever in Philadelphia and the Rise of the First Party System

### MARTIN S. PERNICK

The omens were not auspicious for Philadelphia in the summer of 1793. Unusually large flocks of migrating pigeons filled the daytime sky. By night a comet streaked the heavens. Increased numbers of cats were dying, their bodies putrefying in the streets and sinkholes, as the rains that usually washed them away were replaced by prolonged drought. Most ominously, the swarms of flies seemingly indigenous to the city had been driven off by a dense mass of "moschetoes" that hung over the city like a cloud.[1] Warned by these signs and portents, the learned Philadelphia medical community had prepared itself for the appearance of a somewhat more virulent strain of "autumnal fever" than was usual. By early August, though, the doctors were puzzling over isolated cases of a new disease involving yellowing of the skin and vomiting of an unknown black substance. On August 19, Dr. Benjamin Rush, signer of the Declaration of Independence and dean of Philadelphia medicine, proclaimed that yellow fever had returned to the city for the first time since 1762.

Initial disbelief turned rapidly to panic as the death toll mounted. By the end of the month between 140 and 325 Philadelphians had died of the fever. On one October day, 119 dead were buried. Between August 19 and November 15, 10 to 15 percent of the estimated 45,000 Philadelphians perished, while another 20,000, including most government officials, simply fled.[2] An extralegal committee of citizen volunteers, called upon by the mayor following the hasty departure of the regular municipal officers, gradually brought the panic under control.

MARTIN S. PERNICK is Associate Professor of History at the University of Michigan, Ann Arbor, Michigan.

Revised by author and reprinted with permission from the *William and Mary Quarterly*, 1972, *29*: 559–586.

Growing slowly from a nucleus of ten men who answered Mayor Matthew Clarkson's September 10 call, the committee commandeered the vacant Bush Hill estate for use as a hospital, set up an orphanage, distributed food, firewood, clothes, and medicine to the poor, buried the abandoned corpses, and undertook a complete cleanup of the city.[3]

Good intentions and hard work were not enough; the hospital could do little when no cure was known. Sanitary efforts were random at best when no one understood the cause of the sickness. The city of Philadelphia needed immediate resolution of three crucial medical questions: what caused the fever and how might its spread and recurrence be averted? how should the sick be treated? and should the people evacuate or stay?

Philadelphia was the medical capital of the United States. Franklin's Pennsylvania Hospital, the prestigious College of Physicians, and the American Philosophical Society combined to attract to the city the best of the new nation's scientific and medical talent. But the medical problems posed by yellow fever were simply not solvable by even the best 18th-century physicians — or, more accurately, medical science alone provided no definitive way of choosing from among the scores of conflicting causes, preventives, and cures, each presented as gospel by its learned advocates. This uncertainty provided the opening by which influences initially quite removed from medical science entered the medical debate.[4]

The yellow fever epidemic of 1793 provides an early example of the complex links between health and politics in American society. In addition, the epidemic reveals the respective roles of local and national events in the creation of America's first two-party system.

Philadelphia in 1793 was not only the medical center of America but the political capital of a new republic as well. And in politics as in medicine, the presence of a large body of experts did little to expedite agreement. In fact, 1793 found the political leadership of the nation more divided than at any time in its short past. The year began amid an increasingly bitter verbal duel between Treasury Secretary Alexander Hamilton, writing in John Fenno's *Gazette of the United States*, and Secretary of State Thomas Jefferson, whose views appeared in Philip Freneau's *National Gazette*. The battle, begun over fiscal policy, took on added significance with the news at mid-spring that Revolutionary France had executed America's benefactor, Louis XVI, and had declared war on England. Jefferson and his followers feared English "monarchism" as much as Hamilton and his supporters detested French "anarchy." The arrival of Citizen Genêt, the new French Republican Minister to the United States, inspired sympathetic popular demonstrations in Philadelphia and elsewhere, events organized in part by the newly formed Pennsylvania Democratic Society. The exact purposes of this organization may well have been as unclear to the founders as they are to modern historians, but everyone agreed that it was pro-French and pro-Republican.[5]

In spite of such signs of pro-French sympathy, Jefferson's political standing underwent a marked decline in the summer of 1793. Hamilton gained increased influence over foreign policy within the administration following the April Neutrality Proclamation, while Genêt's rapid success in alienating almost everyone in America further discouraged Jefferson. On July 31, Jefferson notified Washington of his intention to resign by year's end.

Local Philadelphia politics grew more involved following the arrival in early August of over two thousand French refugees from the black revolution in Haiti. Unlike the earlier royalist refugees, the new arrivals included many white radicals and moderates, ousted when the slaves seized control of the revolutionary movement.[6]

Both Hamilton and Jefferson feared dividing the young Republic, but their debate provided the core around which local and congressional factions crystalized to form the first institutional American party system. As Jeffersonians became Democratic-Republicans and Hamiltonians became Federal-

ists, both sought to arouse public interest by taking sides in a variety of local or nonpolitical disputes. Local factions likewise often tried to identify their cause with a national party for ideological, rhetorical, political, or moral support against their local rivals. In either case local antagonisms were deepened and prolonged while the national party gained new grass-roots significance.[7] Not surprisingly, the national parties first found themselves embroiled in local issues in the capital city of Philadelphia. The medical controversies generated by the 1793 epidemic over the cause of the disease, its proper treatment, and the conduct of those caught in the crisis, thereby became an integral chapter in the history of the first party system.

## DIRTY STREETS OR DIRTY FOREIGNERS?: THE CAUSE

Since it was not until 1901 that Walter Reed demonstrated the process by which the *Aëdes aegypti* mosquito transmits yellow fever from an infected person to a healthy one, Philadelphia physicians of 1793 divided bitterly over the cause of the epidemic. Doctors who saw the roots of the disease in domestic causes—the poor sanitation, unhealthy location, or climatic conditions of Philadelphia itself—disputed those who placed the blame on the unhealthy state of the still disembarking refugees and their ships. In fact, both sides were right, since a yellow fever epidemic requires both locally bred mosquitoes and an initial pool of infected persons, such as the exiled Haitians. In 1793, however, there was simply no known medical theory to resolve the dispute.[8] The etiological debate revealed, moreover, a medical community split along partisan political lines. In general, Republican physicians, including the refugee doctors, believed the fever to be local. The "importationists" were almost all nonpartisans or Federalists.

Dr. Michael Leib, a founder of all three branches of the Philadelphia Democratic Society and a member of the key correspondence committee of the "mother society," argued the domestic origin case before the College of Physicians. Joining him was his old professor, Dr. Rush, an outspoken opponent of Hamilton. Rush, a founding fellow of the College, leader of the medical school faculty, and probably the best known physician in Philadelphia, insisted that "miasmata" from local swamps and "effluvia" from unsanitary docks bred the fever. A second member of the Democrats' correspondence committee, Dr. James Hutchinson, who as Secretary of the College and Physician of the Port was responsible for deciding to admit or bar the refugee ships, reported to Pennsylvania Governor Thomas Mifflin on August 26, "It does not seem to be an imported disease; for I have learned of no foreigners or sailors that have hitherto been infected." Dr. Jean Devèze, himself a refugee, attributed importationism to ignorance and party influence.[9]

The advocates of importation included Philadelphia's lone confessed Federalist physician, Dr. Edward Stevens, a future diplomat and close boyhood friend of Hamilton. The other leading importationists were Drs. Adam Kuhn, Isaac Cathrall, and William Currie. Although prominent in the profession, they took no part in party politics in 1793. On November 26, after Hutchinson's death in the epidemic enabled Kuhn and his supporters to gain a majority, the College of Physicians passed a resolution firmly asserting, "No instance has ever occurred of the disease called the *yellow fever*, having been generated in this city, or in any other parts of the United States . . . but there have been frequent instances of its having been imported." The resolution was the work of Drs. Thomas Parke, John Carson, and Samuel P. Griffitts, none of whom was politically active in 1793.[10] Benjamin Rush had resigned from the College a few days earlier. Benjamin Smith Barton was the only Republican physician in Philadelphia to support importationism in this epidemic.[11] (See Table 1.)

Politics entered the issue by different doors with different doctors. As a topic for medical debate "The Origin of Pestilential Fevers" was an old favorite, and several physicians were committed to one side or the other before 1793. One such was Benjamin Rush. His 1789 comments belittling both importationism and its advocates created hostilities which may help explain why few importationists would join Rush in the Jeffersonian councils.[12]

For most physicians, though, the whole issue remained a somewhat remote subject for scholarly speculation until the crisis of 1793 suddenly forced each practitioner to choose a course of immediate action. Many turned for guidance to trusted col-

Table 1

1793 Party Affiliations of Physicians Who Expressed an Opinion on the Cause of Yellow Fever

| | Republicans | Federalists | Uncommitted |
|---|---|---|---|
| Importationists —10 | 1 | 1 | 8 |
| Domestic origin—14 | 6 | 0 | 8 |

Note: Twenty-four Philadelphia physicians, the most prominent third of the practicing healers in town, left evidence of their opinions on the cause of the fever. One-third of this medical elite was actively involved in the earliest stages of party building. The prominence of this elite gave their views social significance despite their lack of statistical significance.

leagues—teachers and friends whose opinions on medical, political, and other matters they had shared in the past.[13] In addition, Republican doctors were the most likely to have come in contact with the localist doctrines which dominated French medicine. In the case of Dr. Hutchinson, politics may have influenced medical decisions more directly. An importationist prior to the epidemic, the Republican port physician apparently switched to localism to avoid closing the city to the French refugees.[14]

Like the physicians, the political leaders of Philadelphia split by party over the cause of the fever. Although Republican editor Freneau vehemently condemned the disputes of the medical men, declaring that "no circumstance has added more to the present calamity," he actually strongly supported a local origin. He made his viewpoint clear in the following poem:

> Doctors raving and disputing,
> Death's pale army still recruiting—
>> What a pother
>> One with t'other!
> Some a-writing, some a-shooting.
>
> Nature's poisons here collected,
> Water, earth, and air infected—
>> O, what pity
>> Such a City,
> Was in such a place erected![15]

On September 23, the *National Gazette* published a discussion of more than a dozen theories of the origin of the disease without once mentioning the possibility of its being imported.[16] In medicine as in politics only one's opposition was seen as the "divisive faction." Local Republican civic leaders like editor Andrew Brown and merchants John Swanwick and Stephen Girard supported Dr. Devèze's explanation that burying the dead inside the city had produced the disease. Jefferson explained to Madison that the fever was "generated in the filth of Water street."[17]

On the other hand, Philadelphia Federalists John Fenno, Oliver Wolcott, Thomas Willing, Benjamin Chew, Levi Hollingsworth, J. B. Bordley, Ebenezer Hazard, Bishop William White, and printer Benjamin Johnson led their party in publicly proclaiming yellow fever a foreign disease.[18] In his days as a Federalist after 1794, William "Peter Porcupine" Cobbett, the Anglo-American pamphleteer, penned a series of libelous attacks on Rush's theories. But in 1793, as a supplicant of the patronage of Secretary Jefferson and a tutor to the refugees, Cobbett spoke of the yellow fever as a typical product of the unhealthy American climate.[19]

More than one-third of the most prominent national and local political leaders in Philadelphia took a public position on the cause of the epidemic. With few exceptions the Republicans backed a domestic source of the fever, while Federalists largely blamed importation. Governor Mifflin, who endorsed importation theories, has been called a Republican although he usually appeared as the nonpartisan "Father of his State." Benjamin Franklin Bache, editor of the Republican *General Advertiser*, believed the disease imported but blamed the *British* West Indies, later calling the fever "a present from the English." The least typical was Republican printer Mathew Carey, who included his native Ireland as well as the French islands among the possible sources of the fever.[20] Timothy Pickering, an intimate friend of Dr. Rush, was probably the only Federalist leader in Philadelphia to claim the yellow fever as a domestic disease.[21]

The party leaders, moreover, moved rapidly to exploit the many political implications they discovered in the medical controversy. Federalists used the importation doctrine to back demands for the quarantine or exclusion of the radical French, and for limitations on trade with the French islands, while Republican merchants saw importationism as a cover for plans to wreck their lucrative trade with the West Indies. Girard and Dr. Devèze denounced the proposed quarantine as "disastrous

to commerce." In June 1798, during the "Quasi-War" with France, the newly drafted quarantine laws were in fact successfully invoked to block the immigration of suspected Haitian subversives.[22]

A novel twist was provided by Dr. Currie's theory that the disease originated on board the French privateer *Sans Culotte*, which brought a prize to Philadelphia in July. Accusing both the French and Port Physician Hutchinson, the Federalists charged that sickness on the ship had been covered up to protect the Republican political and financial stake in her activities. Benjamin Johnson blamed the epidemic on the French "licensed plunderers of the Ocean," adding that "if particular men had done their duty; and had not betrayed more indulgence to French cruizers, than genuine friendship for this city," the disease would have been averted.[23] Federalist charges fed a growing Francophobia. "AMOR PATRIAE" warned Philadelphians not to trust the city's benevolent French physicians. Persistent rumors that the wells had been contaminated preparatory to a French invasion led to threats of mob violence against the hapless refugees.[24]

Although the Federalists talked of closing all trade with the French islands, they seemed far more anxious to arouse public suspicion of the French and the Republicans than to create any precedent for a government embargo on commerce. Indeed, the Federalist merchants feared that localism was part of a Republican conspiracy to discredit Philadelphia and all large commercial centers and to force relocation of the capital in a rural setting. Richard Peters warned Timothy Pickering against Rush's doctrine on October 22: "His Assertion that the Philadelphia Hot beds produced this deadly Plant is . . . a mischievous Opinion . . . and will be eagerly caught at by the Anti-Philadelphians. Stifle this Brat if you can."[25] Rush noted the result by October 28: "A new clamor has been excited against me in which many citizens take a part. I have asserted that the yellow fever was generated in our city. This assertion they say will destroy the character of Philadelphia for healthiness, and drive Congress from it."[26] John Beale Bordley wrote an importationist pamphlet for the admitted purpose of convincing Congress to remain in Philadelphia. Federalist editor John Fenno worried that the domestic origin theory would "not only render multitudes uneasy and interrupt the usual course of business, but injure the interest and reputation of the city in several respects."[27]

Such political fears could easily distort medical objectivity. "Is there a city in the world," asked Levi Hollingsworth, "kept cleaner than Philadelphia?" The College of Physicians answered flatly, "No possible improvement with respect to water or ventilation can make our situation more eligible"—this at a time when Philadelphia had no sewage system, no fresh water supply, and no provision for regular garbage disposal![28]

Republicans did attack large cities as unhealthy, and Jefferson later expressed confidence that the "yellow fever will discourage the growth of great cities in our nation."[29] Yet most Republicans protested that they wanted not to destroy commercial cities but to preserve them through sanitary reform.[30] Federalist fears of a plot to move the capital also proved groundless. In the debates over whether or not Congress could legally meet elsewhere to avoid the fever, the Republicans, for strict constructionist reasons, favored convening in Philadelphia.[31]

The Federalist endorsement of importation proved to be a very effective and popular position as the idea of a native American plague irritated a highly sensitive patriotic nerve. Rush noted that "Loathsome and dangerous diseases have been considered by all nations as of foreign extraction."[32] Importationists made much of the widely held feeling that independent America was the New Eden. Reaching the farthest extreme of this argument, one importationist asserted in 1799 that the doctrine of domestic fevers was "treason," perhaps hoping that the Alien and Sedition Acts gave the Federalists the power to deport foreign diseases along with foreign agitators.[33]

The people of Philadelphia urged their officials to agree on specific actions to prevent the return of yellow fever, but the political implications of the issue made adoption of any single course of action unacceptable. Thus, immediately following the 1793 epidemic, Pennsylvania and other threatened states undertook *both* quarantine and sanitary reform projects. Simple political compromise provided a way around the bitter medical deadlock.[34] Considering the state of medical knowledge in 1793, the imposition of a political settlement may well have been the best result that could have been expected.

In 1793, the division between medicine and theology was still young. Not everyone in Philadelphia believed the cause of the plague was strictly medical; rather, the wrath of the Deity appeared to many as manifest in the fever, and before the debate over the epidemic had ended, theology, like medicine, had become enmeshed in political developments. The devout saw most early American diseases, such as cholera and typhoid, as punishment for the individual sins of vicious immigrants and slothful poor. Unlike these diseases, though, yellow fever was spread not by poor individual hygiene but by infected mosquitoes which could and did bite high and low with complete republican egalitarianism. Some physicians even declared that blacks and the West Indian immigrants were more immune than respectable white Philadelphians. At any rate, the pious saw the yellow fever as a communal punishment rather than as retribution against individual sinners.[35]

The issue that remained, of course, was to identify and root out those communal transgressions which had provoked the pestilence. With no shortage of suggestions as to where the country was going astray, the Republicans first gave political content to the religious debate. At the very height of the plague, Freneau devoted front page coverage to a series of articles and letters which pointed to the pride and vanity of the communal leaders as the major transgression. Mathew Carey joined in the attack. And Benjamin Rush, the Enlightenment man of science, commented in retrospect, "I agree with you in deriving our physical calamities from moral causes. . . . We ascribe all the attributes of the Deity to the name of General Washington. It is considered by our citizens as the bulwark of our nation. God would cease to be what He is, if he did not visit us for these things."[36]

Federalists too put the religious issue in political harness. An official thanksgiving-fast sermon by the Reverend William Smith linked the pestilence with French immorality and with the "wild principles and restless conduct of their partisans here, impatient of all rule and authority."[37] Connecticut Senator Chauncey Goodrich saw the divine anger resulting from Republican adoration of Genêt, while Alexander Graydon recalled the "state of parties in the summer of 1793, when the metropolis of Pennsylvania, then resounding with unhallowed orgies at the dismal butcheries in

France, was visited with a calamity which had much the appearance which heaven sometimes sends to purify the heart."[38]

A peculiar coincidence gave added depth to these speculations, for the fever had miraculously appeared just as Philadelphia completed construction of what one Republican termed its "Synagogue for Satan"—the city's new Chestnut Street Theater. Many in Revolutionary America saw the theater as an extremely complex negative symbol, part bordello and part palace. The new theater, with fluted marble columns and pure golden ornaments, was indeed palatial.[39] While a few Republicans like Swanwick owned stock in the theater company, the major backers were prominent Federalists.[40] They in turn tried to portray opposition to the theater as a Republican scheme to subvert private property. One Francophobe detected the same "rigourous enthusiasm" which spawned the French Revolution motivating the foes of the drama. Opponents of the stage did appeal to Anglophobic, antimonarchical, and Republican imagery to justify their cause, although not all Republicans were antitheater.[41]

Philadelphia's embattled defenders of public virtue had all but given up when the epidemic provided the ammunition for yet another crusade. Sixteen of the city's leading clergymen joined with the Quakers in petitioning the state to shut the new theater. "We conceive that the solemn intimations of Divine Providence in the late distressing calamity which has been experienced in this city, urge upon us in the most forcible manner the duty of reforming every thing which may be offensive to the Supreme Governor of the Universe." Devout Republicans found it significant that "the actors and retainers of the stage, who actually arrived here at a time when the fever raged with the utmost violence," were Englishmen.[42] The opponents of stage plays eventually lost their struggle, even with the arguments gained from the epidemic. The issue, however, helped strengthen the growing bond between Quakers and Republicans in Philadelphia.[43]

## BLEEDING VS. BARK: THE CURE

Medical science today can do little more to cure a case of yellow fever than it could in 1793, a sobering fact that helps explain the continued controversy over the treatment of the disease long after the question of etiology had been shelved. The number of treatments attempted in the sheer desperation of the Philadelphia epidemic was astounding, yet the medical community rapidly split into two main schools. One favored the use of "stimulants"—quinine bark, wine, and cold baths—a method long used in both British and French West Indies. Opposing these "bark and wine murderers," a second group advocated the "new treatment" concocted by Dr. Rush, who believed it advisable to draw an amount of blood which we know today to be in excess of the quantity possessed by most people, and whose doses of mercury caused severe disfiguration of the teeth and skin. But by 18th-century standards his "experimental" approach appeared more advanced than the "traditional" bark cure.[44]

Many factors helped determine which doctors adopted what cure, not the least of which was chance. Rush himself tried the bark and wine method before his "discovery" but lost three of four patients. Another variable was the infamous, tangled infighting among Philadelphia physicians. Almost any medical opinion rendered by Benjamin Rush eventually drew the ridicule of Dr. William Shippen, the man Rush had hauled before a court-martial over their disagreements in the Revolution.[45] Partisan differences were at first unimportant in a doctor's choice of a cure. True, Rush counted among his followers many ardent Republicans such as Dr. Leib, Dr. George Logan, the Quaker pacifist, Dr. Benjamin Say, and most of his former students. However, a large body of Republican "bark and wine doctors" included Hutchinson, Dr. Benjamin Smith Barton, and the French-trained Bush Hill staff under Devèze and Girard. Republican bark doctors did learn the cure from the French refugees, while the Federalist Dr. Stevens and other non-Republican physicians adopted the procedure from the British or Dutch islands, but their actual methods of treating patients were almost identical. Although it was inaccurate, many Philadelphians persisted in the conviction that there was a "Republican cure" and a "Federalist cure."[46]

The man initially responsible for politically polarizing this nonpartisan jumble was Alexander Hamilton. Seeing an opportunity to do a favor for an old friend, Hamilton published a glowing personal tribute to Dr. Stevens, attributing his own recovery to the bark and wine cure. In so doing, Hamilton could not resist a sneer at his old critic, Dr. Rush. Hamilton's tool, Secretary of War Henry Knox, followed, airing his thoughts on Rush a few days later. The local and national Federalist press took the cue and began a barrage of political-sounding attacks on Rush's cure, terminated only by the 1799 libel judgment against Cobbett. Fenno's unkind attempt to derive Rush's bloodletting from that of the French terror resulted in a libel action against him as well, but the case was never tried.[47]

By simply declaring long enough and loud enough that bark and wine was the Federalist cure, these editors were able to make a considerable political issue out of a basically nonpartisan dispute. Their appeal was meant to gain political support among the many users of the mild wine and quinine therapy while personally discrediting Rush. The political element in the attack on bleeding seemed obvious to Rush. "I think it probable that if the new remedies had been introduced by any other person than a decided Democrat and a friend of Madison and Jefferson, they would have met with less opposition from Colonel Hamilton," Rush complained. "Many of us," he later told General Horatio Gates, "have been forced to expiate our sacrifices in the cause of liberty by suffering every species of slander and persecution. I ascribe the opposition to my remedies in the epidemic which desolated our city in 1793 chiefly to an unkind and resentful association of my political principles with my medical character."[48] Rush did not deny the Federalist charge that his cures were associated with his politics. Attacked as a democrat, he replied as a democrat, hoping to rally Republican political support for his medical views. Rush declared his cure the only truly egalitarian form of medicine in that it was easy to master and could be practiced by anyone with little formal training. Putting his beliefs into practice, he trained a group of free blacks as itinerant bleeders during the epidemic and published "do-it-yourself" directions in the newspapers, actions which did not endear him to the guardians of the professional mysteries any more than to the Federalists. Rush declared it unnecessary "to send men educated in colleges . . . to cure . . . pestilential disease," assuring his followers that "men and even women may be employed for that purpose, who have not perverted

their reason by a servile attachment to any system of medicine." "All that is necessary," he added, "might be taught to a boy or girl twelve years old in a few hours."[49]

Rush also adopted the Federalists' derogatory identification of his cures with the French Revolution, affirming "I am in the situation of The French Republic surrounded and invaded by new as well as old enemies, without any other allies." He went so far as to imply that the true treatment, no less than the true politics, could be derived in good democratic fashion: "The people rule here in medicine as well as government." The best cure could be decided by the will of the majority. On October 2, Rush wrote to Elias Boudinot that "Colonel Hamilton's remedies are now as unpopular in our city as his funding system is in Virginia or North Carolina."[50]

Public support of bark and wine by several prominent Federalists gave credence to its reputation as the "Federalist cure." Rush, however, failed in his attempt to rally the Republican leadership behind his "egalitarian" medicine. Prominent Republican leaders largely ignored the issue on which Republican physicians were themselves divided.

No clear political division over the issue of therapy actually existed, despite the highly publicized attempts of Hamilton and Rush to create such a polarization. Republican "bark and wine" physicians denied that bleeding was the Republican cure, but they could not compete for public attention with the colorful and prolific Dr. Benjamin Rush. Many Republican "bark doctors" were refugees, barred from political office and lacking public influence, and Hutchinson's death deprived them of their most prominent and articulate spokesman. The failure of "bark and wine" Republicans to counter the publicity attracted by Hamilton and Rush made the cure of yellow fever seem a clear-cut party issue.[51] Moreover, the injection of politics into this medical debate probably had some adverse side effects. The partisan taint of arguments against mercury and bleeding delayed rejection of the Rush cure long after the medical evidence pointed to its inefficacy and danger.

## TO FLEE OR NOT TO FLEE: THE CREDIT

The first days of the epidemic produced a mad scramble to escape town. Benjamin Rush warned all who could to leave the city; even his bitter rivals Drs. Shippen and Kuhn took his advice this time and quickly departed. The panic was so great that "many people thrust their parents into the streets, as soon as they complained of a headache."[52] Exceptions to the general exodus soon appeared, however. Most of the physicians stuck to their posts. Rush, following his discovery of a "cure," publicly advised everyone to remain in town. The French, familiar with the disease and trained to believe it noncontagious, did not flee. Many shopkeepers and middle-class merchants with no one to look after their affairs, and the poor with no place else to go, stayed as well. A handful of true philanthropists remained. As the epidemic wore on, observers noted that the leaders of each of these groups were often Republicans.[53]

Several Federalists did play major roles in the heroic relief work. Mayor Clarkson organized the citizens' committee while Samuel Coates and John Oldden headed a merchants' distribution organization which handled supplies for the mayor. Coates, an intimate of Rush and Girard, was nonetheless a Federalist and was often criticized by Girard for his Francophobia.[54] Levi Hollingsworth and Caspar W. Morris joined the merchants' group. Clement Humphreys, son of the shipbuilder, remained at his post as a guardian of the poor. Three Federalist clergymen, William Smith, William White, and Robert Blackwell, also remained to comfort the ill. Although these nine men were the only identifiable Federalists at all involved in the organized relief work, an additional five, Jacob Hiltzheimer, Postmaster Timothy Pickering, ex-Postmaster Ebenezer Hazard, Congressman Thomas FitzSimmons, and John Stillé, chose not to join the organized effort but rendered important aid to their families and neighbors individually.[55]

Active Republicans, however, performed the greatest share of the work. Of the 18 men cited in the minutes as the leaders of the citizens' committee, nine were definitely Republicans, one was the brother of an ardent Republican, and seven could not be identified with either party. The mayor was the only Federalist. The Republican leaders of the committee were Vice-chairman Samuel Wetherill, Secretary Caleb Lownes, Stephen Girard of Bush Hill, Israel Israel (orphans), Mathew Carey (printing), Jonathan Dickinson

Sergeant (counsel), James Sharswood (accounts), James Kerr (orphans), and John Connelly (accounts). Treasurer Thomas Wistar was the brother of Republican Dr. Caspar Wistar.[56] The other committeemen were Andrew Adgate (at large), Peter Helm of Bush Hill, Daniel Offley (at large), Joseph Inskeep (at large), John Letchworth (orphans), Samuel Benge (burials), and Henry Deforest (supplies).

Three of the four members of the key correspondence committee which ran the Democratic Society were leaders in fighting the fever. Two, Hutchinson and Jonathan Dickinson Sergeant, lost their lives while caring for the sick. The third was Dr. Leib, who had charge of Bush Hill in the first chaotic days of its existence. Alexander B. Dallas, the fourth member, claimed with some justification that his state office required him to follow the state government to its exile in Germantown.[57] At least 17 men listed as active in the Democratic Society played major roles in aiding the sick. Israel Israel directed the relief and orphanage work of the committee. Well known in Philadelphia for his Revolutionary War exploits and for his antifederalism, Israel was treasurer of the Democratic Society. The president of the society, David Rittenhouse, went on call with his nephew Dr. Barton, arranging for free treatment of the poor. After the death of his son-in-law Sergeant, Rittenhouse left town briefly, but returned before the end of the epidemic to resume his work.[58]

The Quaker Dr. George Logan was an ardent Democrat who had left both medicine and Philadelphia in 1781. Returning now from his retirement at Stenton near Germantown, he served as the committee's inspector at Bush Hill, from where he reported to the world the incredible efforts of the managers, "Citizens Girard and Helm." The one-eyed merchant Girard, who almost alone turned Bush Hill from a pesthouse to a hospital, was also active in the Democratic organization.[59] The labors of Dr. Rush, who formally joined the society in early 1794, were comparable to those of Girard. Visiting hundreds of patients while ill himself, Rush stuck to his post even after the death of his sister. Also members of the Democratic group were John Connelly and James Kerr of the citizens' committee; George Forepaugh, Jeremiah Paul, William Robinson, Sr., James Swaine, and William Watkins of the merchants' committee; volunteer John Barker; and John Swanwick, owner of the committee's orphanage. Others of Republican persuasion cited for their roles were aldermen Hilary Baker and John Barclay, and merchants' committeeman Caspar Snyder.[60]

Among Philadelphia newspapers, only Republican Andrew Brown's *Federal Gazette* appeared throughout the epidemic, keeping the remaining citizens in touch with the relief workers.[61] Freneau, who vowed to publish for as long as possible, held on longer than any editor except Brown. The *National Gazette* last appeared on October 16, a victim of financial losses rather than of editorial dereliction. His work ended, Freneau did not flee the city but remained until mid-December.[62]

The list of Republican heroes also included Frenchmen. In addition to Devèze, all four physicians' aides and most of the staff at Bush Hill were French. The French specialist in tropical medicine, Citizen Robert, hearing of the epidemic while en route to France, rushed to Philadelphia from Boston in what one writer termed a "confirmation of the sincere attachment of the French patriots, to the truly republican Americans!" The largest individual contribution to the relief fund came from Citizen Genêt. Even "THE REPUBLICAN SEAMEN OF FRANCE" got involved, forming Philadelphia's only intact fire company during the epidemic. Freneau credited them with saving the city from the fate of London.[63]

While Republicans dominated the relief work, Federalists often joined the ranks of the refugees, not necessarily from cowardice, as Republicans charged, but rather because of their belief in importation and contagion. No prominent importationist leaders of either party stayed in Philadelphia. The one anticontagionist Federalist official remained; the one importationist Republican fled. Illustrative of the disappearance of Federalists was the case of the Dutch Minister, Francis Van Berkle, who believed himself ill. Since Dr. Stevens had left for New York, Hamilton (from his refuge in Albany) suggested that the minister consult Oliver Wolcott on the use of bark and wine. The minister soon discovered that Wolcott too was gone. Tired of looking for someone to instruct him in the "Federalist cure," Van Berkle was treated by Rush and recovered.[64]

It appeared that the Republicans would receive high praise for their efforts. Benjamin Rush "is be-come the darling of the common people and his humane fortitude and exertions will render him deservedly dear," noted one observer.[65] Bravery and leadership make popular American campaign fare, and the Republicans were not slow to present their political bill for services rendered. Among the first to make an issue of bravery was Jefferson, whose Revolutionary War record had recently come under unkind Federalist scrutiny. His scornful cut at Hamilton as the Treasury Secretary prepared to flee is considered by Dumas Malone to have been Jefferson's most vicious political remark. "His family think him in danger," wrote Jefferson, "and he puts himself so by his excessive alarm. He has been miserable several days before from a firm persuasion he should catch it. A man as timid as he is on the water, as timid on horseback, as timid in sickness, would be a phenomenon if his courage of which he has the reputation in military occasions were genuine. His friends, who have not seen him, suspect it is only an autumnal fever he has." Jefferson also attacked Henry Knox, who had already fled, but after waiting to make sure Hamilton had really gone first, Jefferson himself left town over a week ahead of his planned departure.[66]

Freneau took over the task of castigating the "deserters." His poem, "Orlando's Flight," ridiculed the fugitives:

> On prancing steed, with spunge at nose,
> From town behold Orlando fly;
> Camphor and Tar where'er he goes
> Th' infected shafts of death defy—
>     Safe in an atmosphere of stink,
>     No doctor gets Orlando's chink.

Freneau also implied it was greed that made the fugitives so anxious to preserve themselves. Speaking of the afterworld, he concluded:

> Monarchs are there of little note,
> And Caesar wears a ragged coat.
> . . . . . . . . . . . . . . . . .
> Blame not Orlando if he fled,—
> *So little's got by being dead.*[67]

The last evacuees had not yet returned when a special election brought the heroism issue to the fore. State Senator Samuel Powel, Philadelphia's beloved Revolutionary War mayor, had died of the fever. On December 12, a Republican meeting put forth the name of Israel Israel for Powel's seat. Israel's platform was simple and direct. He was "a gentleman whose philanthropy on a late melancholy occasion is well known, and whose firm and steady attachment to the people will, it is hoped, bring forth the united suffrages of the citizens in his favour."[68] The Federalist response came swiftly. The day after the Israel nomination, Fenno revealed a move to draft Mayor Clarkson as the Federalist choice. In an attempt to outdo the Republicans, Clarkson's backers asserted that "gratitude demands a particular tribute of acknowledgement to him for his assiduity, and perseverance in relieving the distresses of our fellow citizens during the calamity from which we have just emerged."[69] Clarkson, however, was content to be mayor, and the nomination went instead to William Bingham, the extremely wealthy associate of the powerful Willing-Morris partnership. Bingham had followed the progress of the fever from his New Jersey shore retreat. The actual management of his campaign, however, was placed in the hands of relief workers John Oldden and John Stillé. Their efforts apparently countered the appeal of Israel's candidacy, and Bingham won the December 19 contest by a three to two margin.[70]

The return of the "deserters" further complicated Republican use of the heroism issue. While many of the Federalists had fled the fever, most of the evacuees were not Federalists. One-third of all Philadelphians had left, and the majority of the rest remained hidden behind locked doors, venturing out only for necessities. Their initial gratitude toward the members of the committee was mingled with a good deal of shame, guilt, and envy. As one perceptive reviewer noted in commenting on Mathew Carey's account of the epidemic, "To panegyrize our contemporaries, without attracting censure on ourselves, requires a very delicate hand."[71] The Republicans realized that a campaign based solely on praising their own heroics while damning the opposition's defections was politically unwise. They usually attempted to temper their attacks by expressing sympathy with the difficulties encountered by the fugitives, many of whom had been brutally repulsed by the panicked citizens of neighboring cities.[72]

The returnees meanwhile countered criticism with charges of their own, terming the epidemic a "doctors' harvest." The citizens' committee was attacked as too expensive and as growing insolent with power. "Unless the Committee feel *tickled* with

their employment," wrote one critic, "they ought to surrender it to the Guardians of the poor, who are competent to the service, and who will perform it at a *much less expence* and *with far less state*." Rush's black bleeders were easy targets for Federalist charges of profiteering. Actually, the committee and most physicians offered free medical service to the poor, while Rush even distributed free mercury. Yet the boast of Rush's student, Dr. Mease, that the fever had made his fortune for life, and the activities of Samuel Wetherill, whose drug business took precedence over his committee duties, gave the charges just enough credibility to undermine the Republican appeal to public gratitude.[73] A common complaint charged the committeemen with usurping powers reserved for the traditional political elite. "The bulk of them," wrote one resentful critic, "are scarcely known beyond the smoke of their own chimnies."[74] Further, many Philadelphians simply wished to forget the entire painful scene as quickly as possible. The heroes of the epidemic were living reminders of the horror and the suffering. "If the disease has disappeared as it no doubt has, every memento of its existence should disappear with it, that the citizens may once more enjoy repose."[75]

Despite the strenuous efforts of the party organization, Republican heroism was a complete flop as a political issue. A 1797 election in which Israel Israel had defeated Federalist Benjamin Morgan was invalidated when Morgan claimed his backers had been disenfranchised by holding the election while the Federalists were "driven from their homes" by the epidemic of that year. With the fleeing Federalists safely home again, the hapless Israel lost the second election despite heavy contributions from Girard and Sharswood.[76]

## CONCLUSION: HEALTH AS A POLITICAL ISSUE

The yellow fever struck a Federalist Philadelphia in 1793 and left both local and national Federalist rule considerably strengthened. For one thing, the epidemic seriously weakened the national Republican organization. The deaths of Hutchinson and Sergeant eliminated two of the four men responsible for creating and directing new Democratic Society branches. Years later, John Adams declared that these two deaths alone saved the nation from an imminent revolution.[77] The collapse of the *National Gazette* under the financial strain of the epidemic created another void which Bache's *Aurora* could not immediately fill. Even the little-noted death of Citizen Dupont, the French consul, had its political effect, leaving France's critical relations with the United States in the hands of a vice-consul for months until the arrival of a replacement for Genêt.

In issues as well as institutions the Federalists gained, at least in the short run. The Republicans were unable to convert their heavy organizational losses into an effective sympathy vote. By denying any local source of the pestilence, the Federalists won much national chauvinist and local booster support, while their espousal of importationism heightened American Francophobia. In addition, the Federalists managed to identify their opponents with Benjamin Rush's advocacy of a dangerous and controversial remedy. Although Philadelphia Republicans found some additional Quaker support in the theater issue, the national party gained at best a minor new point against large cities.[78]

More important, the epidemic served to introduce new issues and attract new supporters to the two developing parties, thereby extending and broadening the base of the new party system. This development was sometimes local in its origins, as in the debate over the cause of the fever, where the already politically polarized local controversy introduced issues that the national politicians adopted and used. In other issues, such as the bleeding *v.* bark debate, a nonpolarized initial conflict had political meaning imposed from the outside by the intervention of national leaders. Furthermore, the process of giving political significance to social issues was highly selective. The issue which seemed logically closest to politics was that of courage and leadership, but despite the efforts of the local antagonists and the party organization, human feelings of gratitude proved too flimsy a foundation on which to build a political platform.

Neither the risks of disease nor the costs of fighting it are evenly distributed in American society. This inequality, resulting from both biological and social conditions, creates the potential for political division over almost all aspects of public health. But not every health issue actually produces a political conflict. Interest groups overlap in complex ways. Consider, for example, the dilemma facing Federalist merchants, who would gain from a quarantine of the French islands, but simultaneously would suffer from any increase in the rigor of quarantines in general.

Political influence in late 18th-century medicine did not always signify irresponsible meddling. Political compromise permitted concerted public action to fight future epidemics at a time when medical opinion seemed hopelessly deadlocked, although the political significance of the potentially lethal Rush "cure" helped assure its continued use, needlessly endangering the lives of patients.

Finally, not everyone was willing to be drawn into partisan debate over a medical question. Expressing the hope that the next epidemic might be met by the united efforts of "all parties" in the City of Brotherly Love, an anonymous satirist poked fun at both the Federalist and Republican views of the fever:

> Be patient ye vivid sons of mercury with the medical baptisms of your *cold bath brethren*. For had that therapeutic process been tried under the cataract of Niagara, no body can tell the wonders which might have been produced by it . . .
>
> Cease ye yellow fever heroes to censure, those of your brethren whose delicacy of nerves and previous engagements called them suddenly crochet and forceps a la main to Nootka Sound, to catch Otters and Beavers. Be assured, important discoveries have been made by the Jaunt.
>
> Lend a kind ear to the graduates of Montpelier, who inform you that the late disease arose from the burying grounds in the heart of your city, since in France they never bury the dead under Churches, but in balloons high up in the air.[79]
>
> Ye learned and long robed sons of Esculapius, pity and pardon poor Absalom Jones and Richard Allen,[80] two sable Ethiopians, who being ignorant of the Greek and Latin languages, were under the necessity of curing their patients *in English*.[81]

But neither the political nor the medical debates would be silenced so simply.

## NOTES

I would like to thank Eric L. McKitrick for his guidance and encouragement at every stage of this project.

1    J. H. Powell, *Bring Out Your Dead: The Great Plague of Yellow Fever in Philadelphia in 1793* (Philadelphia,

1949), pp. 1–64; Charles E. A. Winslow, *The Conquest of Epidemic Disease: A Chapter in the History of Ideas* (Princeton, 1943), p. 198.

2   Powell, *Bring Out Your Dead,* pp. 8–12, 219, 232. The exact number of deaths is unknown. The figure 4,040, derived from burial lists, includes deaths from all causes in the city but does not include the many fever victims buried elsewhere. The burial lists are appended to Mathew Carey, *A Short Account of the Malignant Fever, . . .* 4th ed. (Philadelphia, 1794). See also Richard H. Shryock, *Medicine and Society in America, 1660–1860* (New York, 1960), pp. 82, 108.

3   Powell, *Bring Out Your Dead,* pp. 143, 242–243.

4   Erwin H. Ackerknecht, "Anticontagionism between 1821 and 1867," *Bull. Hist. Med.,* 1948, *26*: 562–593. An opposing view is J. B. Blake, "Yellow fever in eighteenth century America," *Bull. N.Y. Acad. Med.,* 1968, *44*: 681.

5   Eugene P. Link, *Democratic-Republican Societies, 1790–1800* (New York, 1942); Harry M. Tinkcom, *The Republicans and Federalists in Pennsylvania, 1790–1801: A Study in National Stimulus and Local Response* (Harrisburg, 1950).

6   Frances S. Childs, *French Refugee Life in the United States, 1790–1800: An American Chapter of the French Revolution* (Baltimore, 1940), pp. 22, 103, 142–143, 159.

7   A general picture of the events and mechanisms of party development may be found in Joseph Charles, *The Origins of the American Party System* (New York, 1956); Noble E. Cunningham, Jr., *The Jeffersonian Republicans: The Formation of Party Organization, 1789–1801* (Chapel Hill, 1957); Richard Hofstadter, *The Idea of a Party System: The Rise of Legitimate Opposition in the United States, 1780–1840* (Berkeley and Los Angeles, 1969); and Richard P. McCormick, *The Second American Party System: Party Formation in the Jacksonian Era* (Chapel Hill, 1966).

8   Winslow, *Epidemic Disease,* pp. 195, 200, 231. Related to, but distinct from, the etiology question was the problem of contagion. Almost all importationists believed the fever contagious, but advocates of a local origin differed over whether it could become contagious after appearing. For examples, see David Nassy, *Observations on the Cause, Nature, and Treatment of the Epidemic Disorder Prevalent in Philadelphia* (Philadelphia, 1793), p. 13; Benjamin Rush, *An Enquiry Into the Origin of the Late Epidemic Fever in Philadelphia* (Philadelphia, 1793), p. 14; Benjamin S. Barton, "On yellow fever," n.d. [1806?], Benjamin Smith Barton Papers, Delafield Collection, American Philosophical Society, Philadelphia.

9   Powell, *Bring Out Your Dead,* pp. 43–44; Carey, *Short Account,* p. 12; Benjamin Rush, *An Account of the Bilious Remitting Yellow Fever . . .* (Philadelphia,

1794); *Dictionary of American Biography,* s.v. "Hutchinson, James"; Jean Devèze, *An Enquiry into, and Observations upon; the Causes and Effects of the Epidemic Disease* (Philadelphia, 1794), p. 16; Powell, *Bring Out Your Dead,* pp. 36–44. On the importance of the correspondence committee, see Edward Ford, *David Rittenhouse: Astronomer-Patriot, 1732–1796* (Philadelphia, 1946), p. 190.

10   Records of the College of Physicians, I (1787–1812), 175, Nov. 19, 1793, College of Physicians of Philadelphia; Rush, *Account,* p. 146; Adam Kuhn, Yellow Fever Manuscripts (1794), p. 6, College of Physicians of Philadelphia, Philadelphia; Stacey B. Day, ed., *Edward Stevens: Gastric Physiologist, Physician and American Statesman* (Montreal, 1969); William Currie, *A Treatise on the Synochus Icteroides, Or Yellow Fever . . .* (Philadelphia, 1794), pp. 1, 67, 84; Currie, *An Impartial Review of that Part of Dr. Rush's Late Publication . . . In Which His Opinion is Shewn to be Erroneous; the Importation of the Disease Established; and the Wholesomeness of the City Vindicated* (Philadelphia, 1794), pp. 6–14.

11   Rush, *Account,* p. 146; *Independent Gazetteer* (Philadelphia), Jan. 22, 1794; Benjamin S. Barton to Thomas Pennant, April 11, 1794, Barton Papers. Later epidemics in 1797 and 1798 introduced some blurring of party lines. By 1797, Republican Dr. Caspar Wistar had definitely joined the importationists. See College of Physicians of Philadelphia, *Facts and Observations Relative to the Nature and Origin of the Pestilential Fever . . .* (Philadelphia, 1798), pp. 43, 52; Samuel D. Gross, ed., *Lives of Eminent American Physicians and Surgeons of the Nineteenth Century* (Philadelphia, 1861), pp. 134–135; College of Physicians Records, I, 216, 225, 250. The political allegiance of Dr. William Shippen, Jr., is uncertain. An importationist, he chaired a largely Republican town meeting in 1795 but also appeared in the rolls of the Federalist marching society. See *Independent Gazetteer,* Nov. 30, 1793, July 25, 1795; and General Roll of McPherson's Blues, Hollingsworth Manuscripts, Business Papers Miscellaneous, undated, Historical Society of Pennsylvania, Philadelphia. An unlikely suggestion was made that Shippen did not know who was behind the 1795 meeting, "thus committing himself as a puppet to be moved at the pleasure of very bungling artists." *Gazette of the United States* (Philadelphia), July 25, 1795. Dr. Charles Caldwell continued to champion localism even after his 1796 conversion to Federalism, but in 1793 he was loyal to both the politics and the medicine of Benjamin Rush. See Charles Caldwell, *Autobiography* (Philadelphia, 1855), pp. 174, 182, 254, 267, 278; Caldwell to James Hutchinson, Aug. 1, 1793, Hutchinson Papers, American Philosophical Society.

12  Benjamin Rush, *Medical Inquiries and Observations* (Philadelphia, 1789); Carl Binger, *Revolutionary Doctor: Benjamin Rush, 1746–1813* (New York, 1966), p. 228.

13  Rush, for one, expected just such deference from former students. See *Letters of Benjamin Rush,* ed. L. H. Butterfield, II (Princeton, 1951), 681.

14  Powell feels Hutchinson was "obviously confused." *Bring Out Your Dead,* p. 43. See also n. 23 below.

15  "Pestilence," quoted *ibid.*

16  *National Gazette* (Philadelphia), Sept. 23, 1793.

17  Thomas Jefferson to James Madison, Sept. 1, 1793, in *The Writings of Thomas Jefferson,* ed. Andrew A. Lipscomb and Albert E. Bergh (Washington, D.C., 1903), IX, 214–215; *Federal Gazette* (Philadelphia), Dec. 17, 21, 28, 1793; *Gazette of the United States,* Dec. 18, 1793. Democratic Society leader Israel Israel requested the city to dig sewers following the epidemic. Israel to Clarkson, Jan. 29, 1794, Philadelphia Streets and Alleys Manuscripts, Historical Society of Pennsylvania.

18  For Fenno, see Nathan Goodman, *Benjamin Rush: Physician and Citizen, 1746—1813* (Philadelphia, 1934), p. 198; for Wolcott, see Charles Francis Jenkins, *Washington in Germantown . . .* (Philadelphia, 1905), p. 76; for Willing and Chew, see College of Physicians of Philadelphia, *Additional Facts and Observations Relative to the Nature and Origin of the Pestilential Fever* (Philadelphia, 1806), pp. 10, 11; for Hollingsworth, see "An Old Resident" [Hollingsworth] to David Claypoole, Hollingsworth MSS; for Bordley, see J. B. Bordley, *Yellow Fever* (Philadelphia, 1794); for Hazard, see "Hazard letters," Massachusetts Historical Society, *Collections,* 5th series, III (1877), 338, and Powell, *Bring Out Your Dead,* p. 86; for White, see Bird Wilson, *Memoir of the Life of the Right Reverend William White, D.D., . . .* (Philadelphia, 1839), pp. 158, 288; for Johnson, see Benjamin Johnson, *Account of the Rise, Progress, and Termination of the Malignant Fever* (Philadelphia, 1793), p. 5.

19  Lewis Saul Benjamin [Lewis Melville], *The Life and Letters of William Cobbett in England & America, Based Upon Hitherto Unpublished Family Papers* (New York, 1913), pp. 85–87.

20  For Mifflin, see Powell, *Bring Out Your Dead,* pp. 52–53, Samuel Hazard et al., eds., *Pennsylvania Archives,* 4th series, IV (Harrisburg, 1900), 264–269, and Tinkcom, *Republicans and Federalists,* pp. 72, 112, 219–220; for Bache, see Donald H. Stewart, *The Opposition Press of the Federalist Period* (Albany, 1969), p. 137; for Carey, see Mathew Carey, *Observations on Dr. Rush's Enquiry into the Origin of the Late Epidemic Fever in Philadelphia* (Philadelphia, 1793), and Carey, *Short Account,* p. 67.

21  Charles W. Upham, *The Life of Timothy Pickering,* III (Boston, 1873), 56, 62. Some Federalists from rival cities, such as Harrisburg's Alexander Graydon, encouraged the idea that Philadelphia was an unhealthy place. Alexander Graydon, *Memoirs of a Life* (Harrisburg, 1811), pp. 336–338. However, most Federalist merchants in New York, Baltimore, and Trenton remained importationists, leading the local efforts to cut off the trade of their stricken rival. See *General Advertiser* (Philadelphia), Sept. 18, 20, 23, 1793; and James Weston Livingood, *The Philadelphia-Baltimore Trade Rivalry 1780–1860* (Harrisburg, 1947). Even anticontagionist New York Federalist Noah Webster believed this Philadelphia epidemic contagious. Noah Webster, *A Collection of Papers on the Subject of Bilious Fevers* (New York, 1796), p. 233.

22  Harry Emerson Wildes, *Lonely Midas: The Story of Stephen Girard* (New York, 1943), pp. 121, 126; Albert J. Gares, "Stephen Girard's West Indian trade, 1789–1812," *Penn. Mag. Hist. & Biography,* 1948, *72*: 316; J. Thomas Scharf and Thompson Westcott, *History of Philadelphia, 1609–1884* (Philadelphia, 1884), I, 493.

23  Johnson, *Account,* pp. 5, 9; *Dunlap's American Daily Advertiser* (Philadelphia), Dec. 20, 1793; Rush, *Account,* p. 147. Leib and others defended Hutchinson against the charges raised by the College. *General Advertiser,* Nov. 30, Dec. 10, 1793.

24  *Independent Gazetteer,* Dec. 14, 1793; Henry D. Biddle, ed., *Extracts from the Journal of Elizabeth Drinker* (Philadelphia, 1889), p. 193.

25  Richard Peters to Timothy Pickering, Oct. 22, 1793, Timothy Pickering Papers, Massachusetts Historical Society, Boston, quoted in *Rush Letters,* ed. Butterfield, II, 729–730. Pickering may have shown the letter to Rush. Fearing government restrictions on trade, one Federalist importationist appealed to the benevolence of the merchants and ship captains to impose a voluntary quarantine. "A Philadelphian," in *Occasional Essays on the Yellow Fever . . .* (Philadelphia, 1800), pp. 8–11, 13.

26  Benjamin Rush to Julia Rush, Oct. 28, 1793, in *Rush Letters,* ed. Butterfield, II, 729.

27  Goodman, *Benjamin Rush,* p. 198; Bordley, *Yellow Fever,* p. 1; Blake, "Yellow fever," p. 682.

28  "An Old Resident" to Claypoole, Hollingsworth MSS; College of Physicians, *Facts and Observations,* p. 24.

29  Jefferson to Rush, Sept. 23, 1800, in *Writings of Jefferson,* 10, ed. Lipscomb and Bergh, quoted in Charles N. Glaab, *The American City: A Documentary History* (Homewood, Ill., 1963), p. 52.

30  For example, *Federal Gazette,* Dec. 6, 21, 1793; John Redman Coxe Letters on the Yellow Fever [1794],

p. 139, College of Physicians of Philadelphia; Joseph McFarland, "The epidemic of yellow fever in 1793 and its influence upon Dr. Benjamin Rush," *Med. Life,* 1929, *36*: 468. Both sides in the medical split claimed to be the true friends of commerce. Blake, "Yellow fever," p. 681.

31  Powell, *Bring Out Your Dead,* pp. 260–263. Constitutional principles did not limit the state's power to move its own capital out of Philadelphia in 1799 as a result of the yellow fever. Scharf and Westcott, *Philadelphia,* I, 501.

32  Rush, *Account,* p. 147.

33  College of Physicians, *Facts and Observations,* pp. 15–16; *Rush Letters,* ed. Butterfield, II, 798; Hazard et al., eds., *Pennsylvania Archives,* 4th series, IV, 269.

34  Blake, "Yellow fever," p. 681.

35  For a discussion of the theological perception of cholera, 1832–1866, see Charles E. Rosenberg, *The Cholera Years: The United States in 1832, 1849, and 1866* (Chicago, 1962). See also Shryock, *Medicine and Society,* p. 94; *Rush Letters,* ed. Butterfield, II, 659; Horace W. Smith, *Life and Correspondence of the Rev. William Smith, D.D.,* . . . I (Philadelphia, 1880), 395; *General Advertiser,* Jan. 8, 1794.

36  Rush to William Marshall, Sept. 15, 1798, in *Rush Letters,* ed. Butterfield, II, 807. Rush also blamed party spirit in general. See also *National Gazette,* Oct. 9, 12, 16, 1793; Carey, *Short Account,* p. 10.

37  Smith, *Life of William Smith,* I, p. 392.

38  Graydon, *Memoirs,* p. 335; Stephen G. Kurtz, *The Presidency of John Adams: The Collapse of Federalism, 1795–1800* (Philadelphia, 1957), p. 190; Charles D. Hazen, *Contemporary American Opinion of the French Revolution,* Johns Hopkins University Studies in Historical and Political Science, XVI (Baltimore, 1897), pp. 185–186.

39  *National Gazette,* Oct. 16, 1793; Scharf and Westcott, *Philadelphia,* II, 966–967.

40  Scharf and Westcott, *Philadelphia,* II, 966–967.

41  *Gazette of the United States,* Dec. 19, 28, 1793; *General Advertiser,* Jan. 6, 1794; Arthur Hornblow, *History of the Theatre in America,* I (Philadelphia, 1919), 174–175; *National Gazette,* Oct. 16, 1793.

42  *Gazette of the United States,* Dec. 14, 26, 1793, Feb. 8, 1794; René La Roche, *Yellow Fever* . . . (Philadelphia, 1855), p. 73; William Priest, *Travels in the United States of America* . . . (London, 1802), p. 13; [John Purdon], *A Leisure Hour; or a Series of Poetical Letters, Mostly Written During the Prevalence of the Yellow Fever* (Philadelphia, 1804), p. 27.

43  Several leading Republican literary figures remained aloof from this alliance. Bache, whose son-in-law was an actor, was accused of misrepresenting rank-and-file Republican sentiment on the theater for family reasons. Roger Griswold, *The Republican Court; or, American Society in the Days of Washington* (Philadelphia, 1854), p. 316; *General Advertiser,* Jan. 10, 1794. On January 8, though, Bache attributed his stand to anticlericalism. See also Mathew Carey, *Autobiography* (New York, 1942 [reprint of 1837 ed.]), p. 29.

44  W. H. Hargreaves and R. J. G. Morrison, *The Practice of Tropical Medicine* (London, 1965), pp. 183–185; Powell, *Bring Out Your Dead,* pp. 64, 125, 292. Wine is generally not a stimulant although it was believed to be one. Chris Holmes, "Benjamin Rush and the yellow fever," *Bull. Hist. Med.,* 1966, *40*: 246–262, believes Rush's cures were not lethal, but does not fully distinguish patients like Hazard, who left Rush after one or two treatments, from those who stayed for the full course of bloodletting.

45  David Freeman Hawke, *Benjamin Rush, Revolutionary Gadfly* (Indianapolis, 1971), pp. 208–223, 236–240; Powell, *Bring Out Your Dead,* p. 78; Goodman, *Benjamin Rush,* pp. 90–116.

46  Powell, *Bring Out Your Dead,* pp. 82, 153, 203; George Logan to "Citizen Bache," in *General Advertiser,* Sept. 18, 1793; *The Papers of Alexander Hamilton,* ed. Harold Syrett and Jacob E. Cooke, XV (New York, 1969), 325 n. 1. Say's party affiliation is derived from Tinkcom, *Republicans and Federalists,* p. 240.

47  *Dunlap's American Daily Advertiser,* Sept. 13, 1793; *Hamilton Papers,* ed. Syrett and Cooke, XV, 331–332; Powell, *Bring Out Your Dead,* p. 135; Goodman, *Benjamin Rush,* p. 215; Jenkins, *Washington in Germantown,* p. 25.

48  B. Rush to J. Rush, Oct. 3, 1793, to Horatio Gates, Dec. 26, 1795, to John Dickinson, Oct. 11, 1797, in *Rush Letters,* ed. Butterfield, II, 701, 767, 793; Goodman, *Benjamin Rush,* pp. 203, 209.

49  McFarland, "Yellow fever and Dr. Rush," pp. 486–487; John E. Lane, "Jean Devèze," *Ann. Med. Hist.,* n.s., 1936, *8*: 220; Margaret Woodbury, *Public Opinion in Philadelphia, 1789–1801,* Smith College Studies in History, V (Northampton, Mass., 1920), p. 16; Goodman, *Benjamin Rush,* p. 208. Some Republican bark physicians agreed that Rush's cures were egalitarian but denied that political Republicanism required opposition to medical elitism. See letter of "Citizen Robert, M.D.," *General Advertiser,* Dec. 6, 1793, whose combination of titles reflects his attempt to combine egalitarianism and professional distinctions.

50  Powell, *Bring Out Your Dead,* p. 201; *Rush Letters,* ed. Butterfield, II, 692.

51  McFarland, "Yellow fever and Dr. Rush," p. 462.

52  Goodman, *Benjamin Rush,* p. 183.

53  Stephen Girard to Pierre Changeur & Co., Sept. 11, 1793, Girard Papers, Am. Phil. Soc.; Powell, *Bring Out Your Dead,* pp. 175, 179–180.

54   Powell, *Bring Out Your Dead,* pp. 179, 242. Samuel Coates is not to be confused with William Coates, a founder of the Democratic Society. Henry Simpson, *The Lives of Eminent Philadelphians, Now Deceased* (Philadelphia, 1859), p. 218; *Gazette of the United States,* Dec. 14, 1793.

55   Carey, *Short Account,* pp. 27, 28. Carey seems to slight Federalists in his stories of heroism. For their side, see also *Extracts from the Diary of Jacob Hiltzheimer, of Philadelphia,* ed. Jacob Cox Parsons (Philadelphia, 1893), pp. 195–197; Smith, *Life of William Smith,* I, 379; Upham, *Life of Pickering,* III, 62; "Hazard letters," p. 334; Powell, *Bring Out Your Dead,* p. 138; and Simpson, *Eminent Philadelphians,* pp. 908–922. For party affiliations of Morris (as of 1798), see letter of Nov. 19, 1798, Hollingsworth MSS; of Humphreys, see Scharf and Westcott, *Philadelphia,* I, 490; of Hollingsworth, see David Hackett Fischer, *The Revolution of American Conservatism: The Federalist Party in the Era of Jeffersonian Democracy* (New York, 1965), p. 339; of Hiltzheimer and FitzSimmons, see Tinkcom, *Republicans and Federalists,* pp. 138, 152. In addition, Samuel Pancoast of the merchants' committee was listed as a Federalist by 1817. Scharf and Westcott, *Philadelphia,* I, 588.

56   For Wetherill, see Simpson, *Eminent Philadelphians,* p. 940, and Tinkcom, *Republicans and Federalists,* p. 252; for Lownes, see Scharf and Westcott, *Philadelphia,* I, 477; for Girard, see Link, *Democratic Societies,* pp. 75–76; for Israel, see Powell, *Bring Out Your Dead,* p. 178; for Carey, see Carey, *Autobiography*; for Sergeant, see *Dictionary of American Biography,* s.v. "Sergeant, Jonathan Dickinson"; for Sharswood, see Simpson, *Eminent Philadelphians,* p. 885; for Kerr and Connelly, see Minute Book of the Democratic Society, pp. 29, 47, Historical Society of Pennsylvania, and Scharf and Westcott, *Philadelphia,* I, 507, 588; for Wistar, see Powell, *Bring Out Your Dead,* p. 179. The list of leaders of the committee was compiled from names most frequently cited in *Minutes of the Proceedings of the Committee Appointed on the 14th September, 1793* (Philadelphia, 1848); and Carey, *Short Account,* p. 95.

57   Powell, *Bring Out Your Dead,* pp. 72, 87, 179; Ford, *David Rittenhouse,* p. 190; Kenneth R. Rossman, *Thomas Mifflin and the Politics of the American Revolution* (Chapel Hill, 1952), p. 225.

58   Powell, *Bring Out Your Dead,* p. 177; Ford, *David Rittenhouse,* pp. 190–192.

59   Helm was Girard's assistant in charge of "external affairs." He was a second generation German-American but little else is known of him. The chronology of Bush Hill is as follows: Aug. 31—Mayor authorizes seizure of estate, hospital set up under Leib and others; Sept. 16—Girard and Helm volunteer to manage and administer the hospital for the committee; Sept. 18—Girard appoints Devèze to assist Leib and the medical staff; Sept. 21—Leib resigns in dispute over the proper cure. Powell, *Bring Out Your Dead,* pp. 140–172.

60   Democratic Society Minute Book, pp. 29, 39, 42, 47, 48, 52, 95; Link, *Democratic Societies,* pp. 77, 90; Carey, *Short Account,* pp. 20, 27, 30, 37; Tinkcom, *Republicans and Federalists,* pp. 57, 84, 283. Snyder is identified as of 1799 in Scharf and Westcott, *Philadelphia,* I, 507, 588. There were two John Barclays; this one was president of the Republican Bank of Pennsylvania. Duplication of names makes it impossible to say whether merchants' committeeman William Clifton was the Federalist poet or one of two shopkeepers of that name. Likewise, William Sansom, Guardian of the Poor, may have been either the Federalist or the Republican of that name. Simpson, *Eminent Philadelphians,* p. 210; General Roll of McPherson's Blues, Hollingsworth MSS; J. Hardie, *The Philadelphia Directory and Register . . .* (Philadelphia, 1793), p. 182 and *passim.*

61   Powell, *Bring Out Your Dead,* pp. 85–86. To avoid confusion over the new implications of its old name, the *Federal Gazette* became the *Philadelphia Gazette* on Jan. 1, 1794. Clarence S. Brigham, *History and Bibliography of American Newspapers, 1690–1820,* II (Worcester, Mass., 1947), 91.

62   Lewis Leary, *That Rascal Freneau: A Study in Literary Failure* (New Brunswick, N.J., 1941), pp. 240–246; Dumas Malone, *Jefferson and the Ordeal of Liberty,* Vol. III of *Jefferson and His Time* (Boston, 1962), p. 142.

63   *National Gazette,* Sept. 11, Oct. 9, 1793; Scharf and Westcott, *Philadelphia,* II, 1606; *Minutes of the Committee,* p. 232.

64   Powell's account, *Bring Out Your Dead,* p. 135, differs from Rush's version of the Van Berkle business, B. Rush to J. Rush, Oct. 3, 1793, in *Rush Letters,* ed. Butterfield, II, 701. Wolcott fled with Knox in early September. Jenkins, *Washington in Germantown,* p. 22.

65   Powell, *Bring Out Your Dead,* p. 123.

66   Jefferson to Madison, Sept. 8, 1793, in *The Writings of Thomas Jefferson,* ed. Paul Leicester Ford, VI (New York, 1895), 419; Malone, *Jefferson and the Ordeal of Liberty,* pp. 140–142.

67   *National Gazette,* Sept. 4, 1793. The version in Powell, *Bring Out Your Dead,* p. 240, is not the original 1793 poem but a printed edition of 1795. The original attacks all deserters; the later one absolves all but the fleeing physicians. Condemnation of the fugitives often stressed their wealth. *Gazette of the United States,* letter of Feb. 20, 1794.

68   *Dunlap's American Daily Advertiser,* Dec. 14, 1793; Nathaniel Burt, *The Perennial Philadelphians: The Anat-*

omy of an American Aristocracy (Boston, 1963), pp. 156–157. "Nomination," "platform," etc. are all useful metaphors in spite of the anachronism.

69   *Gazette of the United States,* Dec. 13, 1793.

70   *Ibid.,* Dec. 14, 20, 1793; Robert C. Alberts, *The Golden Voyage: The Life and Times of William Bingham, 1752–1804* (Boston, 1969), p. 246. Out of 14,000 eligible, only 1,282 Philadelphians came out to vote. *Independent Gazetteer,* Dec. 21, 1793.

71   *Dunlap's American Daily Advertiser,* Dec. 14, 1793.

72   *Hamilton Papers,* ed. Syrett and Cooke, XV, 332 n; Carey, *Short Account,* p. 93; Powell, *Bring Out Your Dead,* pp. 216–232.

73   *General Advertiser,* Dec. 2, 1793; *Rush Letters,* ed. Butterfield, II, 736; Johnson, *Account,* p. 28; Powell, *Bring Out Your Dead,* pp. 87, 178. Carey printed rumors of black profiteering similar to Johnson's but he hastily withdrew them. Richard Allen, *Life Experiences and Gospel Labors . . .* (Philadelphia, 1933), pp. 34–35.

74   *General Advertiser,* Dec. 2, 3, 1793; *Federal Gazette,* Dec. 9, 14, 1793.

75   "HOWARD," in *General Advertiser,* Jan. 8, 1794; see also Nov. 27, 1793.

76   Tinkcom, *Republicans and Federalists,* pp. 176–179; John Bach McMaster, *The Life and Times of Stephen Girard, Mariner and Merchant,* I (Philadelphia, 1918), 352. The career of Israel Israel and his role in Philadelphia class politics is traced in John K. Alexander, "The City of Brotherly Fear: the poor in late eighteenth century Philadelphia," in Kenneth T. Jackson and Stanley K. Schultz, comps., *Cities in American History* (New York, 1972), pp. 86–90.

77   *The Works of John Adams . . . ,* ed. Charles Francis Adams, X (Boston, 1856), 47. Jefferson declared the death of Hutchinson to be as great a setback as the Genêt fiasco. Merrill D. Peterson, *Thomas Jefferson and the New Nation: A Biography* (New York, 1970), p. 508.

78   Tinkcom, *Republicans and Federalists,* p. 173.

79   Jean Pierre Blanchard had recently introduced the city to the French hot air balloon.

80   Two of Rush's black apprentices.

81   *Gazette of the United States,* Dec. 23, 1793.

# 26

## Politics and Public Health: Smallpox in Milwaukee, 1894–1895

### JUDITH WALZER LEAVITT

Smallpox was to Milwaukee what cholera and yellow fever were to other 19th-century American cities. It was an infrequent visitor, but when it came, smallpox caused major disruptions of city life and generated fear and panic among the residents. The effects of smallpox epidemics were typically to increase the powers and effectiveness of the Health Department. John Duffy, Charles Rosenberg, and others have indicated this pattern with regard to cholera and yellow fever epidemics.[1] I have found it also explains the impact of smallpox in Milwaukee. As a result of five 19th-century smallpox epidemics, health officials greatly increased their authority to control infectious diseases in Milwaukee.[2]

However, the smallpox epidemic which hit Milwaukee in the summer and fall of 1894 interrupted this pattern. As a direct result of that epidemic, the powers of the Health Department were significantly diminished, and its reputation in the city sank to an all-time low. This 1894 example, I think, serves to dramatize the relationship between politics and public health and to remind us that medical factors do not alone determine the course of public health events.

The 1894 Milwaukee smallpox epidemic illustrates the dependence of 19th-century public health on political circumstances. Moreover, it shows that epidemics could have had—and occasionally did have—retrogressive as well as progressive effects on the development of the public health movement.

A frightening disease, with ugly physical manifestations, smallpox attacked all ages and, exacer-

JUDITH WALZER LEAVITT is Associate Professor of the History of Medicine, History of Science, and Women's Studies, University of Wisconsin, Madison, Wisconsin.

Reprinted with permission from the *Bulletin of the History of Medicine,* 1976, *50*: 553–568.

bated by unsanitary conditions and overcrowding, spread quickly through a city. Victims who did not succumb to the disease were often left disfigured and pockmarked for life. But in the 19th century, smallpox was a preventable disease, since vaccination with cowpox virus was available. Thus one would not expect smallpox still to be a disease of dread. However, although vaccination was quite widely used, it was not universally accepted in the medical community or among the lay public. Most medical practitioners advocated vaccination, but many thought it an inadequate protection against the disease; some antivaccinationists claimed it to be more harmful than the disease itself.[3]

Milwaukee newspapers aired the disagreements within the medical community over vaccination and about treatment of smallpox, and the result was a confusion which seemed to grow as the century wore on. The presence of a large immigrant community in the city, among whom the efficacy of vaccination was most frequently questioned, merely increased dissension.[4]

The infrequent appearance of the disease and the confusion about medical theory account for a large part of the reaction Milwaukeeans had to smallpox. But the particular political circumstances which greeted the outbreak of an epidemic in the city also generated fear. Divided opinion among the people about how to react to the disease, and over whether or not to vaccinate, occasionally furthered already existing political and ethnic divisions in the city. In 1894, the Milwaukee Health Department found it difficult to control a medical situation because of its political ramifications.

Milwaukee in the 1890s was a bustling commercial and industrial city. Its population jumped from 20,000 at mid-century to 115,000 by 1880, and to 285,000 at the turn of the 20th century. By 1910,

Milwaukee was the twelfth largest city in the United States. Contrary to popular belief, its economy was based only partly on beer; other heavy and light industries also flourished.[5] Milwaukee contained members of almost every ethnic group which migrated to this country, with Germans and Poles predominating. Many have noted the German character of 19th-century Milwaukee.[6] Although most of its population lived in single-family, or two- to three-family dwellings, Milwaukee was very much an urban metropolis in the 1890s. Like all other cities in the United States during the period, it wrestled with the problems of housing congestion, street sanitation, and disposal of wastes.

In 1894, a Republican victory at the polls led to the appointment of a new Health Commissioner, Walter Kempster, a Republican and a nationally known physician and psychiatrist. Although best known for his work with the insane, Kempster had spent much time studying how Europeans dealt with contagious diseases, especially cholera, and the new mayor felt that a man of such stature would be an asset to the city.[7]

The Common Council immediately questioned Kempster's appointment. Democrats might have been expected to oppose a Republican appointee as a matter of course; but Kempster's strongest opposition came from fellow Republicans, most vociferously from aldermen Robert Rudolph and Charles Kieckhefer, both representing German wards.[8] Both men criticized the fact that Kempster was new to Milwaukee and unfamiliar with the city and its problems. They opposed his appointment initially because they had supported other local physicians for the job. Kempster's English heritage and national reputation acted against him in the minds of those who sought a familiar, and possibly ethnic, representative of Milwaukee's population. But the majority of the council was willing to give Kempster a chance, and confirmed his appointment by a vote of 23 to 13.[9]

With the nation and the city in the middle of a severe economic depression in 1894, the 26 patronage jobs controlled by the Health Commissioner assumed great significance. Although Kempster was a Republican, he was not susceptible to the influences of fellow party members. In fact, when he announced his appointees, he completely ignored the party's suggested lists. Council members immediately challenged the appointments over which they had consent powers and vetoed some of them, early establishing the pattern which was to typify Kempster's relations with the legislative body.[10]

As a result of this episode, tension existed between the Health Department and the Common Council in June 1894 when the incidence of smallpox began to increase and an epidemic threatened. The atmosphere of cooperation, necessary to cope successfully with an emergency situation, was missing. Smallpox became the weapon with which certain members of the Common Council, led by South Side saloon-keeper Robert Rudolph, fought the Health Commissioner. The Polish and German immigrant groups most hard hit by the epidemic furnished the movement's political strength.

Dr. Kempster's reaction to smallpox in the city was similar to that of health commissioners before him. He at once hired extra physicians to launch a widespread vaccination campaign. He moved swiftly to isolate those patients reported to have the disease by removing them to the Isolation Hospital in the Eleventh Ward, acting under the 1892 ordinance giving him the power to do this forcibly if necessary. And he enforced a strict quarantine on those allowed to remain at home. The department also carried on extensive patient education campaigns and made wide use of the city's disinfecting van.[11]

The reaction of citizens to the Health Department's offensive was initially similar to the response during previous outbreaks. They cooperated with everything but vaccination, which the German and Polish areas of the city resisted. The Health Department had no authority to force vaccinations on anyone who did not want them, although nonvaccinated children could be refused admission to the public schools. Since the epidemic began just when the public schools were closing for the summer, this restraint was not particularly effective.[12]

During June and July, smallpox appeared in all sections of the city, keeping the Health Department busy vaccinating and isolating reported cases. Kempster was confident that his procedures were effective, and that an epidemic would not materialize. But by mid-July it was evident that a significant number of people were not cooperating with the health authorities. Many cases of smallpox went unreported. Discontent with Health Department policy grew when smallpox seemed to localize in the South Side wards. The one hardest hit by the contagion was the Eleventh Ward, site of the Isolation Hospital and home of Alderman Rudolph.

At first Kempster denied that there was a seat of infection in the South Side, but the numerous cases discovered there belied his assertions. Significant numbers of parents refused to allow their children to be examined or vaccinated by health officials, contributing to the rapid spread of the disease.[13] The immediate focus of the people's wrath was the Isolation Hospital in the crowded Eleventh Ward. Despite the renovations that had recently transformed the institution into what health authorities called a "modern facility," residents in the neighborhood still viewed it as a "pest-house" and the source of their trouble. They claimed that it was a "menace to the health of citizens" and a "slaughterhouse" where patients "were not treated like human beings." Health officials maintained that the hospital was in good condition and offered good service to the sick poor who were admitted.[14] Whatever the actual condition of the hospital in July and August 1894, southsiders were convinced that it was a death house for those who went there as patients and that its presence infected the nearby districts.[15]

A crisis was reached on August 5 when a crowd of neighbors successfully resisted an attempt by the Health Department to take a sick two-year-old to the hospital. About 3,000 "furious" people armed with clubs, knives, and stones assembled in front of the child's house. The family had recently lost a child after it had been removed to the hospital, and the mother was frantic with fear and determined not to let the city "kill" (as she put it) another of her children. "I can give it better care and nourishment here than they can give it at the hospital. I will not allow my child to be taken to the hospital." Faced with the violent mob, and unable to control the situation, the ambulance on this occasion beat a hasty retreat.[16].

There is no evidence that Alderman Rudolph was in any way connected with the initial outburst on the night of August 5. But by the next day his name was being intimately linked with the South Side "rioters," and he was participating actively to organize and mold the political force unleashed in his ward. On August 6, he introduced a resolution in the Common Council to remove the power of the Health Commissioner to take patients to the hospital against their will. Although the resolution had no effect against the ordinance which gave the power, its adoption was seen as a vote of support of the southsiders.[17] Rudolph appeared as a leader at public rallies, and on August 7, when a crowd gathered to protest the night burial of a smallpox victim, Rudolph addressed them with a speech that "was not entirely free from incendiarism." With his support, southsiders continued actively to protest Health Department activities.[18]

Dr. Kempster reacted by stiffening the official position, insisting that if smallpox spread it was not due to Health Department negligence but rather to the rioters themselves spreading the contagion through the South Side wards. He carefully defended every argument leveled at the department and told a reporter, "But for politics and bad beer, the matter would never have been heard of."[19] This belittlement of an issue as crucial as life itself to the South Side residents did little to ease tensions between the Health Department and that section of the city. In fact, it emphasized the differences —class and ethnic—between Kempster and the immigrant South Side residents. Showing little compassion, Kempster remained firm during the entire episode, never bending to the southsiders, never recognizing that their concerns may have been legitimate. "I am here to enforce the laws," he said, "and I shall enforce them if I have to break heads to do it. The question of the inhumanity of the laws I have nothing to do with."[20]

The situation on the South Side clearly aided the spread of smallpox in that region of the city. Daily, crowds of people took to the streets, seeking out health officials to harass. Quarantine officials watching guard over houses were frequently the object of the mob's attack. With thousands of people roaming the streets and entering houses infected with smallpox, the contagion was destined to spread throughout the district. Case reports, despite the many concealed from authorities, indicate that the South Side wards 11 and 14 were most severely hit during the summer and fall of 1894 (Fig. 1).[21]

The focus of the crowds' hatred was Dr. Kempster. He symbolized arbitrary governmental authority which was subverting immigrant culture and threatening personal liberty. Calling for his execution, crowds demanded that the "people's

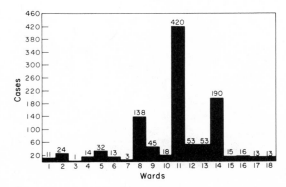

Fig. 1. Milwaukee smallpox epidemic, 1894–1895; ward distribution. Wards 5, 8, 11, 12, 14, and 17 were on the South Side.

rights were paramount and should be protected, if need be, at the point of a pistol."[22] Women played a particularly important part in the disturbances. Since police were reluctant to use their clubs on "feminine shoulders," women were effective at maintaining disorder. Armed with clubs and stones, they assaulted the city police sent to preserve order. They threw stones and scalding water at the ambulance horses in an effort to stop officials from removing any patients. As one newspaper observed the situation: "Mobs of Pomeranian and Polish women armed with baseball bats, potato mashers, clubs, bed slats, salt and pepper, and butcher knives, lay in wait all day for . . . the Isolation Hospital van" (Fig. 2).[23]

City officials met daily to try to determine a course of action which would stem the riots and the spread of smallpox. They consulted the State Board of Health. Despite their efforts, the disturbances continued intermittently through August and into September.[24]

In addition to governmental meetings, South Side citizen groups met to try to regain the image of that section as a peaceable place, safe for business. Deeply regretting "the notoriety which has been recently thrust upon that section of the city," one such meeting blamed the carelessness of the people for spreading the disease. Even the moderate groups, however, were not in sympathy with the Health Department, which, it was felt, had lost the confidence of the people and was thus no longer competent to deal with health emergencies.[25]

The activity in the Eleventh Ward diminished the effectiveness of the Health Department. Kemp-

ster himself admitted that although smallpox had been under control before the riots, quarantine was impossible and the spread of the disease inevitable since the mobs began roaming the streets.[26] Vaccinations, although freely available, were often rejected. During the violence on the South Side the daily work of the Health Department virtually came to a halt. Patients could not be removed to the hospital in the face of weapon-wielding mobs; patients from other wards in the city could not be transported to the hospital through the hostile Eleventh Ward.[27] Kempster was denounced for attempting to remove patients to the hospital, and further denounced when failure to remove such patients resulted in the spread of the epidemic.

To a meeting of concerned physicians and businessmen, he voiced his frustrations:

> The laws are not enforced because the Common Council has prevented me. Not a single proposition that I have made . . . has been acted upon. . . . Proposition after proposition has been made to revise the laws as they now are. This has caused opposition among the people. We come to a house to remove a patient and are resisted. They tell us that their alderman informed them that next week the laws will be changed and they need not go. I have been tied hand and foot with investigations, injunctions and work that is never finished.[28]

At the beginning of September, with the opening of school, the coming of cooler weather, and increased police action against the rioters, the roving mobs on the South Side became less visible. The focus of the anti-Kempster movement changed from street action to the Common Council, as that body took up the battle in earnest.

Alderman Rudolph maintained a hold on his constituency and leadership of the mass movement against the Health Department by his actions and inflammatory rhetoric within the Common Council. There he introduced resolution after resolution and ordinance after ordinance, each one concerned with limiting the power of the Health Department and Walter Kempster. As a member of the Council Health Committee and as a close friend of Council President William G. Rauschenberger, Rudolph had considerable influence over health measures in the council.

Beginning with the measures introduced on August 6 attempting to limit Kempster's power to remove patients to the hospital, Rudolph's actions

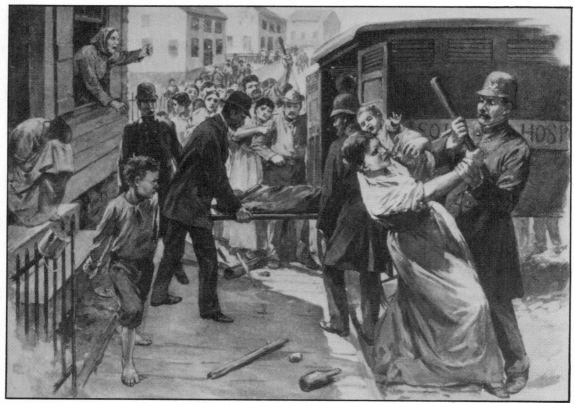

Fig. 2. "Smallpox troubles in Milwaukee." From *Leslie's Weekly Illustrated Newspaper*, Sept. 27, 1894, *79*: 207. I am

*State Historical Society of Wisconsin*

grateful to Martin S. Pernick and Janet S. Numbers for help in locating this illustration.

crescendoed as the epidemic itself increased in intensity. In early September, he introduced an ordinance designed to accomplish what his earlier resolution could not: legally to tie the hands of the Health Commissioner by not allowing him to remove patients without their consent. The ordinance, revised slightly, passed the council and became law.[29]

Part of Rudolph's success in passing this ordinance was due to his scare tactics. The only member of the council in daily touch with the rioters, he promised renewed violence if the council did not pass his measure. He emoted loud and long on the injustices of tearing a child from its mother's breast. And he convinced his fellow politicians that voters would not be happy unless this measure passed. Council President Rauschenberger, who also thought Kempster incapable of handling the epidemic, actively supported Rudolph.[30]

In October, with the epidemic still raging about

the city, Rudolph called for a special investigating committee to inquire into Kempster's activities, listing 34 charges against him.[31] The main charges were that Kempster had been negligent of his duties in the management of the Isolation Hospital, that he showed ignorance of quarantine methods, that patients were removed from their homes when they could have been better taken care of at their residences, and that the Health Department had grown tyrannical.[32] Twenty-eight physicians, including some of the more "prominent" physicians in the city, signed testimonials of misconduct on the part of the Health Commissioner.[33] Rudolph's charges were a serious matter.

Rudolph himself was appointed chairman of the council's committee to investigate the charges. The impeachment proceedings were front-page news in all the city's newspapers. Although most English-language papers declared that the investigation was a "farce" since it was led by so prejudiced a man, even the friendly *Sentinel* agreed that there was a need to clear the air.[34] The German-language press, on the other hand, endorsed Rudolph from the start and fully supported the impeachment proceedings.[35]

Rudolph's allies included the Anti-Vaccination Society, the German-language press, and the South Side activists. There were many physicians among this group. Their leader was Dr. Emil Wahl, a German physician with a successful South Side practice. Dr. Wahl was a member of the Milwaukee Medical Society (although he resigned from that organization when it accepted Kempster as a member), and his accusations that Kempster was incompetent to deal with the epidemic could not be dealt with lightly.[36]

There were genuine differences among physicians about the treatment of smallpox patients, as there had been on the vaccination issue. The division in the medical community was one between men of good faith, similarly trained, who used the tools of their profession to come to opposing conclusions. Dr. Wahl may or may not have been politically motivated to speak publicly against Dr. Kempster, but this does not necessarily mean that his medical disagreements were less real. His arguments were serious ones, which the medical community seriously debated. Wahl's principal complaint was that Kempster was responsible for discharging patients from the hospital while they were still contagious, thus aiding the spread of the disease. The debate centered on the condition of the smallpox pustule at the various stages.

The epidemic reached its height during the month of October, when the impeachment hearings began. South Side physicians, led by Emil Wahl, gave testimony about patients who had been prematurely dismissed from the hospital. Kempster's cross-examination of these witnesses attempted to show their lack of familiarity with the disease and their inability to recognize its contagious states.[37] Witnesses also included South Side families who felt wronged by the Health Department because it had attempted to remove their relatives to the hospital. It was claimed that Kempster had attempted to remove one patient who was not even ill with smallpox. A nurse who had served at the Isolation Hospital charged that the institution was mismanaged, that screens were not kept

on the windows, and that its water supply was not adequate. In answering the charges against him, Kempster continued to deny any wrongdoing. The testimony of many leading physicians, including officers of the State Board of Health, supported him. The Milwaukee Medical Society also backed Kempster during the investigation. The Health Commissioner was obviously better able to withstand the public condemnations because of his medical colleagues' approval.[38]

Judging that nine of the original 34 charges were sustained by the testimony, the investigation committee recommended conviction. Speculation ran high in the city about the council vote on the impeachment question, with newspapers predicting the decision. Daily shifts of various aldermen were front-page headlines. The council heard the relevant testimony for three days and nights consecutively. The exhausted aldermen were eager to be finished with the whole business. As the council neared the vote, its president complained: "I am at a loss to know whether we are attending a circus or a session of the Common Council." Excitement ran high, interruptions were frequent, and disorder was rampant. Finally, in February 1895, with the epidemic not yet over, the council voted 22 to 14 to dismiss the Health Commissioner.[39]

Although the impeachment vote did not divide along party lines, the move against Kempster was nonetheless political. Patronage, class, and ethnic divisions were responsible for a significant part of the opposition to Kempster in the city. Physicians who sought his post or appointments within the Health Department were disappointed and resentful of the man who held office, and Republican politicans were bitter because of their loss of influence in department appointments.[40] From the beginning of his tenure in office, Kempster had labored against a vocal opposition. When the epidemic struck the city, the opposition had a weapon to use to successfully resist the health officer. The issue of the Isolation Hospital was one which carried with it a tradition of anxiety and fear and was easily employed to gather support against Kempster. The issue of forcible removal of children from their homes was one that pulled at the heartstrings of every immigrant parent.

The *Sentinel* termed the movement against Kempster a "cabal," and although it might be hard to document such a conspiracy, there is no ques-

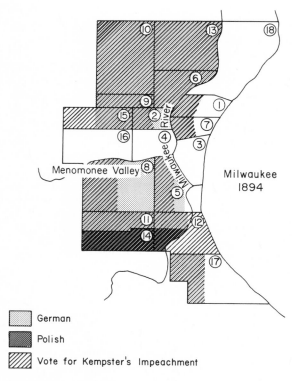

German

Polish

Vote for Kempster's Impeachment

Fig. 3. Ethnic vote for Kempster's impeachment.

tion that Kempster's position in Milwaukee, while it may have been medically sound, was politically untenable. He had few friends and many enemies on the Common Council.[41]

Ethnic divisions in the city were evident from the differences in reactions between the English-language papers which supported Kempster and the German-language press which rejoiced over his dismissal.[42] Analysis of the impeachment vote shows that the ethnic divisions within the city held. Those wards which contained large numbers of German and Polish immigrants, or their descendants, were those which sustained the impeachment vote. Those wards which were largely populated by American-born, or by immigrant groups other than German and Polish, voted for Kempster. Party affiliations did not determine the vote, since both Democrats and Republicans on the council were split. Figure 3 illustrates the close correlation between German and Polish ethnicity and the vote against Kempster.[43]

The smallpox epidemic of 1894 severely divided the city of Milwaukee, causing political conflicts and resentments which were long lived. Most significantly for our interest, it had a retrogressive effect on public health in Milwaukee. Traditionally, epidemics were times when health authori-

MILWAUKEE SMALLPOX EPIDEMIC 1894–1895

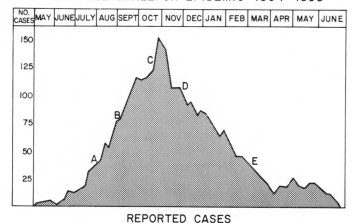

REPORTED CASES

Fig. 4. Cases of smallpox in Milwaukee, 1894–1895, and moves against Kempster.

A. August 6, 1894. Resolution on forcible removal.
B. September 4, 1894. Ordinance on forcible removal.
C. October 15, 1894. Resolution for impeachment in-

vestigation; revised ordinance on forcible removal.
D. November 26, 1894. Revised ordinance on forcible removal passed.
E. February 21, 1895. Common Council impeaches Health Commissioner.

ties increased their powers. This had been true in Milwaukee and in other American cities. In 1894 in Milwaukee the opposite happened. During the height of the epidemic, with fear running high, the council repealed those health measures which were seen as effective in halting the spread of the disease and fired the physician who supported those techniques. As Figure 4 illustrates, the moves against Kempster were all initiated while the epidemic was still raging in the city. Within the space of the ten months from May 1894, when Dr. Kempster took office, to February 1895, when he was dismissed, the Common Council deprived the Health Department of some of the powers important for it to be effective, and ultimately deprived the Health Commissioner of his job. Kempster appealed the impeachment decision and was rein-

stated as Health Commissioner after one year. The episode, however, affected the Health Department permanently. It never regained powers lost during the tumultuous 1894 smallpox epidemic.[44]

Milwaukee's history with the disease illustrates the political nature of the issue of smallpox control. Slowly through the century the Health Department had gained confidence and control over the treatment of smallpox, until by 1894 it felt secure in its powers. But in that year, during a severe epidemic, the Common Council challenged and in part took away the most traditional of all Health Department functions — the ability to control epidemic diseases. Political issues, only some of which were directly related to smallpox, determined how the municipal government handled the medical emergency.

## NOTES

This is a revised version of a paper presented at the annual meeting of the American Association for the History of Medicine, Philadelphia, Pennsylvania, May 1, 1975. The research was aided in part by a Maurice L. Richardson Fellowship from the University of Wisconsin.

1  Charles Rosenberg, studying the effects of cholera epidemics on American cities, noted: "The cholera epidemics of the nineteenth century provided much of the impetus needed to overcome centuries of governmental inertia and indifference in regard to problems of public health. . . . It is not surprising that the growing public health movement found in cholera an effective ally." *The Cholera Years: The United States in 1832, 1849 and 1866* (Chicago: Univ. of Chicago Press, 1962), pp. 2–3. See also John Duffy, who posits that cholera and yellow fever were "important factors in promoting public health measures," because of their "crisis" presentation. "Social impact of disease in the late nineteenth century," *Bull. N.Y. Acad. Med.,* 1971, *47*: 800 [see ch. 29 in this book]. Although Duffy saw smallpox running a poor third to cholera and yellow fever, in Milwaukee smallpox took the place of the former two diseases, which did not threaten the city after 1850. I make the parallel with cholera and yellow fever despite the major differences between those diseases and smallpox, the availability of a preventative for one and not the others. While vaccination raises interesting differences between the examples used here, those differences did not affect the public reaction evoked in each case: fear and panic and an immediate governmental response to alleviate conditions.

2  Smallpox first appeared in Milwaukee in 1843, and reappeared three years later in virulent form. A major epidemic occurred in 1868, immediately after the Board of Health was established, and was responsible for establishing certain power patterns which were to remain throughout the century. During the 1870s Milwaukee suffered two major outbreaks of smallpox. Despite the fact that smallpox was never a major cause of death in Milwaukee, it aroused more interest on the part of the public authorities and was responsible for more public health legislation than any other disease.

3  See Martin Kaufman, "The American antivaccinationists and their arguments," *Bull. Hist. Med.,* 1967, *41*: 463–478. Kaufman describes most antivaccinationists as irregular practitioners, and identifies the movement with sectarian medicine. It is not clear to me that that division holds in Milwaukee, where many regularly trained physicians were hesitant about the protective value of vaccination throughout the 19th century.

4  *Ibid.,* p. 474. Kaufman also noticed the prevalence of strong antivaccinationist sentiment among the immigrants, specifically among the German immigrants. Not only were immigrants in Milwaukee vocal against vaccination, but other governmental health activities also drew their wrath. Placarding a home containing an infectious disease, removing sick to an isolation hospital, requiring private night burials, were all seen by newly arrived Germans and Poles as direct infringements on their personal liberties and were vigorously resisted in Milwaukee. For more on this reaction of Milwaukee im-

migrants, see my *The Healthiest City: Milwaukee and the Politics of Health Reform* (Princeton: Princeton University Press, 1982). The reaction was found throughout the state of Wisconsin. See, for example, the *6th Annual Report of the State Board of Health of Wisconsin, 1881,* pp. 116, 120; and the *15th Annual Report of the State Board of Health of Wisconsin, 1894–1895,* pp. 138–139, 163.

5   For more on Milwaukee's economy see Bayard Still, *Milwaukee: The History of a City* (Madison: The State Historical Society of Wisconsin, 1965), and Roger David Simon, "The expansion of an industrial city: Milwaukee, 1880–1910," (unpublished Ph.D. dissertation, Univ. of Wisconsin-Madison, 1971).

6   On the German population of Milwaukee and its assimilation, see Gerd Korman, *Industrialization, Immigrants and Americanizers: The View from Milwaukee 1866–1921* (Madison: The State Historical Society of Wisconsin, 1967), and Kathleen Neils Conzen, "The German Athens: Milwaukee and the accommodation of its immigrants, 1836–1860" (unpublished Ph.D. dissertation, Univ. of Wisconsin-Madison, 1972).

7   Walter Kempster had only small ties of any kind to the city of Milwaukee. He had a national reputation as physician to the insane and had held posts at the State Lunatic Asylum at Utica, New York, and at the Northern Hospital for the Insane, at Oshkosh, Wisconsin. He had testified for the prosecution in the Guiteau case. He had moved to Milwaukee in 1890, but since that time had been on two missions abroad studying cholera and investigating Jewish emigration from Russia. His tenure in the city of Milwaukee, his critics were quick to point out, had been short indeed. For biographical material on Walter Kempster see the *Dictionary of American Biography* (New York: Charles Scribner's Sons, 1933) X, 324–325; Howard Kelly and Walter Burrage, *American Medical Biographies* (Baltimore: The Norman, Remington Co., 1920), pp. 652–653; and most thoroughly, F. M. Sperry, *A Group of Distinguished Physicians and Surgeons of Milwaukee* (Chicago: J. H. Beers & Co., 1904), pp. 56–69. See also Kempster's obituary, *Milwaukee Sentinel,* Aug. 23, 1918, and the *New York Times,* Aug. 23, 1918, p. 9. Kempster was buried in Arlington National Cemetery.

8   *Milwaukee Sentinel,* April 17, 18, 24, 30, 1894.

9   Eight Republicans opposed and five Democrats supported Kempster. Without Democratic support, the Republican nominee would not have been confirmed. Milwaukee *Common Council Proceedings,* April 30, 1894. See also the *Milwaukee Sentinel,* May 1, 1894.

10  *Milwaukee Sentinel,* June 12, 26, 1894; Milwaukee *Common Council Proceedings,* June 11, 1894, p. 132; May 14, 1894, p. 61.

11  *17th Annual Report of the Milwaukee Health Department, 1894,* pp. 26–32; *19th Annual Report of the Milwaukee Health Department, 1895,* pp. 10–12; *18th and 19th Annual Report of the Health Department, 1895,* pp. 35–39; *Milwaukee Sentinel,* June 28, July 4, 1894. Physicians were urged to cooperate with health officials in reporting the disease. The Health Commissioner closed schools when he thought it necessary. See the *Milwaukee Sentinel,* Sept. 2, 3, Nov. 3, 13, 24, 1894. See also the Milwaukee *School Board Proceedings,* Nov. 6, 1894, pp. 124–125.

12  At least two German-language newspapers argued that vaccination did not protect against smallpox and that its effects were often worse than the disease it was to prevent. The Anti-Vaccination Society disseminated its information through pamphlets widely circulated in three languages. *Milwaukee Sentinel,* Aug. 1, 1894.

13  *Milwaukee Sentinel,* July 23, 1894. See also, July 24, 1894.

14  *Milwaukee Sentinel,* Aug. 3, 4, 6, 1894. The anti-hospital sentiment expressed by residents of the South Side reopened a familiar Milwaukee debate about moving the hospital outside the city limits. The issue flared up, encompassed much time for the city's legal staff, and was finally dropped at the end of the summer. Most physicians were against removal from the city limits, as long-distance travel was not seen as beneficial to an acutely ill patient, nor was it convenient for physicians.

15  The theory of air-borne contagion is not yet disproved as one way in which the smallpox virus might travel. It has also been shown that flies have acted as vectors in spreading the disease. See Cyril W. Dixon, *Smallpox* (London: J & A Churchill, 1962), p. 264. This theory was supported at the time because the Eleventh Ward was, in fact, the main seat of infection in the city. Certainly, popular opinion very strongly blamed the Isolation Hospital for the large number of smallpox cases on the South Side. See the *Milwaukee Sentinel,* Aug. 4, 1894.

16  The mother is quoted in the *Milwaukee Sentinel,* Aug. 6, 1894. For more on the episode, see the *18th and 19th Annual Report of the Milwaukee Health Department, 1895,* pp. 42–43. For a brief popularized account of the riots, see Richard L. Stefanik, "The smallpox riots of 1894," *Historical Messenger,* December 1970, pp. 123–128.

17  Milwaukee *Common Council Proceedings,* Aug. 6, 1894, p. 326. See also the *Milwaukee Sentinel,* Aug. 7, 1894; and the *18th and 19th Annual Report of the Milwaukee Health Department, 1895,* pp. 41–42. The initial ordinance had been passed in reaction to a

cholera scare in the city in 1892, and had never been used.

18 For more on the August 7 rally, see the *Milwaukee Daily News,* a workingman's newspaper, which tended to support the rioters, but not the riots in early August. "There is reason to believe that there has been some basis for the many criticisms . . . made" (Aug. 8, 1894). The *Sentinel,* however, was quick to blame the "ignorance of the people" in not following existing health regulations and in defying authorities (Aug. 8, 1894).

19 *Milwaukee Sentinel,* Aug. 7, 1894.

20 Quoted in the *Milwaukee Daily News,* Aug. 11, 1894.

21 Out of a total of 1,074 cases, 846 were from South Side Wards—half of these were from the Eleventh Ward.

22 *Milwaukee Sentinel,* Aug. 9, 1894.

23 *Milwaukee Sentinel,* Aug. 30, 1894. For more on the role of women in the rioting, see the *Sentinel,* Aug. 10, 12, 1894; and the *Milwaukee Daily News,* Aug. 10, 1894.

24 For details about the involvement of the State Board of Health, see the *Wisconsin State Board of Health Report, 1893–1894,* "Report of the Executive Committee relative to the smallpox situation in the City of Milwaukee," pp. 56–69; U. O. B. Wingate, "Smallpox in Wisconsin from January 1894 to June 1895," *Public Health: Papers and Reports of the American Public Health Association,* 1896, *21*: 268–272; and the *18th and 19th Annual Report of the Milwaukee Health Department, 1895,* pp. 49–58; and the *Milwaukee Sentinel,* Aug. 11, 12, 14, 1894.

25 *Milwaukee Sentinel,* Aug. 12, 14, 1894.

26 *Milwaukee Sentinel,* Aug. 12, 1894.

27 *Evening Wisconsin,* Aug. 29, 1894.

28 Quoted in the *Sentinel,* Oct. 23, 1894.

29 Milwaukee *Common Council Proceedings,* Sept. 4, Oct. 1, Nov. 26, 1894. See a copy of the ordinance as passed in the Appendix to the 1894–1895 *Proceedings,* pp. 22–23. Section I provided: "The commissioner of health shall not remove to any Isolation Hospital in said city any child or person suffering from any such disease who can be nursed and cared for during such illness in his or her home during the continuance of the disease except upon the recommendation and advice of the said commissioner of health or one of the assistant commissioners of health, and the physician, if any, attending upon such child or person, not being a member of the health department of said city; and in case such commissioner, or assistant commissioner and such physician shall be unable to agree as to the advisability of removing such child or person, then they shall call in and appoint another physician not a member of the health department, and the deci-

sion of the majority of such physicians and commissioner or assistant commissioner shall be decisive of the question. The third physician called in, as above provided, shall not receive or be entitled to any fees from the city for consultation or service in the decision of the case submitted to such board of physicians." The conditions were so burdensome they effectively tied the hands of a health commissioner attempting to act swiftly to stem an epidemic.

30 *Milwaukee Sentinel,* Sept. 4, 5, Oct. 2, 6, 7, 9, Dec. 2, 1894. *Evening Wisconsin,* Oct. 8, 1894. See also *18th and 19th Annual Report of the Milwaukee Health Department, 1895,* p. 69; and the Milwaukee *Common Council Proceedings,* Sept. 4, 1894.

31 Milwaukee *Common Council Proceedings,* Oct. 15, 1894, pp. 524–531. Although the two actions discussed here, ordinances for the removal of patients and impeachment, were not the only ones Alderman Rudolph initiated against the Health Commissioner, they were the most important, and thus form the focus of the discussion here. For additional measures the council considered at Rudolph's initiation, see *Common Council Proceedings,* Aug. 20, 1894, pp. 364–365; Sept. 4, 1894, pp. 374–375; Oct. 15, 1894, p. 497; Oct. 29, 1894, p. 571; Nov. 12, 1894, p. 583. See also the *Milwaukee Sentinel,* Aug. 21, Sept. 1, Oct. 2, 13, 1894.

32 *Milwaukee Sentinel,* Oct. 16, 1894.

33 Of the 28, at least 19 were members of the local medical society, the State Medical Association or the American Medical Association. See the membership list of the Milwaukee Medical Society and the local A.M.A. members in the archives of the Milwaukee Academy of Medicine. The membership list of the State Medical Society was in the *Wisconsin Medical Journal,* 1903–1904, pp. 196–208. At least two of the physicians had been brought to court by Kempster, charged with not reporting smallpox, which might account for their hostile position.

34 See the *Milwaukee Sentinel, Daily News,* and *Evening Wisconsin, passim,* Oct. 15, 1894, to Feb. 21, 1895. See, for example, editorial of Jan. 5, 1895, in the *Sentinel* entitled, "The farce continued." Other newspapers voiced similar sentiments. The (Milwaukee) *Catholic Citizen* ridiculed the matter of putting the "prosecuting attorney on the bench as the judge of the case" (Oct. 20, 1894).

35 See, for example, *Seebote* and *Herold, passim,* in these months.

36 For biographical material on Emil Wahl, see Louis Frank, *The Medical History of Milwaukee 1834–1914* (Milwaukee: Germania Press, 1915), p. 72. He appears on the membership list of the Milwaukee Medical Society, having joined the organization in

1888. For more on Wahl's resignation, see the Milwaukee Medical Society minutes, Jan. 22, 1895, and Feb. 12, 1895, in the archives of the Milwaukee Academy of Medicine.

37  *Milwaukee Sentinel,* Nov. 15, 16, 17, 28, 29; Dec. 4, 5, 1894; Jan. 4–16, 1895. See also the *Milwaukee Journal,* Jan. 4–10, 1895.

38  At a joint meeting, Medical Society members and business leaders hissed Rudolph's name while loudly cheering Kempster's. See the *Sentinel,* Oct. 23, 1894. The transcripts of the impeachment proceedings are, unfortunately, lost, and it is impossible to discern the technical aspects of the medical debate from the newspaper accounts.

39  For the press assessment of how the vote would be, see the *Milwaukee Sentinel,* Feb. 14, 15, 16, 18, 1895; *Milwaukee Journal,* Feb. 18, 1895; and the *Daily News,* Feb. 18, 1895. See a description of the final session in the *Milwaukee Journal,* Feb. 21, 1895; *Milwaukee Sentinel,* Feb. 21, 1895.

40  For contemporary arguments along these lines, see the *Milwaukee Sentinel,* Aug. 30, 31, Sept. 2, 4, 1894, Feb. 20, 22, 1895, Jan. 21, 1896; *Daily News,* Aug. 31,

1894; *Milwaukee Journal,* Feb. 19, 1895; *Catholic Citizen,* Sept. 8, 1894.

41  *Milwaukee Sentinel,* Feb. 22, 1895.

42  See, for example, the editorial in the *Herold,* Feb. 22, 1895, in which it was noted: "The decision of the Common Council . . . will be received by the great majority of the population with satisfaction. It is the confirmation of many months' experience and the conviction that [Kempster] is not the right man to execute those measures necessary in the case of an epidemic. . . . [He] is not master of the situation and could not awaken the general trust which is, after all, in such a case, a necessary prerequisite." I am grateful to Edith Hoshino Altbach for help in translating this editorial.

43  The sources of ethnicity were the *Eleventh United State Census,* 1890, and the 1895 *Wisconsin State Census.* Precise population figures by ethnic group were not available by ward.

44  See the *Milwaukee Sentinel,* Jan. 18, 1896. For a copy of the judge's decision, see the *18th and 19th Annual Report, 1895,* pp. 81–85.

# Public Health Reform

America's urban health problems reached frightening proportions during the middle years of the 19th century. Mortality rates in cities like New York, Boston, and Philadelphia rose alarmingly, as infectious diseases raged out of control. Hoards of immigrants crowded into ill-ventilated tenements and basement hovels, while workers of all ages toiled long hours in stifling sweatshops. Although Americans living below the subsistence level were the most vulnerable, the public health movement arose primarily from concerns of the middle and upper classes.

Among the many factors motivating public health reformers in the 1840s was pietism, described by Charles E. Rosenberg and Carroll Smith-Rosenberg. This evangelical dedication to helping others, also evident in contemporary temperance and abolitionist crusades, often gave public health reform a religious flavor.

The American movement also benefited from the English experience with sanitary reform, although our country's political institutions created unique problems. Gert H. Brieger describes the political struggle in New York to establish a permanent, effective board of health, which culminated in 1866 with the creation of the Metropolitan Board of Health, the first of its kind in America. Within a year of its birth this organization successfully met its first challenge in reducing the death rate during a cholera epidemic.

Following New York's lead, other cities and states established their own boards, and for a brief period, from 1879 to 1883, there was even a National Board of Health. But the public health movement generally remained a municipal or state affair, led by public-spirited physicians, sanitarians, engineers, nurses, and philanthropic groups. By the 1870s their efforts seemed to be paying off, as urban death rates declined and allocations for public health stabilized.

The most significant spurs to reform were the frequent epidemics that brought terror and death to American cities in the 18th and 19th centuries. Positively, they stimulated public health activities and the development of ameliorative institutions. John Duffy illustrates this point by showing how yellow fever and cholera stirred cities to spend money for such needed, yet expensive, projects as sewerage, water-supply systems, and garbage-disposal works.

Many factors determined whether an epidemic would have positive or negative impact and whether support for public health issues would benefit or suffer. Existing medical knowledge defined the limits of health activity, but that alone did not determine action. Because appropriations had to pass through city councils and thus be debated in the public arena, politicians had to be convinced that health measures were both expedient and popular. Economic considerations, class and ethnicity, timing with regard to elections, and personalities all played a part in their decisions and determined how a particular city would respond to a given threat to the public health. Gretchen A. Condran, Henry Williams, and Rose A. Cheney analyze the effects of public-health measures on lowering urban death rates.

Today, nonmedical factors continue to affect the success of public health activities, even in situations where medicine has proven efficacious. Penicillin, for example, can cure most forms of syphilis and gonorrhea, yet sexually transmitted diseases exist in epidemic proportions. Individual modesty or fear, sexual morality, the reluctance of physicians to report cases, and the question of individual rights all influence the incidence and spread of these diseases. Medicine does not act in a vacuum.

# 27

## Pietism and the Origins of the American Public Health Movement: A Note on John H. Griscom and Robert M. Hartley

### CHARLES E. ROSENBERG AND CARROLL SMITH-ROSENBERG

In 1842 Robert M. Hartley, a pious and charitable New Yorker, helped found the New York Association for Improving the Condition of the Poor. That same year John H. Griscom, M.D., City Inspector, submitted to New York's Common Council an elaborately critical report on the city's sanitary condition. These two events initiated the first more-than-episodic public health movement in any American city; there is a distinct continuity in men and ideas between these events in 1842 and the better-known public health agitation of the 60s.

During the decades before the Civil War, New York seemed the filthiest and least healthy of American cities. In the 1840s and early 1850s the two New Yorkers most concerned with the need for reforming such baleful conditions were the abovementioned John H. Griscom and Robert Hartley—the first a name familiar to students of the history of public health, the second very likely unknown. These men were in some ways dissimilar: one was a physician, the other a businessman turned innovator in social welfare; one a Quaker, the other an orthodox Presbyterian. In other ways they had much in common. For the medical historian, their most pertinent similarity lies in both having become involved in public health reform as a result, essentially, of their response to an intense pietism widespread in their generation.

That evangelical religion had a broad impact in ante-bellum America has become a historical com-

monplace.[1] It is the intention of this paper to suggest that such spiritual dedication played an important role in helping to create a concern for health conditions in the nation's cities. The vast majority of respectable urban Americans—including physicians—found no great difficulty in ignoring the medieval filth and misery which surrounded them. English and French crusaders for public health reform found only a handful of North American advocates before the late 1850s. The motivations which inspired America's pioneer sanitarians cannot therefore be explained alone in terms of European influences or as an inevitable, almost instinctive, rejection of intolerable conditions. The following pages attempt no comprehensive study of either Hartley or Griscom, but hope only to suggest the place of religious motives in shaping their dedication to social reform—as such pietistic convictions did in inspiring the work of virtually every urban philanthropist in this period.

### I

To historians of American public health and American urban history, John H. Griscom is known primarily as the author of an eloquent pamphlet describing the *Sanitary Condition of the Laboring Population of New York* (1845).[2] Yet this is only a small part of his efforts in the cause of public health. Beginning with his tenure as New York's City Inspector—the community's principal health officer—in 1842 and culminating with his presidency of the Third National Quarantine and Sanitary Convention in 1859, Griscom labored constantly to alert his fellow New Yorkers to the need for sanitary reform. Griscom was for a number of years almost alone among New York physicians in

CHARLES E. ROSENBERG is Professor of History and Sociology of Science at the University of Pennsylvania, Philadelphia, Pennsylvania.

CARROLL SMITH-ROSENBERG is Professor of History, University of Pennsylvania, Philadelphia, Pennsylvania.

Reprinted with permission from the *Journal of the History of Medicine and Allied Sciences*, 1968, *23*: 16–35.

his crusade.[3] This reformist impulse was indeed so atypical in the medical world of the 1840s that it seems logical to explain Griscom's involvement in public health matters not in terms of his role as a physician, but in terms of his being his father's son.

The senior John Griscom was a Quaker educator and philanthropist who exemplified in his long career of benevolence a characteristically American respect for science and learning coupled with an intense pietism. Griscom was born in 1774 into an established Quaker family in New Jersey. He studied briefly in Philadelphia, then turned to secondary school teaching in Burlington, New Jersey. Griscom was remarkably successful, and at the invitation of a number of wealthy New Yorkers he moved in 1807 to the emerging metropolis and began to conduct a private school. This was the beginning of more than a half-century of ceaseless benevolence.[4] In addition to his teaching, Griscom was, for example, instrumental in founding the House of Refuge for destitute and vagrant children and a Society for the Prevention of Pauperism —as well as a half-dozen similar philanthropies. He was very much a part of New York's interdenominational evangelical establishment; though a Quaker, he worked closely with Methodists, with Episcopalians, with Presbyterians, to found and manage some of the city's most ambitious charities.[5]

In one area, however, Griscom's activities were quite individualistic. He was fascinated by science generally and chemistry specifically. The Quaker schoolmaster was one of the first Americans successfully to attempt the popularization of chemistry; he spoke at schools and lyceums, to mechanics groups, and gave public lectures.[6] Such scientific proselytizing implied no concession to materialism. Quite the contrary: Griscom's world was of a piece and the study of nature could, he assumed, only illuminate God's greatness. Griscom assumed indeed that any and all learning must inevitably have a spiritual effect. "It seems to me almost an axiomatic truth," he explained, "that sound learning and science do, by a natural law, gravitate towards virtue."[7] And as a man of piety he never shirked his duty of serving as an evangel of science, helping to make his fellow Americans at once more learned and moral.

Griscom soon became one of the handful of re-

spectable New Yorkers alarmed by the misery of so many among the city's poor. In his work with school-age children and especially as a result of his years with the House of Refuge and the Society for the Prevention of Pauperism, Griscom accumulated detailed knowledge of the conditions in which his less fortunate fellow New Yorkers lived. With such broadly social concerns, and in a society in which scientific knowledge was uncommon, Griscom was gradually drawn into areas which seem to the 20th-century reader specifically medical. In 1822, for example, he became embroiled— as a reigning expert on chemistry and thus on disinfection—in debate over the best means of preventing the spread of yellow fever. In similar fashion, Griscom was called upon to act as an adviser on ventilation.[8] Yellow fever, ventilation, science education, and, most important, the condition of the poor—these were to be the central concerns in the life of his physician son.[9]

John H. Griscom was born in 1809 and attended his father's New York school. Not surprisingly, with the elder Griscom so well connected in New York's scientific and philanthropic circles, the younger traveled the path of accepted success in New York medicine. He attended several full sessions of the Rutgers Medical College, where his father served as Professor of Chemistry and Natural Philosophy, and studied successively under two eminent preceptors, John D. Godman and Valentine Mott. After the final collapse of the Rutgers School in 1830, Griscom attended the University of Pennsylvania School of Medicine, graduating in 1832. While he was still a medical student, he had been a walker in the New York Hospital. Returning to New York from Philadelphia, he was awarded an appointment at the New York Dispensary. In 1842 Griscom was also made attending physician at the Eastern Dispensary and a year later received a coveted appointment as attending physician at New York Hospital. Griscom was a founding member of both the New York Medical and Surgical Society and the New York Academy of Medicine. When the academy was organized in 1847, Griscom served on five of its committees the first year, an unmistakable indication—as both common sense and political scientists tell us—of establishment membership.[10]

In addition to his responsibilities as a practitioner, Griscom found time to express a passion for intellectual improvement similar to that which had marked his father's career. The younger Griscom began in the late 1830s to devote a good deal of time to popular education in physiology and hygiene. He wrote several school texts, and soon began to offer public lectures. Fundamental improvement in the health of Americans would depend ultimately, he always held, upon disseminating the truths of hygiene at all levels throughout the community; there was no subject so important and so unfortunately neglected in the curriculum. "The general introduction of this subject," he wrote in 1844, "as a branch of school learning, would, I hesitate not to say, have a greater meliorating influence upon the human condition, than any other." Griscom also believed that hygiene and physiology had a spiritual as well as material content. What subject, for example, could more effectively demonstrate to children their total dependence upon the Lord and the need for obeying His admirably contrived laws? "Indulgence in a vicious or immoral course of life," Griscom assured his young readers, "is sure to prove destructive to health."[11] An understanding of anatomy and physiology would, moreover, in addition to preserving health and morality, draw the mind upwards towards the Contriver of this marvelous "animal mechanism."

Griscom drew habitually upon arguments from design. New York's mortality rates, for example, could not be a normal part of God's world; could He have planned so inefficient a system? A goodly portion of the sickness which afflicted men, Griscom argued, resulted not from some mysterious and ineluctable dispensation of Providence, but from man's own ignorance. (And in the moral calculus of the Griscoms, sin and ignorance unimproved were hardly distinguishable.) Were men only to utilize properly the fresh air, the pure water, the intelligence granted them by the Lord, they would escape unnecessary sickness and premature death. Yet air, water, food — the necessities of life — became all too often the channels through which disease attacked. "Left to the care of nature herself," Griscom lectured, "these would be far less frequently, to man, the sources of disease; but by his own wilfullness and intermeddling, and sad to say, by his own ignorance, he creates the poison which he presents to his own lips."[12] Like many of his contemporaries, Griscom emphasized the unnatural quality of city life, the essentially more

healthful — because more natural — life of the savage. One need only compare the rude health of the American Indian with Griscom's wan and narrow-chested fellow New Yorkers.[13] The contrast was easily explained: the savage lived a simple life, in unthinking harmony with the bounties supplied abundantly by the Lord. The ignorance and cupidity of civilized man, on the other hand, everywhere polluted the sources for a healthful life.

This emphasis was consistent with Griscom's essentially optimistic and melioristic tone; civilized life was not inevitably or necessarily unhealthy. To remedy its evils, one need only apply knowledge already available; ventilation was a case in point. The true fault lay not in the existence of cities as such, but in man's obstinate failure to use his intelligence in making city life as healthy as it might be. In this sense, Griscom was certain, such neglects were culpable, an affront to God. "Cleanliness," he noted in 1850, "is said to be 'next to godliness,' and if, after admitting this, we reflect that cleanliness can not exist without ventilation, we must then look upon the latter as not only a *moral* but *religious* duty." What was needed, Griscom urged, was a "*sanatory* regeneration of society."[14]

But, it may be objected, all these arguments were quite commonplace, formulae so traditionalistic that it would be unsafe to assume from them any overwhelming degree of pietism in their user. This may, to some extent, be conceded; but Griscom's lasting significance does not rest upon the formal content of his writings. His historical reputation is based on the Quaker physician's tenacious commitment to bettering the living conditions of deprived New Yorkers. For this was a period when such concerns were atypical in the medical profession, when the filling of public health posts was often a badge of professional inadequacy or second-rate careerism. It does not seem likely that the well-connected Griscom was simply an opportunist seeking notoriety and the sinecure of a political appointment.[15] And if this is not the case, the only apparent motivation for his untiring concern was religious — for a truly secular humanitarianism was still essentially alien to Griscom's time and social class. Even in his explicitly detailed appeals for public health reorganization, Griscom displayed a persistent tone of moral concern, a guiding dependence upon moral imperatives in shaping his understanding of individual behavior and the place which such reform might play in the upgrading of civic virtue.

Most famous of these appeals is his *Sanitary Condition of the Laboring Population of New York*, delivered in December of 1844 as a public lecture and published soon after. (This pamphlet was in its turn an expansion and elaboration of remarks Griscom had appended to his 1842 report as City Inspector).[16] The Quaker physician emphasized the contrast between the city's essentially healthful physical setting and its disgracefully high mortality rate. There was an unmistakable connection between New York's excessive premature deaths and the miserable condition of the city's tenements. Most deplorable was the plight of thousands who inhabited underground apartments, prey to cellar dampness — even flooding — and poor ventilation. As he describes such conditions, Griscom's decorous prose suggests the emotional impact of the squalor he has seen. "It is almost impossible," he explained, "when contemplating the circumstances and conditions of the poor beings who inhabit these holes, to maintain the proper degree of calmness requisite for thorough inspection, and the exercise of a sound judgment, respecting them."[17] The only solution lay in the use of the state's regulatory powers; New York City needed a board of health endowed with broad powers and staffed by properly trained medical men.[18] Griscom reiterated such arguments for two decades — at legislative hearings, in journal articles, at meetings of the New York Academy of Medicine and the American Medical Association.

Public health reform would result not only in healthier New Yorkers, but in more moral and law-abiding ones. John H. Griscom's world, like his father's, was an organic one. Physical health and living conditions, morality and religion were a tightly knit series of causes and effects. The cellar resident, no matter how pious or industrious at first, could not long remain a productive, church-going member of society. Damp, ill-ventilated apartments soon brought disease, depressed vital energies, and, inevitably, the "moral tone" as well. Unemployment, neglect of person and God soon followed. Such debilitated slum-dwellers turned then to alcohol for the physiological stimulation lacking in their unhospitable environment; the picture of the filthy, drunken, immoral pauper was complete. "From a low state of general health," Griscom explained,

whether in an individual or in numbers, proceed diminished energy of body and of mind, and a vitiated moral perception, the frequent precursor of habits and deeds, which give employment to the officers of police, and the ministers of justice. . . . The coincidence, or parallelism, of moral degradation and physical disease, is plainly apparent to an experienced observer.[19]

How, for example, could man's innate love of modesty and decorum manifest itself in New York's reeking tenements? Was it surprising that incest, prostitution, and venereal disease should thrive in districts where families had to perform all their biological functions in one small and crowded room? Just as man has an innate feeling for morality, he had an instinctive feeling for order and cleanliness; but, Griscom asked, how could these homely virtues be encouraged in such circumstances? Rents were so high and accommodations so shoddy that even with a steady job and the best of will, working men found it almost impossible to find decent quarters for their families.[20] Man's natural capacity for virtue, like his natural state of health, was every day corrupted — by individual sin and ignorance and by the inequities of social organization.

And the atmosphere, the most universal of God's blessings, was, lamentably, in cities everywhere polluted. Not only did a vitiated atmosphere deplete the slum-dweller's vital powers, it served as a medium for the spread of disease. Epidemic and "miasmatic" diseases — cholera, yellow fever, malaria — were, of course, presumed to be spread through the atmosphere. Griscom believed, however, that even those diseases normally assumed to be contagious might in confined circumstances also be air-borne. "The contagious viri of small-pox, measles, scarlet fever, and all others of that class," Griscom explained, "are also admitted to be communicated through the intermedium of the atmosphere. . . ."[21] The more contaminated the atmosphere, the more concentrated the infectious principle — and the more likely one was to contract it. In crowded tenements all these circumstances coincided; diseases normally noncontagious might often become so, while the slum-dwellers, with vital energies chronically reduced by breathing such vitiated air, succumbed readily whenever they were unfortunate enough to come in contact with "contagious viri." It was only to be expected that Griscom should have emphasized the evils of a vitiated atmosphere and the need for improved systems of ventilation in his calls for reform.[22] Not only was ventilation a fashionable cause, it provided a scientifically reassuring vehicle for Griscom's need to instruct and improve.

Griscom could at first muster scant support in his attempts to gather data on slum conditions and in demanding their reform. Both in his 1842 report as City Inspector and in his *Sanitary Condition of the Laboring Population* Griscom relied heavily upon the testimony of missionaries of the New York City Tract Society. For they, with the city's dispensary physicians, were the only emissaries of respectable society to the tenement districts in which the poor lived and died.[23] Griscom's dependence upon the help of city missionaries indicates not only something of his personal ties, but something of the origins of a growing awareness of slum conditions among proper and articulate New Yorkers. It is no accident that public health reformers in this generation spoke so often and so casually of the need for health missionaries and the distribution of health tracts. The reviewer of Griscom's *Sanitary Condition* in the *New York Journal of Medicine* actually suggested, by way of conclusion, that it be reprinted and distributed by the City Tract Society.[24] In ideas, in actions, in associations, Griscom consistently displayed the pietistic origin of his concern for public health.

In subsequent years, as increasing numbers of physicians became interested in public health problems, this motivating pattern of religiously oriented humanitarianism persisted. Stephen Smith and his wife, for example, were both active in the affairs of the American Female Guardian Society, an organization occupying a "left-wing" position in the evangelical united front. John Ordronaux, another prominent writer on public health matters, urged in his 1866 anniversary discourse to the New York Academy of Medicine that the American Tract Society print and distribute health tracts among the poor:

> Let the poor be taught that there is religion in cleanliness, in ventilation, and in good food; let them but once be induced to put these lessons into practice, and we may rest assured their spiritual culture and moral elevation will be rendered all the more easy and certain.

"Disease, like sin," he explained, "is permitted to exist; but conscience and revelation on the one hand, and reason and science on the other, are the kindred means with which God has armed us against them."[25]

## II

More influential than Griscom in illuminating the misery and sickness which existed in New York of the 1840s was his contemporary, Robert M. Hartley. Hartley was a man of great vigor and tenacity —and, as a principal organizer and long-time director of the New York Association for Improving the Condition of the Poor, is ordinarily considered the shaper of America's first protosocial welfare agency. One of the most significant of Hartley's accomplishments was his leadership of the association's pioneer involvement in tenement and public health reform, an involvement which in point of time exactly paralleled Griscom's.

Despite Hartley's self-consciously pragmatic attempts to professionalize charity, the history of the A.I.C.P. and Hartley's own life illustrate how directly the origins of his social activism were rooted in the evangelical enthusiasm of his youth. Robert Milham Hartley was born in England in 1796 and came to the United States as a three-year-old with his merchant father. The family settled in western New York state, in an area known to historians and contemporaries as the Burned-Over District, for the intensity of the religious revivals which swept through it. Like his father, young Hartley went into business, making a mercantile career in New York City. But as in the case of many of his contemporaries, the competitive urgings of commerce did not fill his life. As a boy, Hartley experienced a conversion to evangelical Protestantism and even before arriving in New York City, while still a clerk in upstate New York, he organized prayer meetings and crusaded for proper Sabbath observance. Soon after moving to New York City, Hartley became active in the affairs of his Presbyterian church, serving as an elder and assuming leadership in the church's program of house-to-house missionary visiting. Hartley also began to play an active role in the work of the New York City Tract Society. In 1829 he helped organize the New York City Temperance Society and in 1833 became its corresponding secretary and agent. Hartley was instrumental in formulating the latter society's policy of total abstinence — a novelty at a time when temperance still meant only temperance.[26]

The perfectionism implied in Hartley's advocacy of total abstinence was a characteristic of the late 1820s and early 1830s, a period of increasingly millennial enthusiasm. Hartley's spiritual life was informed by this intense pietism throughout his career, even when dedicated as an older man to ostensibly secular goals (as the rational distribution of charity and the construction of model tenements). Fortunately for the historian, Hartley kept a diary which demonstrates clearly the continuity of his spiritual commitment. The entry for October 15, 1845, for example, reads:

> Revised a plan for the press, long under consideration, to remodel all the city dispensaries so as to distribute the physicians and the medical depots generally over the city. And now, O my soul, how hast thou this day withstood the assaults of an evil world? Answer ere thou sinkest to the insensibility of sleep, as under the searching eye of him with whom thou has to do.

And that for March 19, 1856:

> I am, on a review, much dissatisfied with my labors to-day. I have done but little of that I designed to do. Truly I am an unprofitable servant; yet God mercifully forbears to punish. O for a higher wisdom than my own to direct the labors of my calling! At evening attended a sanitary lecture at the Cooper Institute. To-day my mind has been pervaded with a deep seriousness, and a desire to dwell on spiritual things.

Such sentiments were habitual with the one-time merchant who could, by 1856, nevertheless write that sanitary reform was "the basis of most other reform in this city." There was not, nor could there be, any conflict between Hartley's vigorous pragmatism and intense pietism; the spiritual energies of his youth had been gradually rechanneled so as to shape and motivate his career of overtly secular benevolence. His pious activism had always to be maximized; it could alone placate his consciousness of sin and spiritual imperfection. "My failures," Hartley wrote when past 70, "I believe were less owing to insuperable difficulties, than to my lack of earnestness and energy."[27] The contemplative life had few appeals for the pious in Jacksonian America.

These spiritual compulsions and the slum con-

tacts they engendered had made Hartley and a number of like-minded evangelicals aware of their city's unsavory health conditions well before the formation of the A.I.C.P. in 1842. By the mid 1830s, for example, the New York City Tract Society, of which Hartley had been a member since 1827, began with New York's other city missions to take notice of the sickness and poverty encountered by their missionaries and volunteer tract distributors. Conditions already bad were harshly exacerbated by the panic of 1837 and the lengthy depression which followed; with growing frequency, the annual reports of these evangelical societies lamented in detail the misery of the city's slums. It had begun to seem increasingly unlikely that the souls of the poor could be saved while their bodies remained in such wretchedness.[28] Hartley's temperance work too, though it may seem today a moral, if not moralistic, concern, drew him increasingly into an understanding of the brutal facts of slum life.

It was, indeed, through temperance that Hartley first became involved with a specific public health problem. New York's infant mortality rate was remarkably high — and by the mid-1830s, Hartley had become aware of what he considered a central role played by contaminated milk in swelling these dismaying statistics. He was particularly indignant when investigations showed that a good portion of the city's milk supply came from animals closely confined in filthy and unventilated stalls, and — worst of all — fed exclusively on distillery swill. In the winter of 1836–37, Hartley wrote a series of articles exposing these evils, and in 1842 a full-length treatise on the subject.[29]

Hartley's discussion of the milk problem displays a characteristic 19th-century mixture of pragmatic scientism, religious metaphor doing duty as medical logic, and unmistakable piety. Arguments from Liebig nestle comfortably against those drawn from moral imperative and providential design. Hartley appealed, as did Griscom, to the ultimate value of the natural — read godly — in condemning the unhealthfulness of the milk produced in such grossly unnatural conditions. Cows kept without exercise, in filthy and unventilated stables, without room even to turn about, fed on hot and reeking swill — such animals could be expected to live but a short time and to produce milk as foul as their own conditions and diet. Could men of good will fold their arms and blame the death of so many innocents upon some inscrutable and unavoidable dispensation? "Can such be the purpose of the benevolent Creator?" Hartley, like Griscom, asked fellow New Yorkers.

> Is so large a number of His rational offspring born with such feeble powers of vitality that life necessarily becomes extinct on the threshold of existence? Such conclusions, being inconsistent with the teachings of his Word and Providence, must be rejected as impious and absurd.

And to an activist like Hartley, the conclusion was unmistakable: no truly pious New Yorker should purchase milk from this tainted source. "Can you continue so, and feel that you have discharged your duty to God, to your families and to the community? Are you not bound by the most powerful obligations to wash your hands from all participation in so great an evil?"[30]

It takes no great sophistication to discern the moralism, the temperance zeal in Hartley's overtly pragmatic concern for pure milk. And one could, indeed, make a great deal of the function played by images of pollution, of unnatural alcohol defiling that most natural of goods, God's pure milk (as one could with Griscom's discussion of the manner in which men violated the air they breathed).[31] Their habitual dependence upon such emotion-laden metaphors does not prove Hartley or Griscom to have been pious obscurantists; they were simply utilizing a traditional idiom in rationalizing and dramatizing a deeply held philanthropic commitment. (This was in a period, it must be recalled, when existing etiological knowledge seemed only to underscore the unity between moral and medical truths expressed by such time-honored images and admonitions.) The distinction between that which we regard as pragmatic environmentalism and that which we dismiss as mere moralism is, in regard to the public health movement of the 1840s and 50s, far more confusing than enlightening. Both styles of thought supplemented each other, interacting with the energies of pietism to motivate and broaden the concern of a man like Hartley with the human problems of his city.

Hartley's interest in public health only began with his crusade for pure milk. As corresponding secretary and agent of the A.I.C.P., Hartley soon involved himself and the association he guided in a varied group of measures aimed at improving the health of New Yorkers. For Hartley, like Griscom, assumed that man could be neither provident nor moral without health. As one surveys American cities in the 1840s and early 1850s, it soon becomes apparent that the A.I.C.P. had indeed the most coherent and far-seeing public health program of any benevolent group — while medical societies still concerned themselves only marginally with such matters.

The association's managers were certain of the means by which the city's health conditions could be improved; the provision of decent housing was an indispensable first step. As early as 1846, only two years after the organization had begun independent life, its directors voted to form a committee to investigate New York's slums. The committee issued its report the following year; the city's tenements, they concluded, were utterly inadequate to the preservation of either human health or Christian morality. Echoing Griscom's arguments of 1842, the association's committee contended that New York's crowded, filthy, and ill-ventilated tenements eroded not only good health and moral standards, but also self-respect and religious sentiment. Man, a weakened creature at best, needed a decent environment in order to preserve his industriousness, cleanliness, and morality. This environment, the committee reported to their fellow New Yorkers, could not be found in the city's ever-widening slums. The committee concluded by warning the association firmly: if they hoped to reduce the amount of poverty in New York and improve the morale of the poor, they must first reform tenement conditions.[32]

> Great value should be attached to this much-desired reform, seeing it lies at the basis of other reforms; and as the health and morals of thousands are injured or destroyed by the influence of circumstances around them, an improvement of the circumstances in connection with other appropriate means, afford the only rational hope of effectively elevating their character and condition, and of relieving the city from numerous evils which now exist.

Following European precedents, Hartley and the association turned first to private investment. Model tenements could be constructed, buildings which would provide light and air and still bring a 6 percent return to the Christian capitalists who, it was hoped, would finance their construction. Despite years of effort, however, and the launching of one substantial experiment, these plans never came to fruition.[33] By the mid-1850s, the association, still dedicated to the amelioration of tenement housing, had turned largely to legislative solutions; only the power of the state could end the worst of such abuses — and thus allow the possibility of physical and moral regeneration.[34]

Most notably, the A.I.C.P. sponsored an ambitious study of New York's housing conditions, a study far more detailed than Griscom's earlier report. The committee presented a detailed, ward-by-ward description of New York's slums. A model of lucidity for its time, this document remained until the mid-60s a source of data for American housing reformers and public health workers.[35] Throughout the 1850s, in legislative investigations, in medical articles and reports, in the activities of the New York Sanitary Association and the National Quarantine and Sanitary Conventions, the findings of the A.I.C.P. played a significant role in demonstrating the need for improved housing in safeguarding the health of the city's working population.[36]

In their broad concern for New York's "dependent classes," the A.I.C.P. did not limit its health program to demands for housing reform. It endorsed an eclectic range of public health measures, including the provision of medical care for the indigent. No sooner, indeed, had the A.I.C.P. been founded than it began to investigate the health of the poor and the adequacy of medical care available. In 1845, even before the appearance of its first annual report, the Association published Hartley's *A Plan for the Better Distribution of Medical Attendance*, a proposal for the increased provision of out-patient care. Within six years, the A.I.C.P. established two new medical dispensaries. Association visitors worked closely with dispensary physicians, bringing them to the sick poor, even distributing medicines from central depositories. Throughout the 1850s and 60s, the A.I.C.P. continued to concern itself with such practical health needs. In 1852 it opened a Bath and Wash House, where for a minimal charge (imposed to prevent pauperization of the users) the poor could bathe and wash their clothing. This was New York's first public bath. In 1862, as well, the association's leg-islative efforts at last won a state law regulating the production and sale of milk. During these same years the A.I.C.P. also supported such general public health measures as the improvement of the city's sewers, the regulation of slaughter houses and bone-boiling establishments, and the prevention of tenement dwellers from keeping pigs, goats, and cows in their apartments. It fought among a growing number of allies and with final success — in 1866 — to secure an effective, professionally staffed metropolitan Board of Health.[37]

III

The preceding pages have not sought to contend that all Americans who called in the 1840s and 50s for public health reform were "secularized" evangelists, but rather to argue that a certain number, especially among this pioneer generation, found a central motivation for their driving activism in a pervading spirit of millennial piety. English example and influence were certainly influential, indeed crucial; the writings of Hartley and Griscom reflected again and again their familiarity with contemporary English public health appeals. Yet the question remains: why were these men — unlike the great majority of their medical contemporaries — so receptive to the ideas of the pioneer English sanitarians? The only plausible explanation lies, we have suggested, in their religiously based commitment to saving and helping the unfortunate, in their assumption that an intimate relationship existed between environment, health, and morals.

Perhaps, finally, it might be argued that "pietistic" or "evangelical" is not quite the right word to describe the motivations of men so different as the orthodox Hartley and the Quaker Griscom. And it must be confessed that they differed markedly in their attitude toward the poor and the poverty both sought to alleviate. (Griscom, for example, was at heart an environmental determinist, concerned far more with the implacably forbidding conditions of the slum than with the sins of those who inhabited them. Hartley, on the other hand, never escaped the conviction that original sin was the ultimate cause of all human misery, despite his understanding of the environmental factors which seemed often to cause and always to exacerbate the demoralization of poverty).[38] Yet these individual differences suggest all the more unmistakably the overarching commonality of feeling which bound Griscom and Hartley together, an urgent need to help and in helping to convert — whether one understands the term conversion in the narrowly orthodox sense of predestined salvation, or in the humanistic sense which characterized the Griscom family's millennial faith in education, in science, and in moral improvement. It meant, in operational terms, a need to reach out to the disadvantaged, an inability to tolerate wrongs which might through one's efforts be ameliorated.

## NOTES

1   The now-classic discussion of the influence of pietism in American history is that by H. Richard Niebuhr, *The Kingdom of God in America* (New York: Harper & Bros., 1937). W. G. McLoughlin has provided a more recent synthetic discussion of "Pietism and the American character," *Am. Quart.*, 1965, *17*: 163–186. The present study uses the term "pietism" within a specifically Christian context; McLoughlin employs the term in a much broader sense, to describe almost all behavior dictated in any way by moral imperatives. Among the most influential of recent monographic discussions of the social effects of pietism in ante-bellum America are Whitney Cross, *The Burned-Over District. The Social and Intellectual History of Enthusiastic Religion in Western New York, 1800–1850* (Ithaca: Cornell Univ. Press, 1950); T. L. Smith, *Revivalism and Social Reform in Mid-Nineteenth-Century America* (New York and Nashville: Abingdon, 1957).

2   *The Sanitary Condition of the Laboring Population of New York. With Suggestions for Its Improvement. A Discourse (with Additions) Delivered on the 30th December, 1844, at the Repository of the American Institute* (New York: Harper & Bros., 1845). Compare the discussion of this pamphlet by George Rosen, *A History of Public Health* (New York: MD Publications, c. 1958), pp. 237–239. Rosen contends (p. 238) that "this study already contains in essence the principles and objectives that were to characterize the American sanitary reform movement for the next 30 years."

3   This generalization is based partially on a search for items of public health concern in half a dozen American medical journals between 1843 and 1847. The comparative lack of concern is unmistakable and emphasized by the English origin of many of those items found directly relating to public health. We should like to thank Steven J. Peitzman, a student at the University of Pennsylvania, for his help in this search. With the 1850s, the interest of American physicians began to increase.

4   The most important source of information for Griscom's life is the memoir by his son: J. H. Griscom, *Memoir of John Griscom, LL.D., Late Professor of Chemistry and Natural Philosophy; with an Account of the New York High School; Society for the Prevention of Pauperism;*

*the House of Refuge; and Other Institutions. Compiled from an autobiography, and other sources* (New York: Robert Carter and Brothers, 1859). Cf. E. F. Smith, "John Griscom," *D.A.B.*, VIII, 7. The manuscript division of the New York Public Library contains an important collection of Griscom's incoming correspondence. For the background of Quaker pietism and benevolence, see S. V. James, *A People among Peoples: Quaker Benevolence in Eighteenth-Century America* (Cambridge, Mass.: Harvard Univ. Press, 1963).

5   Formal theological positions were remarkably unimportant in comparison with the common dedication of such men to spiritual activism and social improvement. Griscom, a Quaker, could write of Thomas Chalmers, a Scotch Presbyterian: "It would be difficult to name any writer of the past or present century, entitled to a higher rank . . . as a defender and expounder of theological truth." *Memoir*, p. 379. Chalmers was, significantly, a pioneer in social welfare as well as a prominent theologian and popularizer of natural theology.

6   A recent student of science in Jeffersonian America has described Griscom's chemical lectures as atypically successful and long-lived. J. C. Greene, "Science and the public in the age of Jefferson," *Isis*, 1958, *49*: 20.

7   From a letter of Griscom's, Aug. 27, 1847. *Memoir*, p. 365. Cf. Jos. Murray, Jr., to Griscom, Feb. 13, 1817, Griscom Correspondence, NYPL.

8   On ventilation, see Henry Vethake to Griscom, Nov. 27, 1819; Jacob Bigelow to Griscom, Oct. 29, 1822, Griscom Correspondence. On Griscom's yellow fever interests, see James Hardie, *An Account of the Yellow Fever Which Occurred in the City of New York, in the Year 1822* . . . (New York: Samuel Marks, 1822), pp. 51, 71; New York City, Board of Health, *A History of the Proceedings of the Board of Health, of the City of New York, in the Summer and Fall of 1822* . . . (New York: P. & H. Van Pelt, 1823), pp. 230–242. As early as 1807, David Hosack had written to Griscom, asking for an explanation of factors effecting putrefaction and their possible relationship to disease etiology. Hosack to Griscom, Oct. 23, 1809, Hosack Letter-Book, Rare Book Room, New York Academy of Medicine.

9   Unfortunately, there seem to have survived almost no documents illustrating the younger Griscom's personal life. Perhaps most significant in illuminating Griscom's spiritual life is his careful memoir of his father; its tone leaves little doubt of the son's pietistic orientation. There are a half-dozen Griscom letters in the Gulian Verplanck Papers at the New-York Historical Society. The Municipal Archives and Records Center, 38 William Street, contains many documents signed by Griscom in the papers of the Commissioners of Emigration; these are, however, routine notations relating to the bonding of handicapped immigrants. (Griscom was "secular agent" of the Commissioner from 1848 to 1851.) A search of the rough minutes and Filed and Approved Papers of the Common Council at the archives disclosed no materials relating directly to Griscom's tenure as City Inspector.

10  Philip Van Ingen, *The New York Academy of Medicine. Its First Hundred Years* (New York: Columbia Univ. Press, 1949), p. 20. Van Ingen also notes that Griscom was among the first group of trustees elected when the Academy was chartered (p. 43). For other biographical material, see S. W. Francis, *Biographical Sketches of Distinguished Living New York Physicians* (New York: George P. Putnam, 1867), pp. 45–59; [Philip Van Ingen], *A Brief Account of the First One Hundred Years of the New York Medical and Surgical Society* ([New York]: Privately printed, 1946), p. 43, which notes that Griscom resigned from the society as a protest against the expulsion of Horace Green; "John H. Griscom (1809–1874)," *Dictionary of American Medical Biography,* ed. Howard A. Kelly and Walter Burrage (New York and London: D. Appleton Co., 1928), pp. 501–502; "New York Medical and Surgical Society. First 100 years. Biographies. Vol. II," Rare Book Room, New York Academy of Medicine, pp. 475–484. This typed sketch is the most detailed account available of Griscom's life.

11  "Our Creator afflicts us with diseases," Griscom elaborated, "that we may know how frail and dependent we are. But he has also given us a knowledge of the laws which regulate our growth, and our lives, so that by attending to them, and living purely and uprightly, we may avoid those diseases, in a great degree." Griscom, *First Lessons in Human Physiology; To Which Are Added Brief Rules of Health. For the Use of Schools,* 6th ed. (New York: Roe Lockwood & Son, 1847), pp. 132–133. A principal motive in his writing of texts for the study of such comparatively novel subjects, Griscom explained to parents, "has been the desire to render the study of our frames subservient to moral improvement, by furnishing the young reader with incontestible evidence of a Great First Cause." *Animal Mechanism and Physiology; Being a Plain and Familiar Exposition of the Structure and Functions of the Human System . . .* (New York: Harper and Bros., 1839), p. vii. All of Griscom's specific appeals for public health reform called at least in passing for efforts to raise the level of public knowledge; he urged, for example, at one point the establishment of a "Hygiological Society" to be composed of physicians and laymen and dedicated to the spread of hygienic truths. *Anniversary Discourse. Before the New York Academy of Medicine. Delivered in Clinton Hall, November 22d, 1854* (New York: R. Craighead, 1855), p. 52.

12  Griscom, *Improvements of the Public Health, and the Establishment of a Sanitary Police in the City of New York* (Albany: C. Van Benthuysen, 1857), p. 3. Such seemingly primitivistic appeals to the contrast between the health of the rural, even savage, life and urban conditions are to be found in virtually all of Griscom's writings. Like natural theology itself, such ideas were almost universal at this time. For a discussion of the emotional resonance in this period between the idea of sin and the unnatural, virtue and the natural, see C. E. Rosenberg, *The Cholera Years: The United States, 1832, 1849, and 1866* (Chicago: Univ. of Chicago Press, 1962), p. 132 and *passim.*

13  In addition to his frequent reiteration of the standard warnings of his generation against tightly-laced corsets and alcohol, Griscom wrote books on the problems of ventilation and—in amusingly apocalyptic tones—the evils of tobacco. *The Use of Tobacco, and the Evils, Physical, Moral, and Social, Resulting Therefrom* (New York: G. P. Putnam & Son, 1868); *The Uses and Abuses of Air: Showing Its Influence in Sustaining Life, and Producing Disease . . .* (New York: Redfield, 1850).

14  Griscom, *Uses and Abuses of Air,* pp. 137 n, 143.

15  Such allegations were made in editorials in D. M. Reese's *American Medical Gazette,* accusing Griscom of a 20-year dedication to the hope of feeding from the "public crib." "That consumption hospital," *ibid.,* 1857, *8*: 112–113; "Medical politics," *ibid.,* 113. Van Ingen's history of the New York Academy of Medicine notes Griscom had been involved in reprimanding Reese for allegedly unethical conduct. Van Ingen, *New York Academy of Medicine,* pp. 90–91, 115–116. An anonymous reviewer was also harshly critical of an 1842 pamphlet by Griscom on spinal deformity, implying that it was the work of a quack and written to attract "business." *N.Y. Med. Gaz.,* 1842, *2*: 179–182. This is the only evidence we have found indicating that Griscom may have been inspired by sordid motives.

16  New York City, *Annual Report of the Interments in the*

*City and County of New-York, for the Year 1842, with Remarks Thereon, And a Brief View of the Sanitary Condition of the City* (New York: James Van Norden, 1843). This report had been ordered printed in "four times the usual number." The source of Griscom's political influence in 1842 and thus the explanation of his appointment as City Inspector is, in the absence of manuscript evidence, obscure.

17   Griscom, *Sanitary Condition*, p. 8. Like many of his contemporaries, Griscom habitually emphasized the economic gains to be realized through public health reform; one feels, however, that such hard-headed appeals were simply arguments and rationalizations for a more basic humanitarian commitment.

18   There was no American equivalent of the Chadwickian hostility to physicians among lay advocates of public health. Griscom based all of his proposals upon the impossibility of any but physicians properly fulfilling the duties of a health officer; in keeping with his emphasis was Griscom's assumption that existing medical knowledge was adequate to the explanation and thus prevention of a good portion of the sickness which burdened the city. In 1842, Griscom outlined his essential organizational point of view in regard to New York's Board of Health. New York City, Board of Aldermen, *Communication from the City Inspector, Recommending a Reorganization of the Health Police*, April 24, 1843. Doc. No. 111, pp. 1314–1320.

19   The first portion of this quotation is from Griscom, *Sanitary Condition*, p. 1, the second from Griscom's *Annual Report for 1842*, p. 173.

20   Griscom was also consistently critical of both the exploitive behavior of many of the city's property-holders and the culpable failure of many among the wealthy to ventilate their mansions and observe moderation in eating and drinking—all sins more deserving of condemnation than the almost involuntary misdeeds of the poor. Cf. *Sanitary Condition*, p. 20.

21   Griscom, *Uses and Abuses of Air*, p. 92. The etiological position assumed by Griscom—quite common in the 1840s—was termed by contemporaries "contingent-contagionism" the conviction, that is, that many infectious diseases were contagious only in such confined quarters as hospital wards and slum apartments. This belief provided an excellent vehicle for the expression of social criticism as well as explaining some of the logical dilemmas implicit in either contagionism or noncontagionism.

22   It is tempting, moreover, to interpret Griscom's rejection of early ideas of the specific and particularate etiology of epidemic disease within the same humanitarian framework. Like many other public health leaders of his first generation—Edwin Snow

of Providence and H. G. Clark of Boston, for example—Griscom found it difficult to modify his earlier emphasis upon the importance of local conditions in creating the necessary environment for epidemic disease. For an emphasis upon local causes implied a system in which man's own actions and volitions were the ultimate and most meaningful cause of the pestilence which afflicted him; to place the blame for an epidemic upon some impersonal and specific contagion—as John Snow seemed to do in the case of cholera—was to create an etiological scheme in which Griscom's habitual demands for environmental reform would be deprived of their immediacy. In 1866, for example, Griscom argued that the presence of cholera on a ship in quarantine was due not to some specific and unavoidable contagion, but to the ship's filthy condition. If the ship had been equally filthy and there had been no cholera influence present, ship fever would have resulted; if the ship had been clean there would have been neither cholera nor typhus. Griscom, "The where, the when, the why, and the how, of the first appearance and greatest prevalence of cholera in cities," *Bull. N.Y. Acad. Med.*, 1866, *3*: 6–26, and his comments at page 49–50. His bias in favor of an etiology which justified sanitary reform is equally apparent in his discussion of yellow fever; he argued, for example, that it was of little practical significance whether the city's filthy docks and slips had given rise to yellow fever or simply provided "a richly manured soil in which the germs of that disease, introduced from abroad, would grow with redoubled vigor. . . . It is enough to know that such conditions are inimical to human life, and should never be permitted." *A History, Chronological and Circumstantial, of the Visitations of Yellow Fever in New York City . . .* (New York: Hall, Clayton & Co., 1858), p. 21. Cf. Rosenberg, *The Cholera Years*, p. 196.

23   For the testimony of these city missionaries, see *Sanitary Condition*, pp. 24–38; New York, *Annual Report of Interments, 1842*, pp. 167–171. More than a few prominent New York clergymen became active in medical and public health affairs—Henry Bellows, for example, and William Muhlenberg. (Bellows, of course, directed the Sanitary Commission during the Civil War, while Muhlenberg founded St. Luke's Hospital.) Cf. Ann Ayres, *The Life and Work of William Augustus Muhlenberg* (New York: Harper & Bros., 1880); W. Q. Maxwell, *Lincoln's Fifth Wheel: The Political History of the United States Sanitary Commission* (New York: Longmans, Green & Co., 1956). Perhaps most professional in his career as city missionary-*cum*-public health expert was S. B. Halliday, active for a half-century in the sav-

ing of souls and the improvement of health conditions. It is quite clear that the original motivations for Halliday's concern with environmental reform — nurtured during decades of work for a succession of New York religious charities — lay in his conversion during the revivalistic enthusiasm of the early 1830s. Cf. S. B. Halliday, *Lost and Found; or Life Among the Poor* (New York: Blakeman & Mason, 1859); Carroll S. Rosenberg, "Protestants and Five Pointers: The Five Points House of Industry, 1850–1870," *N.-Y. Hist. Soc. Quart.*, 1964, *48*: 347 and *passim*. The relationship between the city mission movement and the growing demand for environmental reform is a complex one. For a more detailed account, see Carroll S. Rosenberg, "Evangelicalism and the New City. The city mission movement in New York, 1812–1870" (Ph.D. dissertation, Columbia Univ., 1968).

24    *N.Y. J. Med.*, 1845, *4*: 30. In a city with a paucity of institutional structures and organizational models, it was natural that Griscom should have drawn upon the personnel and pattern of activities of the city missions — just as he depended upon the city's dispensaries. In almost all his proposals for board of health reorganization, Griscom suggested that the dispensary physicians, the only medical men who understood tenement conditions, be made district health officers.

25    John Ordronaux, *Prophylaxis, an Anniversary Oration Delivered before the New York Academy of Medicine, Wednesday, Dec. 19th, 1866* (New York: Bailliere Brothers, 1867), pp. 16, 68.

26    Both in his purely evangelical work and in his temperance agitation, Hartley was a consistent advocate of the need for methodical house-to-house visitation; it was such visiting which, for the first time, brought numbers of middle-class New Yorkers into contact with slum conditions. The basic source for Hartley's life is a *Memorial of Robert Milham Hartley. Edited by his son, Isaac Smithson Hartley, D.D.* (Utica, N.Y.: Printed, not published, 1882). The preceding paragraph is synthesized from his detailed biography. For evaluations of Hartley's place in the development of American social welfare, see R. H. Bremner, *From the Depths. The Discovery of Poverty in the United States* (New York: New York Univ. Press, c. 1956), pp. 35–38; Roy Lubove, "The New York Association for Improving the Condition of the Poor: the formative years," *N.-Y. Hist. Soc. Quart.*, 1959, *43*: 307–27. The most important source for Hartley's ideas and activities are the annual reports of the A.I.C.P. for its first three decades; there are also some valuable surviving manuscript sources — including the minutes of the association's Board of Managers — at the Community Service Society, 105

E. 22nd Street, New York. For the city mission background of Hartley's early work and the significance both practical and theological of house-to-house visiting, see Carroll S. Rosenberg, "Evangelicalism and the New City."

27    Hartley, *Memorial*, pp. 229, 288, 297, respectively for the quoted passages. These are typical of many similar entries.

28    The institutional history of the A.I.C.P., like Hartley's personal biography, demonstrates an evolution from pietistic beginnings to a more secular benevolence. Though ordinarily considered a pragmatic — if in some ways moralistic and status-oriented — response to urban conditions, the association actually began as an outgrowth of the New York City Tract Society. This organization had, by the early 1840s, found itself so preoccupied with the economic needs of the poor that its managers feared their primary objective of converting all New Yorkers to evangelical Protestantism might be lost in the demands of day-to-day meliorism. Hence their establishment of a separate organization, the A.I.C.P., to deal with the material ills of the poor. (John H. Griscom was a member of the association's first executive committee, as well as serving as a volunteer visitor and committee member for his district.) Though the A.I.C.P.'s object was not formally the salvation of souls, the moral and psychological views of poverty entertained by the spokesmen of this new organization were identical with those expressed for many years by New York's evangelical leaders. For a detailed treatment of these developments, see Carroll S. Rosenberg, "Evangelicalism and the New City," chs. 6, 10. The founding of the A.I.C.P. by the Tract Society can be traced in the archives of the latter group, now the New York City Mission Society, 105 E. 22d Street.

29    R. M. Hartley, *An Historical, Scientific and Practical Essay on Milk as an Article of Human Sustenance; with a Consideration of the Effects Consequent upon the Unnatural Methods of Producing It for the Supply of Large Cities* (New York: Jonathan Leavitt, 1842).

30    *Ibid.*, pp. 235, 331. Cf. pp. 29–30, 128, 144–145, 208, 212, 232. Hartley's argument from design was, of course, a commonplace in this generation, among physicians as well as laymen and the clergy. This was vigorously illustrated by Dr. A. K. Gardner, a prominent specialist in diseases of women and children, when testifying at a hearing in 1858 and recalling the condition of swill-fed cows he had seen: "And I drew the conclusion that they were not in a state of nature; and the next conclusion that I drew was, that cows not in a natural condition, could not give milk of a natural character. . . . I then considered that if God made the milk in a certain way,

that it could not be improved upon; and if any milk was totally opposite from the natural milk, God's milk, that it must be totally wrong." New York City Board of Health, *Majority and Minority Reports of the Select Committee of the Board of Health, Appointed to Investigate the Character and Condition of the Sources from Which Cow's Milk Is Derived, for Sale in the City of New York* (New York: Charles W. Baker, 1858), pp. 169–170.

31   For an important discussion of the background of such images of "infection" and the gradual and complex secularization of this concept, see Owsei Temkin, "An historical analysis of the concept of infection," in *Studies in Intellectual History* (Baltimore: Johns Hopkins Press, 1953), pp. 123–147, esp. pp. 139–144. See also the discussion of the interaction between scientific thought and religious values provided by L. G. Stevenson in two significant articles: "Science down the drain. On the hostility of certain sanitarians to animal experimentation, bacteriology and immunology," *Bull. Hist. Med.,* 1955, *29:* 1–26, esp. pp. 3–4n.; and "Religious elements in the background of the British anti-vivisection movement," *Yale J. Biol. & Med.,* 1956, *29:* 125–127.

32   New York Association for Improving the Condition of the Poor, *4th Annual Report,* 1847, p. 23; *3rd Annual Report,* 1846, p. 22.

33   R. H. Bremner has written an account of the A.I.C.P.'s one substantial experiment in this area: "The big flat: history of a New York tenement house," *Am. Hist. Rev.,* 1958, *64:* 54–62. Cf. A.I.C.P., *5th Annual Report,* 1848, pp. 18–19; *10th Annual Report,* 1853, pp. 26–27; Board of Managers, Minutes, April 10, 1854, Community Service Society.

34   It was always assumed, of course, that such reforms would have an inevitable spiritual effect. At the eleventh annual meeting of the A.I.C.P., for example, the influential clergyman T. L. Cuyler, made this point of view explicit in praising the association's just-completed housing report. "The sanitary statements of the Report," he proposed, "show that where cleanliness and ventilation are neglected, disease and mortality are proportionately increased. And where the body is unclean, and the dwelling wretched, there is commonly a correspondingly moral degradation. . . . Sanitary reform," Cuyler urged, "is intimately connected with the spread of true religion. The dwellings of the poor are to be looked after as well as their souls," N.Y.A.I.C.P., *11th Annual Report, 1854,* p. 6. The other principal speaker at this meeting was the Reverend Henry Bellows, later—as we have noted—prominent for his work with the Sanitary Commission during the Civil War. Both Cuyler and Bellows were also active in the New York Sanitary Association.

35   N.Y.A.I.C.P., *First Report of a Committee on the Sanitary Condition of the Poor in the City of New York* (New York: John F. Trow, 1853). Though less famous than the Shattuck Report of 1850, this document seems to have been quoted with equal frequency in the dozen years after its publication. Also revealing is the detailed discussion of this report the succeeding year in the association's *11th Annual Report, 1854,* pp. 19–29. Hartley, who wrote all the association's annual reports, significantly began his discussion with a quotation from Thomas Chalmers: "That all our sufferings and evils (so far as they exceed those inseparable from a finite and imperfect nature) may be traced to ignorance or neglect of those laws of nature which God has established for our good, and displayed for our instruction." *Ibid.,* p. 19. Beginning with the mid-1850s and through the establishment of the Metropolitan Board of Health in 1866, the A.I.C.P. reports regularly called for state intervention in New York's housing and sanitary affairs.

36   Long-time A.I.C.P. supporters were, for example, influential in the New York Sanitary Association (founded 1859), though the association itself was modeled after the British Health of Towns Associations, while similar ties existed between the A.I.C.P. and the Citizens' Association. For a discussion of the events leading to the passage of the Metropolitan Board of Health Bill and the place of these organizations, see G. H. Brieger, "Sanitary reform in New York City: Stephen Smith and the passage of the Metropolitan Health Bill," *Bull. Hist. Med.,* 1966, *40:* 407–429. [See ch. 28 in this book.] For an example of the prominence of A.I.C.P. findings in contemporary public health debate, see New York State, Senate, *Report of the Select Committee Appointed to Investigate the Health Department of the City of New York. In Senate, Feb. 3, 1859. Document No. 49* [Albany, 1859]. The committee's conclusions simply echo the Hartley-Griscom position in calling for state action and in blaming much of the city's pauperism and ill-health on poor housing, pp. 13–16.

37   N.Y.A.I.C.P., *A Plan for Better Distribution of Medical Attendance and Medicines for the Indigent Sick, by the Public Dispensaries in the City of New York* (New York, 1845). On dispensaries see A.I.C.P., *8th Annual Report, 1851,* pp. 20–22; *9th Annual Report, 1852,* pp. 38–39. The two dispensaries were the DeMilt and the Northeastern. There was some controversy as to how much the A.I.C.P. actually had to do with the DeMilt Dispensary after Hartley arranged the meetings which led to its establishment. DeMilt Dispensary in the City of New York, *25th Annual Report, 1875,* pp. 25–28. More relevant, however, is the philanthropic career of F. E. Mather, a promi-

nent New Yorker and president of the DeMilt Dispensary for its first quarter-century. He became involved in such public health matters through the A.I.C.P. and later served as president of the New York Sanitary Association and attended the National Sanitary and Quarantine Conventions. On public baths, see N.Y.A.I.C.P., *9th Annual Report, 1852,* pp. 39–40. N.Y.A.I.C.P., *19th Annual Report, 1862,* pp. 54–58, reprints the text of the act against adulteration of milk. For the history of the Society for the Ruptured and Crippled, see *ibid.*, 38–43; Fenwick Beekman, *The Hospital for the Ruptured and Crippled. A Historical Sketch* . . . (New York: Printed, not published, 1939). Hartley took a personal interest in the establishment of the Presbyterian Hospital and served for eight years as its secretary. *Memorial,* p. 484.

38   Griscom retained his formal adherence to the Society of Friends, "whose tenets," he explained late in life, "are regarded by me as most in accordance with Scripture teachings, as the most liberal in sentiment, and most truly democratic in practice of all sects." Francis, *Biographical Sketches,* p. 54. We have been unable to determine whether Griscom was an orthodox or Hicksite Quaker. His humanitarian environmentalism is, indeed, Griscom's most significant — and endearing — characteristic. He even blamed poor ventilation for the sluggish behavior of school children who normally received the rod instead of the fresh air they actually needed. *Uses and Abuses of Air,* p. 51. Hartley is consistently harsher than Griscom in his social and individual judgments — a harshness intensified by his rigid Manchestrian views.

# 28

## Sanitary Reform in New York City: Stephen Smith and the Passage of the Metropolitan Health Bill

### GERT H. BRIEGER

### I

"Frenzy in the South," proclaimed the bold headline of the *New York Times* on March 10, 1865. These were the last days of the long and bitter struggle, and New Yorkers welcomed the news. Each day they read about Grant and Sheridan in Virginia and of Sherman's impressive march up through the Carolinas. On March 16, however, a different subject dominated the first two pages of the paper. Instead of the usual fare of war news, the *Times* provided its readers with the testimony of Dr. Stephen Smith presented before a joint committee of the New York State Legislature. He had given evidence about the sanitary conditions of New York City and on the urgent need for new health laws. Smith gave a stinging indictment of the municipal authorities responsible for the public health and described the miserable conditions of the city's streets and tenements. This testimony, based on a massive effort by a large group of reform-dedicated physicians, was the culmination of years of effort by numerous citizens of America's major metropolis.[1]

The horrible conditions which existed at the close of the Civil War were not peculiar to New York or to that period. As Ford has pointed out, the relationship between cellar-dwellings and disease production in New York had been discussed as early as the 1790s.[2] In 1820 David Hosack told the medical students of the College of Physicians and Surgeons that the filth in various parts of the city

was marked and that amelioration could probably not be achieved without the aid of the state legislature.[3] Benjamin W. McCready, in 1837, pointed to poor housing and insufficient space as a major source of ill-health among the workers.[4] In 1842, John H. Griscom, one of the truly important figures in the story of sanitary reform, appended to his annual report of the City Inspector's office a pamphlet entitled "A Brief View of the Sanitary Condition of the City," in which he described living conditions and the destitution and misery of cellar-dwellers. He urged upon the Common Council the necessity of better housing laws.[5]

In December 1844, Griscom delivered a discourse at the American Institute which he published during the next year as *The Sanitary Condition of the Laboring Population of New York*. He reported the health problems which faced many tenement-dwelling New Yorkers, and he urged "SANITARY REFORM." He was anxious to profit from the experience of English and French sanitarians, and their influence is evident in the text as well as the title.[6]

Griscom was one of the first to show that the system of subtenancy and the rental extortions of the sublandlord were among the principal causes of misery of so many of the city's poor. This system enabled the owner of one or several houses to rent them to a sublandlord, who in turn divided them into as many apartments as possible. He then extracted as much rent as he could, often from helpless immigrants. By making few repairs and providing little maintenance he realized a great profit. Often he owned the local store as well and fixed prices at relatively high levels. The working classes were virtually restricted to lower Manhattan because there was no means of inexpensive,

GERT H. BRIEGER is William H. Welch Professor and Director of the Institute of the History of Medicine at the Johns Hopkins University School of Medicine, Baltimore, Maryland.

Reprinted with permission from the *Bulletin of the History of Medicine*, 1966, *40*: 407–429.

rapid transportation which would have freed them from the packed tenement conditions.[7]

Griscom also clearly described the evils of cellar-dwellings, often soggy and lacking ventilation. Many of the cellar-apartments were below sea level. When high tides came, the rooms were submerged! During heavy rains, the streets drained into the cellars. The cellar-dwellers, or Troglodytes as they were often called, lived and slept on planks suspended well above the floors.

In contrast to McCready, who seems to have practiced and taught medicine in comparative quiet, Griscom continued active agitation for improved public health laws. He was one of the first to stress that the physicians in the public dispensaries of the city would be ideally suited for the jobs of health wardens or sanitary inspectors.[8] He was the first witness before the Select Committee of the New York Senate appointed in 1858 to investigate the health department of New York City. He then sat with the committee during its interrogation of over 20 witnesses, often interjecting lively questions and barbed remarks.[9]

This committee was appointed to investigate the "assertion that great defects exist, and great improvements are practicable in the health department and sanitary laws of the city of New York."[10] Three major questions were asked: (1) Whether the allegations were true that New York had a higher ratio of mortality than other large cities. (2) If true, what were the causes of this excess mortality. (3) What were the possible remedies.[11]

Almost unanimously the witnesses gave an affirmative answer to the first question. As to the causes, this report established what was to become a constantly recurring refrain. Almost all the witnesses ascribed the excessive mortality to overcrowded tenement houses, improper light, ventilation, and food, filthy streets, insufficient sewerage, and an almost total lack of a regularly constituted and effective department of health.

Contrary to the arguments put forward by the City Inspector, Mr. Morton, the committee stated that a properly constituted health department would require the talents of the best educated men, well versed in the recent advances of medical science. Not since 1844 had a physician been City Inspector. "A man when he wants his watch repaired," argued Dr. John McNulty, "does not take it to a shoemaker. . . ."[12]

The City Inspector and his men disagreed. Mr. Richard Downing, Superintendent of Sanitary Inspection, claimed that knowledge of the law, not medicine, was necessary. It did not require medical knowledge, he said, to smell an odor or to recognize a filthy street.[13] Mr. Morton added his feeling that physicians would not do the job; they would think it undignified to "go running through tenement houses and sticking their noses down privies, to see if they were healthy or not. . . ."[14]

For two years prior to the Senate committee's investigation, the leading medical society, the New York Academy of Medicine, petitioned the legislature for modifications of the health laws. In 1856 the academy sent a memorial to Albany which stated that "a large portion of the annual mortality of this city results from diseases, whose causes are more or less within our control, but which are totally unchecked by any public administration of proper sanitary precautions, and that from this neglect, in addition to a very great and unnecessary loss of life, the city and State endure an incalculable detriment to their commercial and moral interests."[15] No bill was passed at the 1857 session.[16] Nor was a renewal of the petition successful the following year.

In the meantime, however, the legislature did pass the Metropolitan Police Bill, in 1857, an important model and precedent for future health legislation. By transferring to state control the city's police force, the Republican state legislature created a new police district comprising the counties of New York, Kings, Richmond, and Westchester. The Board of Police was to consist of five commissioners, plus the mayors of New York and Brooklyn. New York's Mayor Fernando Wood resisted the new law and kept control of his original municipal force — most of whom had voted for him on the Democratic ticket. Only after rioting in the streets with the municipal faction, the arrest of Mayor Wood, and the use of the state militia, did the Metropolitan Police finally win their right to act as the city's legally constituted guardians of the peace.[17]

A recent historian of this episode pointed out how the situation was complicated by a growing political and social cleavage between New York City and the rest of the state.[18] Each mayor, in his annual messages of the succeeding years, used the argument that local problems, such as sanitation, should be kept under local control. Thus the sanitary reform measures, suggested repeatedly between 1856 and 1866 by the leading physicians of New York, took on increasingly complex political overtones. Health bill advocates found themselves fighting, not only for good health and efficient sanitary administration, but against political corruption and the control of Tammany Hall over the city.[19]

In the meantime, the New York Sanitary Association had been founded in January 1859. The members immediately took up the fight for the health bill before the legislature, then in session. John Griscom and Elisha Harris were officers of the group, and Stephen Smith, Joseph M. Smith, and Peter Cooper were among the members of the council.[20]

That winter the association impressed upon the legislators the urgent need for a health bill. They used established arguments: New York's ratio of mortality was greater than that of most cities in the United States and western Europe; those diseases which most contributed to this mortality were due to the absence of proper sanitary administrations and were just those diseases thought to be preventable; New York had three separate health authorities, none of which functioned properly. These were the Board of Health, composed of the Mayor, Aldermen, and Councilmen and rarely in session; the Commissioners of Health, including the Mayor, the Presidents of the Boards of Aldermen and Councilmen, the Resident Physician, and Health Officer of the Port; and the City Inspector's Department.[21] The Sanitary Association pointed out that there were about 112 individuals directly and indirectly supposedly concerned for the health of the people, but "that there is not one who feels it to be required of him to take note of, or to use any effort whatever to check the immense amount of disease. . . ."[22]

Once again the story was the same. Their bill failed to pass.

By the end of 1860, the Sanitary Association could say that its meetings had been well attended and that it considered itself a permanent organization. It continued to act as a lobby group in Albany. The membership increased to over 250, representing the professions of law, medicine, education, and divinity.[23]

As late as 1862 the group continued to hear interesting papers, but the pressures of the war seem to have caused a cessation of its activities sometime in that year.[24]

While I have concerned myself primarily with matters of the public health, problems of personal health were not ignored. The sanitarians had the twin aims of improving the health laws and of educating the people, especially the poor, in the ways of proper hygiene. This, indeed, was also the aim of the numerous philanthropic organizations that flourished in New York at mid-century. The popular magazines and the newspapers often contained articles on health or advice on matters pertaining to diet or epidemics. One author, in 1856, thought that Americans should be the healthiest people in the world. If they were not, it was due to the hectic pace of life, with too much work and too little play.[25]

Medical teachers did not neglect the subject of hygiene, although often admitting that, in this area, ". . . the profession of medicine has hitherto grievously failed"[26] — this, even though the medical profession had expended an incredible amount of time and talent upon the subject of public and private hygiene in the quarter century before the Civil War.[27] And so, too, many doctors believed that hygiene and not quarantine was the true law of health.[28]

## II

When the *New York Journal of Medicine* ceased publication in 1860, Stephen Smith shifted his editorial chair to the newly established *American Medical Times*, and he began four years of vigorous crusading in a large variety of areas. The older journal had contained few editorial comments in its bimonthly numbers, while its successor, a weekly, published lengthy editorials in every issue. In his writings he concerned himself with the role of medicine and the medical profession in society, including frequent expositions on wartime problems.[29]

Since Smith was a New Yorker, and because his journal was published in that city and presumably found most of its readers there, he usually devoted himself to local sanitary problems — primarily the need for legislative reform and the necessity for vigorous action on the part of the medical profession. In his first editorial in the new journal he set forth many of the precepts he planned to follow. He singled out the subject of hygiene to receive vigilant and faithful attention.[30] In the third number he elaborated on these ideas and stated his intention periodically to examine the more important questions relating to sanitary and quarantine systems of American cities and particularly the role and duty of the medical profession.[31] Despite the potential usefulness of his public health editorials nationally, he consistently focused on New York City.

During the summer of 1860 things looked bleak indeed. The country was threatened by division, political feelings ran high, and local sanitary problems continued to increase. More and more immigrants had to be fed and housed as each month passed. Smith shared the pessimistic mood of late summer when he noted that amidst legislative corruption it was not at all certain that improved health laws could be obtained: "And such are the necessities of the people, such the jeopardy of life and health as well as commercial interests, that our population cannot safely await the good time coming, when good laws and municipal reform shall effect the sanitary improvements now demanded. From various quarters the question comes up — What shall be done?"[32]

His answer was clear: he believed that more pressing than questions of quarantine were those relating to civic hygiene. More attention had to be devoted to municipal sanitary arrangements, especially to those of New York.[33]

The cause of sanitary reform moved forward slowly during the Civil War. Although official population figures showed a slight decrease in the 1865 census as compared with 1860, the city's municipal problems became worse.[34] Stokes noted that the city's growth during the war had been checked, but not stopped entirely. Fewer buildings were erected and the misery of crowded tenements grew. The increase in production and the resultant higher wages probably did elevate the general standard of living, but often prices increased too so the poorest classes were left with a net loss.[35] The poor did not share in the profits of rising real estate values and the general business expansion — in fact these things operated to their disadvantage. The increase in luxury which "struck every observer" falls short of describing the condition of more than half of the population — the tenement dwellers.[36]

Although wages rose, prices rose faster. Eggs, 15 cents in 1861, rose to 25 cents by the end of 1863; potatoes went from $1.50 to $2.25 per bushel during the same period. The increase in wages was generally about 25 percent, or less than half the increase of prices.[37]

Citizens interested in sanitary reform worked on through the war years. They helped introduce a bill into the state legislature each winter, but it failed to pass with each succeeding session. The daily papers and popular journals continued to clamor for both municipal and sanitary reform, building up to quite a pitch in the year prior to the success of 1866 — the Metropolitan Health Bill.

The medical press was also active, especially the influential *American Medical Times*. Others, besides Stephen Smith, participated in the effort; but it is on Smith's role I wish to focus. I should note that his work in the early 1860s was of much broader scope than my emphasis on sanitation would indicate.

Prior to 1864, Smith's efforts in behalf of a Metropolitan Health Bill were confined chiefly to the numerous editorials praising each bill, exhorting his fellow physicians to exert influence upon the legislature, and bemoaning the lack of a properly constituted health department in the city.

In December 1860, he asked: Will the next legislature provide a sanitary code for the city?[38] He pointed out that more than a fourth of the state's population resided in New York and Brooklyn. He noted that it was widely acknowledged that these million and a quarter people were "living under one of the most corrupt and corrupting municipal governments in the civilized world, and that reform without the interposition of State legislation is impractical." To call the existing Health Department by that name was a misnomer. "It does little for health, but much for disease and death."[39]

Early in 1861, Smith aimed his editorial guns in a violent attack on the City Inspector, who was to become a favorite target for the next five years.[40]

The City Inspector was really the only active health official in New York. It is true that there was a Physician of the Port and a Resident Physician, who, with the Mayor and Presidents of the Boards of Councilmen and Aldermen, constituted a Commission of Health. In fact, however, in matters other than quarantine, it was mainly the City Inspector and his 44 health wardens who looked after the sanitation of the city.[41]

In his report for 1860, the inspector, Mr. Daniel E. Delavan, a two-year incumbent in the post, claimed a healthy condition for New York when compared to European cities.[42] What problems there were he attributed mainly to immigrants. His report admitted many of the sanitary problems of New York and he gave some reasons for them. In the first place, he was very critical of the medical profession for their failure to cooperate in the proper registration of vital statistics. Thus he noted the paradox of "opposition among the very class whose leading spirits have been most active for some years past in this city in urging the cause of sanitary reform."[43] He admitted to the filthy condition of the streets, stating that the Common Council had removed $50,000 from his budget and that in November 1860 money for street cleaning ran out; 300 miles of paved streets was a lot to sweep.[44] Mr. Delavan also was opposed to having the state legislature do for the citizens what they could best do for themselves. With a final thrust aimed at those working for reform, he said, "Nor is it necessary for the further efficiency of this department that it should become the nursery of students of medicine. . . ."[45]

Smith dealt harshly with this report. He noted that it contained ". . . its usual variety of loose and often absurd statements in regard to the public health, and deductions, the result of the most profound ignorance of sanitary science."[46] He objected mostly to the assertion that New York was a healthy city. The ratio of 1 death in 36 of its population made the mortality rate the highest of civilized cities.

Early in 1862, Smith bemoaned the singular indifference, which he felt was evident in the city, toward the fearful living conditions of most of its people.[47] The *Medical and Surgical Reporter* of Philadelphia agreed and said that the Augean stable had to be cleansed and a Hercules of sanitary science was needed to do the job.[48]

In February 1862 Smith became more optimistic about the possibility of a health bill. There was good evidence at last that a reorganization of the health department was to take place. Perhaps he saw a turning point in the road to victory when he noted that, "the question which is presented this winter is not, Shall there be a reform, but, What shall be its character?"[49]

Optimism was short-lived. In early May he be-

gan an editorial plaintively announcing the adjournment of the legislature without the enactment of a health bill. The metropolitan concept introduced into the proposed bill was distasteful to the mayor. Smith decided that Mayor Opdyke had really joined the "Ring" and thereby had aided the defeat of "this most righteous measure."[50]

Others, too, "confessed to a very great disappointment" at the failure of the bill. The *Medical and Surgical Reporter* entitled its editorial, "Health Bills and a Diseased Body Politic." "Politicians, those curses of our country . . ." doubtless were to blame, said the *Reporter*.[51] And so again New York was left to its own sanitary devices, devices that were due to receive shocking public description and denunciation in the succeeding few years.

In what had become a cycle of editorial moods, Smith seemed most discouraged toward the end of 1862. It was an extremely busy year for him, personally. Besides the weekly editorial writing and editing of the *Medical Times*, he wrote a manual for military surgeons, used in the Civil War; he continued active teaching and practice at the Bellevue Hospital and its new Medical College, where he was the first Professor of the Principles of Surgery; and he served a stint in the military hospitals of Virginia as an acting assistant surgeon. But the sanitary reform of New York was still a pressing concern for him.

In November he wrote that prospects for a bill seemed discouraging, that many had been led to believe that subsequent efforts would lead nowhere and hence should be abandoned indefinitely. Smith disagreed. While thousands of New Yorkers were dying annually of what he firmly believed were preventable diseases, and while half the city's population lived in the cheerless, sunless, and airless tenements, it was unthinkable to yield in the struggle. Ceaseless agitation would be required. His feelings were perhaps neatly summed up when he noted in November of 1862, "we should not, however, lose sight of the fact that we are striving to accomplish a reform which in importance and in magnitude rises superior to all civil, social, religious, or political questions of the time."[52] Allowing for the exaggeration and zeal of the reformer, this statement still, I believe, illustrates the extent of his commitment to sanitary reform, especially in view of the state of the nation's political and economic health.

He described the efforts he envisioned from legislative enactments: First, they should protect the
citizen, especially the impoverished one, from disease and thereby lengthen life; second, they would
develop a strong and healthy generation of citizens; and third, all health reforms would add
greatly to the sum of human happiness. So fully
impressed was he with the importance of sanitary
reform that he felt, even though the prospect of
success was not as great as it had been the year
before, "we ought to put forth increased energy instead of relaxing our efforts."[53]

Public apathy was a major obstacle in the path
of sanitary reform. This unconcern was as prevalent in much of the medical profession as it seems
to have been in the general public. Numerous writers appealed to the educated, the rich, the influential, to raise their voices in protest. *Harper's Weekly*
noted, for instance, "There is certainly no city in
the world where intelligent and decent people surrender themselves to a band of knaves with such
good humor as in New York."[54] The *Medical Times*
noted that: "The country is horrified when a thousand fall victims in an ill-fought battle, but in this
city 10,000 die annually of diseases which the city
authorities have the power to remove, and no one
is shocked."[55]

December 12, 1863, marked a turning point. On
that day a group of the leading lawyers and merchants of the city, including Peter Cooper, John
Jacob Astor, Jr., August Belmont, and Hamilton
Fish, formed the Citizens' Association. They were
organized "for purposes of public usefulness."[56]

At an association meeting two months later, a
committee was formed to solicit from the medical
profession the "fullest and most reliable information relative to the public health." Shortly, 24 of the
city's leading medical men received a letter from
the association—among them: Valentine Mott,
Willard Parker, Stephen Smith, John H. Griscom,
Elisha Harris, Austin Flint, Frank H. Hamilton,
and Gurdon Buck.

Only a week later, on March 9, the physicians
answered the committee's request for information.
The doctors pointed out that although New York
with its many natural advantages ought to be one
of the healthiest cities, the exact reverse was the
case. They believed the high mortality rate was a
reliable index of the city's miserable health conditions. They provided comparative statistics: mor-

tality in New York was 1 in every 35.7 of the population, while in Philadelphia it was 1 in 43.6, in
Boston 1 in 41.2, and in Hartford as low as 1 in
54.8. The city fared poorly in comparison to London and Liverpool as well. They pointed to Lyon
Playfair's figures in Great Britain, which showed
that for every death there were at least 28 cases
of illness.[57]

In the meantime, the Citizens' Association
busied itself with the task of lobbying for the health
bill then being considered in Albany. Representatives appeared before the legislature on March 15
and 16, only to meet resistance from both Democratic and Republican members. The former regarded the sweeping measures proposed under a
metropolitan, nonpolitical health department as
being aimed at their friends, which indeed it was.
The Republicans were reluctant to interfere in city
affairs, thereby hurting their chances in the upcoming presidential election that fall. The members of the Citizens' Association found, according
to Stephen Smith, that to many members of the
legislature, "the death of five thousand citizens was
not so serious as the possibility of a presidential
defeat."[58]

It must have been clear, at this point, to the Citizens' Association and the friends of sanitary reform, that what they really needed was a set of clear
and extensive facts about the health conditions of
the city—facts that would overcome the inertia of
some legislators and facts which would once and
for all clearly disprove the data which the City Inspector's Office had for so long been bringing to
Albany to controvert any proposal for better laws.

A Council of Hygiene and Public Health was
formed in April within the Citizens' Association.
Its president was Joseph M. Smith, a prominent
physician and writer who had made a monumen-
tal study of the epidemics of New York State.[59]
Elisha Harris, a close friend and neighbor of Stephen Smith, was made secretary. The council consisted of 16 physicians, many of whom had been
recipients and signers of the letters noted above.[60]

To gather the necessary facts about the true
health and sanitary conditions of New York and
its three-quarters of a million residents, an extensive survey was planned. This survey was organized
and directed primarily by Stephen Smith.[61] It was
to become, according to numerous commenters,
the most complete sanitary survey ever made, and

certainly an important landmark in the history of public health in America.

The survey began early in May, got under full swing by July, and was completed by mid-November.[62] The city was divided into 31 districts, each inspected thoroughly by a physician. It was intended, by means of the survey, to arrive at "positive knowledge of the amount of preventible disease existing in New York, the location of insalubrious quarters, the peculiar habitats of typhus, smallpox, . . . and the conditions on which the alarming prevalence of these diseases depend."[63] A month later, in late July, Smith noted, "It is nothing less than a full and accurate inquiry into the causes of disease in this city by competent medical men."[64] And thus it should also be credited as a landmark in the history of epidemiology.

Although there were numerous etiological theories current in 1864, in the sanitarians' view the environment played the most important part, especially the so-called localizing causes, or those which promoted the prevalence of disease in particular localities. Each of the 31 inspectors reported on his district and described his findings mainly in terms of cleanliness and filth.[65]

The inspectors were, for the most part, young physicians who were employed by one of the public (charity supported) dispensaries of the city. They were ideally qualified, for their patients mostly came from the poorer districts; moreover, they had had experience in visiting the tenements. They were given only token compensation ($40 per month) for their labor. Their reports, charts, maps, and diagrams filled 17 folio volumes. On his return from his work on behalf of the U.S. Sanitary Commission, Dr. Harris edited the 360-page report and added a 143-page introduction. The report was published in April 1865. The reviews of the book were uniformly laudatory, and many pointed out the great importance of the survey and the *Report* for the future of sanitary government in New York.[66]

The *Report* has been frequently cited in discussions of American public health and of housing problems. Indeed, it deserves to be ranked very high among primary documents, not only in the history of public health reform but in epidemiology as well. Furthermore, it affords an extremely detailed look at some aspects of the way of life in each of the wards of New York in 1864, and it should be of great interest in the study of urban history.

Epidemiology has been defined as "the study of the distribution and determinants of disease prevalence in man."[67] According to this concept, then, the *Report* belongs among the most important of 19th century epidemiological studies. It contains graphic, statistical, and descriptive information on population, number and size of tenement houses, prevailing diseases, schools, churches, stores, slaughter-houses, factories, brothels, drinking establishments, sewerage, streets, and topography.

Its impact was manifold. Certainly it did not "drop stillborn from the printer's hand," as had been the case with the Shattuck *Report* 15 years earlier. Instead, as Kramer has pointed out for the Chadwick *Report*, it was a document that was alive; it aroused indignation and wonderment; it had emotional appeal beyond its intellectual content. And it led to effective legislation.[68]

Besides the descriptions of overflowing privies with their nauseous odors, garbage, offal, ashes, and generally dirty streets, the inspectors also wrote about slaughterhouses, fat- and bone-boiling establishments, and stables, all dispersed among the tenements. The streets were the main focus of complaint from the magazines and newspapers of the day as well. Youngsters, it is said, could easily earn nickels by standing along Broadway and sweeping a path through the muck for those who wanted to cross.[69] On Thirty-ninth Street, the inspector reported that blood and liquid animal remains flowed for two blocks from a slaughterhouse to the river.[70] Another great source of nuisance was the wooden garbage box. These usually rotted, allowing liquid contents to flow out. It seems they also provided a ready source of wood for political bonfires.[71]

Occasionally the survey itself was responsible for immediate improvements. In parts of the third district the inspector noted progress with each succeeding visit he made.[72]

It was armed with the data from this comprehensive epidemiological study of New York City that Stephen Smith appeared before the legislature in Albany on February 13, 1865. The report had not yet been published, but Smith in his testimony, to which I alluded at the opening of this paper, quoted widely from it. He spoke before the joint committee of the Senate and Assembly, presided over by Andrew D. White. The committee had already heard testimony from Mr. Dorman B. Eaton on the legal aspects of the proposed bill.[73] Smith told them that he and the Citizens' Association had been inspired and aided by the work of similar organizations in Great Britain, notably the Health of Towns Association.

He further told the legislators that the best method of arriving at a complete understanding of the existing causes of disease was by a house-to-house inspection. Since it was disease that was the object of study, it could only have been carried out properly by sufficiently trained men, viz., physicians.

He described conditions in general terms of cleanliness, stating that the degree of public health of a town was to be measured by its cleanliness and that in no way was the sanitary government of New York to be commended. He called the City Inspector's department a "gigantic imposture." The 22 health wardens and an equal number of assistants were grossly ignorant of sanitary matters, but that was to be expected in view of their backgrounds, since they were liquor store owners, local politicians, stonemasons, and carpenters. Not only were they ignorant of medical matters, but Smith also accused them of unwillingness to visit houses where known cases of disease existed. He told of one health warden who sent for an attendant of a smallpox patient in an upper room. Ordering the attendant not to approach too closely, he then advised: "Burn camphor on the stove, and hang bags of camphor about the necks of the children." Smith then asked the members of the Senate and Assembly:

> To what depth of humiliation must that community have descended, which tolerates as its sanitary officers men who are not only utterly disqualified by education, business, and moral character, but who have not even the poor qualification of courage to perform their duties?

He ended his long testimony with the recommendation that New York heed the experience of other large cities in establishing a well-organized health board. That board, he opined, should be independent of politics and above partisan control. Furthermore the board must combine administrative ability with a knowledge of disease and its prevention. For this reason he felt that the composition of the board should include medical and nonmedical members. His testimony, although well organized and at times forceful as well as eloquent, was not original. It represented the consensus of most of his coworkers. It is to his credit, however, that the problems of sanitary reform were continually held up before the medical profession through his editorials in the *American Medical Times* and now were brought before the general public, with the aid of the *New York Times*. Equally to his credit was it that he had helped to write the medical portion of the proposed bill and, together with Dorman B. Eaton, a lawyer and a keen student of sanitary laws, had drafted the final version.

Why the *Times* hesitated for over a month before publishing his speech I cannot explain with certainty. It is entirely possible that when the testimony was given on February 13, the prospect of legislation was bright; but that by March 16, when the *Times* printed the speech, the bill was already in dire straits.[74] Henry Raymond and the *Times* were deeply committed to a health reform measure, as is attested by frequent editorials during the winter of 1865 and again during the next session in 1866. It may well be that the *Times* felt that publication of the facts would serve to bring pressure to bear upon the reluctant legislators.[75] That it did not achieve this result is a matter of record. But now the issues and the facts were clearly before the public. Because part of the Citizens' Association survey was published in the *Times* it achieved a wider public circulation for writing on the subject of sanitation than had ever been the case before. This was a milestone in New York history.

Unfortunately, Smith's testimony in February, its publication in March, and the subsequent appearance of the printed *Report* were not enough to sway the lawmakers in Albany. Frequent editorials in the *Times*, the *Tribune*, and the *Citizen*, a weekly paper founded by the Citizens' Association in 1864, did not seem to help either.

On January 16, 1865, the *Times* noted that typhus and smallpox were running rife. The "ignorant men called 'Health Wardens'" were receiving annually an aggregate of nearly $50,000, but in the opinion of the newspaper, "The only persons who are doing anything for the public health are the agents of the Citizens' Association."

On March 3, the *Tribune* reported the continuing discussion in Albany and the testimony that had been given for the bill by the members of the Citizens' Association and against it by Francis I. A. Boole, the City Inspector; Lewis A. Sayre, the resident physician; and Cyrus Ramsey, the Registrar in the City Inspector's department. According to the *Tribune*, Ramsey attempted ineffectually to controvert the statements made by Smith, Eaton, and the friends of reform. The *Tribune*, somewhat incredulously, noted that Ramsey was driven to extremes in support of the existing corrupt system when he even went so far as to ridicule the idea that cleanliness was an important source of health.[76]

As March progressed, the *Times* pointed out that the Democratic members in the legislature hung together on every question, but not the Republicans. The health bill had, despite pleas from many sides, once again become a political and partisan issue.[77] The *Tribune* said, "To lose the rich *placer* of the City Inspector's department is to cut the winds of scores of active workers, whose only duty is to sign the payrolls and work for the party that gives them fat sinecures."[78]

On April 12, three days after Appomattox, the bill finally came out of committee into the House. Two days later, amid "perfect bedlam," it was defeated. Most New Yorkers, however, were probably much too dazed and saddened to read the account from Albany on the morning of April 15. The headline that day proclaimed "Awful Event."[79] It is not likely that in the days following the tragic and shocking death of Lincoln, those who had labored so hard that year for a health bill had any time for grief on its account.

In 1865 cholera threatened New York again, and the press of the city became increasingly alarmed over the prospects of another epidemic. The summer passed, however, and with a sigh of relief those concerned felt that with the approaching cold season the city would be safe, at least temporarily. But the need for legislative action became more acute.[80]

On November 9, the *Nation* claimed that New York was nearly as filthy as the Asiatic towns from which the cholera came.

> It is awful yet comical to learn that the Board of Health, which at such a crisis ought to reign supreme, is such a disreputable body that, nobody having the power to adjourn it if once organized, the Mayor is afraid to call it together.[81]

The *Times*, a day later, noted that the Mayor considered the cholera the lesser of the two evils, and so left the Board alone.[82]

As 1866 opened, Mayor John T. Hoffman, a Tammany leader, stated in his first message to the Common Council that the Board of Commissioners of Health, would be "able to accomplish all that may be required of it." He was against a metropolitan bill, and he used the old argument that such a bill would be an interference with the municipal rights of New York.[83] The *Times* retorted that the only branches of the city government managed with honesty were Central Park, the Police Department, and the charities on Blackwell's Island—all created by the state legislature. As for the *Times*, it felt that, "We would prefer to live under a 'Legislative Commission' to dying prematurely and painfully under the pure Democratic rule of a city constituency."[84]

All through January and February the *Times*, and occasionally the *Tribune*, continued to press for a bill. After a complicated fight between the Senate, which passed a bill including the names of four physicians who were to be commissioners, and the Assembly, which wanted to allow the governor to name the members of the board, the whole thing was nearly scuttled once again.[85] Success was finally achieved on February 15. The Assembly passed an amended bill allowing the governor to name the commissioners. With the aid of an impassioned speech by Senator Andrew D. White, using some of the testimony Stephen Smith had presented the previous year, the Conference Committee of the two houses settled their differences and received assurances from Governor Fenton that none of his appointments would be on a political basis.[86] On February 21, 1866, the *Times* felt that the final victory for a health bill was not to be passed over without public notice. The dedicated physicians and philanthropists who, for ten years, had come each winter to Albany received due praise.

The official date of passage was February 26, and the title of the law was "An Act to Create A Metropolitan Sanitary District and Board of Health therein for the Preservation of Life and Health and to Prevent the Spread of Disease."[87]

The law, which in essence had been drafted by Stephen Smith and Dorman B. Eaton the year before, created a health department for the metropolitan area of New York. The new Metropolitan Board of Health, as it was called, was given extremely broad powers to make laws, to carry them out, and to sit in judgment of them, all at the same time. Questions of constitutionality would soon arise.[88]

The general implications of this bill of 1866 are several. It was undoubtedly a major triumph in the history of public health, as noted by Rosen.[89] Locally it served to give a great city the beginning of really effective sanitary government, carried out by professionals. Furthermore, as a major piece of reform legislation it may have been one of the beginning moves against a thread of corruption so strong that it was not broken until the Tweed "Ring" was finally deposed in the early 1870s. The Reverend Samuel Osgood may have had the health bill in mind when he said:

> Careful legislation, with intelligent suffrage and a city government more on the plan of the national, and taking from the Common Council its temptations to base jobs, will set us right, and free us from being subject to the dynasty of dirt and sovereignty of sots.[90]

On a broader scale, the sanitary reform of New York City had several more specific results. In the first place it was the first comprehensive health legislation of its kind in the United States, and later it was to serve as a model for numerous local and state bills. In this respect too the reform movement seems to have united the sanitary interests of numerous physicians and laymen alike. Sanitary science was becoming a specialty in this country, as in Europe. The work in New York also led to the formation of the most important national health group, the American Public Health Association. Stephen Smith, who was one of the prime movers in its founding and its first president, gave credit to his work for the Metropolitan Health Bill and later as a commissioner on the board for providing their inception of the A.P.H.A. in 1872.[91]

Finally, the sanitary reform work in New York also played a role in the changing status or image of the physician and of medicine as a whole. Kramer has noted that before public health could be undertaken, medicine had to put its house in order.[92] But the reverse may have been even more the case: Effective sanitary legislation and the organization of competent health departments played a great part in helping medicine to reestablish the much needed order in the house.

## NOTES

A portion of this paper was presented to The Johns Hopkins Medical History Club, March 14, 1966, and at the Hixon Hour, University of Kansas Medical Center, April 18, 1966. It is part of a larger project, a biographical study of Stephen Smith, in which I am presently engaged. See *Bull. Hist. Med.,* 1965, *39:* 85.

This investigation was supported by U.S. Public Health Service Training Grant number 9T1-LM-105-06.

1   Smith had presented the evidence to the legislative committee on Feb. 13, 1865. It was published in the *New York Times* a month later and was reprinted in Stephen Smith, *The City That Was* (New York: Allaben, 1911), ch. 4. The latter version contained only very minor changes.

2   James Ford, *Slums and Housing, with Special Reference to New York City, History, Conditions, Policy,* 2 vols. (Cambridge, Mass.: Harvard Univ. Press, 1936), I, 17-204. Ford describes many of the early health ordinances. The amount of space he has devoted to sanitary matters is an indication of the close relationship of health and housing. There are a number of other works that deal with health conditions and sanitary laws prior to 1866. A few examples are Susan Wade Peabody, "Historical study of legislation regarding public health in the states of New York and Massachusetts," *J. Infect. Dis.,* 1909, Suppl. No. 4, 156 pp.; Charles F. Bolduan, "Over a century of health administration in New York City," *Department of Health Monograph Series,* No. 13, 1916; John Blake, "Historical study of the development of the New York City Department of Health," typescript, *c.* 1952, 128 pp.; Charles E. Rosenberg, *The Cholera Years: The United States in 1832, 1849, and 1866* (Chicago: Univ. of Chicago Press, 1962); George Rosen, "Public health problems in New York City during the nineteenth century," *N.Y. St. J. Med.,* 1950, *50:* 73-78; and Howard D. Kramer, "Early municipal and state boards of health," *Bull. Hist. Med.,* 1950, *24:* 503-509.

I should also say at the outset that the city did have a health organization during the years prior to the Metropolitan Health Bill of 1866. A history of the department is in the process of being compiled by Professor John Duffy, who will give in great detail what I have perhaps too much simplified in this paper. [Editors' note: Since the original publication of this article, Duffy's book has been published: John Duffy, *A History of Public Health in New York City,* 2 vols. (New York: Russell Sage Foundation, 1968–1974).] It was the "felt reality" of the time, however, according to many physicians, that New York did not indeed have a health department worthy of that name. *Reports, Resolutions, and Proceedings of the Commissioners of Health of the City of New York for the Years 1856–1859* (New York: Clark, 1860), reveals that meetings were frequent, sometimes even daily, but that mostly they dealt with quarantine matters and occasionally with removal of nuisances.

3   David Hosack, "Observations on the means of improving the medical police of the city of New York," in *Essays on Various Subjects of Medical Science,* 2 vols. (New York: Seymour, 1824), II, 9–86.

4   Benjamin W. McCready, *On the Influence of Trades, Professions, and Occupations in the United States, in the Production of Disease,* ed. Genevieve Miller (Baltimore: Johns Hopkins Press, 1943), pp. 41–45.

5   John H. Griscom, *Annual Report of the Interments in the City and County of New York for the Year 1842, with Remarks Therein, And a Brief View of the Sanitary Condition of the City* (New York, 1843). See also Lawrence Veiller, "Tenement house reform in New York City, 1834–1900," in *The Tenement House Problem,* ed. Robert W. DeForest and Lawrence Veiller, 2 vols. (New York: Macmillan, 1903), I, 71–75, in which Veiller has included long quotes from Griscom.

6   Not only were New Yorkers influenced and inspired by the work of the Parisian and London sanitarians, but there were frequent allusions to the mortality rates in these cities, as compared to New York. New York usually fared second best. See also "Health: New York versus London," *Hunt's Merchant's Magazine,* 1863, *48*: 120–124; and "Health of New York, Philadelphia, and Baltimore, for 1860," *Am. Med. Monthly,* 1861, *15*: 312–316. It was especially galling to New Yorkers that the over-all mortality rate of the United States was far lower than that of England (15 per 1000 *v.* 23 per 1000) yet in New York City it was much higher (36 per 1000). See *Report of the Committee on the Incorporation of Cities and Villages, on the bill entitled "An Act concerning the Public Health of the counties of New York, Kings, and Richmond,"* New York State Legislature, Assembly Doc. No. 129, 1860.

7   The problem of tenements and housing reform has been fully dealt with by others. The role of housing in sanitary reform was a central one. See for instance, Ford, *Slums and Housing;* DeForest and Veiller, *The Tenement House Problem;* Gordon Atkins, *Health, Housing, and Poverty in New York City 1865–*

*1898* (Ann Arbor: Edwards, 1947), which includes a good discussion of the sanitary reform of 1866. Roy Lubove, *The Progressives and the Slums* (Pittsburgh: Univ. of Pittsburgh Press, 1962), also deals with the formation of the Metropolitan Board of Health.

8   John H. Griscom, "Improvements of the public health, and the establishment of a sanitary police in the city of New York," *Tr. Med. Soc. St. N.Y.,* 1857, pp. 107–123.

9   *Report of the Select Committee Appointed to Investigate the Health Department of the City of New York,* New York State Legislature, Senate Doc. No. 49, 1859.

10   *Ibid.,* p. 1.

11   *Ibid.,* p. 3.

12   *Ibid.,* p. 52.

13   *Ibid.,* pp. 156–157.

14   *Ibid.,* p. 174.

15   New York State Legislature, Assembly Doc. No. 129, p. 1.

16   Not only was the bill refused, but, to add to the problems of sanitation, the City Inspector was at that time given supervision of street cleaning. As the New York Sanitary Association pointed out later, this was added to his already grossly neglected sanitary duties. *Reports of the Sanitary Association of the City of New York* (New York, 1859), p. 7.

17   See Denis T. Lynch, *"Boss" Tweed, the Story of a Grim Generation* (New York: Boni and Liverwright, 1927), pp. 187–199; Samuel A. Pleasants, *Fernando Wood of New York* (New York: Columbia Univ. Studies in History, Economics and Public Law, No. 536, 1948), ch. 5; James F. Richardson, "Mayor Fernando Wood and the New York Police force, 1855–1857," *N.-Y. Hist. Soc. Quart.,* 1966, *50*: 5–40.

18   Richardson, "Mayor Fernando Wood," p. 6.

19   Those interested in sanitary reform seem to have been well aware of their enemies. Stephen Smith frequently described corrupt practices such as the bribery to which the Tammany-controlled City Inspector's Office allegedly resorted. The 1857 bill had been "effectually defeated by the paid agents of corrupt officials who succeeded, at a late period of the session, in sequestering or destroying all traces of the bill, both manuscript and printed." *Am. Med. Times,* 1860, *1*: 423. It must also be noted that the friends of sanitary reform early realized that a health department with jurisdiction merely over New York, and not including Brooklyn or the other surrounding communities, would have been of little avail. The large interchange of people each day made the metropolitan concept a necessity. See "New York Health Bills," *Am. Med. Times,* 1862, *4*: 70–71. For a brief, general description of New York City government, see Seth Low, *New York in 1850*

*and in 1890* (New York: New-York Historical Society, 1892).

20    N.Y. Sanitary Association, *Report.* Elisha Harris must have been everybody's favorite secretary. He held that job in the Sanitary Association, and later in the Council of Hygiene, the U.S. Sanitary Commission, and the American Public Health Association. See also, Wilson G. Smillie, *Public Health, Its Promise for the Future* (New York: Macmillan, 1955), pp. 289–290.

21    N.Y. Sanitary Association, *Report,* pp. 11–13.

22    *Ibid.,* p. 13.

23    *Second Annual Report of the N.Y. Sanitary Association for the year ending December 1860* (New York, 1860), pp. 1–23.

24    Louis Elsberg's "The domain of medical police," *Am. Med. Monthly,* 1862, *17*: 321–337, was delivered before the Association. This concept of medical police was a prominent idea in the writings of John Griscom too. See George Rosen, "The fate of the concept of medical police 1780–1890," *Centaurus,* 1957, *5*: 97–113. Actually the term "sanitary police" might be more applicable to the goals of the New York sanitarians. According to Shattuck, in the term "medical police," cure of disease is implied; while in the idea of "sanitary police" prevention is stressed. Lemuel Shattuck, *Report of the Sanitary Commission of Massachusetts 1850* (repr.; Cambridge, Mass.: Harvard Univ. Press, 1948).

25    [Robert Tomes], "Why we get sick," *Harper's Monthly,* 1856, *13*: 642–647. The author noted that, "A host of diseases of the heart, the brain, nerves, and stomach, which exhaust the doctor's skill and fill his pockets, came in with modern civilization. To these diseases the Americans are far more subject than any other people . . . ," p. 642.

26    Frank H. Hamilton, "Hygiene," *N.Y. J. Med.,* 1859, *7*: 60–74, p. 60. Hamilton, a renowned surgeon, had been Stephen Smith's teacher and preceptor and remained a close friend in later years.

27    *Ibid.,* p. 63.

28    "Quarantine and Hygiene," *North Am. Rev.,* 1860, *91*: 438–491, p. 491.

29    Although Elisha Harris and George Shrady were assistant editors, I have ascribed the editorials to Smith, throughout. Harris actually resigned in 1861 because of increasing work with the U.S. Sanitary Commission. Shrady apparently did most of the reports of medical society meetings. Furthermore, Smith published many of the editorials in his book *Doctor in Medicine and Other Papers on Professional Subjects* (New York: Wood, 1872), thereby claiming authorship for those included. In various letters to his wife, to be dealt with in a future study, Smith complained of the wearying task of his weekly editorials. In this paper I am concerned only with those editorials that dealt with sanitary reform.

30    *Am. Med. Times,* 1860, *1*: 15. Howard D. Kramer, "The beginnings of the public health movement in the United States," *Bull. Hist. Med.,* 1947, *21*: 352–376, gives Smith and the *American Medical Times* a great deal of credit for bringing about reform, p. 375. Also Kramer, "Early municipal and state boards."

31    "Our sanitary defences," *Am. Med. Times,* 1860, *1*: 46–47.

32    *Ibid.,* p. 100.

33    *Ibid.,* 1861, *2*: 47–48.

34    For a general discussion see Emerson D. Fite, *Social and Industrial Conditions in the North During the Civil War* (New York: Macmillan, 1910), p. 229.

35    I. N. Phelps Stokes, *The Iconography of Manhattan Island,* 6 vols. (New York, 1895–1928), III, 736–756; Milledge L. Bonham, Jr., "New York and the Civil War," in *History of the State of New York,* 10 vols., ed. Alexander C. Flick (New York: Columbia Univ. Press, 1933–1937), VII, 99–135.

36    Allan Nevins, *The Evening Post, A Century of Journalism* (New York: Boni and Liverwright, 1922), p. 364.

37    Fite, *Social and Industrial Conditions,* p. 184. Also Edgar W. Martin, *The Standard of Living in 1860* (Chicago: Univ. of Chicago Press, 1942), contains many useful data.

38    "Health Laws," *Am. Med. Times,* 1860, *1*: 423–424.

39    *Ibid.*

40    "Health of New York in 1860," *Am. Med. Times,* 1861, *2*: 63–64.

41    See *Proceedings of a Select Committee of The Senate . . . Appointed to Investigate Various Departments of the City of New York,* New York State Legislature, Senate Doc. No. 38, Feb. 9, 1865. In this 612-page report, which dealt only with the City Inspector's department, there is a wealth of information. Testimony revealed the buying and selling of jobs and the incompetence of the health wardens. The duties of the 22 wardens and an equal number of assistants were to report nuisances, inspect buildings, privies, and cesspools, report all diseases, and to prevent accumulation of garbage and offal on the streets and sidewalks (p. 345). Several health wardens admitted they did not go personally to see cases of disease. They generally admitted that some smallpox existed and "a few fevers," when in fact smallpox, typhus, typhoid, cholera infantum, and scarlatina were widespread (pp. 455–456). Several of the wardens also admitted that they "devoted" a month's pay—but usually claimed ignorance of the fact it was used to aid defeat of health bills in Albany (pp. 462, 467).

42    *Annual Report of the City Inspector . . . for the Year End-*

*ing December 31, 1860* (New York: Board of Aldermen, Doc. No. 5, 1861), p. 10.

43 *Ibid.,* pp. 16–17.

44 *Ibid.,* pp. 19–22.

45 *Ibid.,* p. 60.

46 *Am. Med. Times,* 1861, *2:* 63.

47 "Sanitary legislation," *Am. Med. Times,* 1862, *4:* 28–29.

48 *Med. & Surg. Reptr.,* 1862, *7:* 349–351.

49 "New York health bills," *Am. Med. Times,* 1862, *4:* 70.

50 "Failure of the health bill," *ibid.,* pp. 250–251.

51 *Med. & Surg. Reptr.,* 1862, *8:* 124–125.

52 "The prospect of health-reform in New York," *Am. Med. Times,* 1862, *5:* 276.

53 *Ibid.,* p. 277.

54 *Harper's Weekly,* 1863, *7:* 786.

55 "Sanitary interests in New York," *Am. Med. Times,* 1863, *6:* 21–22.

56 For a description of the founding of the Citizens' Association, see Edward C. Mack, *Peter Cooper, Citizen of New York* (New York: Duell, Sloan, Pearce, 1949), ch. 19. See also the *New York Citizen,* Aug. 13, 1864.

57 These two letters may be found in *Report of the Council of Hygiene and Public Health of the Citizens' Association of New York, Upon the Sanitary Condition of the City* (New York: Appleton, 1865), pp. ix–xiii.

58 "Citizens' Association and health reform," *Am. Med. Times,* 1864, *8:* 200. Also at the beginning of 1864 there was an investigation into the affairs of the City Inspector's department. Smith published excerpts from a letter written by Thomas N. Carr, who had been superintendent of street cleaning. Carr said that New York simply had no sanitary department worthy of the name. He felt that the only concern the City Inspector had was for the streets. Carr continued: "On an examination of the annual sanitary reports of England or France, the mind is astonished by the vastness of research, investigation, and scientific elaboration which these reports contain, and yet, strange to say, street cleaning, instead of being the all absorbing feature of these documents, is not even mentioned." *Am. Med. Times,* 1864, *8:* 57.

59 Joseph M. Smith, "Report on the medical topography and epidemics of New York," *Tr. A.M.A.,* 1860, *13:* 81–269.

60 In 1865 Smith became the secretary. For the names of the members of the council, see the first part of the introduction to the *Report.*

61 The evidence concerning Smith's role lies mostly within his own writings, especially *The City That Was.* Charles F. Chandler, however, also gave Smith credit for organizing the survey. See *Stephen Smith: Addresses in Recognition of His Public Services on the Occasion of His Eighty-Eighth Birthday* (New York: New York Academy of Medicine, 1911), p. 19, in which Chandler, then an old man himself, noted, "This work was organized and supervised to its completion by Dr. Stephen Smith." In 1864 Joseph M. Smith, the president of the council, was 75 years old. Elisha Harris, the secretary, was mainly occupied by the U.S. Sanitary Commission.

62 *New York Times,* March 16, 1865, or *The City That Was,* p. 57.

63 *Am. Med. Times,* 1864, *8:* 307. The *New York Tribune,* June 3, 1864, had great praise for the efforts of the Citizens' Association.

64 *Am. Med. Times,* 1866, *9:* 47.

65 There is a long discussion of etiological factors in disease in the introductory portion of the *Report,* pp. xlvii–lxviii. See also Richard H. Shryock, "The origins and significance of the public health movement in the United States," *Ann. Med. Hist.,* 1929, *1:* 645–665, especially pp. 650–652; Charles E. Rosenberg, "The cause of cholera: aspects of etiological thought in nineteenth century America," *Bull. Hist. Med.,* 1960, *34:* 331–354, and his *The Cholera Years;* and John Simon, *Filth Diseases and Their Prevention,* 1st Am. ed. (Boston: Campbell, 1876).

66 The *New York Times* on July 7, 1865, said: "No volume of intenser interest has ever seen the light in this city. . . ." See also *Nation,* 1865, *1:* 250; *Am. J. Med. Sci.,* 1865, *100:* 419–428.

67 Brian MacMahon, Thomas F. Pugh, and Johannes Ipsen, *Epidemiologic Methods* (Boston: Little, Brown, 1960), p. 3.

68 Kramer, "Beginnings," pp. 361–362. There were occasional descriptions of living conditions among the poor in the general press. See, for instance, Samuel B. Halliday, *The Lost and Found; or Life Among the Poor* (New York: Blakeman & Mason, 1859). Halliday was a member of the N.Y. Sanitary Association. Soon after the survey of the Citizens' Association was published there was a vivid article in the *Nation* by Bayard Taylor, entitled "A descent into the depths," 1866, *2:* 302–304. Although I have focused attention on the two societies in which Smith played a role, this is not to say that they were the only ones active in sanitary reform at this time. The A.I.C.P. and the various missions and tract societies were also active. The A.I.C.P *Report* for 1853 contains a long discussion of sanitary needs. Its founder and leading spirit, Robert M. Hartley, was well known for his crusade against swill milk. See Roy Lubove, "The New York Association for Improving the Condition of the Poor: the formative years," *N.-Y. Hist. Soc. Quart.,* 1959, *43:* 307–327; and Atkins, *Health, Housing, and Poverty.* Carroll S. Rosenberg's "Protestants and Five Pointers: The Five Points House of Industry, 1850–1870," *N.-Y.*

*Hist. Soc. Quart.*, 1964, *48*: 327–347, describes New York's most notorious slum and efforts toward amelioration. Also Allan Nevins has drawn attention to the reformers in his "The golden thread in the history of New York," *N.-Y. Hist. Soc. Quart.,* 1955, *39*: 5–22.

69    Israel Weinstein, "Eighty years of public health in New York City," *Bull. N.Y. Acad. Med.,* 1947, *23*: 221–237.

70    *Citizens' Association Report,* pp. 261–262.

71    *Ibid.,* p. 285; and *Annual Report of the City Inspector . . . for the Year Ending December 31, 1861* (New York: Board of Aldermen, Doc. no. 4, 1862), pp. 21–23.

72    *Citizens' Association Report,* p. 42.

73    Smith, *City That Was,* p. 46; Andrew Dickson White, *Autobiography,* 2 vols. (New York: Century, 1905), I, 107–110. White reported the oft-quoted testimony of one of the city's health wardens, who, when asked the meaning of the word "hygiene," answered that it referred to bad smells arising from standing water. White also sat on a Senate committee during the investigation of the City Inspector's department early in 1865. Despite the pleas of the Citizens' Association, City Inspector Boole was not dismissed. See Stokes, *Iconography,* V, 1912; and Senate Doc. No. 38, 1865, p. 467. Eaton's testimony was given Feb. 2, 1865, and was published by "Friends of the Bill" later that year. Together with an appendix, his remarks take up 56 printed pages. *Remarks of D. B. Eaton, Esq., at a Joint Meeting of the Committees of the Senate and Assembly* (New York: Nesbitt, 1865).

74    On March 10 and 11, 1865, the *Times* noted that opposition was brewing from quarters formerly friendly to the bill. The paper warned that delay in passage of the bill was dangerous, so late in the session. Smith gave a great deal of credit to Henry J. Raymond, editor of the *Times,* calling him an ardent reformer. *City That Was,* p. 173.

75    That some of the legislators were impressed by the testimony was attested to by at least one member of Smith's audience. After hearing the description of sweatshop conditions in the tenements and of clothing, in the process of manufacture, draped over cribs of children with active smallpox, one of the committee supposedly said to Smith: "Why I bought underwear at one of those stores a few days ago, and I believe I have got smallpox, for I begin to itch all over." *City That Was,* p. 156. It should be stressed that this episode was 46 years in the past when the book was published.

76    Ramsey was a physician but seems to have been completely under Tammany sway. Lewis A. Sayre was the Resident Physician of New York, as well

as a leading teacher of orthopedic surgery. His difference of opinion with the members of the Citizens' Association seems, on the surface, to have been on intellectual grounds. Smith, who was a fellow faculty member of Sayre's at Bellevue, had once called the latter's job (as Resident Physician) a sinecure. *Am. Med. Times,* 1862, *4*: 252. It is, of course, quite possible that Sayre's own vested interests prompted his belief in the status quo. His salary was about $5,000 per year.

77    *New York Times,* March 20, 1865.

78    *New York Tribune,* March 20, 1865.

79    *New York Times,* April 13, 15, 17; *New York Tribune,* April 15. The *Times* on April 17 noted three reasons for the defeat of the bill: Several Union (Republican) members were absent owing to illness; several others were unwilling to create another commission for the Governor; and City Inspector F.I.A. Boole had spent nearly the whole winter in Albany, armed with sufficient funds to kill the bill. This occurred in an Assembly in which the Republicans had a majority of 24. For a discussion of Boole, see Gustavus Myers, *The History of Tammany Hall* (New York: Boni and Liverwright, 1917), pp. 205–208. An informative discussion of the state political situation at this time may be found in Homer A. Stebbins, *A Political History of the State of New York 1865–1869* (New York: Columbia Univ. Studies in History, Economics and Public Law, No. 55, 1913).

80    *New York Times,* Oct. 31, Nov. 9, 1865; *Nation,* 1865, *1*: 609.

81    *Nation,* 1865, *1*: 577.

82    Quoted by Rosenberg, *Cholera Years,* p. 186. See also Smith, *City That Was,* p. 166.

83    The speech is printed in the *New York Times,* Jan. 3, 1866.

84    *Ibid.,* Jan. 7, 1866.

85    *Ibid.,* Feb. 7, 1866.

86    *Ibid.,* Feb. 16, 20, 1866.

87    *Laws of New York, 1866,* Ch. 74 (reprinted by Bergen & Tripp, Printers, 1866).

88    Smith described Eaton's role and his activities in other spheres in chapter 6 of *The City That Was.* This book, incidentally, was dedicated to the memory of Dorman B. Eaton. Eaton was perhaps best known for his work in civil service reform. See Ari Hoogenboom, *Outlawing The Spoils: A History of the Civil Service Reform Movement, 1865–1883* (Urbana: Univ. of Illinois Press, 1961). Eaton was credited by Smith with having written the legal aspects of that bill. Eaton's views can be seen in his "The essential conditions of good sanitary administration," *Reports and Papers, American Public Health Association,* 1874–1875, *2*: 498–514. He was a student of English sanitary law and patterned the New York bill on what he

had learned in England. See Dorman B. Eaton, *Sanitary Regulations in England and New York* (New York: Amerman, 1872). See also Stephen Smith, "Development of American public health endeavor," *Am. J. Public Hlth.*, 1915, *5*: 1115–1119; Stephen Smith, "The origin and organization of the Department of Health of the City of New York," *Med. Rec.*, 1918, *93*: 1115–1117; and his "The history of public health, 1871–1921," in *A Half Century of Public Health*, ed. M. P. Ravenel (New York: A.P.H.A., 1921), pp. 1–12; especially pp. 4–10 deal with the Metropolitan Health Bill.

89  George Rosen, *A History of Public Health* (New York: MD, 1958), p. 247.

90  Samuel Osgood, *New York in the Nineteenth Century* (New York: New-York Historical Society, 1866), pp. 40–41. See also a review of numerous documents of the Citizens' Association, including the *Report of the Council of Hygiene*, by James Parton, "The government of the City of New York," *North Am. Rev.*, 1866, *103*: 413–465. Deserving more work is an analysis of those who were involved in the health reform movement. What were their backgrounds, their motives, and how large a part did they actually play? Also, how was the health reform movement, if indeed one can call it a movement at all, related to other reforms and reformers of the time? Health legislation played an important role in the general amelioration of the urban environment and in the development of cities. This too is an aspect of 19th-century public health that deserves much more study. See particularly Charles N. Glaab, *The American City, A Documentary Study* (Homewood: Dorsey, 1963). Also Arthur M. Schlesinger, "The city in American history," *Miss. Valley Hist. Rev.*, 1940, *27*: 43–66, and Blake McKelvey, *The Urbanization of America 1860–1915* (New Brunswick: Rutgers Univ. Press, 1963).

91  Stephen Smith, "American public health endeavor," p. 1117. Eaton and Elisha Harris were also active in the early work of the A.P.H.A.

92  Kramer, "Beginnings," p. 370.

# 29

## Social Impact of Disease in the Late 19th Century

### JOHN DUFFY

The late 19th century witnessed the bacteriological revolution, without doubt one of the most significant events in the history of medicine. Prior to this, epidemic and endemic diseases were as inexplicable and mysterious to man as they had been to his most primitive forebears. A few empirical discoveries, such as vaccination for smallpox, had led to some improvement in conditions of health, but the origin and transmission of diseases were as obscure as ever. Acrimonious debates characterized medical meetings as late as the 1880s as theory vied with theory, and theorist with theorist. The greatest advance in knowledge of infectious diseases until then had come from the general recognition that such diseases flourished in filthy, overcrowded conditions. This development, for which the medical profession deserved only partial credit, resulted in the movement for sanitation, which began reducing the urban death rate well before bacteriology provided health officials with a sound rationale.

Although the movement for public and personal hygiene was firmly established in the second half of the 19th century, and Pasteur, Koch, and their colleagues were unraveling the tangled skein of bacteriology, communicable diseases still remained the leading health problem. The health records of every city show that tuberculosis, diphtheria, scarlet fever, whooping cough, enteric disorders, measles, smallpox, and even malaria were endemic. Infant mortality—largely attributed to such vague causes as summer fever and diarrhea, teething, colic, and convulsions—was a major component of the high total death rate. The loss of so many children,

JOHN DUFFY is Priscilla Alden Burke Professor Emeritus of History, University of Maryland, College Park, Maryland.

Reprinted with permission from the *Bulletin of the New York Academy of Medicine*, 1971, 47: 797–811.

however, was accepted as the inexorable working of fate.

Smallpox, the one disease for which a fairly effective preventive measure was available, should have created no difficulty, yet it continued to flare up in every American city. A series of outbreaks in New York City during the 1870s caused 805 deaths in 1871, 929 in 1872, 484 in 1874, and 1,280 in 1875.[1] During three of these same years the annual death toll from smallpox in New Orleans was more than 500, and Dr. Joseph Jones, president of the Louisiana State Board of Health, later declared that 6,432 residents of New Orleans had died of smallpox in the years from 1863 to 1883. As late as the winter of 1899–1900, 3 of 12 medical students at Tulane University infected during a widespread outbreak died of the disease.[2]

Compared with other communicable infections such as diphtheria, for which little could be done, smallpox was only a minor cause of death. Diphtheria, a fearful disorder with an equally high fatality rate, was a major epidemic disease throughout most of this period. Earlier, during the 1850s and 1860s, it had been merely one of many children's complaints, but its incidence took a startling upturn in the 1870s. From 1866 to 1872 diphtheria deaths in New York averaged about 325 per year. In 1873 the figure jumped to 1,151, increased to more than 1,600 in 1874, and then reached a new high of 2,329 in 1875. From 1880 to 1896 the annual deaths from diphtheria never fell below 1,000; on three occasions the total was well in excess of 2,000. The peak period for diphtheria in New York City came during the 1890s, the years when throat cultures and antitoxin therapy were introduced. New York's problems with diphtheria were in no sense unique.[3] In New Orleans a health official informed a joint meeting of the city's two medical societies in 1887 that diphtheria had long existed there, but never before had it been "so widespread and abundant as now."[4] By this date diphtheria had spread throughout America, ravaging town and country alike. Since many deaths from diphtheria went unrecorded, and the hundreds of infant deaths attributed to croup and other vague causes undoubtedly included some cases of diphtheria, the actual toll was probably larger than the statistics of mortality show.

The most surprising aspect of diphtheria was that it aroused so little concern. One of the few newspaper editorials about it came after an 1873–1874 epidemic which killed 1,344 people in New York City. On this occasion the editor of the *New York Times* declared: "Had a tithe of the number died from anything resembling cholera or yellow fever we should have had a public scare which would have compelled such a cleaning out of tenements, flushing of sewers, and clearing away of street filth as had not been witnessed for many years."[5] Occasional discussions can be found in medical journals and transactions of societies but these centered chiefly around methods of treatment. The casual public reaction to diphtheria contrasts sharply with the attitude of colonists a century or so earlier. When a virulent form of the disease suddenly burst upon western Europe and the American colonies in the 1730s, it aroused widespread apprehension. By the 1870s, however, diphtheria was a familiar disorder to which the population had become accustomed, and its annual toll among the young had come to be taken as a matter of course. The doctors could do little about it, and the public attitude was one of resignation.

This same fatalistic attitude also characterized the public reaction to scarlet fever, tuberculosis, typhoid, and the other perennial disorders. Dr. Abraham Jacobi, reporting for the Committee on Hygiene of the New York County Medical Society, pointed out that between 1866 and 1890 about 43,000 residents of New York had died of diphtheria and croup and that more than 18,000 had succumbed to scarlet fever. Despite this enormous mortality, the city had made virtually no public provision for the sick. Nine years before, in 1882, he continued, the municipal hospital facilities were so crowded with cases of smallpox, typhus, and typhoid that there had been no room for patients with diphtheria or scarlet fever. Since that time

nothing had been done except to open one hospital with 70 beds. Almost in despair, Dr. Jacobi exclaimed: "Seventy beds, and twenty-five hundred cases are permitted to die annually."[6] Dr. Jacobi's statement takes on added significance when one considers that New York City had one of the best health departments in the United States.

In terms of mortality, two diseases, phthisis, or consumption (tuberculosis of the lungs), and pneumonia, should have caused the greatest outcry. Both, however, were considered "constitutional" diseases, and their very frequence dispelled the fears one might expect to be associated with them. In 1870 tuberculosis of the lungs was responsible for about 4,000 deaths in New York City; this figure rose steadily in the ensuing years until about 1890, when almost 5,500 deaths were reported. Deaths from pneumonia rose even more sharply — from 1,836 in 1870 to 6,487 in 1893. Despite their enormous death toll, these familiar and chronic complaints lacked the drama of the great pestilences, and they went largely unnoticed by the general public.[7]

Although most of these statistics have been drawn from New York and New Orleans, the conditions that they reflect prevailed in all major American cities. New Orleans and other southern urban areas differed from the North only with respect to malaria and yellow fever. As in the North, tuberculosis and the respiratory diseases were the number one killers, while diphtheria, scarlet fever, smallpox, measles, and other disorders contributed to the general mortality.

Although gradually receding southward, malaria was a major problem in the United States throughout the 19th century. In New York City 457 deaths were attributed to malaria during 1881, and it was 1895 before the city's annual number of deaths from the disease fell below 100.[8] In terms of total mortality, malaria was of little significance to New York and most northern cities, but it was a major factor in the South. In 1888 Dr. Stanford Chaillé surveyed the causes of death in New Orleans and concluded that tuberculosis, malaria, and dysentery were the chief culprits. Bearing out Dr. Chaillé's statement, the records of the New Orleans Charity Hospital for 1883 show that 45 percent of the 8,000 patients admitted were treated for malaria. But malaria, too, was an old and familiar complaint, and in those areas where it was endemic its recurrence each spring and fall was accepted almost as inevitably as the seasonal cycle itself.[9]

In sharp contrast to this casual acceptance of the diseases mentioned thus far was the public reaction to Asiatic cholera and yellow fever. Although both disorders had reached their peak in the 1850s and henceforth were only a minor cause of morbidity and mortality, they dominated newspaper stories relating to health, preoccupied a good share of the time of the medical profession, and were important factors in promoting public health measures. Had either disease gained a permanent foothold in the United States, it might well have been among the ranking causes of mortality and morbidity, but at the same time it would have become familiar and in the process would have lost its capacity to inspire terror. As it was, outbreaks of cholera in any part of the world or the appearance of a case of cholera or yellow fever in quarantine was enough to arouse the newspapers, medical societies, and civic authorities in every American port.

Of the two diseases, yellow fever had a much longer history in the United States. It first appeared in the late 17th century in Boston and then plagued every American port from Boston southward until the beginning of the 19th century. After a series of major epidemics from 1793 to 1805, the northeastern section of the United States was virtually free of the disease. Attacks on the South Atlantic and Gulf Coast areas, however, intensified in the first half of the 19th century and reached their peak in the 1850s. The number and intensity of the outbreaks, with one or two exceptions, tapered off sharply after the Civil War, although the disease continued to be a real threat to every southern port.[10]

Yellow fever is a fatal and frightening disease; its attacks on the cities of the eastern seaboard from 1793 to 1805 left a vivid imprint upon the public mind. Throughout the remainder of the century, memories of this pestilence were constantly revived by grim accounts of the recurrent outbreaks in southern ports. Moreover, the disease was endemic in the West Indies, and it was a rare summer when one or more cases were not discovered by northern quarantine officials. In 1856 lax enforcement of quarantine laws resulted in more than 500 cases of yellow fever on Staten Island and the western end of Long Island. The New York City quarantine station was located on Staten Island at this time, and outraged local residents barricaded all entrances to it. When the New York authorities responded in 1857 by buying a new site several miles away, an armed mob vandalized the buildings. The following summer, when additional yellow fever patients were landed, another mob burned the quarantine hospital to the ground. Determined opposition by local citizens at all proposed new sites forced the quarantine officials to buy an old steamer to use as a floating hospital for yellow fever.[11] Although the fever never gained a foothold in Manhattan, every summer New York newspapers carried stories of its ravages in the South, and they rarely failed to editorialize upon its danger whenever cases were reported on incoming vessels.

In southern ports it was not necessary to revive old memories, since most residents had experienced close contact with the disease. In 1866–1867 the fever struck coastal towns from Wilmington and New Bern in North Carolina all the way to Brownsville, Texas. Desultory attacks continued until 1878, when the disease was once again widespread. On this occasion it traveled up the Mississippi Valley as far as St. Louis, Chattanooga, and Louisville. Aside from a major outbreak in Florida during 1888, only scattered cases were reported until 1897–1899 and 1905, when minor epidemics occurred in New Orleans and the surrounding areas. The 1878 outbreak, by far the most severe in the postwar years, resulted in 27,000 cases and over 4,000 deaths in New Orleans and wiped out almost 10 percent of the populations of Memphis and Vicksburg.[12]

Considering these statistics, it is not to be wondered that rumors of yellow jack or the "saffron scourge," as it was sometimes called in New Orleans, was enough to cause panic. When a reported outbreak of yellow fever in Ocean Springs, Mississippi, in 1897 led the New Orleans Board of Health to proclaim a quarantine against all Gulf Coast towns, a panic-stricken mob of New Orleans residents vacationing in one of the resorts seized control of a train and brought it to the Louisiana state line. Here the train was held up until the health officials, recognizing the hungry and desperate condition of the passengers, reluctantly permitted them to enter New Orleans. This act of mercy by the Board of Health was assailed bitterly and was a factor in the subsequent resignation of the entire board. [13]

When the disease appeared in New Orleans, the mayor arranged for one of the schools to be used as a temporary yellow fever hospital. The following night an armed mob, objecting to the presence of a hospital in their neighborhood, set fire to the building. When firemen arrived, onlookers cut the hoses, precipitating a fight between the mob and the firemen and policemen. Even as late as 1905 the reaction to the presence of yellow fever was one of profound shock. The president of the local medical society in New Orleans wrote: "When the first knowledge reached our city of the presence of this dread disease in our midst, there was almost a panic — stocks and bonds went begging, a pall seemed to be thrown on all things, a general exodus of those who could afford it took place, and the commercial interests seem paralyzed."[14]

Asiatic cholera, the most feared of all diseases in the 19th century, arrived in the western world as a by-product of the industrial revolution. Because of its short incubation period and rapid course, the disease was restricted to the Far East almost until the advent of steam power and rapid transportation. At the same time, industrialism brought massive urbanization with all its concomitant problems: crowded slums, limited and contaminated water supplies, hopelessly ineffectual methods for eliminating sewage and garbage, and city governments ill-equipped to deal with the explosive growth of population. Thus the industrial revolution provided both the rapid transportation necessary for spreading the disease and seed beds where it could flourish in the crowded cities.

Improvements in communication contributed further to enhancing the role played by cholera, for no disease in American history was so widely heralded at its first appearance (1832). The introduction of cheap newspapers and journals had made it possible for the American public to follow the disastrous course of this pestilence as it advanced through Russia, eastern Europe, and pushed northwestward to the Atlantic. The accounts of its destructive progress built up growing apprehensions which were intensified by urgent warnings from health authorities and medical societies that the filthy state of American communities had already set the stage for explosive outbursts of disease. Cholera struck the United States first in 1832 and returned in 1848–1849. On both occasions it swept through cities and towns within a few weeks, killing thousands. In 1866 and 1873 the disease again threatened, but prompt sanitary measures limited its effect. Without knowing precisely why, health authorities recognized that the infection was spread through the feces of infected persons, and they resorted successfully to disinfecting procedures.[15]

Unlike yellow fever, which periodically demonstrated the reality of its threat, Asiatic cholera was never more than a potential danger in the years which followed the Civil War, yet it received an inordinate amount of attention from newspapers and journals in all sections of the United States. Most of the civic cleanups and sanitary campaigns were sparked by what was considered to be the imminent danger from this disease. It shared with yellow fever the capacity for creating panic and brutalizing decent citizens. Victims of Asiatic cholera were often dumped ashore by crews and passengers of river boats, much to the dismay of local residents, who occasionally left them there to die. When the disease appeared in Pittsburgh in 1849 and the Sisters of Mercy opened their hospital to its victims, meetings were held by indignant neighborhood residents and local newspaper correspondents attacked the sisters bitterly. In nearby Allegheny the same situation held true for the Reverend Passavant when he, too, offered help to cholera patients.[16]

The reaction of Americans to a threatened cholera outbreak in 1873 shows how the apprehensions aroused by earlier epidemics carried over into the postwar years. As the disease began spreading into Europe, the newspapers were filled with cholera stories, and the *New York Times* editorialized on "cholera panics." The editor of a medical journal declared that in the United States cholera was the "all-absorbing topic." Responding to demands from newspapers and medical societies, the New York City Health Department promptly began a major effort to alleviate the worst sanitary conditions within the city.[17]

A few years later, when cholera broke out in Toulon and Marseilles, American newspapers once again carried daily front-page reports of the disease. In July 1884 President Chester Arthur reflected national concern by issuing a proclamation warning state officials to be on guard. Throughout the following winter cholera continued to pre-occupy public attention. In January a group of New York businessmen organized the Sanitary Protective Society to mobilize all existing health agencies within the city. As the public clamor for action increased, the city board of health secured a special appropriation of $50,000. When the expected epidemic did not materialize, the board was given permission to retain the fund for future use. The following year Asiatic cholera was reported in Italy, and President S. Grover Cleveland was requested to prohibit all Italian immigration until the danger was over.[18]

The last major cholera scare came in 1892. Once again a state of alarm characterized the entire American seaboard. Daily front-page stories reported enormous casualties in Russia and hinted of comparable figures in western European cities. Municipal authorities, collaborating with health officials, initiated massive sanitary campaigns, checked on food and water supplies, and made preparations for the expected assault. In New York the city health department retained its summer corps of 50 physicians on an emergency basis; the St. John's Guild lent its "floating hospital" for the use of cholera cases; J. P. Morgan offered the use of a steamship to house cabin passengers from immigrant vessels during the quarantine period; and the directors of St. Mark's Hospital organized a volunteer medical and nursing corps. On the national scene President Benjamin Harrison responded to the crisis by ordering all immigrant vessels to perform a minimum 20-day quarantine. To facilitate the procedure of quarantine, the state of New York leased buildings on Fire Island for the use of healthy cabin passengers during the quarantine period. On hearing this news, the local board of health promptly deputized all citizens and prepared to resist. An armed mob lined the pier, and it was not until the governor mobilized the National Guard that the mob dispersed and passengers were able to land without being molested.[19]

Since most societies tend to operate on a crisis basis, the diseases which were most effective in precipitating social change were those with the greatest shock value. In this category it is clear that Asiatic cholera and yellow fever stood by themselves, with smallpox a poor third, and the other disorders ranking well behind. The outbreaks of

yellow fever which struck the eastern seaboard from 1793 to 1795 had the immediate effect of bringing into existence temporary boards of health, which had surprisingly wide powers. In New York City, for example, the Board of Health was given the authority and funds to evacuate large sections of the city and to provide food, housing, and medical care for the poor. A permanent result of these outbreaks was the creation of the office of City Inspector, a forerunner of New York's health department. Throughout the century yellow fever scares continued to give impetus to health reform. The outbreaks in the 1850s in New Orleans and the southern states had repercussions in every eastern port and greatly strengthened the position of reformers fighting for permanent boards of health.

In the southern states, which bore the brunt of the attacks in the 19th century, yellow fever provided the chief stimulus to health reform. Two major epidemics in Louisiana in 1853 and 1854, the first of which killed almost 9,000 residents of New Orleans and the second another 2,500, were directly responsible for the creation of the Louisiana State Board of Health, the first such agency in the United States.[20] Successive epidemics strengthened this board until 1897, when the consternation aroused by the reappearance of yellow fever after an absence of several years forced the members of the board to resign and led to a reorganization of the state board and the establishment of a separate board of health for New Orleans. In 1878 the disastrous outbreak, which affected almost every major town on the South Atlantic and Gulf coasts and spread far up the Mississippi Valley, aroused the entire nation. In Memphis, a city which had not recovered from the Civil War, the loss of 3,500 residents to yellow fever brought a major social and political upheaval.[21] On the national scene, Congress reacted by passing the first national quarantine act. As the full impact of the 1878 epidemic was felt, health reformers were able to secure from Congress a second measure creating the National Board of Health. Neither of these laws proved effective; the quarantine law was weak, and the National Board of Health, after a stormy existence, virtually disappeared in 1883 when Congress eliminated its appropriation. Nonetheless, during its brief lifetime the National Board of Health did help to arouse a public health consciousness, and it paved the way for the creation of the United States Public Health Service a few years later.

Asiatic cholera, because it constituted a threat to all areas, was possibly even more significant than yellow fever. The first two waves of this disorder, 1832–1835 and 1848–1855, struck at the coastal cities and then followed the unexcelled waterways of North America. In their wake they left not only a trail of death and suffering but also a host of temporary health boards. During the first attack on Pittsburgh, for example, a ten-man sanitary board was appointed and given an appropriation of $10,000. The following year the funds were reduced to $6,000 and, as the threat of cholera receded, the board disappeared and the funds for sanitation were virtually eliminated from the municipal budget.[22] The second wave of Asiatic cholera at the mid-century coincided with the emerging sanitary movement and the peak years of yellow fever. The two diseases were largely responsible for the organization of the National Sanitary Conventions which met from 1856 to 1860. These gatherings of state and municipal health officials and representatives of medical societies were the first attempts to devise national quarantine and public health programs, and they helped lay the basis for the subsequent establishment of the American Public Health Association.

The second and third waves of Asiatic cholera played a significant role in the establishment of the Health Department of New York City. More than 5,000 New Yorkers died of cholera during 1849 and several hundred more died of it in 1854. Since sanitationists argued that cholera was the product of crowding, and the filth-and-quarantine faction believed that it was a specific communicable disease which could be kept out of the city, cholera supplied both factions in the health movement with ammunition in their effort to obtain a permanent health agency for the city. In the years following the cholera outbreaks of 1849–1854, campaigns to educate the public gradually gained momentum. Several health bills for New York City were introduced into the state legislature during the early 1860s but they all failed. At this stage the third epidemic wave of Asiatic cholera appeared, and its threat in the winter of 1865–66 led to the passage of a Metropolitan Board of Health Act for New York City. The first problem confronting the Metropolitan Board was to deal with the imminent

danger from cholera. An energetic sanitary campaign combined with rigid isolation, quarantine, and disinfection measures kept the number of cases to a minimum. This 1866 attack on the United States was relatively mild and probably would have had a minor effect on New York City. New Yorkers, remembering the 5,000 deaths a few years earlier, gave full credit to the Metropolitan Board of Health. This auspicious start left a residue of good will which resulted in strong public support for the health department for many years.[23]

Repeated cholera scares continued to remind New York officials and the general public of the need for a strong health department, but it was not until 1892 that the disorder again made a permanent impact on the city. The widespread alarm touched off by cholera in that year has already been mentioned. For several years prior to it Drs. Hermann M. Biggs and T. Mitchell Prudden had been advocating the establishment of a bacteriological laboratory. Capitalizing on the general apprehension, Dr. Biggs won his point with the city Board of Estimate, and, in September 1892, New York City established the first laboratory to be used for the routine diagnosis of disease.

Possibly more important than the direct effect of epidemic diseases upon social and political reform was their indirect impact. The middle and upper classes sought to insulate themselves from the deplorable condition of the working class, but for those members who encountered the appalling infant mortality and the ravages of disease among the lower economic groups the experience was often traumatic. Moreover, as conditions in the urban slums worsened, the diseases of the poor could not be contained, and public health became a matter of concern for all the people.

Members of the medical profession were among the first to encounter the disease and misery of the poor. It was recognized that clinics and dispensaries catering to the poor were essential to medical training and research, and young physicians and surgeons were thrown into direct contact with the realities of poverty. Not surprisingly, in America physicians were among the leading advocates of public health. More significantly, since the integral relation between poverty and disease was all too obvious, they were also among the leaders of social reform.

During the terrible epidemics of Asiatic cholera and yellow fever, volunteer groups of all sorts came in contact with dire poverty, and many individuals seeking to help the deserving poor gradually came to realize that even the undeserving poor were the product of their brutalizing environment. In the South a notable example of the volunteer groups was the Howard Association, named after John Howard, the famous English reformer. Originating in New Orleans during a yellow fever epidemic in 1837, its program gradually spread to other southern cities and towns. The members were young businessmen who volunteered their services during major epidemics. The Howards, as they were called, organized massive relief programs to provide medical care for the sick poor and housing and food for their families. The willingness of these men to volunteer for work with the Howard Association evidences some degree of social conscience, but their intimate contact with poverty created a new awareness of social needs.

As far back as the 16th century it had been argued that a country's population was a major form of wealth. By the mid-19th century demography was emerging as a science, and improvements in the collection of vital statistics began to reveal the high morbidity and mortality rates in urban areas. One of the major arguments used by health and social reformers was the economic cost of sickness and death. Estimating the productivity per adult worker, they calculated the loss of productivity caused by the many deaths and added to it the cost of medical care for the sick. The validity of this argument was demonstrated clearly by the repeated epidemics of yellow fever which effectively closed down southern cities, and brought all economic activities to a halt. Throughout the 19th century most physicians and laymen believed that epidemic diseases were either propagated or nurtured in conditions of dirt and overcrowding. This environmental concept led to an assault on the atrocious tenement conditions, nuisance trades, deplorable working conditions, and other abuses.

Late in the century the bacteriological revolution turned the medical profession away from environmentalism and focused its attention upon pathogenic organisms. The germ theory had the beneficent effect of awakening the upper classes to the realization that bacteria were no respecters of economic or social position and that a man's health

was dependent to some extent on the health of his fellowmen. The knowledge that the diseases of the workers who sewed clothes in their filthy tenement homes or who processed food could be spread to decent, clean, and respectable citizens served as a powerful incentive to the reform of public health. Since public health could not be separated from social conditions, the net result was an attack on poverty.

The best evidence that a concern for public health underlay much of the effort for social reform is to be found in the multiplicity of volunteer sanitary associations which sprang up in the late 19th century. In every city private groups worked to establish or improve water and sewerage systems, to clean streets, to provide pure milk for the infant poor, to remedy abuses in municipal hospitals and other institutions, and to establish dispensaries, clinics, and hospitals. Examples of these groups in New York City were the Association for Improving the Condition of the Poor, the New York Sanitary Reform Society, the Ladies Health Protective Association, the St. John's Guild, the Sanitary Protective League, the Sanitary Aid Society, and the New York Society for the Prevention of Contagious Diseases. Of the many voluntary organizations operating in New York during this period, some sought only one immediate objective and disbanded after a brief existence, others created organizations that survived for many years. What they all shared in common was the belief that a healthy population was basic to a sound society.

In glancing back over the 19th century one can safely conclude that the rapid expansion of urban areas provided fertile grounds for communicable diseases, and that these diseases were both a cause and effect of the desperate poverty which characterized so many of the cities. At the same time the frightening sickness and death rates drew attention to the deplorable condition of the poor. Dramatic outbreaks of yellow fever and cholera profoundly stirred public opinion and directly and indirectly contributed to the growth of public health institutions. Meanwhile statistical evidence was developing which showed an even heavier toll from chronic and endemic disorders. The net effect, as shown by even the most cursory reading of late-19th-century newspapers, was that public health and sanitary reform became major public issues. And for nearly all social reformers, whether their concern was with infant welfare, tenement conditions, or even political reform, the elimination of sickness and disease became a major aim.

## NOTES

1   See the *Annual Report of the New York City Health Department, 1871–75* (the title varies, sometimes designated as the *Annual Report of the Board of Health . . .*).

2   *The Rudolph Matas History of Medicine in Louisiana,* ed. J. Duffy, 2 vols. (Baton Rouge, 1958), II, 438, 442–443.

3   *Annual Report N.Y.C. Health Dept., 1866–1896.*

4   *New Orleans Med. & Surg. J.,* 1887–1888, *15:* 470–474.

5   *New York Times,* July 14, 1874.

6   A. Jacobi, "The unsanitary condition of the primary schools of the City of New York," *Sanitarian,* 1892, *28:* 331–324.

7   *Annual Report N.Y.C. Health Dept. 1870–1893.*

8   *Ibid.*

9   S. E. Chaillé, "Life and death rates; New Orleans and other cities compared," *New Orleans Med. & Surg. J.,* 1888–1889, *16:* 85–100. *Ibid.,* 1884–1885, *12:* 716–717.

10   J. Duffy, "Yellow fever in the continental United States during the nineteenth century," *Bull. N.Y. Acad. Med.,* 1968, *54:* 687–701.

11   J. Duffy, *A History of Public Health in New York City, 1625–1866* (New York, 1968), pp. 101–123, 440–460.

12   Duffy, "Yellow fever in the continental United States," pp. 639–696.

13   *The Rudolph Matas History of Medicine in Louisiana,* ed. Duffy, II, 430.

14   G. Augustin, *History of Yellow Fever* (New Orleans, 1909), pp. 1061–1062.

15   For an excellent account, see C. E. Rosenberg, *The Cholera Years: The United States in 1832, 1849 and 1866* (Chicago, 1962).

16   J. Duffy, "The impact of Asiatic cholera on Pittsburgh, Wheeling, and Charleston," *Western Penn. Hist. Mag.,* 1964, *58:* 199–211.

17   *Sanitarian,* 1873, *1:* 228–229.

18   This material was taken from chapter 7 of the author's second volume on the public health history of New York City: *A History of Public Health in New York City, 1866–1966* (New York, 1974).

19   *Ibid.*

20   J. Duffy, *Sword of Pestilence: The New Orleans Yellow Fever Epidemic of 1853* (Baton Rouge, 1966), pp. 139, 167.

21   J. H. Ellis, "Memphis' sanitary revolution, 1880–1890," *Tenn. Hist. Quart.,* 1964, *23:* 59–72.

22   Duffy, "Impact of Asiatic cholera on Pittsburgh, Wheeling, and Charleston," pp. 202–203.

23   Duffy, *History of Public Health in New York City, 1625–1866,* pp. 441–446.

# 30

## The Decline in Mortality in Philadelphia
## from 1870 to 1930: The Role of Municipal Services

GRETCHEN A. CONDRAN, HENRY WILLIAMS, AND ROSE A. CHENEY

The Christmas season of 1880 should have been a happy occasion for Charles and Caroline Kautz. Charles, a German immigrant in his mid-40s, had operated a three-person bakery in the Moyamensing section of Philadelphia over a decade. Caroline, several years his junior and his wife of over 15 years, had married him during her teens and soon assumed the responsibilities of parenthood. Though Pennsylvania born, Caroline also came from German stock and, with her husband, worshiped at a local German Lutheran church. Caroline and Charles Kautz and their three sons and three daughters must have eagerly anticipated a joyous holiday celebration.

But it was not their fate to enjoy this Christmas. In 3½ weeks from late November to mid-December, smallpox took the lives of five of the six Kautz children. Six-year-old Clara died on November 20, followed by Albert (aged 2) two weeks later, then Edward (aged 4) on December 10, Charles (aged 8) on December 11, and Bertha (aged 10) on December 14. Only 12-year-old Sophia survived. Burial in the Lutheran church cemetery followed each of the deaths in numbing succession.

GRETCHEN A. CONDRAN is Research Associate Professor in the Population Studies Center at the University of Pennsylvania, Philadelphia, Pennsylvania.
HENRY WILLIAMS is Associate Director of the Philadelphia Social History Project at the University of Pennsylvania, Philadelphia, Pennsylvania.
ROSE CHENEY is Statistician/Demographer at the Philadelphia Health Management Corporation and a doctoral candidate in the Population Studies Center at the University of Pennsylvania, Philadelphia, Pennsylvania.

Reprinted with permission from *The Pennsylvania Magazine of History and Biography,* Medical Philadelphia Issue, April 1984, *108*: 153–177.

The tragedies that befell the Kautzes over a century ago illustrate in a concrete way part of the enormous gap separating the 20th and the 19th centuries in America. Epidemic diseases, childhood death, and low adult life expectancies dominated life. Indeed, in the space of a decade, the Kautzes had witnessed smallpox epidemics in Philadelphia in 1871–1872 and 1876 prior to the 1880–1881 epidemic that devastated their family. The difference between the two centuries is often measured in terms of the rapid diffusion of communications, transportation, and machine technologies throughout our society. These forces, without doubt, make our lives much different. But they are no more important to us than the lengthening of adult life and the elimination both of frequent early death and the constant anticipation of epidemic disease. Recurrent smallpox epidemics, for example, which in Philadelphia alone took 4,464 lives in 1871 and 1872 and 1,760 lives in 1880 and 1881, seem to be remnants of a distant past.[1] Illnesses that rarely confront us today were frequently present only a century ago.[2]

Yet, as significant as the reduction in mortality has been, scholars still search for the reasons for the "mortality transition." Rising personal income, improved diet, better sanitation and personal hygiene, public health activities, advancing medical technology are offered as competing, complementary, or interacting explanations.[3] How any or all of these factors affect the propensity for a disease to be present in the environment (exposure), or for a given population to avoid infection from a disease which is present (resistance), or for survival when individuals contract a disease (case survival) is also open to considerable debate.

Although the origins and sources of the mortality transition are not fully understood, scholars have developed a commonly accepted portrait of the change. It occurred during the 19th and early 20th centuries in most of Europe, the United States, Canada, Australia, and New Zealand. In American cities, for example, mortality levels were high at the beginning of the 19th century and remained high for most of the century. Although mortality rates for some age groups and from some diseases (e.g., cholera and typhus) began declining earlier, a substantial and sustained decline in overall mortality levels did not begin until late in the 19th century.[4]

The changes in mortality rates in Philadelphia closely paralleled in both timing and magnitude those in other large cities of the United States and in urban areas in other industrializing nations.[5] These trends can be traced fairly well after 1860 when the official registration of deaths with the issuance of a death certificate began. The deaths were aggregated and published in annual reports of the Board of Health and included in the mayor's yearly report. The published data provide a classification of the deaths by age and cause for the total population of the city. In addition, deaths by cause are published for the wards within the city.

Using an average of these registration data for three years surrounding each federal decennial census date from 1870 to 1930 and base population figures from the decennial censuses, one can observe the pattern of mortality change.[6] The description of changing mortality is expressed in two ways: as the probability that an individual in a particular age group will die during a given five-year age period and as the expectation of life at selected ages. For each year, the expectation of life for a given age is the average number of years that would be lived by a hypothetical group of persons who reached that age in the year and who were subjected to that year's probabilities of dying at each subsequent age.

The magnitude of the overall mortality decline in Philadelphia is apparent for all age groups (see Table 1). In 1870, for example, about 175 of every 1,000 children born never survived to their first birthday. By 1930, fewer than 75 of every 1,000 infants perished during the first year of life — a decline of about 175 percent in the probability of dying.

Table 1
Life Table Probabilities of Dying ($q_x$ x 1000) and Expectations of Life at Selected Ages, Philadelphia, 1870 to 1930

| Age | 1870 | 1880 | 1890 | 1900 | 1910 | 1920 | 1930 |
|---|---|---|---|---|---|---|---|
| *Probability of Dying ($q_x$ x 1000)* | | | | | | | |
| 0–1* | 174.0 | 159.7 | 152.9 | 136.5 | 119.7 | 95.5 | 74.9 |
| 1–5 | 141.9 | 120.6 | 111.1 | 89.3 | 68.5 | 40.8 | 23.1 |
| 5–10 | 41.9 | 37.8 | 36.8 | 28.3 | 19.8 | 17.6 | 10.9 |
| 10–15 | 19.8 | 19.2 | 17.0 | 16.9 | 11.9 | 11.2 | 7.7 |
| 15–20 | 32.9 | 30.0 | 28.7 | 31.2 | 21.6 | 17.9 | 12.5 |
| 20–30 | 114.2 | 97.8 | 82.3 | 71.7 | 55.7 | 53.8 | 19.2 |
| 30–40 | 117.9 | 109.7 | 96.3 | 95.6 | 84.5 | 68.8 | 28.8 |
| 40–50 | 133.7 | 131.9 | 127.3 | 127.2 | 117.1 | 98.4 | 50.4 |
| 50–60 | 194.5 | 183.5 | 190.9 | 198.2 | 194.4 | 169.7 | 99.6 |
| 60–70 | 319.7 | 303.0 | 326.5 | 350.5 | 354.7 | 314.9 | 182.9 |
| *Expectation of Life* | | | | | | | |
| $e_0$ | 39.6 | 42.3 | 43.7 | 45.8 | 49.6 | 54.4 | 57.9 |
| $e_1$ | 46.8 | 49.3 | 50.5 | 52.0 | 55.4 | 59.1 | 61.5 |
| $e_5$ | 50.4 | 51.8 | 52.6 | 52.9 | 55.3 | 57.6 | 58.9 |
| $e_{20}$ | 39.8 | 41.0 | 41.6 | 41.6 | 43.0 | 45.0 | 45.6 |

*Estimated by fitting Coale and Demeny South Model Life tables to $_4q_1$.
Source: Gretchen A. Condran and Rose A. Cheney, "Mortality Trends in Philadelphia: Age- and Cause-Specific Death Rates 1870–1930," *Demography*, 1982, *9* (No. 1): 100.

Indeed, the late 19th century was still a difficult time for all children. Over a third of all infants born in 1870 died before they were ten. Sixty years later, about a tenth did not survive to that age, a substantial improvement in life chances. Young adults also suffered from a harsh mortality regime in 1870—114 of every 1,000 individuals reaching age 20 never lived to age 30—but by 1930 fewer than 20 of 1,000 20-year-olds died within ten years. The elderly also enjoyed a moderation in their mortality rates. In 1870, about 320 of every 1,000 individuals reaching 60 years of age died within the next decade; by 1930, the corresponding figure was 183.

The declines in infant mortality were particularly important for raising life expectancies between 1870 and 1930. At birth in 1870 an individual could expect on average to reach age 40; by 1930, an infant could expect to reach age 58—an increase in life expectancy of about 46 percent. The impact of the mortality transition, however, was not as substantial for those who could survive their childhood and adolescent years. In 1870, for example, individuals who made it to age 20 could on average expect to see age 60; by 1930, the group of young adults might expect to celebrate their 66th birthday—an increase of life expectancy of but 15 percent. Clearly, the major consequence of the transition was to increase the numbers who survived infancy and childhood. Those who had already reached adulthood gained fewer additional years of life.

Although mortality rates declined for each age group between 1870 and 1930, the timing of the reduction differed by group (see Table 1). Childhood and infant mortality levels declined throughout each of the six decades, but the declines were uneven. The expectation of life at birth and at age one in Philadelphia rose almost three years between 1870 and 1880, but increased at a slower rate between 1880 and 1900. After 1900, the rate of improvement in mortality levels increased again.

On the other hand, substantial declines in adult mortality did not occur in Philadelphia until after the turn of the century, except for 20-to-29-year-olds. This group exhibited the highest rates of death from tuberculosis, and declines in its overall death rates occurred steadily from 1870 to 1930, largely because the deaths from tuberculosis were declining. In contrast to the other groups, the elderly actually exhibited rising mortality rates until the 1910–1920 decade, but then a precipitous drop to 1930.

Cause-of-death data provide the first clues to the explanation of these trends and age-group differentials, but these data must be used with caution. A correct assessment of the levels of a disease in a population is dependent upon the consistency of classification schemes and reporting procedures over time. In Philadelphia, data are available from 1870 to 1930 but are not of uniform quality for the entire period. Between 1870 and 1900, the number of causes of death reported by the Bureau of Health steadily increased. Much of the increase resulted from changes in diagnostic ability and the replacement of general cause-of-death categories with more specific descriptions of the sources of mortality. In 1904, the Bureau of Health began to group individual causes into broader nosological headings.[7]

Thirteen causes of death can be followed with reasonable certainty from 1870 to 1930. Although these infectious diseases represent but a minority of all causes of death reported in Philadelphia, they account for 45 percent of all deaths occurring in 1870, about 40 percent of those in 1900, and about 24 percent of those in 1930. As we will see, these declining proportions indicate that increasing control of infectious disease played a significant role in the overall mortality decline. Even for these selected causes of death, however, causes for which diagnosis was probably very accurate throughout the period must be separated from those in which trends may be obscured by changes in diagnosis over time (see Table 2). The mortality rates for each disease are standardized on the age distribution of Philadelphia's population in 1870 and, therefore, the rates for each cause are those which would have occurred if the age distribution of Philadelphia's population had not changed in the time period.

The group of infectious diseases for which diagnosis was very good showed a spectacular decline over the period. In 1870, about 600 of every 100,000 Philadelphians died from these causes; 60 years later fewer than 80 did. Scarlet fever, smallpox, typhoid, and diphtheria, all major killers in 1870, were virtually eliminated as causes of death by 1930. The timing in declines differed by specific disease, however. Most of the individual disease categories declined between 1870 and 1900 and

Table 2
Percent Contribution of Causes of Death to
Overall Decline in Age-Standardized Death Rates
Philadelphia, 1870, 1900, and 1930

| Causes of Death | Percent Decline Explained by Cause* | | |
|---|---|---|---|
| | 1870–1930 | 1870–1900 | 1900–1930 |
| Infectious — | | | |
| specific diagnosis | 52.1 | 64.7 | 44.5 |
| Diphtheria and croup | 5.4 | − 5.1 | 11.8 |
| Erysipelas | 0.5 | 0.8 | 0.3 |
| Malaria | 0.4 | 0.8 | 0.3 |
| Measles | 0.7 | 0.8 | 0.6 |
| Scarlet fever | 8.8 | 18.5 | 2.8 |
| Smallpox | 8.5 | 21.5 | 0.6 |
| Tuberculosis | 22.5 | 26.8 | 19.8 |
| Typhoid | 4.6 | 1.1 | 6.8 |
| Whooping cough | 0.7 | − 0.6 | 1.5 |
| Primarily Infectious — | | | |
| diagnosis less specific | 14.1 | − 1.3 | 23.5 |
| Diarrheal diseases | 16.4 | 19.8 | 14.3 |
| Epidemic meningitis | 0.0 | 0.1 | 0.0 |
| Influenza | − 1.5 | − 2.8 | − 0.7 |
| Pneumonia | − 0.8 | −18.4 | 10.0 |
| Residual | 33.7 | 36.6 | 32.0 |

*The percent decline was calculated using 1900 and 1930
   death rates standardized on the age distribution of
   the 1870 Philadelphia population.

Source: Gretchen A. Condran and Rose A. Cheney,
   "Mortality Trends in Philadelphia: Age- and Cause-
   Specific Death Rates 1870–1930," *Demography*, 1982,
   9 (No. 1): 103.

continued to decline between 1900 and 1930, but
diphtheria and whooping cough exhibited declines
only after 1900.

The second group of diseases, those whose diagnoses were more problematic in the 19th and
early 20th centuries, showed less clear downward
trends than the more easily diagnosed causes of
death. Death rates from diarrheal diseases declined
throughout the period, although the decline was
much greater after 1900 than before. Epidemic
meningitis changed little between 1870 and 1930,
while influenza death rates rose for both 30-year

periods. Pneumonia death rates increased substantially between 1870 and 1900 but demonstrated a
large decline in the next 30 years. The fairly steady
decline which occurred in the residual category of
cause of death is difficult to interpret. This category contains many different causes of death, including all those that are ill-defined such as marasmus and debility. Therefore, actual changes in the
death rates cannot be distinguished from improvements in the diagnosis over time.

Examining the contribution of the 13 cause-of-
death categories to the overall decline in mortality
establishes that the control of these infectious diseases was the most important component of the
mortality transition (see Table 2). The percentage
of the total decline in mortality due to each cause
of death was calculated for the whole period from
1870 to 1930 and for each of the two 30-year periods separately. Over the 60-year period, two-thirds
of the mortality transition is accounted for by the
decline in the combined 13 disease categories alone.
Over half of the total reduction is explained solely
by decreases in diseases subject to specific diagnoses. These diseases were particularly responsible
for the decline from 1870 to 1900, but also contributed heavily to mortality decline after the turn
of the century. In contrast, mortality rates from
the group of infectious diseases which were less
easily diagnosed actually rose until 1900, but became a significant part of the overall decline afterward.

The fluctuations in the trends of particular diseases bring us closer to the mechanisms governing the transition. For both time periods, tuberculosis explained the largest percentage of the decline
in the age-standardized death rates. It accounted
for 26.8 percent of the decline in mortality from
1870 to 1900, 19.8 percent of the decline from 1900
to 1930, and over 22 percent for the entire six decades. Decreasing death rates from diarrheal diseases explain about 16 percent of the mortality decline from 1870 to 1930, contributing slightly more
to the overall decline during the initial 30 years.
The severity of scarlet fever and smallpox epidemics declined so much from 1870 to 1900 that
they represent the third and fourth most significant contributions. After 1900, however, they were
no longer important causes of death, and they no
longer contributed to the decline in mortality.
Other diseases actually increased in destructive-

ness before becoming sources of the mortality decline. Deaths due to diphtheria and, particularly, to pneumonia rose between 1870 and 1900, but these diseases became important sources of mortality decline between 1900 and 1930. Quite clearly, the mortality transition was largely a consequence of the reduction in fatalities from infectious diseases. Why did this reduction occur?

Much of the demographic literature seeking to explain the mortality transition asserts that in the past mortality declines in more developed areas resulted from economic growth and changes in living standards and that the importation of modern technology has been responsible for recent mortality reductions in less-developed areas.[8] This contention is generally true, but it remains a general hypothesis implying specific relationships which have yet to be empirically verified. The specific determinants of declines in mortality remain a central question in studying the demographic changes of industrialized nations, historically, and of developing nations, presently.

Thomas McKeown and his colleagues[9] have emphasized the importance of economic development and accompanying increases in food supplies and per capita income as sources of the historical decline in mortality in the West. From an examination of the diseases which contributed to the decline in mortality in England and Wales during the 19th century, the McKeown group concludes that the major influence on declining death rates was the rising standard of living, the most significant feature of which was an improvement in diet. They argue that improvements in hygiene and public sanitation had some impact on mortality rates after 1850 and that minor changes in overall mortality levels resulted from a favorable shift in the relationship between micro-organisms and the human hosts. Advancing medical technology had but a limited impact on mortality decline. According to McKeown, therapies made no contribution and immunization accounted for only a small part of the reduction in the death rates before 1935. A comparison of other studies with that of McKeown is hampered by variations in the research methods and classification schemes used to elaborate the determinants of mortality decline. Regardless of the broad categories used, however, the literature suggests that the factors responsible for the spectacular decline in mortality which occurred in late 19th- and early 20th-century Europe and the United States were numerous and complex. The importance of each factor has, by no means, been firmly established.[10] In many previous discussions, economic development has been considered mainly in terms of increases in per capita income and has been related to mortality through advances in nutrition.[11] However, economic development and industrialization encompass not only additions to per capita income, but also technological changes, increases in knowledge (including medical knowledge), mass education, urbanization, and changes in the social organization of both governmental and other groups. All these aspects of economic development affect mortality levels by influencing a number of other factors which more immediately determine mortality levels: density, crowding, immigration, water supplies, food purity, per capita food supplies, expenditures on public health, and personal hygiene practices.

Many of these phenomena are related to each other, often in complicated ways. Explanations of the decline of mortality usually juxtapose the variables relating to changes in income, medical technology, public health activity, or the environment. Such explanations should be replaced by a model which sees income changes operating through a number of these variables. Increased per capita income leads to increases in the purchase of health-enhancing goods—especially better food and better housing. It also potentially improves an individual's health by increasing his access to medical care and services and, on a more aggregate level, by increasing the funds available for public expenditures on health activities. At the same time, many of the intermediate variables which influenced mortality were probably also affected by aspects of economic development other than the change in per capita income. Improvements in nutrition resulted from changes in per capita income but also from technological changes, particularly those in transportation and food processing.

Because the decline in mortality was largely a result of a decline in infectious diseases, we can begin an explanation of mortality decline with the relatively simple notion that the chances of dying from a particular disease depend on three things: the exposure of a population to the disease; the population's resistance to the disease; and, once the disease is contracted, the ability of the people to survive its effects. Although these three are not easily distinguished empirically within populations, they can help us to organize some of the more easily identified variables which have affected mortality levels. [12]

In general, the decline in mortality prior to 1930 resulted largely from a decrease in exposure, and/or an increase in resistance, so that individuals were less likely to die from a given disease because they were less likely to contract it in the first place. This is not to say that there were no improvements in survival rates once a disease was contracted. Some researchers, for example, argue that improvements in case survival were a major part of the decline in the death rate from diphtheria. [13] Our analysis will concentrate on the prevention of illness, largely because it appears to have been a more significant factor in the early mortality decline than efforts to treat illness once it occurred.

Disease prevention resulted from a series of explicit public and private efforts in conjunction with economic forces that were beyond the public's immediate control. It is unwise to single out any particular factor as central to disease control, though we can conclude that a rising standard of living, promoted by rapid economic development, was a significant cause of this phenomenon.

The history of tuberculosis, the disease most important to mortality decline in Philadelphia, illustrates well the difficulties in explaining why the exposure of a given population to a particular disease declined. Overt efforts to contain this disease were not especially effective, largely because medical and public officials debated its contagious nature until nearly the turn of the century and took virtually no effective actions to limit it before 1930. [14] Nevertheless, its decline as a source of mortality is evident, both during the late 19th century, when little was known about this debilitating affliction, and during the first 30 years of the 20th century, when tuberculosis was at last recognized as a contagious disease. Explanations citing improvement in diet resulting from economic advance and the growing resistance of populations to the disease as a consequence of exposure both suggest possible answers, but it is clear that explicit attempts at containment do not account for its decline. [15]

Other diseases were effectively limited by direct and knowledgeable action, particularly by public health authorities. The emergence of the public health bureaucracy is an important aspect of the process of economic development and population growth. In Philadelphia from 1870 to 1930, the government apparatus concerned with the health and welfare of the population considerably expanded its scope. The growth of its power and influence helped produce lower mortality rates from a number of specific causes of death. Initially, the public health sector had an impact on medical science through the institution of data collection systems which informed the activities and pronouncements of public health officials. Later, as in other cities, public health efforts were concentrated primarily on reducing the population's exposure to disease by decreasing the number of pathogens in the environment. Public health activities encompassing quarantines, disinfection, purification of water supplies, and advocacy of particular child care practices all focused on prevention of illness, a focus that has to some extent been lost in the more recent emphasis on antibiotics and high technology medical treatment. Even in the instances where medical treatment played a central role in disease control, as with smallpox, public campaigns were largely responsible for promoting such medical remedies as vaccination. [16]

The history of public health activities in the 19th and early 20th centuries has been written for a number of cities and our aim is not to add Philadelphia to these histories. Rather, we seek to illuminate the connections between those activities and the shifts in mortality levels outlined above. To do that, we will focus on two causes of death on which public health activities were focused. By concentrating on one city and, at times, on small sections of Philadelphia, we will attempt to establish patterns and explanations that might apply to other urban areas during their mortality transitions.

The most dramatic impact of the city's activity can be observed in the efforts to combat high death rates from typhoid fever by cleaning up city water supplies. The pollution of water supplies quite often accompanied city growth. Impure water was not a problem in every large city, but Philadelphia shared with many cities the pollution of a central water system. The centralization of water systems allowed typhoid fever, transmitted through human excreta, to spread throughout the city.

As early as 1860, the Bureau of Health found two problems with the water supply system in Philadelphia. First, especially in summer, the quantity was inadequate to meet the needs of the population. The Bureau of Health argued that the shortage of water had adverse consequences, because more water was needed both for personal hygiene and to clean streets and sewers. In addition, the water supply was being polluted.[17] In 1861, the annual report of the Bureau of Health contained a scathing account of the pollutants of the water supply.[18] The city received water from several water stations, but all water came ultimately from the Schuylkill and Delaware rivers. According to the Bureau of Health, the Schuylkill was being polluted by sulphate of iron from coal mines, by the infusion of refuse dyes and wastes from the various factories on the eastern bank, and, most objectionable of all, by the emptying of city sewers into the river. The sewers received drainage from the streets and were connected to privies and cesspools.[19] The Delaware River was even more foul. In 1874, the Bureau of Health suggested that the Delaware be terminated as a source of water in favor of the Schuylkill, which, by that time, was protected from some pollutants.[20] The city had acquired land along both sides of the river for park land to prevent further growth of pollution-producing industries along the river banks.[21]

The pollution problems remained, however, and city officials linked impure water with diseases, particularly typhoid fever. Filtration of the water supply was first broached as early as 1853 but not implemented until after the turn of the century.[22] At the time filtration was begun, the city was divided into six water districts that received water from different waterworks. The timing of the introduction of water filters differed across the six districts. The death rates from typhoid fever from 1890 to 1920 have been calculated for each of the water districts and are shown in Fig. 1. The graph points out the importance of water filtration in combating the disease. The Roxborough (1902) and Belmont (1904) districts were the first to receive filtered water. In these two districts, the 1905–1906 typhoid epidemic that showed up in the other four water districts did not occur. The Tor-

resdale district had high rates of typhoid in 1905, 1906, and 1907 but showed a precipitous decline by 1908. Its water filtration system was put into operation in 1907. By the end of 1908, 56 percent of the city's water was being filtered. Subsequently, filtered water was supplied to the East Park, Queen Lane, and Fairmount water districts so that on March 1, 1909, "the entire city was supplied with filtered water." No epidemics of typhoid fever occurred after the filtration began.[23]

For the city as a whole the picture is clear. The year 1906 is the peak typhoid year for the city—over 1,000 deaths occurred in just one year. Epidemics had occurred with regularity before that. The number of deaths grew in each epidemic as the city's population grew and as an increasing proportion of the city's population was exposed to the polluted water supply. Epidemics ceased in 1906, for by the time the next epidemic would have likely occurred, the water supply was filtered.

While it was agreed that the purification of the polluted water supply affected the death rate from typhoid fever, contemporaries were intrigued by the notion, supported by data in several cities, that the death rates from diseases other than typhoid fever would decline following the purification of public water supplies. The idea arose from the work of two individuals, Hiram F. Mills of Lawrence, Massachusetts, and J. J. Reincke of Hamburg, Germany. In 1893–1894, they observed that the purification of polluted water supplies in Lawrence and Hamburg produced a significant decline in the general death rate. The relationship was named the "Mills-Reincke phenomenon." It was tested on a number of other cities by Allen Hazen, who in 1904 reached the conclusion that "where one death from typhoid fever has been avoided by the use of better water, a certain number of deaths, probably two or three, from other causes have been avoided." He hypothesized that the decline in the overall death rate following the water purification would be two or three times greater than that from the decline in typhoid fever alone.[24]

Although some of the excess decline in the overall death rates observed by Mills, Reincke, and Hazen was attributable to changes in other waterborne diseases, it was not totally accounted for by these. Changes in typhoid rates were related to pneumonia, tuberculosis, and other diseases which were not water-borne. In Philadelphia, during the period when water filtration was introduced, there was no constant multiplicative relationship between the decline in typhoid death rates and the decline in death rates from other causes. The existence of six water districts with differences in the timing of filtration affords us an opportunity to examine more carefully the relationship between the conditions of the water supplied to the population and the deaths from diseases other than typhoid. The water district data for Philadelphia show very little evidence of the Mills-Reincke phenomenon.

None of the causes of death which we examined showed the decline coincidental to water filtration which is seen in the typhoid fever death rates. There was little or no association between deaths from typhoid fever and deaths from tuberculosis or pneumonia, the leading causes of adult mortality. More surprisingly, however, even diseases like infant and childhood diarrhea, dysentery, and enteritis, which might be water-borne, did not decline in water districts immediately following filtration. Water filtration did put an end to epidemic

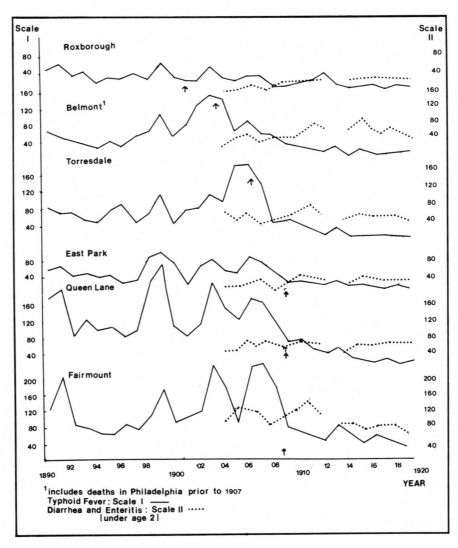

Fig. 1: Deaths from typhoid fever in Philadelphia water districts, 1890–1920.

outbreaks of typhoid fever, but it did not go beyond that.

The major cause of death among infants and young children was diarrheal disease. In these age groups, diarrhea is generally precipitated by contaminated food or water supplies and/or malnutrition. The immediate cause of death is dehydration, which occurs most quickly in very young infants with low body weights.[25] In 19th-century Philadelphia, there was a definite seasonal pattern to infant and childhood diarrheal deaths, the frequency having been much greater in the summer months.[26]

The decline in diarrheal death rates for the city as a whole is shown in Fig. 2. Mortality rates from infant and childhood diarrhea declined from the mid-1870s to 1900. An upsurge appeared shortly after 1900 and was followed by a relatively steep decline. The rise after 1900 corresponds to a shift in the classification scheme of causes of death, and therefore is likely to be an artifact of the changing nosology. The best estimate of the trend in infant and childhood diarrheal death rates is that they continued downward throughout the first decade of the 20th century and that the decline became steeper sometime about 1910. The sharp downward trend beginning about 1910 would be consistent with the positive influence of water filtration on the occurrence of the disease. However, as we have stated in the previous section, it is clear that the source of the decline was not the shifts in the water supply. Fig. 1, which contains the typhoid fever deaths, includes the numbers of deaths from infant and childhood diarrhea. There is no evidence of a decline in these deaths resulting from filtration of the city's water supply. The factors influencing the levels of mortality from diarrhea in the early years of life must be sought elsewhere.

The Bureau of Health in Philadelphia undertook three activities directed particularly at reducing infant and early childhood mortality rates. The first of these was the issuance of pamphlets on the care and feeding of children. In the mid-to-late 1870s, 40,000 copies of a circular urging mothers to breastfeed their babies and to postpone weaning until after the summer months were distributed. For mothers who did not breastfeed, the pamphlets suggested that clean bottles be used in feeding infants.[27] The advice contained in the pamphlet was sound. From the scanty data available, it appears

that breast-fed babies had lower death rates from diarrheal diseases than did babies fed animal milk. The question which cannot be answered is whether the advice was heeded by enough mothers to have produced a decline in mortality rates. Changes in the seasonal pattern of diarrheal diseases suggests that the advice was heeded and may have resulted in an attenuation of the summer peak of mortality among one-year-olds prior to 1880, but a seasonal pattern, particularly for infants, continued until 1920.[28]

The impact created by the establishment of a Child Hygiene Bureau can be somewhat more easily assessed. The bureau was organized in 1910 and located child hygiene clinics in 8 wards between 1910 and 1914 and in 19 wards between 1915 and 1918.[29] Trends in death rates based on births for child hygiene districts are shown in Fig. 3. Wards were selected as sites of clinics because of the high infant and childhood death rates. Therefore, the wards with clinics had higher infant diarrheal death rates before the clinics opened than wards without clinics. The wards with clinics, however, showed declines in diarrheal death rates which were steeper than those without clinics, so that by 1930, the infant diarrheal rates in the latter were higher than those in the former. Also noticeable in Fig. 3 is that while infant diarrheal death rates were declining for all wards for the time period from 1904 to 1920, clinics appear to have accelerated the decline in the wards that had them.

Finally, the Bureau of Health worked long to improve the quality of the milk being fed to children in the city. In 1889, City Council created the post of inspector of milk to insure the wholesomeness of milk in the city. This appointment, however, by no means solved the problems.[30] Between 1890 and 1914, difficult legislative struggles were waged for the city councilmen's votes on various regulations affecting the milk supply. Milk producers favored little or no regulation, while the Bureau of Health argued that the poor quality of the milk supply had adverse health consequences and that regulation of the producers was needed.[31]

There were a number of problems with the milk supplied to the city. First, it was often skimmed and/or had added water. As a consequence, babies and young children fed the milk were likely to be inadequately nourished. Second, the milk itself was impure. Sloppy handling resulted in pollutants that

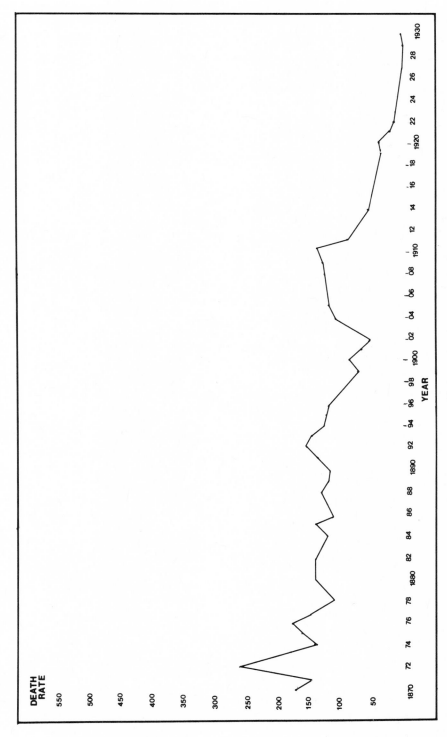

Fig. 2: Death rates from diarrheal diseases under age two (2), Philadelphia, 1870–1930 (death rates per 1,000 total population).

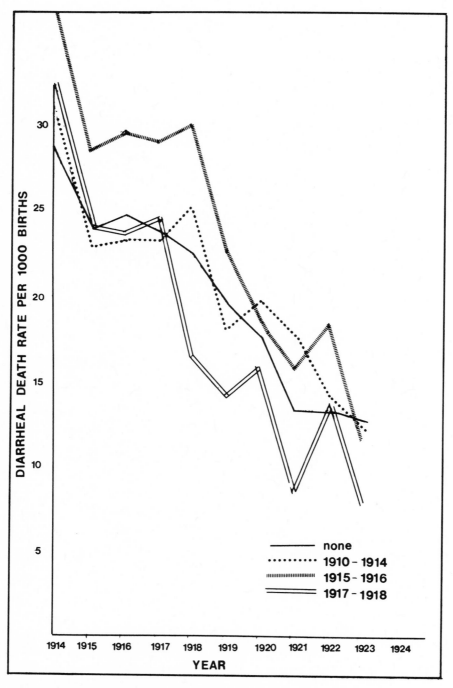

Fig. 3: Infant diarrheal death rates in wards classified by timing of child hygiene programs, Philadelphia, 1914–1923.

entered the milk, and lack of refrigeration, especially in the summer, resulted in the growth of bacteria. Third, some of the milk was obtained from tubercular cows and was a source of nonrespiratory tuberculosis in the population. The last problem seems not to have been severe; a system of inspecting herds for tuberculosis was instituted quite early. The first two problems with the milk supply were likely to have directly affected the incidence of diarrheal diseases in infants and young children. Bureau of Health efforts to prevent the adulteration of milk were only moderately successful between 1890 and 1895. In 1895, the inspector was given authority to check the bacteriological content of the milk.[32] Both home and commercial pasteurization of milk was being done by 1905.[33] As the result of legislation going into effect in 1911, milk was condemned and destroyed if its temperature was below standard. In that year alone almost 29,000 quarts of milk failed to meet the standard.[34] On July 1, 1914, an ordinance requiring all milk in the city to be pasteurized was passed.[35]

Limited statistics available on the quality of the milk supply indicate that improvements occurred over time. Between 1889 and 1893, an average of 8.5 percent of inspected milk was found to be skimmed or watered. During the next five years that percentage had dropped to 3.3. From 1899 through 1903, an average of about 1.5 percent was skimmed or watered, and for two five-year periods after that, average yearly percentages dropped to .5 and .2 percent. Statistics from 1899 to 1911 on the bacteriological content of milk show a much less consistent downward trend. A substantial drop occurred between 1908 and 1909 and in the years following.[36] These improvements happened before universal pasteurization became law. In summary, improvements in the milk supply came largely after the turn of the century, but were substantial enough to have accelerated the decline in infant and childhood diarrhea.

The decline in mortality experienced by Western industrialized nations in the late 19th and early 20th centuries creates a major historical question. As illustrated by our case study of Philadelphia, life expectancies at birth significantly increased and propensities to die from infectious disease, particularly tuberculosis and infant diarrhea, decreased during the period from 1870 to 1930. Certain epidemic diseases, notably typhoid fever, smallpox, and scarlet fever, virtually disappeared as causes of death. Of particular importance was the sharp drop in the frequency of infant and childhood death, which propelled the marked increase in life expectancies. The circumstances surrounding the deaths of the Kautz children 100 years ago have long been gone from the Western world.

The reasons for this remarkable change remain elusive. We can say with some assurance that mortality declines occurred because the population became less exposed and more resistant to infectious disease, rather than because medical technology increased chances of survival once a disease was contracted. But explaining this reduced exposure and greater resistance is difficult.

Certainly, no single factor can account for the mortality transition. Our brief discussion of the diseases central to the mortality decline indicates a multitude of possibilities. Tuberculosis, for example, declined in impact for no clearly discernible reason, although improved diet and growing resistance among the population to the disease were probable factors. Smallpox was eradicated through a combination of advancing medical technology and governmental crusades promoting vaccination. Typhoid fever was eliminated by water filtration, and infant and childhood diarrheal deaths were sharply decreased by several factors, including public dissemination of information about the diseases, the establishment of locally based child hygiene clinics, and improvement in the quality of milk.

Underlying the overall transition was a general improvement in living standards, concurrent with rapid economic development. Economic advance in itself, however, would not have produced the evident declines in death rates of certain diseases without the efforts of public officials who proposed, debated, and carried out many actions to further the health of their community. Typhoid fever, smallpox, and infant and childhood diarrhea, in particular, were severely curtailed by their activities.

Governmental intervention in Philadelphia occurred in spite of opposition from various special interest groups and constant bickering between the Board of Health and City Council. Regulation often came, too, with officials possessing only limited knowledge about the health problems against which their efforts were directed. But its impact was not small. Considering only typhoid fever, diarrheal diseases, and smallpox, direct public health activities probably account for almost one-third of the mortality decline in Philadelphia between 1870 and 1930. And this conservative estimate ignores possible indirect effects on other diseases.

Scepticism voiced today about the role of government too often neglects the very beneficial impact public agencies have made in the lives of their citizenry, particularly in the field of public health.

Many commentators also mistakenly think of public intervention and regulation as phenomena associated with the expansion of government in the 1930s. Yet by 1930 infectious epidemic disease and exceedingly high mortality rates had been brought largely under control with the direct assistance of a well-established municipal services bureaucracy. The health issues we face today are not the same as those a century ago, but we would be prudent to recognize past successes and how they were achieved.

## NOTES

This research was done at the Philadelphia Social History Project, Theodore Hershberg, director, with support from the Center for Population Research, National Institute of Child Health and Human Development (RO 1HD 12413). The PSHP gratefully acknowledges the funding it has received from the following federal agencies: the National Institute of Mental Health; the National Science Foundation; and the National Endowment for the Humanities.

We also wish to thank William Kreider, Jeffrey Seaman, Wayne Dunlap, and Mara Weitzman for computer support, and Alicia Gilham for graphics and typing.

1   City of Philadelphia, *First Annual Message of Edwin S. Stuart, Mayor of the City of Philadelphia, with Annual Report of Abraham M. Beitler and the Annual Report of the Board of Health for the year ending December 31, 1891* (Philadelphia, 1892), p. 508.

2   In a recent review of Robert Gottfried's book on the Black Death, William H. McNeill takes a much longer view of how "the disappearance of epidemic disease as a serious factor in human life . . . separate[s] us from our ancestors." See "The plague of plagues," *N.Y. Rev. Books,* July 21, 1983, *30*: 28–29.

3   See for example: Thomas McKeown, *The Modern Rise of Population* (New York, 1976), pp. 128–142; Thomas McKeown and R. G. Record, "Reasons for the decline of mortality in England and Wales during the nineteenth century," *Population Stud.,* July 1962, *16*: (No. 2): 94–122; Samuel H. Preston and Etienne van de Walle, "Urban French mortality in the nineteenth century," *Population Stud.*, July 1978, *32* (No. 2): 275–297; Gretchen A. Condran and Rose A. Cheney, "Mortality trends in Philadelphia: age- and cause-specific death rates 1870–1930," *Demography*, Feb. 1982, *9* (No. 1): 97–123.

4   Gretchen A. Condran and Eileen Crimmins, "Mortality differentials between rural and urban areas of states in the northeastern United States, 1890–

1900," *J. Hist. Geography,* Apr. 1980, *6* (No. 2): 179–202; Robert Higgs, "Mortality in rural america, 1870–1920: estimates and conjectures," *Explorations Econ. Hist.,* 1973, *10* (No. 2): 177–193.

5   Condran and Cheney, "Mortality trends in Philadelphia," pp. 98–99.

6   The values of $_1q_0$ in Table 1 were estimated using the values of $_4q_1$ fitted to South Model Life tables. For a full explanation of the estimating procedure, see Condran and Cheney, "Mortality trends in Philadelphia," pp. 91–102.

7   City of Philadelphia, *Annual Report of the Bureau of Health of the City of Philadelphia for the year ending December 31, 1904* (Philadelphia, 1905), pp. 236–267.

8   Abdel R. Omran, "The epidemiological transition: a theory of the epidemiology of population change," *Milbank Mem. Fund Quart.,* 1971, *49* (No. 4, Part 1): 509–538; United Nations, *Population Bulletin of the United Nations, no. 6 (with special reference to the situation and recent trends of mortality in the world)* (New York, 1963), pp. 9–10; Kingsley Davis, "The amazing decline of mortality in underdeveloped areas," *Am. Econ. Rev.,* 1956, *46*: 305–318; George Stolnitz, "A century of international mortality trends," *Population Stud.,* July 1955, *9* (No. 1): 24–55.

9   McKeown, *The Modern Rise of Population,* p. 153; McKeown and Record, "Reasons for the decline of mortality," pp. 94–122; Thomas McKeown and R. G. Brown, "Medical evidence related to English population changes in the eighteenth century," *Population Stud.,* 1955, *9*: 119–141.

10   For a listing of factors influencing mortality levels, see United Nations, *The Determinants and Consequences of Population Trends* (New York, 1973), pp. 86–91.

11   McKeown, *The Modern Rise of Population,* pp. 153–154.

12   Eileen M. Crimmins and Gretchen A. Condran, "Mortality variation in U.S. cities in 1900: a two-level explanation by cause-of-death and underlying factors," *Soc. Sci. Hist.,* Winter, 1983, *7* (No. 1): 31–59.

13    See, for example, John Duffy, *A History of Public Health in New York City 1866–1966* (New York, 1974), p. 157.

14    City of Philadelphia, *First Annual Message of Charles F. Warwick, Mayor of the City of Philadelphia, with Annual Reports of Abraham M. Beitler and of the Board of Health for the year ending December 31, 1895* (Philadelphia, 1896), p. 80; City of Philadelphia, *Fourth Annual Message of Edwin S. Stuart, Mayor of the City of Philadelphia, with Annual Reports of Abraham M. Beitler and of the Board of Health for the year ending December 31, 1894* (Philadelphia, 1895), pp. 72–78.

15    See, for example, Edgar Sydenstriker, *Health and Environment* (New York, 1933), pp. 120–121; E. R. N. Grigg, "The arcana of tuberculosis" Part I, *Am. Rev. Tuberculosis & Pulmonary Dis.*, 1958, *78* (No. 2): 151–172.

16    McKeown, *The Modern Rise of Population*, p. 99; City of Philadelphia, *First Annual Message of Charles Warwick, 1895*, pp. 83–84; Preston and van de Walle, "Urban French mortality," p. 282.

17    City of Philadelphia, *Report of the Department of Health for 1860* (Philadelphia, 1861), pp. 39–41.

18    City of Philadelphia, *Report of the Board of Health of the City and Port of Philadelphia to the Mayor for 1861* (Philadelphia, 1862), pp. 16–17.

19    *Ibid*.

20    City of Philadelphia, *Report of the Board of Health of the City and Port of Philadelphia to the Mayor for the year 1874* (Philadelphia, 1875), pp. 45–47.

21    City of Philadelphia, *Report of the Board of Health of the City and Port of Philadelphia to the Mayor for the year 1872* (Philadelphia, 1873), pp. 99–101.

22    James C. Booth and T. H. Garrett, *Report of the Philadelphia Watering Committee . . . on Filtration . . . on Schuylkill Water* (Philadelphia, 1854).

23    City of Philadelphia, *Annual Report of the Bureau of Water for the year 1902* (Philadelphia, 1903), p. 94, found in *Fourth Annual Message of Samuel H. Ashbridge, Mayor of the City of Philadelphia, Vol. II;* City of Philadelphia, *Annual Report of the Bureau of Water for the year 1904* (Philadelphia, 1905), p. 69, found in *Second Annual Message of John Weaver, Mayor of the City of Philadelphia, Vol. II;* City of Philadelphia, *Annual Report of the Bureau of Water for the year 1907* (Philadelphia, 1908), p. 47, found in *First Annual Message of John E. Reyburn, Mayor of the City of Philadelphia, Vol. II;* City of Philadelphia, *Annual Report of the Bureau of Water for the year 1908* (Philadelphia, 1909), p. 50, found in *Second Annual Message of John E. Reyburn, Mayor of the City of Philadelphia, Vol. II*; City of Philadelphia, *Annual Report of the Bureau of Water for the year 1909* (Philadelphia, 1910), p. 47 (quotation), found in *Third Annual Message of John E. Reyburn, Mayor of the City of Philadelphia, Vol. II*. Although

the entire city received filtered water in 1909, problems with supplying the Queen Lane district meant that a dependable supply was not finally insured until 1911. See City of Philadelphia, *Annual Reports of the Director of the Department of Public Health and Charities and of the Chief of the Bureau of Health for the year ending December 31, 1911* (Philadelphia, 1912), p. 17.

24    W. T. Sedgwick and J. Scott MacNutt, "On the Mills-Reincke phenomenon and Hazen's theorem concerning the decrease in mortality from diseases other than typhoid fever following the purification of public water-supplies," *J. Infect. Dis.*, Aug. 1910, *7* (No. 4): 489–563.

25    Samuel H. Preston, *Mortality Patterns in National Populations: With Special Reference to Recorded Causes of Death* (New York, 1976), p. 38.

26    Rose A. Cheney, "Seasonal infant and childhood mortality in Philadelphia, 1865–1920," *J. Interdisc. Hist.*, Winter 1984, *14* (No. 3): 561–562.

27    City of Philadelphia, *Report of the Board of Health for the year 1874,* pp. 397–402.

28    Cheney, "Seasonal infant and childhood mortality," pp. 578–579.

29    City of Philadelphia, *Third Annual Message of Harry A. Markey, Mayor of Philadelphia, containing the reports of the various Departments of the City of Philadelphia for the year ending December 31, 1930* (Philadelphia, 1931), p. 391; City of Philadelphia, *Second Annual Message of Harry A. Markey, Mayor of Philadelphia, containing the reports of the various Departments of the City of Philadelphia, for the year ending December 31, 1929* (Philadelphia, 1930), pp. 233–238, 397; City of Philadelphia, *Annual Report of the Bureau of Health for the year ending December 31, 1923* (Philadelphia, 1924), p. 11; City of Philadelphia, *Annual Report of the Bureau of Health for the year ending December 31, 1922* (Philadelphia, 1923), p. 83.

30    City of Philadelphia, *Second Annual Message of Edwin H. Fitler, Mayor of the City of Philadelphia, with Annual Report of William S. Stokeley and Annual Report of the Bureau of Health for the year ending December 31, 1888* (Philadelphia, 1889), pp. 19–20.

31    A record of the battles waged can be found in the Annual Reports of the Bureau of Health for the years from 1890 to 1914.

32    City of Philadelphia, *First Annual Message of Charles F. Warwick, Mayor of the City of Philadelphia, with Annual Reports of Abraham M. Beitler and the Board of Health for the year ending December 31, 1895* (Philadelphia, 1896), p. 140.

33    City of Philadelphia, *Third Annual Message of John Weaver, Mayor of the City of Philadelphia, with the Annual Reports of the Director of the Department of Public Health and Charities and the Chief of the Bureau of Health*

*for the year ending December 31, 1905* (Philadelphia, 1906), pp. 214–215.

34   City of Philadelphia, *Annual Reports of the Director of the Department of Public Health and Charities and of the Chief of the Bureau of Health for the year ending December 31, 1911* (Philadelphia, 1912), pp. 21–23.

35   City of Philadelphia, *Fourth Annual Message of Rudolph Blankenburg, Mayor of Philadelphia, Vol. III* (Philadelphia, 1915), p. 4.

36   The statistics presented are from the Annual Reports of the Bureau of Health for the years from 1889 to 1913.

# HEALTH AND THE ENVIRONMENT

Most 19th-century physicians attributed rising mortality rates in American cities to the filthy urban environment. The popular "miasmatic" theory, linking dirt with disease, motivated much public health activity: street cleaning, garbage collection and disposal, water and sewer systems, and food regulation.

Control over milk supplies emerged as a serious problem in the 1840s and continued to plague cities until the widespread adoption of pasteurization in the 1920s. Cities also attempted to regulate ice cream shops, bakeries, and slaughterhouses. But few municipalities were able effectively to control meat packing before 1906. With the establishment of health department laboratories and the passage of the Pure Food and Drugs Act, food control became systematic.

Polluted water sources presented another public health problem. In 1801 Philadelphia opened its municipal water system, designed to bring fresh country water into the city. This action helped to save Philadelphia from devastation by cholera in 1832. New York and Boston, recognizing the benefits, followed suit, and other cities across the country copied the eastern model. Chicago, although located at the edge of Lake Michigan, an ample body of water, faced a peculiar problem because of the city's flat terrain. Louis P. Cain describes the lengths to which that city went to supply its inhabitants with water. The Chicago hero Ellis Sylvester Chesbrough, like other engineers, achieved national prominence for his urban sanitation efforts.

Engineers, plumbers, and other nonmedical sanitarians contributed as much to the public health movement as physicians. The medical profession may have perceived the necessity of sanitation, but engineers provided the technical expertise needed to execute the massive urban cleanups. James H. Cassedy explores the methods and influence of one filth-oriented sanitation expert during the early days of the bacteriologic era.

In the 20th century sanitation lost its dominant position in the public health movement. The germ theory changed the focus of health activity from cleaning the environment to tracking down specific bacteria, shifting disease control from the streets to the laboratory. Today, however, in a world beset with new environmental problems, such as those described by James C. Whorton, sanitation is once again assuming a central role.

# 31

## Raising and Watering a City:
## Ellis Sylvester Chesbrough and Chicago's First Sanitation System

LOUIS P. CAIN

The engineers responsible for invention and mechanization in agriculture, manufacturing, and transportation are prominent historical figures, but few people are aware of the men who pioneered the sanitation systems so crucial to urbanization. As cities grew, their initial approaches to waste disposal and water supply proved unacceptable. As early as 1798 Benjamin Latrobe noted in his journal that the fresh groundwater which located the site of Philadelphia was befouled by the city's increasing population concentration. In Latrobe's opinion, Philadelphia's existing water-supply strategy was a major source of disease. Even before he assumed the responsibility for the city's new waterworks, Latrobe was convinced of the project's utility: "The great scheme of bringing the water of the Schuylkill to Philadelphia to supply the city is now become an object of immense importance, . . . though it is at present neglected from a failure of funds. The evil, however, which it is intended collaterally to correct is so serious and of such magnitude as to call loudly upon all who are inhabitants of Philadelphia for their utmost exertions to complete it."[1]

The emerging concentrations of population and manufacturing in the 19th century necessitated a reexamination of sanitation strategies. With urbanization, the haphazard approaches of the past could not guarantee pure water supplies and adequate waste disposal. Urban growth inevitably required the implementation of sanitation systems, and these systems, in turn, permitted further growth.

LOUIS P. CAIN is Professor of Economics, Loyola University of Chicago, Chicago, Illinois.

Reprinted with permission from *Technology and Culture*, 1972, *13*: 353–372. Copyright 1972 by the Society for the History of Technology, and published by the University of Chicago Press.

Students of Chicago's formative decades inevitably encounter the name of Ellis Sylvester Chesbrough; by studying Chesbrough, a student can focus on the truly unique character and contribution of Chicago's sanitation system. Chesbrough's works were the innovations most responsible for Chicago's unrestricted urban growth; they freed the city from the limitations imposed by an unfavorable natural topography. A flat, nonporous terrain, slightly elevated from Lake Michigan and the Chicago River, made drainage and absorption nearly impossible. In rainy weather, the topsoil became swamplike. Urban growth required a drainage system which could remove both surface water and household wastes. The natural depository for such a drainage system was Lake Michigan; however, the lake was simultaneously the city's natural water-supply source. Lake water had to be conserved if it was to be potable, and this meant it had to be protected from urban wastes. Fortunately, beginning in the 1850s, Chicago's city fathers recognized pollution as a serious threat to the city's health and took immediate action. This paper investigates how Chesbrough responded to Chicago's anomalous water-supply and waste-disposal needs in the 1850s and 1860s, and inquires into his engineering education to discover the antecedents of his innovative ideas.

### I

Ellis Sylvester Chesbrough was born of Puritan ancestry in Baltimore County, Maryland, in July 1813. An unsuccessful business venture exhausted the family's means and suspended young Sylvester's education, and so, at nine years of age, he went to work. Between his ninth and fifteenth birthdays

Chesbrough spent only a year in a classroom, but he did find time outside his counting-house duties to pursue his studies. Chesbrough acquired most of his basic education without the benefit of formal training or a regular teacher, and the same was true of his engineering education.

In 1828 Chesbrough's father took a job with a railroad engineering company employed by the Baltimore and Ohio Railroad Company. Through the father's influence, the son gained employment as a chainman with a similar company engaged in preliminary surveying work in and about Baltimore.[2] Chesbrough's company was under Lieutenant Joshua Barney, U.S. Army, and most of the engineers were army officers, many of them graduates of the U.S. Military Academy's practical, as opposed to theoretical, engineering course.[3] Chesbrough was fortunate in being affiliated with several of the army's most prominent engineers. In 1830–31 he worked as an assistant engineer to Colonel Stephen H. Long.[4] Near the end of 1831, Chesbrough joined the engineering corps of Captain William Gibbs McNeill, where he served immediately under Lieutenant George W. Whistler.[5]

The Panic of 1837 and the resulting depression dealt a hard blow to the country's internal improvement's bubble, and Chesbrough, like many other engineers, found himself out of work as the flow of funds dried up in the early 1840s. He went to his father's residence in Providence, Rhode Island, where, during the winter of 1842, he spent his leisure time in the workshop of a nearby railroad learning the practical use of tools. The following year he purchased a farm adjacent to one owned by his father in Niagara County, New York. His venture into farming was mercifully brief; after an unsuccessful year, Chesbrough gladly returned to engineering.

In 1846 Chesbrough was offered the position of chief engineer on the Boston Water Works' West Division. This position completed his engineering education. Up to this time, all his experience was related to railroad engineering, and he had mastered many civil engineering essentials, such as grading, tunneling, and surveying. Chesbrough was reluctant to accept the Boston position because he considered himself unacquainted with hydraulic engineering. His friends and Boston's water commissioners implored him to accept the position, and, after being assured John Jervis's counsel, Chesbrough assented.

There was good reason for Chesbrough to consider an association with Jervis valuable. Jervis had been active in every phase of engineering, particularly those dealing with hydraulics. Jervis was a product of the New York canal system and had learned hydraulic engineering on the job by working on the Erie Canal. In 1846 Jervis was appointed consulting engineer on the Boston Water Works, with Chesbrough the chief engineer. Jervis had the responsibility for designing both the Cochituate Aqueduct and the Brookline Reservoir; Chesbrough, the responsibility for supervising the execution of Jervis's plans.[6] In 1850 Chesbrough became sole commissioner of Boston's water works, and a year later, he became Boston's first city engineer.

The United States' early experience with internal improvements and the education of engineers coalesced in Chesbrough's career. He learned civil engineering from some of the army's most competent engineers. He learned hydraulic engineering from Jervis, perhaps the most competent engineer trained by the New York canal system. The education and experience which Chesbrough utilized in freeing Chicago from its topographical liabilities and in implementing an effective sanitation system grew out of his first-hand experience with many of the country's internal improvements.

## II

In the early 1850s Chicago's random waste disposal methods led to a succession of cholera and dysentery epidemics. The Illinois legislature created the Chicago Board of Sewerage Commissioners on February 14, 1855, to combat what was generally conceded to be an intolerable situation.[7] The commissioners sought "the most competent engineer of the time who was available for the position of chief engineer."[8] Their selection, E. Sylvester Chesbrough, resigned his position as Boston's city engineer and came to Chicago.[9] Immediately after accepting the position, Chesbrough submitted a report in which he outlined his plan for a sewerage system designed to solve Chicago's drainage and waste-disposal problem. His plan represents the first comprehensive sewerage system undertaken by any major city in the United States. He had learned about sewer construction, grading, and "building-raising" from different sources. Now he merged them and "pulled Chicago out of the mud."

Prior to Chesbrough's arrival, Chicago's sewerage commissioners solicited the public for plans and suggestions. Thirty-nine proposals were received, and, although the board claimed Chesbrough utilized many of these suggestions, he did not use any of the proposals in its entirety.[10] Chesbrough's task was to construct a sewerage system whose main objective was to "improve and preserve" the city's health. In his opinion, the existing privy vaults and drainage sluices were "abominations that should be swept away as speedily as possible," and that "to construct the vaults as they should be, and maintain them even in a comparatively inoffensive condition, would be more expensive than to construct an entire system of sewerage for no other purpose, if the past experience of London and other large cities was any guide for the future of Chicago."[11]

Chesbrough's 1855 report to the Board of Sewerage Commissioners made several references to the sewers of New York, Boston, and Philadelphia. Additionally, the report showed that Chesbrough was familiar, through his reading, with the sewers of London, Paris, and other European cities. It is important to remember, however, that not one U.S. city at that time had a comprehensive sewerage system, even though most had sewers. Consequently, Chesbrough had to rely on his training and intuition in assessing sewerage system alternatives.

Chesbrough's 1855 report considered four possibilities: (1) drainage directly into the Chicago River and then into Lake Michigan; (2) drainage directly into Lake Michigan; (3) drainage into artificial reservoirs to be pumped and used as fertilizer (sewage farming); and (4) drainage directly into the Chicago River, and then by a proposed steamboat canal into the Des Plaines River. Although this fourth possibility was the method which Chicago eventually adopted (the Chicago Sanitary District's Sanitary and Ship Canal), the city's 80,000 inhabitants in 1855 did not warrant the expense which this alternative involved.

Chesbrough recommended the first plan.[12] This is not to say he failed to realize that his preferred method was a potential health hazard, particularly during the warmer months, and might obstruct river navigation by making the waterways shal-

lower.[13] Chesbrough discussed the objections to his recommended alternative:

> It is proposed to remove the first [health hazard] by pouring into the river from the lake a sufficient body of pure water into the North and South Branches to prevent offensive or injurious exhalations. . . . The latter objection [obstruct navigation] is believed to be groundless, because the substances to be conveyed through the sewers to the river could in no case be heavier than the soil of this vicinity, but would generally be much lighter. While these substances might, to some extent, be deposited there when there is little or no current, they would, during the seasons of rain and flood, be swept on by the same force that has hitherto preserved the depth of the river.[14]

Apparently, Chesbrough did not realize that spring freshets and floods might force the sewers' accumulations into the lake in such a way as to pollute the city's water supply. This is somewhat surprising, as the basic sanitation principle of the day was to locate the eventual sewage outlet as far from the water-supply source as possible.

Chesbrough had three objections to the second possibility, drainage directly into Lake Michigan. First, it would require a greater sewer length and, consequently, would incur greater cost. Second, he supposed that this plan would seriously affect the water supply, if any sewer outlets were located near the pumping station. At this time, Chicago's water-supply intake was located a short distance offshore at the Chicago Avenue lakefront, approximately one-half mile north of the Chicago River's mouth. Chesbrough did not elaborate on this objection. Third, he felt drainage into the lake would create difficulties in preventing sewer outlet injury during stormy weather, or snow and ice obstruction during winter.[15]

Sewer farming was rejected in part because of the uncertainty whether future fertilizer demand would be sufficient to cover distribution costs. Further, Chesbrough was uncertain as to both the needed reservoir capacity and the expense of building the necessary reservoirs. Finally, Chesbrough thought there would be a great health hazard created by foul odors emanating from sewage spread over a wide surface.

Chesbrough termed the use of a steamboat canal, not yet constructed to flush the sewage into the Des Plaines River, the fourth possibility, "too remote." Although he was aware of the "evils" which would result when raw sewage passed into Lake Michigan, Chesbrough felt it impossible to create an outlet to the southwest. Brown claims, however, that "he appears to have believed that this would be the ultimate solution of the sewerage problem," as, in fact, it was.[16]

> With regard to the fourth plan . . . which would divert a large and constantly flowing stream from Lake Michigan into the Illinois River, it is too remote a contingency to be relied upon for present purposes; besides the cost of it, or any other similar channel in that direction, sufficient to drain off the sewage of the city, would be not only far more than the present sewerage law provides for, but more than would be necessary to construct the sewers for five times the present population. Should the proposed steam-boat canal ever be made for commercial purposes the plan now recommended would be about as well adapted to such a state of things, as it is to the present.[17]

Certainly his plan was readily adaptable to such a scheme. The Sanitary District of Chicago was created in 1889 for the express purpose of implementing this fourth possibility. The Sanitary District then constructed the "proposed steamboat canal," which unquestionably was beyond the means of Chicagoans in 1855.

In December 1855 Chesbrough submitted his plan for Chicago's sewage disposal and drainage. Under this plan, all of the sewage of Chicago's west division, all the sewage of the north division except for the lakefront area, and about one-half the sewage of the south division was deposited in the Chicago River. This sewage passed from the river into Lake Michigan. The dividing line in the south division was State Street; the area east of State Street drained directly into the lake. As the area east of State Street was primarily residential, Chicago's business district was sewered into the river. This district, west of State Street, included the majority of Chicago's packinghouses, distilleries, and hotels. Thus, the river received large quantities of pollutants daily.[18]

The sewers themselves were outstanding phenomena. Brick sewers, three to six feet in diameter, were laid above the ground down the center of the street. Chicago's topography, being unusually flat, was unfavorable to sewer construction. The Chi-

cago River banks were only two feet above the water level. Near the river's north and south branches, the ground level reached a maximum of 10 to 12 feet above the lake. In reality, the task of constructing underground sewers required raising the city.[19] From the beginning, Chesbrough insisted that a high grade was necessary for proper drainage and dry streets. Chicago lacked this high grade, and, thus, the decision to raise the city's level, concomitant with sewer installation, was one which solved the waste disposal and drainage problem in the context of Chicago's existing topography and future necessities.[20]

The Chesbrough plan called for an intercepting sewer system which emptied into the Chicago River. The sewers were to be constructed on the combined system; that is, they would collect sewage from both buildings and streets. This was consistent with the best contemporary thinking and practice. As sewer construction progressed away from the river, the streets had to be raised beneath the sewers. After the sewers were laid, earth was filled in around them, entirely covering them. The packed-down fill provided roadbeds for new, higher streets. These streets were rounded in the center, with gutter apertures leading to the sewer. Such streets would stay dry and could be paved, as contrasted to the mud which had plagued the city previously.

A second facet of Chesbrough's sewerage plan involved dredging the Chicago River. The river had been dredged previously, but it was still too small to handle the anticipated sewage load. Chesbrough planned to widen and deepen the river, as well as to straighten its meandering course. Contracts for this work had been let to the partnership of John P. Chapin and Harry Fox. It was Fox who suggested using the dredgings from the river as fill around the sewers.[21]

It is interesting to digress on the consequences of Chesbrough's plan to raise the city. Where vacant lots existed, they were filled to the new level. A few old frame buildings were torn down, and the lots filled. It proved relatively easy to raise frame buildings to the new level, if the owners could afford it. The city's newer buildings were brick and stone, however, and they were constructed on the old level. These newer buildings would not be torn down, and many of Chicago's homes and offices were to be left "in the hole."

When new buildings and sidewalks were constructed on the higher level, Chicago increasingly became a city built on two levels.[22] Legal attempts to maintain the lower level were uniformly settled in favor of the city and its new level.[23]

The raising of brick buildings proved to be a difficult proposition. George Pullman, who later became famous for his "Palace cars," devised and instituted a method to raise brick buildings.[24] Pullman first used his method in connection with the Erie Canal enlargement of the 1850s, so Chesbrough would have known that the problems concomitant with raising the city's grade were surmountable. One of Pullman's biographers described his activities during those years:

> He made contracts with the State of New York for raising buildings on the line of the enlargement of the Erie Canal, which occupied about four years in their completion. At the end of that time, in 1859, he removed to Chicago, and almost immediately entered upon the work, then just begun, of bringing our city up to grade by the raising of many of our most prominent brick and marble structures, including the Matteson and Tremont Houses, together with many of our heaviest South Water street blocks. He was one of the contractors for raising by one operation, the massive buildings of the entire Lake street front of the block between Clark and LaSalle streets, including the Marine Bank and several of our largest stores, the business of all these continuing almost unimpeded during the process — a feat, in its class, probably without a parallel in the world.[25]

The Tremont Hotel was the first brick building which Pullman raised in Chicago. Soon his method was utilized to raise all Chicago's brick buildings from their former muddy level. The work required years. No one knows the cost, but it has been estimated at $10,000,000.[26]

In December 1856 the sewerage commissioners sent Chesbrough to visit several European cities in order to discover if their sewage disposal techniques were relevant to Chicago's needs.[27] Chicago was taking an open-minded approach to this question, and, evidently, the city was prepared to adopt an unconventional approach if it proved to be the best solution. The report of this trip, which Chesbrough submitted in 1858, represents one of the first sanitary engineering treatises.[28] Ches-

brough visited and reported on the sewerage of Liverpool, Manchester, Rugby, London, Amsterdam, Hamburg, Paris, Worthing, Croydon, Leicester, Edinburgh, Glasgow, and Carlisle. He concluded that none of these cities furnished an exact criterion to judge the effects of disposing sewage directly into the Chicago River, but he felt their collective experience suggested that it probably would be necessary to keep the river free of sewage accumulations.

Chesbrough ended his report by relating the European experience to Chicago's sewerage needs. Two points which Chesbrough made in this concluding section are worthy of special mention.[29] The first is the experience of Worthing, "a small watering town on the southern coast of England." At one time this town of 5,000 had drained directly into the sea, "but owing to offensive smells caused by this practice, and the consequent injury to the reputation of town as a watering place, upon which its prosperity very much depends," Worthing decided to find an alternative sewerage scheme.[30] Chesbrough concluded that Worthing's experience "shows that the mere discharge of filth into the sea gives no security against its being cast back in a more offensive state than ever, especially when the prevailing winds are toward shore," and that this suggests "the possibility of creating on the lake shore as great a nuisance as would be taken from the river."[31]

Second, Chesbrough included a prophetic paragraph which could serve as a summary to Chicago's sanitary history for a half-century thereafter:

> Under these circumstances it seems advisable to do nothing with regard to relieving the river at present, nor towards carrying out that portion of the plan which provides for forcing water from the lake into it, during the summer months. Should the Canal Company [the Illinois and Michigan Canal] not be obliged to pump enough during warm weather to keep the river from being offensive, it is understood that they would pump as much as they could for a reasonable compensation. This would furnish some criterion by which to judge of the probable effect of a still greater quantity driven in from the lake, according to the plan. The thorough [*sic*] cut for a steamboat canal, to the Illinois River, which the demands of commerce are calling more and more loudly for, if ever constructed, would give as perfect relief to Chicago as is proposed for London by the latest intercepting scheme.[32]

The Chicago River's south branch became quite polluted shortly after sewage was admitted into it. The Illinois and Michigan Canal's pumps, however, utilized south branch water to provide the canal's summit level, and, consequently, the pumps relieved a portion of the river's pollution load. The real significance of Chesbrough's statement lies in the fact that, as early as 1858, Chicagoans recognized the Illinois and Michigan Canal's sewage disposal potential.[33] In following years, the canal's pumps were used regularly to relieve the pollution load. Further, the canal itself was deepened and additional pumps were installed to increase the canal's capacity for handling sewage. Finally, the Chicago Sanitary District was formed in order to construct a new and enlarged canal to service Chicago's waste disposal needs, as Chesbrough had prophesied.

In 1861 the Board of Public Works was formed by incorporating the duties of the Board of Sewerage Commissioners, the Board of Water Commissioners, and other miscellaneous departments. Chesbrough was named chief engineer of this new board and, consequently, inherited the water-supply problem in addition to the waste-disposal problem. His inheritance was the "vicious circle" created by Lake Michigan's dual role as water supplier and eventual waste disposer.

## III

Chicago's continued population growth through the decade of the 1850s, the new sewerage works, and the expansion of packinghouses and distilleries had increased the number of pollutants drained into the Chicago River. Lake Michigan soon became fouled by the river's influx, and Chicagoans began to complain of the public water supply's offensiveness and pollution. The existing water intake was a wooden pipe which extended a few hundred feet out into Lake Michigan, one-half mile north of the Chicago River's mouth. In 1859, one of Chicago's water commissioners "proposed to sink a wrought iron pipe . . . one mile out into the lake, to obtain the supply from a point which could not be affected by the river."[34] Chesbrough was asked to study and report on the commissioner's plan, and to do the same on "erecting additional pumping works, in such locality as shall secure a supply of pure water."

Chesbrough's report discussed several methods without making a specific recommendation. Even at this early date, however, he considered a tunnel under the lake to be the most desirable alternative. Chesbrough was not afraid to combine grading, tunneling, and hydraulic principles to create a new water-supply system. When he later offered plans for a lake tunnel, his innovative proposal drew considerable opposition at the start and unmitigated acclaim when it proved successful.

Shortly after its formation in 1861, the Board of Public Works adopted as its goal the acquisition of an unpolluted water supply. Consequently, the board requested Chesbrough to make a canvass of the various water-supply possibilities and to investigate several filtration methods. Chesbrough dismissed the existing filtration methods as inadequate; his studied opinion was that the tunnel method was the most desirable:

> The engineer of the Board [E. S. Chesbrough], after much doubt and careful examination of the whole subject, became more inclined to the tunnel plan than any other, as combining great directness to the nearest inexhaustible supply of pure water, with permanency of structure and ease of maintenance. The possibility, and, in the estimation of many, the probability of meeting insuperable difficulties in the nature of soil, or storms, or ice on the lake, were fully considered. One by one the objections appeared to be overcome, either by providing against them, or discovering that they had no real foundation.[35]

Chesbrough continued to explore the tunnel plan's potential. When he had worked out the details, a proposal was submitted to several engineers, all of whom considered the tunnel plan to be feasible. Nevertheless, the 1861 board was against adopting the project. After a new board was elected and additional soil examinations had been made, Chesbrough's water-supply tunnel plan was adopted. The new board reported:

> What is most to be desired by the city is, that the supply should be drawn from the deep water of the lake, two miles out from the present Water Works. . . . The careful investigation of the subject has satisfied us sufficiently to say, that with our present knowledge, we consider it practicable to extend a tunnel of five feet diameter the required distance under the bed of the lake, the mouth or inlet to such a conduit being the out-

most shaft, protected by a pier [crib], which will be used in the construction of the tunnel.[36]

In their 1863 report, the Board of Public Works noted that three projects had been considered, any one of which would have afforded Chicago a healthier and better protected water supply. These were (1) a two-mile lake tunnel, (2) a filtering or settling basin, and (3) a one-mile lake tunnel located five miles to the north.[37] The board had two principal objections to the second plan. First, they commented:

> For settling and filtering the water from sediment, we are of the opinion that the basin would be found effective, and would continue to be so, but that for filtration it is not safe to rely upon it. There have been filtering basins of the character in other places. Some of them appear to have continued to work well during long use, and others have failed and become useless.[38]

Second, the board objected to the basin scheme because the water supply intakes would still be in the shallow water close to shore, and would not be located in a deeper point where the water was considered to be better.

Chesbrough's 1863 report acknowledged that the board had considered the three most promising possibilities and had rejected one; he was to assess the remaining two. Almost immediately he dismissed, on the grounds of greater cost, any project which required moving the existing water works, such as the board's third proposal:

> Other projects, such as erecting a new pumping works at Winnetka, or going to Crystal Lake and bringing a supply thence by simple gravitation, as is done for cities of New York, Boston, Baltimore, and Albany, have been considered, but their great cost, as compared with that of obtaining an abundant supply of good and wholesome water at points much nearer the city, is deemed a sufficient apology for not discussing their details here.[39]

Chesbrough concerned himself only with those plans which would bring water from a point two miles east of the existing Chicago Avenue Water Works, and there were two of these:

> Of the plans proposed for obtaining water from the lake, where it will be free from not only the wash of the shore, but from the effects of the river,

two classes only have been considered; one, an *iron pipe with flexible joints*; and the other, *a tunnel under the bottom of the lake*.[40]

Although the cost of the iron pipe project was slightly less than the tunnel project, Chesbrough chose between them on other than an initial cost basis:[41]

> In consequence of the possibility of such a pipe being injured by anchors, by the sinking of a heavily loaded vessel over it, or by the effect of an unusual current in the lake moving it from its place, it has been thought preferable to attempt the construction of a tunnel under the bottom of the lake.[42]

His research had convinced him that the tunnel's construction would be less difficult than was generally supposed. Lill and Diversey's brewery, adjacent to the water works, was the site of artesian borings which showed that, between 25 and 100 feet deep, the ground at the lake shore was a clay which was also found on the lake bottom where the water was 25 feet deep. A tunnel could easily be constructed in this type of clay, if it were continuous. Chesbrough was confident that the clay was continuous, but he admitted he was uncertain whether beds of sand might not be interspersed with the clay.[43]

The lake shaft was to be formed by sinking iron cylinders to the desired depth. Chesbrough noted that this was not a difficult problem in that the pneumatic process had been successfully employed on "the Theiss bridge in Hungary, and the railroad bridge across the Savannah River . . . and recently the Harlem bridge in New York."[44]

In giving cost estimates for the tunnel project's component parts, Chesbrough clearly showed the sources of his research. The principal source was the Thames tunnel, and Chesbrough noted that the first thoughts of most people were the great construction difficulties and "enormous" costs which had been encountered on the Thames project. He was quick to refute these thoughts and countered that "as we have every reason to believe, the clay formation here would shield us from such inroads of water as were met within the Thames tunnel operation."[45] In estimating excavation costs, Chesbrough made the same point: "There is good reason to believe that nothing in the soil here would be more difficult than that through which the sewers of London are sometimes tunneled."[46]

Chesbrough also used the Thames experience, plus that of the Boston Water Works tunnel, to estimate masonry costs. Cribs had been used principally in pier and breakwater construction, and Chesbrough based his crib cost estimates on figures which had been made for a proposed breakwater in Michigan City, Indiana, at the bottom of Lake Michigan.

After reaching his cost estimate for masonry and excavation, Chesbrough compared it with figures which had been reached for other major tunnel projects.[47] In particular, Chesbrough referred to reports from (1) the commissioner of the Troy and Greenfield Railroad, and (2) the Hoosac Tunnel. Included in the commissioner's report was the report of Charles Storrow, who had been sent to investigate European tunnels. Because the tunnels which Storrow had studied were for railroads, they were all much larger than the one which Chesbrough was planning. Therefore, Chesbrough estimated the cost of each tunnel had it been constructed with a five-foot width. From these estimates, he concluded that his cost estimate for the proposed water tunnel was reasonable.

The engineering achievement involved in constructing the water-supply system was no less significant than that represented by Chesbrough's sewer system. As conceived, the task was to dig a shaft near the lake shore to a depth significantly below the lake bottom and then burrow two miles beneath the lake. A similar shaft was to be dug at the lake end and was to be protected by a crib. The engineering problem was to connect the shore and lake points by a straight line 69 feet below the surface of Lake Michigan. Contemporary compasses could not be used since, below ground level, local attraction rendered them inaccurate. To a worker in the tunnel, the only place where the direction of the line drawn between the two shafts could be observed was at the top of either shaft. Consequently, when the engineers attempted to run the tunnel's axis parallel to this imaginary line on the lake's surface, they ran into difficulties affecting the turn from shaft to tunnel.[48]

When the lake shaft was completed, workers were lowered to begin burrowing westward to meet with the other workers burrowing eastward. The tunnel was sloped two feet per mile from the lake end to the shore so that it could be emptied should repairs prove necessary; the water would be shut off at the lake end. Although the methods were primitive — the tunnel was dug entirely by manual labor — it was claimed that the workers caused the two tunnel sections to meet within one inch of achieving a perfectly smooth wall.[49]

Chesbrough's engineering competence was coupled with a sense of economic reality, and these traits combined to insure the reputation he earned in Chicago. His 1863 report contained a section on "plans for improving the Chicago river." Chesbrough knew that moving the water-supply intake farther into the lake would not improve the river's offensive condition. In the 1855 sewerage report, he had argued that flushing canals would be necessary in both the north and south branches to purify the river, and he restated this position in several reports thereafter. By raising the issue once again, Chesbrough not only demonstrated the completeness of his approach, but also what one memorialist called "the characteristic firmness of conviction and modest persistence of Mr. Chesbrough."[50]

As before, Chesbrough's methodology was to enumerate and evaluate the possibilities for improving the river: (1) north and south branch flushing canals, (2) Des Plaines River diversion into the south branch, and (3) drainage southwest into the Illinois River Valley. The first was preferred because Chesbrough felt it was "undoubtedly feasible, would be completely under the control of the city, and there is every reason to believe [it] would be effectual."[51] He considered the second plan "defective" in that the Des Plaines River's flow was least when the Chicago River's pollution was greatest. Although Chesbrough correctly assumed that the third project would be the ultimate solution, he rejected it as "requiring much larger means than the Board can at present control."[52] Chesbrough's attention to Chicagoans' ability to pay established him as a practical man and lent credence to his innovative ideas. His consideration of a sanitary canal connecting the Chicago and Illinois Rivers indicates Chesbrough had learned that water-supply and waste-disposal problems are interdependent and must be solved simultaneously.

IV

Chicago is an urban center which had, and still has, serious water pollution problems. Lake Michigan's present pollution problem is primarily the result of industrial discharge in the Calumet and Indiana Harbor areas and the discharge of inadequately treated sewage by the North Shore Sanitary District (Lake County, Illinois) and several Wisconsin cities. Under normal circumstances, the Metropolitan Sanitary District of Greater Chicago diverts the sewage and the treated effluent from Lake Michigan. Presently, Chicago is meeting its responsibility with respect to Lake Michigan pollution. On the other hand, both the Chicago River and the Illinois River valley are polluted because some industries in the Chicago area still discharge their wastes into the water and the Sanitary District falls short of 100 percent treatment. Approximately 10 percent of the sewage goes untreated at this time, but it is the district's stated objective to achieve 100 percent treatment in the 1970s.[53] While these few sentences oversimplify a very complex situation, the outline is apparent. Chicago must seek outside help to reduce Lake Michigan pollution and the consequent threat to the city's water supply. Chicago and its Cook County suburbs, by themselves, could significantly reduce pollution in the Chicago, Des Plaines, and Illinois rivers.

When faced with Lake Michigan and Chicago River pollution in the 1850s and 1860s, Chicagoans had sought the best solutions available. Cost considerations had entered the argument only in deciding among equally effective methods; Chicagoans were not reluctant to pay the price necessary to secure sanitary conditions. They indebted the city through bond issues and themselves through tax assessments in order to finance these public works. Muddy streets and impure water were manifest physical representations of the city's problems, and solutions to these benefitted the city's residents, individually and collectively. The public's acceptance of an increased tax burden to finance these works must be viewed as public recognition of the problems' dimensions. If the city's water supply had not been conserved, and if the

city's natural topography had not been improved, Chicago's urban growth would have been severely limited.

When the pollution problem is explored in a historical context, students will find that the objectives which Chesbrough sought — minimize pollution and obtain a pure water supply — are the same as today's objectives. Nineteenth-century engineers, however, were not faced with the imminent "death" of large bodies of water; they were faced only with protecting urban populations from polluted water supplies.

In studying Chesbrough's works in Chicago, one gets the impression that today's pollution problem is not the result of ignorance as to pollution's effects, but ignorance as to how deadly the pollution load has become. In many cases, techniques first utilized in the 1850s and 1860s are still used today. Although these techniques no longer solve the problems for which they were intended, their inadequacies did not become apparent until recently. Perhaps this is because the demands on these techniques were much less heavy during the earlier period than they now are. Perhaps it is because the engineers of Chesbrough's generation made such dramatic innovations that the declining effectiveness of these techniques and improvements just recently became evident to sanitary engineers and laymen. Or perhaps it is because the 20th-century sanitary engineers who recognize the problem are unable to communicate the necessity for action. While the technology and technicians have been available, an uninformed and apathetic public has not invested sufficient capital in pollution control. Whatever the case, through inaction, the cost of proper treatment has reached a price which may be greater than the public is willing to pay. Unfortunately, the 20th century has been unable to find a sanitary engineer with the same farsightedness in his method, and resoluteness in seeing his proposals adopted, as that characteristic of Ellis Sylvester Chesbrough.

## NOTES

1   Benjamin Henry Latrobe, *The Journal of Latrobe* (New York, 1905), p. 98.

2   The engineering education of E. S. Chesbrough began in this company, and he quickly proved an apt student. See *Biographical Sketches of the Leading Men of Chicago,* written by the Best Talent of the Northwest (Chicago, 1868), p. 192; see also *Proc. Am. Soc. Civil Engrs.,* November 1889, *15*: 161.

3   See Daniel H. Calhoun, *American Civil Engineer: Origins and Conflict* (Cambridge, Mass., 1960), p. 38;

and Forest Hill, *Roads, Rails and Waterways* (Norman, Okla., 1957), pp. 12 ff.

4  Of particular interest to Chesbrough's later career is the fact that Long had carried out extensive exploratory surveys in the West. In 1816 Long was asked to report to the federal government on the physiographic features in the region of a proposed canal between Lake Michigan and the Illinois River. Although it is only speculation, one wonders how much knowledge of Chicago's topographical peculiarities Long passed on to Chesbrough. It is known that Long prepared detailed reports of his visit to Chicago. See Richard George Wood, *Stephen Harriman Long* (Glendale, Calif., 1966).

5  The major supply of engineers developed from what Calhoun called "the persisting pattern of on-the-job training." The supply provided by the leading scholastic source, the U.S. Military Academy, and the leading civilian source, the New York State canal system, was insufficient. The engineers of that day were active builders; thus, some form of on-the-job training had to be inaugurated to increase the supply and meet the demand. What developed was a hierarchical engineering corps. Lacking any formal education, Chesbrough learned every phase of his job by working his way up the civil engineering hierarchy.

In addition to the books by Hill and Calhoun (see n. 3 above), other recent books which discuss the oral transmission of engineering knowledge are Stephen Salsbury, *The State, the Investor, and the Railroad: The Boston and Albany, 1825–1867* (Cambridge, Mass., 1967); Harry N. Scheiber, *Ohio Canal Era* (Athens, Ohio, 1969); and Ronald E. Shaw, *Erie Water West* (Lexington, Ky., 1966).

6  Chesbrough's role in the Cochituate works is mentioned in a study of the waterworks of Boston, New York, Philadelphia, and Baltimore by Nelson M. Blake (*Water for the Cities* [Syracuse, 1956]).

7  The board was empowered to (1) supervise the drainage and sewage disposal of Chicago's three natural divisions; (2) plan a coordinated system for the future; and (3) issue bonds, purchase lots, and erect buildings implementing their plan. The board's actions were made subject to the Chicago City Council's approval. The act is summarized in several works including G. P. Brown, *Drainage Channel and Waterway* (Chicago, 1894), p. 50.

8  A. T. Andreas, *History of Chicago from the Earliest Period to the Present Time* (Chicago, 1884), I, 191; Bessie Louis Pierce, *A History of Chicago* (New York, 1940), II, 330; Soper, Watson, and Martin, *A Report to the Chicago Real Estate Board on the Disposal of the Sewage and Protection of the Water Supply of Chicago,*

*Illinois* (Chicago, 1915), p. 69, hereafter referred to as the *C.R.E.B. Report.*

9  It is quite possible that Jervis played a significant role in Chicago's choice, for during the early 1850s Jervis was professionally engaged in the Chicago area. Chicago's city fathers would have been aware of Jervis's engineering reputation, and it is probable that he was consulted regarding chief engineer candidates. Because he had worked with Chesbrough just prior to this, it is likely that Jervis gave Chesbrough an excellent recommendation.

In 1881 Chesbrough, serving as consulting engineer of the New Croton Aqueduct, employed Jervis, who discussed the work with Chesbrough daily. This indicates the esteem in which Chesbrough held Jervis, for Jervis was then 86 years old. Chesbrough, at 68 years of age, belonged to another generation.

10  Although the commissioners' report mentions the public's proposals, it does not indicate what they were, or even which parts of Chesbrough's plan were adapted from these suggestions.

11  Brown, *Drainage Channel*, p. 53.

12  *Report and Plan of Sewerage for the City of Chicago, Illinois,* adopted by the Board of Sewerage Commissioners, Dec. 31, 1855, hereafter referred to as the *1855 Report.* Also quoted in *C.R.E.B. Report,* p. 71. Chesbrough had a systematic approach to costs, but a very general approach to benefits. This evidently was consistent with the approach adopted on other U.S. internal improvement projects. See Lawrence G. Hines, "The early nineteenth century internal improvement reports and the philosophy of public investment," *J. Econ. Issues,* December 1968, *2:* 384–392.

13  Chesbrough planned to pump sufficient lake water into the north and south branches of the Chicago River to flush offensive solid pollutants. He also proposed flushing the sewers as well. See reprinted article, Langdon Pearse, "Chicago's quest for potable water," *Water and Sewage Works,* May 1955, *3.*

14  *1855 Report.* Also quoted in Andreas, *History of Chicago,* I, 191.

15  *C.R.E.B. Report,* p. 72; Pearse, "Chicago's quest," p. 3.

16  Brown, *Drainage Channel,* p. 53. To be precise, the Sanitary District's Sanitary and Ship Canal was the last step in Chicago's adoption of the dilution method. Ultimately, Chicago's growth was sufficient to require sewage treatment in addition to dilution.

17  *1855 Report.* Also quoted in Brown, *Drainage Channel,* p. 55.

18  R. Isham Randolph, "A history of sanitation in Chicago," *J. Western Soc. Engrs.,* October 1939, *44:*

229; Richard S. Kirby and Philip G. Laurson, *The Early Years of Modern Civil Engineering* (New Haven, 1932), p. 234; George W. Rafter and M. N. Baker, *Sewage Disposal in the United States* (New York, 1894), pp. 169–170.

19  *C.R.E.B. Report,* p. 69.

20  The grade which the city council adopted was lower than Chesbrough advocated, but it was sufficiently high to permit the construction of 7–8 foot cellars. The council's decision was to raise the grade to 10 feet on streets adjacent to the river; Chesbrough's higher grade was rejected because the city fathers felt there would be difficulties in locating sufficient fill. See *C.R.E.B. Report,* p. 70.

21  *Biographical Sketches,* p. 482. Fox's company was responsible for almost every topographical improvement in the Chicago area. The company deepened the Chicago River, developed the Chicago Harbor, installed road and railroad bridges, dredged the Illinois and Michigan Canal, and then performed similar services throughout the Midwest.

22  Randolph, "Sanitation in Chicago," p. 229. For many years, some sewers lay wholly above the ground, at the same level or higher than adjoining buildings.

23  "Up from the mud: an account of how Chicago's streets and buildings were raised," compiled by Workers of the Writer's Program, W.P.A. in Illinois for Board of Education, 1941. The raising of cities was relatively common. It was pointed out to me that all of downtown Atlanta was "raised" by the construction of roadways.

24  *Ibid.*

25  *Biographical Sketches,* p. 472. See also Seymour Currey, *Chicago: Its History and Its Builders* (Chicago, 1962), Vol. III; and Stanley Buder, *Pullman: An Experiment in Industrial Order and Community Planning, 1880–1930* (New York, 1967).

26  Lloyd Wendt and Herman Kogan, *Give the Lady What She Wants* (Chicago, 1952), p. 57. Wendt and Kogan do not say how they arrived at this number, and give no reference. Pullman reportedly received $45,000 for raising the Tremont Hotel. At $45,000 per brick building, $10,000,000 will raise over 200 buildings. This is probably an overestimate of the number of buildings raised, but the large number of other expenditures, including Chicago River dredging and legal expenditures, suggest that the $10,000,000 figure is an underestimate.

27  *Report of the Results of Examinations Made in Relation to Sewerage in Several European Cities, in the Winter of 1856–57,* published in Chicago by the Board of Sewerage Commissioners (1858), p. 3, hereafter referred to as the *1858 Report.* See also Randolph,

"Sanitation in Chicago," p. 229; Brown, *Drainage Channel,* p. 57.

28  *1858 Report,* p. 92. Chesbrough's memorialist in the *Proc. Am. Soc. Civil Engrs.* (November 1889, *15*: 162), unhesitatingly assessed the significance of Chesbrough's European trip report: "The importance of this report and the influence it exerted . . . can hardly be estimated. At the time the report was written, there was not a town or city in the United States that had been sewered in any manner worthy of being called a system. This being, perhaps, the first really exhaustive study which the subject had received on this side of the water, and Chicago being the first city to adopt a systematic sewerage system, the Chicago system soon became famous and Mr. Chesbrough, for twenty-five years, was the recognized head of sanitary engineering in this country." Modern usage would limit the term "sanitary engineer" to those men involved with water and sewage treatment. Apparently, the American Society of Civil Engineers at that time considered a sanitary engineer to be a man involved with sanitation works. Thus, while Chesbrough was not concerned with sanitary engineering as that discipline is currently defined, he must be considered a precursor of the modern sanitary engineer and, in fact, was called one by his peers and contemporaries.

29  On this trip Chesbrough visited Zaardam, near Amsterdam, to investigate the possibility of using windmills to pump flushing water for Chicago's sewers; he decided in favor of steam pumps (*1858 Report,* p. 29).

30  *1858 Report,* p. 39.

31  *Ibid.,* p. 93.

32  *Ibid.,* p. 94.

33  Nevertheless, in 1863, the Board of Public Works issued a report on purifying the Chicago River. This is discussed in Brown, *Drainage Channel,* ch. 6. The report recommended the construction of flushing canals along the lines of Fullerton Avenue and Sixteenth Street. Therefore, although the Illinois and Michigan Canal's potential was realized, city officials evidently were not ready to pursue it.

34  Brown, *Drainage Channel,* p. 32.

35  Reported in Brown, *Drainage Channel,* p. 33.

36  *Second Annual Report of the Board of Public Works to the Common Council of the City of Chicago* (April 1, 1863), p. 5, hereafter referred to as *1863 Report.*

37  Cost estimates for each of the projects were as follows: 2-mile lake tunnel exclusive of light house, $307,552; a filtering or settling basin, $300,575; a 1-mile lake tunnel 5 miles to the north, $380,000 (*ibid.,* p. 9).

38  *Ibid.,* p. 8.

39  *Ibid.,* p. 39.

40  *Ibid.*

41  Chesbrough roughly estimated the iron pipe scheme to cost $250,000. The choice seems to have been made on the basis of expected cost. *Ibid.,* pp. 40–41.

42  *Ibid.,* p. 41.

43  *Ibid.*

44  *Ibid.* Originally, Chesbrough planned on four shafts.

45  *Ibid.,* p. 43.

46  *Ibid.,* p. 45.

47  Chesbrough estimated the cost to be $13.54 per linear foot. *Ibid.,* p. 48.

48  J. M. Wing, *The Tunnels and Water System of Chicago* (Chicago, 1874), p. 33.

49  *Ibid.,* p. 76.

50  *Proc. Am. Soc. Civil Engrs.,* November 1889, *15*: 162.

51  *1863 Report,* p. 57. Chesbrough was concerned with a definite planning period which seems to reflect a longer time than the Marshallian short run, and a shorter time than the Marshallian long run.

52  *Ibid.*

53  It can now (1985) be noted that the district failed to achieve this objective.

# 32

## The Flamboyant Colonel Waring: An Anticontagionist Holds the American Stage in the Age of Pasteur and Koch

### JAMES H. CASSEDY

Despite the dramatic European discoveries of the 1870s and 1880s in the medical sciences, the contagionist findings of the dawning age of bacteriology had little substantial impact upon the American medical profession or upon American sanitary practices until the 1890s and afterward. To be sure, occasional pioneer laboratory investigators like George Sternberg, Daniel Salmon, and Theobald Smith were active and were making significant contributions before 1890. Likewise, professors like William H. Welch and T. Mitchell Prudden were slowly spreading the news from Europe through academic circles. Also, a handful of far-seeing health officers like Charles V. Chapin of Providence and Hermann M. Biggs of New York were already looking into the potent implications of the newly proved germ theory for their day-to-day sanitary work. Yet, these pioneers did not find quick success or ready acceptance in the United States for their contagionist conclusions. On the contrary, for most of the last quarter of the 19th century it was the concept of anticontagionism which continued to hold the dominant position in the thinking of American doctors and sanitarians. In the period just preceding its complete eclipse, anticontagionism was enjoying its greatest vogue.[1]

The most conspicuous leader of American anticontagionism during this time was the colorful Colonel George E. Waring, Jr. (1833–1898). A persuasive publicist, Waring became the leading propagandist for the country-wide adoption of every kind of basic sanitary facility, private and public. An

JAMES H. CASSEDY is Historian, History of Medicine Division, National Library of Medicine, Bethesda, Maryland.

Reprinted with permission from *Bulletin of the History of Medicine,* 1962, *36*: 163–176.

energetic and inventive engineer, he became one of the key individuals in the raising of sanitary engineering in the United States to the dignity of a profession. Not a physician, he nevertheless shaped American medical thinking of the period more than almost any doctor did.

Like Edwin Chadwick, Lemuel Shattuck, and certain other 19th-century sanitarians, Waring came into the public health movement by the side door, from an occupation in which he was not originally very much concerned with sanitation. Chadwick had first been a Poor Law bureaucrat, Shattuck a teacher and amateur genealogist. Waring started out as a farmer. After getting what training in agricultural chemistry and engineering was available in ante-bellum Poughkeepsie, New York, he toured Vermont and Maine lecturing upon scientific agriculture. Then, for a few years he was manager of Horace Greeley's farm at Chappaqua, New York. In 1857, when Frederick Law Olmsted and Calvert Vaux planned and started the construction of New York City's great Central Park, Waring joined their staff as an agricultural and drainage engineer. He stayed with this pioneer project through its virtual completion in 1861, at which time he was swept up in the Civil War. He spent four years as a cavalry officer in the Union army.

After the war Waring returned to his career as a scientific farmer, chiefly near Newport, Rhode Island. Elaborating upon his experience in this field, in a series of widely circulated technical books, he developed a reputation as an expert on scientific agriculture.[2] Waring also wrote popular horse stories.[3] As he began to enjoy a substantial income, he started going off on the European tours which were so fashionable. Then, in vivid travel accounts, which were published in *Scribner's* and the *Atlantic Monthly*, he told stay-at-home Americans about the things he had seen in Europe.[4] By the mid-1870s Waring was well-known to the American general reading public as well as to people in agricultural and engineering circles.

Waring's connection with the public health movement dates from the same immediate postwar period. Stimulated by his reading about the important achievements of English engineers and sanitarians since the 1840s, Waring gradually, as an adjunct to his work in agricultural drainage, became occupied with the whole broad range of problems associated with sanitary engineering. As his activities in this area multiplied, he found the most fertile sort of field for the exercise of both his engineering and his writing talents.

In 1867 Waring published the first of what would become a long list of popular and amazingly influential books, pamphlets, and articles upon various aspects of sanitation. This earliest sanitary publication from his pen, *Draining for Profit and Draining for Health*, was as strongly tinged with the materialism of the Gilded Age as it was with the idealism of the sanitary movement. With the work, however, Waring became established as a successful practical sanitarian.

To retain this reputation and to extend it still further, Waring had to be and was a persuasive sanitary salesman. One of his few failures in this capacity, however, came during this early period. In 1868 he acquired a financial interest in a British-designed earth closet. After getting his old friend Frederick Law Olmsted to help him make some modifications, Waring set about to sell it in the United States. Promotion of the earth closet involved making the most vigorous denunciation of the competing water closet. This Waring did by vividly painting the dangers to health from "sewer gas," the odor which often rose from defective water closets.[5] Despite his extensive propaganda, however, the earth closet did not have a large American sale. Rural people were satisfied with their privy vaults. On the other hand, those city Americans who were beginning to get away from the ancient privies were increasingly insisting upon water closets. This was particularly so as more water closets came on the market and as cities began to get adequate public water supplies. Waring, quickly sensing this trend, bowed to the

inevitable and soon gave up his interest in earth closets.

With no apparent serious pangs of principle, Waring now shifted his sales argument so that, from being one of its most outspoken critics, he became the most fervent advocate in America for the universal adoption of the water closet. The important point for him now was not only that the privy vault had to go, but that the water closet had to be properly built and correctly installed. Broadening out quickly, Waring became an ardent crusader against all of the perils to health which were then thought to exist with the presence in the home of faulty bathroom plumbing and in the community of inadequate sewerage systems.

By the mid-1870s this crusade was having considerable influence. In 1875 and 1876 he published, in the *Atlantic Monthly* and *Scribner's*, several series of popular articles on the sanitation and sewerage of houses and towns.[6] Henry I. Bowditch of Boston, himself among the most eminent of American sanitarians, was somewhat taken back by the "infinite gusto" with which Waring discussed such subjects on those traditionally polite pages.[7] But the readers of these magazines were convinced and shaken by this strenuous advocacy of sanitary works and better plumbing. In fact, as one highly qualified observer reported, Waring, in these articles, made New Englanders so vividly aware of the dangers to their health of sewer gas that they "feared it perhaps more than they did the Evil One."[8]

Sewer gas thus became to many Americans, as well as to many Europeans and Englishmen of the late 19th century, what miasmata had been to the people of many previous centuries. It came to be regarded as the source of virtually every communicable disease with the notable exception of smallpox. This was essentially the same traditional anticontagionist faith in the filth theory of disease and in environmental sanitation as that upon which Americans had relied since Noah Webster and Benjamin Rush had enunciated the principles before 1800. This was part and parcel of the same "sanitary idea" which Edwin Chadwick and Southwood Smith had devised in England in the 1840s. With cities becoming rapidly larger and progressively dirtier after the Civil War, and with the water closets of the day giving off as much odor as the privies, the anticontagionist sewer gas theory was highly plausible. In fact, as presented by the engineer-publicist Waring, it became as much a part of the armament of the late 19th century American anticontagionist as the "sanitary idea" itself or as the famous "groundwater theory" of disease of the great German scientist Max von Pettenkofer.

Waring's confident rationale of the causation of disease long carried more conviction for Americans than any of the arguments which the squabbling medical profession presented. In fact, during much of this period, a large part of that profession enthusiastically endorsed his views and accepted his leadership. This is not to say that Waring was an original thinker. Rather, he was the synthesizer and popularizer of the views of others. For example, from British medical literature and public health reports of the 1860s, he drew out material for a discussion of the so-called "filth diseases" which was widely circulated five years before John Simon elaborated his famous report on the same subject.[9] For this and other works, in order to bolster his attack on sewer gas (and, of course, to promote the sale of plumbing fixtures), Waring found some of his best arguments in the anticontagionist "pythogenic theory" of the prominent English clinician Dr. Charles Murchison.[10] In 1878, in order specifically to prove that typhoid fever was of spontaneous origin rather than contagious, Waring drew heavily not only upon the writings of Murchison but also on those of Chadwick and Pettenkofer. The resulting essay won for him the annual Fiske Fund Prize of the Rhode Island Medical Society.[11] Such an award, of course, reveals a great deal about the state of empirical medicine at that period. It also points up strongly the extent to which medical theory was then intertwined with the energetic but often dogmatic and a priori propagandizing of the engineer.[12]

In this 1878 essay, Waring argued persuasively, William Budd, Lister, and Koch notwithstanding, that there was "strong presumptive evidence of the correctness of Dr. Murchison's theory of a possible *de novo* origin," not only for typhoid fever but for almost all communicable diseases. He went on to trace disease outbreaks to such causes as a foul-smelling house drain or the proximity of a stagnant ditch. The poison itself, he said, might be due to "the exhalations of decomposing matters in dung-heaps, pig-sties, privy vaults, cellars, cesspools, drains, and sewers; or it may be due (according to Pettenkofer) to the development of the poison deep in the ground, and its escape in an active condition in ground exhalations." The remedy, of course, as he saw it, was obvious, particularly after the successes of the British sanitary revolution. This meant the removal of all of the sources of bad air, particularly through the installation of proper sanitary fixtures—drains, water closets, sinks, cesspools, sewers—all efficiently designed and provided with the elaborate valves necessary to keep sewer gas from coming up into houses. "Those more serious defects which come of ignorantly arranged plumbing work," Waring concluded, "are responsible not only for most of the zymotic diseases appearing in the better class of houses, but in like degree for the generally ailing condition of so many of those who pass most of their days and nights in these houses."[13]

The sanitation of the individual house which Waring advocated was, however, only part of the story. In order fully to prevent disease, according to the sanitary idea (which was also the ancient Hippocratean ideal of pure air, pure water, and pure soil), the entire community had to be cleansed. In the late 19th century several Americans were working on the problems this involved. Pioneers in the water purification experiments of these years included men like James B. Kirkwood of St. Louis, William R. Nichols of the Massachusetts Institute of Technology, the Lawrence investigators of slow sand filtration, and the Providence and Louisville investigators of mechanical filtration. In the evolution of modern sewage and refuse removal techniques, on the other hand, there were such important pioneers as Rudolph Hering of New York, Hiram Mills and his Lawrence associates, Samuel Gray and other Providence sanitarians—and Waring.

The sewerage systems of American cities before the Civil War almost without exception were haphazard and primitive affairs, little more than elongated open drains. This situation continued up to 1880 in most places, despite the development of scientific principles of sewer design and construction in England by Robert Rawlinson around 1850 and the beginning soon afterwards of modern systems in several large European cities. Engineers in Brooklyn, Chicago, Providence, and Boston had, by the 70s, drawn up good plans for sewers in those cities, but the construction of even these was hardly under way.[14] It took a yellow fever epidemic and the salesmanship of George E. Waring to get American sewer construction really under way.

In 1878 the city of Memphis, Tennessee, was decimated by the worst of a series of devastating yellow fever epidemics. Out of a population of some 40,000 to 50,000, over half, who had heard the chilling news that the disease was coming up the Mississippi River, fled the city. Among those who stayed on, nearly all developed yellow fever, and around 5,000 died from it. Some sanitarians pointed to the catastrophe as an argument for stricter quarantine measures. Waring, however, was one of a number who saw the epidemic as proof that quarantine, which had been tried for years, was not the answer to yellow fever. Beyond any doubt, he pointed out, the reason for the epidemic lay in the incredibly filthy condition of the city, and the only way to prevent future devastation was to institute thorough measures of internal sanitation immediately.

During the wave of public horror which followed the epidemic, President Hayes appointed Waring as one of three special commissioners who were to cooperate with the newly established National Board of Health in devising a plan for the sanitary improvement of Memphis. Never at a loss, Waring was ready with a plan, and he lost no time persuading the rest of the commission and the board to accept it. He then hired himself out to the city of Memphis to carry out a large part of the plan, the building of a complete sewerage system. Waring's energetic carrying out of this project during 1880 was a dramatic demonstration of modern sanitary engineering in the service of the sanitary idea. It provided a powerful impetus to the launching of sewer construction projects in all sizes of communities across the United States.

The Memphis episode was a fortuitous element in Waring's sanitary crusade. Apart from this, however, the episode led to something of a controversy among American engineers as to the respective merits of the two principal kinds of sewerage systems. Waring was the champion of the "separate" system, such as he had installed in Memphis. Not original with Waring, the separate system had been advocated in England by Edwin Chadwick as early as 1842 as a sanitary necessity. During the 1870s, however, Waring had obtained the American rights

to the system and had made certain modifications which he had patented. He thus had a substantial personal financial stake in this system, just as earlier he had had a stake in earth closets.[15]

The separate sewerage system, as opposed to the combined system, kept rain water apart from sewage and waste matter. Waring argued for the system such advantages as ease of ventilation, an absence of manholes, the use of smaller pipes, cheapness, and healthfulness.[16] Some other engineers argued equally forcefully the advantages of the combined system. When the argument came to a head in 1880, the American Public Health Association sent the respected engineer Rudolph Hering to Europe to investigate accepted European designs and principles of sewer construction. Hering's thorough report largely settled the controversy. It showed that combined systems were cheaper in densely populated areas such as large cities, while separate systems were cheaper in less settled areas. Technically and from the point of view of health, both were essentially sound.

Hering's report was an important factor in placing American sewer design from this time forward upon an increasingly rational basis. This did not mean, however, that Waring's interests suffered from the report. On the contrary, Waring had received much publicity for his separate or "Memphis" system, and he capitalized upon it to the full. He flooded the market with reports, brochures, and learned papers about the Memphis system and went as far afield as England to talk to sanitarians about his successes.[17] Presumably yellow fever, as a result of this work, had been banished from Memphis.

From this time on, Waring had more professional work than he could handle. He was in great demand as consulting engineer to sewerage projects, not only all over the United States but in Paris, The Hague, and other European cities. He was called in to advise on the sanitary condition of the White House. He was designated a special agent in charge of municipal social statistics for the Tenth Census.

Waring also played a prominent, if unenviable, part in the ill-fated National Board of Health. Elected secretary of that body, he had early recognized the danger to the board from the bitter opposition of Dr. John Hamilton of the Marine Hospital Service. When Congress met in 1884 to decide whether or not to continue the board, Waring testified vigorously in its behalf and against Hamilton's opposition to federal sanitary activity. But Hamilton had played his hand well in getting congressional support, and in this fight he turned out to be the stronger of the two. Never adequately supported, never fully understood by the democracy, and too far ahead of its times, the board was now allowed by Congress to pass out of existence.[18]

In and out of Newport, Rhode Island, during these years, Waring occasionally found time in which to experiment. In one of his experiments which had some significance, he pointed out the role which aeration could play in the processing of sewage.[19] But Waring did not fit well into the part of the patient, careful researcher. More than experimentation, he liked direct action of the sort that he had known ever since his cavalry service in the Civil War. He also liked to associate with the great and near great.

In Newport, therefore, he reveled in his role as sanitary shepherd for the vacation villas of the wealthy tycoons of American business and finance. His exact position was that of Consulting Engineer of the Sanitary Protection Association of Newport. This was a private group, founded in 1878, whose members subscribed for regular expert sanitary inspection and maintenance for their estates. It was an unusual private sanitary initiative, one which was taken in the absence of adequate public sanitary facilities. Waring did much, through his prestige as well as his actual participation, to make the organization a success. Although it had a European model, it was the first of its kind in the United States. During the 1880s and '90s, private groups in a number of other American cities — Brooklyn, Lynn, Trenton, Montreal, and Savannah, among others — followed this Newport initiative and founded similar cooperative sanitary organizations.[20]

Whatever sort of project Waring turned his hand to, he got things done, because he was a forceful and energetic person. He was a man of ingenuity and daring who was completely at home among the strongwilled individualists of these late 19th-century decades. He was also a man who had much of the showmanship and not a little of the sense of civic responsibility which Theodore Roosevelt was already beginning to display. All of these traits were displayed in abundance from 1895 to 1898,

when Waring was Commissioner of Street Cleaning for New York City under the anti-Tammany administration of Mayor Strong. As commissioner, Waring aggressively and quickly changed New York streets from among the dirtiest in the world to among the cleanest. To do this, he first formed an advisory committee of civic-minded citizens to help him survey the conditions and to advise him as to remedies. Then he set out to reorganize his department in order to raise its morale and efficiency. He took the personnel out of politics, put them all into white duck uniforms, and then put them on a career basis, with a for then novel Board of Arbitration to settle routine employee problems. He renovated the department's street-cleaning and garbage-collecting equipment. To obtain efficiency in his operation, he insisted that New Yorkers separate their refuse into three categories: garbage, ashes, and rubbish. Finally, in the East Side slum areas, he organized dozens of boys' and girls' clubs, whose members were to promote the city's cleanliness by reporting rubbish thrown into the streets and by themselves conducting cleanups of school yards and tenements. The children met in weekly meetings, wore special badges, and marched proudly with the regular street-cleaning battalions in the annual parade of New York's "white wings" or "white angels," an event which Waring had begun.

Some of these innovations did not last beyond Waring's term as Street Commissioner. The basic changes, however, constituted a permanent improvement of New York's street cleaning and garbage collection services. This provided a notable example for other cities and towns across the United States.[21]

Waring cleaned up the streets of New York in the name of health, just as his previous work had been in the name of health. To the anticontagionists of the day, he had long since become the highest type of hero of his age, the "apostle of cleanliness, the scourge of dirt."[22] For them, what he had done in New York was an essential step in applying the sanitary idea to the city. They followed him all the way in his Chadwickian belief that any kind of filth, anything that was dirty, was a dangerous source of possible disease and must be removed.

There were also others in New York during the 90s who were concerned with the prevention of disease. But these persons did not approach the problem through street cleaning. These others were contagionists who were caught up in the early enthusiasm of the age of bacteriology. T. Mitchell Prudden was one of the teachers who was showing the new generation of medical students the dangers of germs. Hermann M. Biggs was fighting tuberculosis through anti-spitting ordinances, careful medical inspection, and adequate hospitalization. William H. Park had been devising laboratory tests to determine the presence in individuals of the germs of diphtheria. In 1893 the New York City Department of Health built a diagnostic laboratory so it could make these tests on a routine basis. It also began to manufacture the new antitoxin to try to prevent and cure diphtheria.

All of these activities were beginning to undermine the position of New York anticontagionists. But New York was a large place. There was still plenty of room, during the 1890s, for both camps, for both beliefs. In fact, this was true not just in New York but everywhere, at least as long as yellow fever remained a mysterious disease apparently caused, so far as anyone could tell, by spontaneous generation in filth. The resolution of this mystery soon after 1900 constitutes an ironic final commentary upon Waring's career.

In 1898, with the return of Tammany Hall to power in New York City, Waring was out of a job. This was the year of the Spanish-American War. After the cessation of hostilities in Cuba, the United States army commanders were gravely concerned with dangers from yellow fever to the troops who would for several years have to occupy Havana and other cities of the island. To meet this serious threat from disease, the army enlisted an outside commission of experts to select camp sites and make suggestions for their proper sanitation. The commission was also charged with making a thorough investigation of the sanitary condition of Havana and other Cuban cities and recommending the measures necessary to stamp out yellow fever and other communicable diseases.

Waring was chosen chairman of the commission and went to Cuba early in October of 1898. In his short stay of just under three weeks he learned everything that he wanted to know. It was, of course, no news to anyone that Havana was one of the filthiest cities in the western hemisphere. Waring merely confirmed that there were virtually no sewers; that garbage, rubbish, and feces were thrown freely into the streets; that public markets were nauseatingly foul; that house privies were so neglected that their contents frequently flowed over into yards and wells; that the street cleaning department had virtually no money; and that there was no systematic plan for garbage collection or disposal. He noted that there was a good water supply to the city but that there were extensive marshes which promoted bad malarial conditions.

To Waring, the answer to these conditions was an obvious one. For the sum of ten million dollars, he said, he could eliminate yellow fever from Havana. He would construct a complete sewerage system, pave all of the streets, drain all of the marshes. He would build a municipal garbage incinerator, establish sanitary markets and abattoirs, eliminate all privy vaults, and introduce water closets universally. He would reorganize the department of public cleansing and put it upon an efficient basis.[23]

His survey completed, Waring left Cuba before the end of October. On the way back to the United States he wrote up the first draft of his report and recommendations. The day after his arrival in New York he fell ill. Four days later, he died of yellow fever.

Many people mourned Waring's untimely end. One observer argued that he had been a victim of American expansionism. Another wrote, still more aptly, that "his death at the hands of the king of dirt diseases gives a mournful but most impressive emphasis to the lesson which he taught so earnestly of the kinship of dirt and disease."[24] Feeling much the same way as this second commentator, the army commanders in Cuba acted quickly upon Waring's recommendations. Everything that he had considered necessary for the health of the troops was done. In the process Havana was changed in a few months from one of the dirtiest into one of the cleanest cities in the Americas. It was a transformation which excited the admiration of the world. It was widely hailed, moreover, as a great triumph for the anticontagionist viewpoint, for the sanitary idea. The success of Memphis was clearly being repeated in Havana.

Unfortunately for the partisans of anticontagionism, despite all that had been done, yellow fever remained rampant in Havana. As never before, people began to realize that, despite its many salutary effects, cleanliness by itself was not the answer. The army now had to start all over again. This time, however, it chose a totally different kind of approach. Now it was the Yellow Fever Commission, under the laboratory-oriented Major Walter Reed, which moved in. Quickly, the commission sifted the available facts and theories, and ultimately it took up the little-regarded mosquito hypothesis of Carlos Finlay. Inevitably, new heroes, who exposed themselves alternately to filth and to mosquito bites, were made in the control wards of the commission. And, inexorably, the participants moved forward to a conclusion. Filth as such as shown to play no causative role in the disease. Instead, the mosquito known as the stegomyia was correctly singled out and proven to be the carrier of the yellow fever poison. Finally, then, it was up to William Crawford Gorgas and his engineers to search out and destroy every breeding place of the stegomyia. This done, yellow fever was eradicated and the American forces were safe in Havana.[25]

Even before the Reed Commission's findings were published, alert and scientifically trained health officers of the new era (Charles V. Chapin of Providence stood out among them) were already proclaiming "the end of the filth theory of disease."[26] But the commission's work drove the "coffin nail" into the remnants of the anticontagionists' belief. After 1900, no great new champion of the filth theory emerged in the United States to take Waring's place. The laboratory researchers and scientific public health men of the age of bacteriology in a few years enjoyed an almost complete dominance in national public health circles. The filth theorists who remained, a dogmatic and narrowly unprogressive minority for the most part, could only mutter ineffectually and fade into the backwash of the public health movement. There, at local levels, as Martin Arrowsmith would find out, they delayed the spread of the new scientific doctrines and techniques for some years. But they would never emerge from the backwash. Waring had died just in time, while he still had valid reason to think that he was right. His followers found themselves in the untenable position of holding inflexibly to an idea which had been shown to be only half right. Filth in the form of human excrement certainly caused disease, but the laboratory men pointed out that there was no direct connection between infectious disease and such general dirty things as decaying potatoes, bad smells, untidy streets, or trash in vacant lots.

With his view discredited, Waring quickly came to be remembered by the laboratory men chiefly as one of those who, despite the more accurate knowledge about the infectious diseases which flowered after 1875, had still clung to the crude ideas of an earlier age.[27] In the far-sweeping age of bacteriology, the engineer could no longer influence medical theory as Waring had done unless he were also a precise laboratory scientist.

Most of the laboratory men of the early 20th century could not see that Waring, like his master Edwin Chadwick and the other filth theorists, had in fact made a great contribution to mankind in carrying through with the sanitary idea. They could not see that the insistence upon sewers, pure water, water closets, and clean streets for our cities was a major civilizing influence. During the early reign of the laboratory men, the vague general approach to disease through the eradication of dirt on the basis of a priori reasoning was considered to be incompatible with the precise a posteriori approach of specific measures for particular diseases.[28] It would be 20 or 30 years or more before health officials could begin again to see value to the public health in both approaches. With such a revised perspective, there would be a better chance, perhaps, for an effective social medicine to take hold.

## NOTES

1   This is by no means an original finding. The student of this subject will already be familiar with articles by such authors as Erwin Ackerknecht and Phyllis A. Richmond.

2   *Elements of Agriculture,* originally published in 1854 as a "book for young farmers," was reissued in 1868. In 1869 Waring published a revision of W. S. Court-

ney's, *The Farmers' and Mechanics' Manual. Waring's Book of the Farm*, which first appeared in 1877, went through several editions. In 1881, he published *The Saddle Horse*, a training and riding guide.

3   See, for instance, *Whip and Spur* (1875), *Ruby* (1883), and *Vix* (1883).

4   As subsequently published in book form, these in-

cluded *A Farmer's Vacation* (1876), *The Bride of the Rhine* (1878), and *Tyrol and the Skirt of the Alps* (1880).

5  G. E. Waring, Jr., *Earth Closets: How to Make Them and How to Use Them* (New York: Tribune Association, 1868); and *Earth Closets and Earth Sewage* (New York: Tribune Association, 1870).

6  These articles were quickly collected and published in book form; *The Sanitary Drainage of Houses and Towns* (New York: Hurd and Houghton; Cambridge, Mass.: Riverside Press, 1876) was the most influential and went through several editions. Others included *The Sanitary Condition of City and Country Dwelling Houses* (New York: D. Van Nostrand Co., 1877) and *Village Improvements and Farm Villages* (Boston: J. R. Osgood & Co., 1877).

7  Henry I. Bowditch, *Public Hygiene in America* (Boston: Little, Brown, 1877), *passim*.

8  Charles V. Chapin, "Science and public health," in *Papers of Charles V. Chapin, M.D.,* (New York: Commonwealth Fund; London: Oxford Univ. Press, 1934), p. 50.

9  Waring, *Earth Closets and Earth Sewage, passim*; John Simon, *Filth Diseases and Their Prevention* (Boston: J. Campbell, 1876).

10  Murchison's most famous work was *A Treatise on the Continued Fevers of Great Britain* (London: Parker, Son, and Bourn, 1862).

11  Waring, "The causation of typhoid fever," in *First Annual Report of the State Board of Health of the State of Rhode Island* (Providence, 1879), pp. 159–173.

12  Almost 20 years later Waring was still accorded an honored place in American medical circles. In 1896, for instance, he delivered the "annual address in medicine" at Yale University, a talk on the subject of "The proper disposal of sewage."

13  Waring, "Causation of typhoid fever," pp. 159, 161, 163, 172.

14  For further historical details on these developments, see Rudolph Hering, "Sewage and solid refuse removal," in *A Half Century of Public Health,* ed. M. P. Ravenel (New York: American Public Health Association, 1921), pp. 181–196; G. W. Fuller et al., "Historic review of the development of sanitary engineering in the United States during the past one hundred and fifty years: a symposium," *Tr. Am. Soc. Civil Engrs.,* 1928, *92*: 1207–1324; and W. P. Gerhard, "A half century of sanitation," *Am. Architect & Bldg. News,* 1899, *63* (Nos. 1209, Feb. 25; 1210, March 4; 1211, March 11): 61–63, 67–69, 75–76.

15  Gerhard, "A half century of sanitation," p. 67.

16  Waring, "The sewering and draining of cities," *Public Health: Papers and Reports,* 1880, *5*: 35–40.

17  Gerhard, "A half century of sanitation," *passim*.

18  For a further account of this controversy, see Wilson G. Smillie, *Public Health: Its Promise for the Future* (New York: Macmillan, 1955), pp. 337–338.

19  Kenneth Allen, "Remarks," in Fuller et al., "Historic review," p. 1294; also Waring, *The Purification of Sewage by Forced Aeration* (Newport, R.I.: F. W. Marshall, 1895).

20  See Horatio R. Storer, "Sanitary protection in Newport," *Public Health: Papers and Reports,* 1881, *6*: 209–216.

21  For details of Waring's work in New York, the reader may consult the various meagre biographical sources, most important of which are the following three articles: "George E. Waring, Jr.," *D.A.B.,* XIX, 456–457; William Potts, "George Edwin Waring, Jr.," obit. in *The Charities Review* (N.Y.), 1898, *8*: 461–468; and Albert Shaw, *Life of Col. George E. Waring, Jr.* (New York: Patriotic League, 1899). Despite its title, the Shaw pamphlet is far from a thorough biography. Rather, it consists of a short (10 page) tribute, together with excerpts from several newspaper obituaries. More valuably, however, it includes a résumé of Waring's uncompleted report on Havana, together with a short paper written by Waring in 1897, "New York, AD 1997—a prophecy." This last is a short but interesting projection into the future, somewhat in the tradition of *Utopia, New Atlantis,* or more particularly, Benjamin Richardson's *Hygeia: A City of Health,* which had been having a considerable vogue for two decades among both contagionists and anticontagionists.

22  Quoted in Shaw, *Life of Col. Waring, Jr.,* p. 31. Also see Potts, "George Edwin Waring, Jr.," p. 462.

23  For details of Waring's report on Havana, see résumé in Shaw, *Life of Col. Waring, Jr., passim.*

24  Quoted, *ibid.,* pp. 30, 31.

25  For the full dramatic story of the Reed Commission and its work, there is still no better source than Howard Kelly, *Walter Reed and Yellow Fever* (New York: McClure, Phillips & Co., 1906).

26  Charles V. Chapin, "The end of the filth theory of disease," *Popular Science Monthly,* 1902, *60*: 234–239.

27  *Ibid.,* p. 239.

28  See James H. Cassedy, "Dr. Charles V. Chapin and the modern public health movement" (Ph.D. dissertation, Brown Univ., 1959), ch. 17.

# 33

## Insecticide Spray Residues and Public Health, 1865–1938

### JAMES C. WHORTON

The current controversy over the threat to public health posed by pesticide residues on foods is commonly assumed to have been initiated by the 1962 publication of Rachel Carson's *Silent Spring*. One student of the subject has even divided the history of crop pest control into two eras — BC, Before Carson, and AC, After Carson — and suggested that only during these latter days has man realized "that pesticides were not the panacea heralding the millennium."[1] Chemical insecticides, however, primarily in the form of inorganic arsenic compounds, had been the subject of debate for nearly a century before the Carson attack on the misuse of organic pesticides. The importance of this debate, though, is not confined to its having served as a prologue to *Silent Spring*. The history of the problem of insecticide residues during the late 19th and early 20th centuries serves a broader function as an illustration of the special difficulties associated with the recognition and regulation of public health hazards caused by chemical contamination of the human environment.

### I

Insects have always competed with man for the fruits of his agricultural labors, though perhaps never more successfully than in 19th-century America.[2] The rapid opening of huge areas of land to agriculture and the introduction of labor-saving machinery both encouraged the transformation of America's subsistence farmers into businessmen profiting from the large-scale cultivation of specific products. The extensive monoculture which came

JAMES C. WHORTON is Professor of Biomedical History at the University of Washington, Seattle, Washington.

Reprinted with permission from the *Bulletin of the History of Medicine*, 1971, *45*: 219–241.

to characterize American agriculture during the second half of the 19th century, however, soon proved to be a two-edged sword, for the covering of vast fields with a single crop also provided insect pests of that crop with an abundant food supply and stimulated insect proliferation. As a consequence, the pages of American agricultural journals of that day were filled with the lamentations of farmers defeated by such unlikely sounding enemies as the codling moth, the Rocky Mountain locust, and the Colorado potato beetle.

Agricultural defeat seemed at first inevitable, for the sudden increase in insect numbers had rendered the farmer's primitive defenses obsolete. The young science of economic entomology, moreover, whose business it was to advise agriculturalists how to combat insect depredations, was similarly unprepared for the intensified insect offensive. Thus even into the 1860s, by which time farmers were desperate for improved "insect remedies," entomologists were still praising Harris's 20-year-old manual as the best source of information on the destruction of insect pests.[3] Harris's remedies, however, were almost exclusively slow and laborious variations of hunting or luring the insects and then crushing them by hand. More imaginative techniques were occasionally suggested, but even these were generally inefficient physical methods. Thus Townend Glover, the first economic entomologist to be employed by the United States government, recommended that infested plants be syringed with whale oil soap and that the insects which fell from the slippery leaves then be stamped to death.[4]

Chemical methods of insect control had been used sporadically since antiquity and had attracted some attention from 19th-century American entomologists,[5] but on the whole, economic entomologists shared the opinion of the editor of the *Practical Entomologist*, that "if the work of destroying Insects is to be accomplished satisfactorily, we feel confident that it will have to be the result of no chemical preparations, but of simple means, directed by a knowledge of the history and habits of the depredators."[6] Thus when the Colorado potato beetle began its destructive eastward advance during the 1860s, professional entomologists placed their hopes for halting its march on physical techniques. They were particularly enthusiastic about the development of a horsedrawn vehicle designed to dislodge beetles from potato plants and crush them under heavy rollers. This mechanical marvel even moved one prominent entomologist to observe that "the world certainly does move," and then to ask proudly, "Who would have believed fifty years ago, that in the year 1867 we should be slaying Bugs by Horse-power?"[7] The gentleman's astonishment at the progress of technology would have been even greater, one suspects, had he been aware that in the very year of his writing, in response to the excesses of the same potato beetle, there was being introduced a method of insect control which would shortly outmode even "Horse-power."

By the mid-1860s, it was evident to many farmers that the traditional approach to pest control was no longer adequate, and it was simply a matter of time before someone would realize that poisoning potato beetles *en masse* might be more effective and less time-consuming than crushing them individually. There is no record of the earliest testing of this theory,[8] but by the autumn of 1868 the editors of the *American Agriculturalist* were warning their subscribers of some "unsafe advice":

> The following is going the rounds of the press. "Sure death to Potato Bugs: Take 1 lb. Paris green, 2 lbs. pulverized lime. Mix together, and sprinkle the vines." We consider this unsafe, as there is no intimation of the fact, not generally known, that Paris green is a compound of arsenic and copper [copper aceto-arsenite], and a deadly poison. Such things should never be recommended without a full statement of their properties, so that one may know with what he is dealing. The poison would be very likely to kill the potato bugs, but how about the vines?[9]

In spite of this warning, use of the new method spread quickly. Within the next decade, Paris green, a common, inexpensive pigment, was being applied, both as a powder and as a water spray, to many crops other than potatoes. During the 1880s, Paris green was rivaled in popularity by London purple, an arsenical by-product of the aniline dye industry, though the close of the century saw both these poisons being replaced in the farmer's favor by lead arsenate. This last compound of two toxic metals was to remain the most popular of all insecticides until the release of DDT for public consumption after World War II.

The eventual success of the arsenical insecticides should nevertheless not be allowed to obscure the initial hesitancy of the agricultural community to use them. Many farmers, in fact, shunned Paris green at first, fearing that the poison might not confine its action to the beetles. As the *American Agriculturalist's* warning indicates, however, much of this early reluctance to use arsenic as an insecticide stemmed from misgivings about its possible economic drawbacks, rather than from hygienic considerations. Thus it was feared that arsenicals might injure plant foliage, which indeed proved to be the case,[10] though this problem was easily overcome by diluting the arsenic with larger quantities of lime, flour, or ashes for dry application, and with more water for sprays. There was agricultural anxiety as well over the effects of arsenic on soil fertility, especially after Glover reported in 1870 that his preliminary experiments conducted at the Department of Agriculture indicated that arsenic in the soil interfered with plant growth.[11] The more complete experiments of William McMurtrie, the Department's chemist, however, suggested that harmful soil concentrations of arsenic could not be reached in actual practice,[12] and the question of arsenical poisoning of soils was dismissed, only to be reasserted 30 years later.[13] The poisoning of their livestock was also feared by farmers, and apparently with good reason, for more than a decade after the introduction of Paris green as an insecticide, agricultural journals were still complaining that "'familiarity has bred contempt' for this dangerous substance, and there have been more horses, cows, pigs and fowls lost by poisoning [during the past season] than ever before."[14] All these cases, however, could be blamed on gross carelessness, such as the leaving of used containers of Paris green in areas frequented by farm animals. Such accidents could easily be avoided, but there were other sources of exposure less amenable to control. In particular, many fruit growers had to graze livestock in their orchards but were afraid the animals might be poisoned by eating the grass beneath trees sprayed with arsenicals. This apprehension was relieved by A. J. Cook, entomologist at Michigan Agriculture College and perhaps the leading propagandist for the safety of arsenical insecticides. Cook sprayed one of his fruit trees with double-strength London purple, allowed it to drip dry onto the grass below, then cut the grass and fed it to his own horse.[15] The beast survived, in apparently good health, as did a sheep on which the experiment was repeated.

Thus by 1890, agricultural scientists had established to their satisfaction that arsenical insecticides, when properly used,[16] would not harm crops or livestock. Farmers, however, had not been so preoccupied with their produce and animals that they had overlooked the danger to themselves. Late in the century, the entomologist C. H. Fernald recalled that many farmers had initially refused to use arsenicals for fear of poisoning themselves and their families:

> There was bitter opposition to the use of these insecticides for a long time, and the reports of cases of poisoning, which were said to have occurred at that time, were startling in the extreme. It was even claimed that potatoes would absorb the poison to such an extent that the tubers would carry poisonous doses, so that after each meal it would be necessary to take an antidote for the poison.[17]

Most of this opposition was short-lived, however, for the exigencies of insect control could be satisfied only by arsenic. Sooner or later, most farmers embraced the persuasion of S. L. Allen, who "was quite afraid to use it, until I found something must be done, or we would lose our whole crop, and until after trying a few rows, and watching the effect and making calculations of the chance of poisoning."[18] Farmers were encouraged in their adoption of this attitude by the agricultural press, which proclaimed that "no other poison than arsenic in some form is effective, or applicable on the large scale," while denying that arsenicals had caused any "authentic case of . . . injury."[19]

Similar assurances of safety issued from scientific sources. In his study of arsenical soils, for instance, McMurtrie concluded that potatoes do not absorb arsenic from the soil,[20] an observation corroborated by the experiments of the chemist Kedzie.[21] As the application of arsenicals was extended to crops other than potatoes, however, fears of poisoning developed anew, for the treated produce was no longer underground, where it could be poisoned only by absorbing arsenic from the soil. Most fruits and vegetables were exposed directly to arsenical sprays and had, in fact, to be covered with the spray in order to be protected. Such protection could be self-defeating, though, if the apple was saved from the worm only to be poisoned by arsenic, so the question of the level of arsenic residues on sprayed produce assumed great significance for 19th-century entomologists. Of the resultant attempts to determine these levels, the most influential was that of Cook, who concluded in 1880 that arsenical sprays of normal concentration were completely removed from fruit by wind and rain within three weeks after application.[22] Hence it seemed safe to eat arsenically treated fruit that had not been picked shortly after spraying, though Cook suggested that fruit should nevertheless be washed thoroughly before being eaten.

Cook's cautious optimism was shared by his fellow entomologists, for although not all of the other studies of arsenical residues concurred in the observation that arsenic was completely removed by weathering, they did generally agree that, even when present, residues were too small to be harmful.[23] The produce subjected to chemical analysis, however, had been sprayed according to entomological recommendations for strength of spray and frequency of application, recommendations which were not necessarily followed outside agricultural experiment stations. American farmers, after all, have always been notoriously independent, and when faced with a threat to their crops they might be expected to rely more on their own judgment than on that of some experiment station theoretician presumably unacquainted with the practical hardships of husbandry. Consequently entomological complaints of farmers spraying too heavily and too often were not uncommon. One entomologist grumbled that although his state experiment station had never recommended more than three arsenical sprayings per season, it was a common practice among farmers in his state to spray as many as nine times![24] Another reported that more than one farmer had personally confided that his philosophy of spraying was "that if twice a month is good, four or five times as often would be a great deal better."[25]

Thus it was recognized by entomologists that marketed produce might carry residues of arsenic greater than the low levels found in their controlled experiments. This possibility seemed to be no cause for alarm, however, for it could easily be calculated that even if none of the insecticide from the heaviest spraying was removed by weathering, the quantity of arsenic adhering to the surface of an apple would still be far below the lethal dose of two to three grains, and "a person would be obliged to eat at one meal eight or ten barrels of . . . fruit in order to consume enough arsenic to cause any injury."[26] Agricultural scientists were concerned only with the question of acute arsenical poisoning, and the possibility of chronic arsenicism was not seriously considered except by Kedzie, who agreed that "any of the doses of arsenic . . . found in a pound of these fruits might be swallowed without endangering life by such single dose," but who also feared that "it is the repeated doses, day by day . . . that might produce slow poisoning and the gradual undermining of the health without obvious cause."[27]

Yet if the hazard of chronic arsenic poisoning was not generally appreciated in agricultural circles, it was a subject of much interest to the medical profession. Arsenic had been used medicinally since antiquity, but it achieved its peak of therapeutic popularity during the 19th century, when it came to be employed, especially in the form of Fowler's solution, in the treatment of almost all skin diseases and, at one time or another, it appears, for virtually every other type of ailment as well. Arsenic's rise in medical favor, however, was paralleled by a growing store of evidence that the drug was being abused, and that its prolonged administration might lead to chronic skin and nervous disorders in some patients,[28] and even to skin cancer in others.[29] Physicians were aware, furthermore, that exposure to arsenic was not limited to patients under the watchful eye of a doctor. The fame of Fowler's solution as a specific for skin ailments, for example, had suggested to several imaginative entrepreneurs the inclusion of arsenic in cosmetic products such as the "sulphide of arsenicum," which promised to give ladies complexions "to rival the lily and the rose."[30] Domestic contact

with arsenic, however, was not reserved exclusively for the fairer sex, for the pigments Paris green and Scheele's green (copper arsenite) were used to color a wide variety of products ranging from house paints to water colors, fabrics, candles, food wrappers, construction papers used in kindergartens, playing cards, concert tickets, artificial flowers, even confectionery! All of these items attracted medical criticism as potential sources of arsenic poisoning, but the greatest concern of all was expressed over the use of arsenical pigments in wall papers. Numerous cases of both acute and chronic arsenicism were traced to green wallpapers from which the poison had been released as a dust and as the gas ethyl arsine.[31]

In view of this medical concern for the chronic effects of arsenical medicines and manufactures, it might be expected both that agriculturalists would have reevaluated their position on the safety of arsenical residues and that the medical profession would have criticized the unrestricted application of arsenic to food crops. With the previously cited exception of Kedzie, however, agricultural scientists failed to appreciate the hazard of chronic arsenicism and, well into the 20th century, were still defending arsenical sprays on the grounds that they left residues smaller than the standard medical dose of arsenic and therefore could not be harmful.[32] Such arguments should have provoked refutations from physicians, but the medical profession maintained a virtually unbroken silence on the question of arsenical insecticides.[33] This silence was perhaps due in part to medical ignorance of agricultural practice, for the campaign against other arsenical contaminants, as well as for sanitary reform generally, was led by urbanites concerned with the health problems of the cities. Such men might have been unaware of the use of arsenic as an insecticide and surely would have been more inclined to look for food adulterants in processed items than in nature's own, presumably unalloyed, produce.

It is suspected, however, that the medical profession's reticence on the subject of arsenical insecticides was due less to lack of familiarity with rural customs than to uncertainty about arsenic toxicology. The fears of epidemic chronic arsenical poisoning expressed by some physicians had to compete with the belief held by others that small amounts of arsenic were harmless, and even that continued exposure to low levels of the poison could produce immunity. This latter belief was associated with the tradition of the Styrian arsenic-eaters, the peasants of southeastern Austria who, since mid-century, had gained ever-increasing medical renown for their practice of regularly consuming normally lethal quantities of arsenic with impunity. The Styrians claimed to be able to develop a tolerance for the poison by taking it first in small amounts and then gradually increasing the dosage, while the benefits of this bizarre dietary supplement were believed to be improved complexion, greater stamina, and increased sexual appetite. Although these claims were initially received with scepticism,[34] verification of the Styrians' ability to survive massive doses of arsenic[35] eventually converted many doctors to a belief in the possibility of habituation to arsenic and gained for that substance a reputation as a healthful stimulant.[36] Consequently, criticism of arsenical wallpapers and similar items often provoked only such cavalier responses as that made by the editors of the *Medical Record*, who observed that "the conclusion to be drawn . . . is obviously that it is inexpedient to eat wallpaper unless one . . . is in need of a strong tonic."[37] Others, observing that most of the leaders of the antiarsenic campaign were residents of Boston, saw in "arseniophobia" simply the latest expression of Yankee eccentricity. "There seems to be an appalling possibility," one New York physician despaired, "that Massachusetts is being systematically poisoned by an inoculable, malignantly infective, and extremely prevalent form of arsenical poisoning. We rejoice to learn that the Legislature and State Board of Health are at work upon the question."[38]

In an atmosphere in which even the well-documented hazard of arsenical wallpapers was given no more serious reception than this, it is hardly surprising that the matter of insecticide residues, supposed to contain considerably less arsenic than most wallpapers, was almost completely ignored by the medical profession. Only the Boston physician W. B. Hills seems to have publicly criticized the use of arsenical insecticides, and even his opposition was less than vigorous. Detecting large quantities of copper and arsenic in the urine of one of his patients, and unable to find any other source for these metals, Hills suggested that the patient's illness had been caused by Paris green

residues and further cautioned that "we may have, in the free use of Paris green in the garden and field, one explanation of the frequent occurrence of arsenic in the system."[39]

Hills' mild reproach was not the only instance, however, of medical opposition to chemical pesticides. During the autumn of 1891, agents of the New York City Board of Health confiscated and destroyed considerable quantities of Hudson Valley grapes bearing residues of Bordeaux mixture, a fungicide composed largely of copper sulfate.[40] Agricultural scientists uniformly denounced the action, charging that the condemned fruit had contained so little copper that "one would need to eat from one-half to one ton of these grapes, stems, skins and all, to obtain the least injurious effect."[41] B. T. Galloway, Chief of the Division of Vegetable Pathology, United States Department of Agriculture, hastened to New York to conduct a personal investigation of the affair and subsequently criticized the Board of Health for making "a mountain out of a molehill."[42] This judgment was exploited by the popular press, which took the Board to task for its irresponsible action causing serious economic losses to the state's vineyardists. Other agriculturalists also rallied to the defense of their industry, and the subsequent literary barrage in support of the safety of copper fungicides (and often of arsenical insecticides as well)[43] completed the defeat of the New York Board of Health. This public humiliation of the Board, though perhaps deserved, was nevertheless unfortunate, for it undoubtedly dampened any enthusiasm others might have felt for criticizing arsenical insecticides. As has been suggested, however, even without the New York débâcle, there could have been few physicians eager to attack arsenicals. Of those aware of the use of such insecticides, none could have contradicted the agriculturalists' contention that there existed no substantiated reports of severe illness or death caused by the consumption of sprayed produce, and the proper reply that chronic, rather than acute, poisoning represented the true arsenical hazard was disputed by elements within the medical profession itself. If arsenic residues were causing only mild illness, furthermore, the phenomenon might easily be overlooked, either by the victim, who might dismiss the early symptoms as the inevitable toll exacted by the stresses of modern life, or by his physician, who, according to Putnam,[44] was too often unfamiliar with the symptoms of chronic arsenicism.

Agricultural assurances that arsenical insecticides presented no threat to health thus went effectively unopposed, and by the close of the century the nation's farmers no longer felt any qualms about accepting advice such as that of the entomologist E. G. Packard to "Spray, O Spray:"

> Spray, farmers, spray with care,
> Spray the apple, peach and pear;
> Spray for scab, and spray for blight,
> Spray, O spray, and do it right. . . .
>
> Spray your grapes, spray them well,
> Make first class what you've to sell,
> The very best is none too good,
> You can have it, if you would.
>
> Spray your roses, for the slug,
> Spray the fat potato bug;
> Spray your cantaloupes, spray them thin,
> You must fight if you would win.
>
> Spray for blight, and spray for rot,
> Take good care of what you've got;
> Spray farmers, spray with care,
> Spray, O spray the buglets there.[45]

## II

Packard's paean to poison exemplifies the naive enthusiasm for arsenical sprays which characterized economic entomology during the opening decades of this century,[46] an enthusiasm which was further encouraged by improvements in insecticide technology. By the early 1900s, lead arsenate had largely replaced Paris green and London purple, because it was less soluble than the older compounds and therefore not as readily removed from produce by the action of rain and wind. Increased adherence, interpreted as prolonged protection, was also achieved by the addition of adhesive agents to spray mixtures and by the use of improved pumps capable of applying the spray at much higher pressures. Thus 19th-century confidence that arsenic residues would be quickly removed by weathering gave way to 20th-century boasts such as "after the second spraying one year in the Yakima Valley [of Washington] three inches of rain fell in a few hours, yet where arsenate of lead was used there was no need of re-applying the spray."[47] The necessary concomitant

of this entomological progress, of course, was a similar progress in the level of arsenic residues on sprayed produce, but the potential danger of this trend continued to be ignored, in spite of the fact that the opening year of the century had provided a sensational demonstration of the harmful consequences of long-term exposure to small quantities of arsenic.

During the fall and winter of 1900, an epidemic of peripheral neuritis, an ailment long endemic to the area, broke out among the poorer classes of Manchester, England. Traced to the contamination of cheap beer with arsenic, the epidemic resulted in 70 deaths, more than 6,000 illnesses, and the appointment of a Royal Commission to investigate the danger of arsenical contamination of foods in general. This Commission, chaired by the venerable Lord Kelvin, for more than two years met regularly to collect and evaluate scientific testimony on the hazard of arsenical contamination of food and drink, and finally concluded that:

> the evidence we have received fully justifies us in pronouncing certain quantities of arsenic in beer and in other foods as liable to be deleterious, and at the same time capable of exclusion, with comparative ease, by the careful manufacturer. In our view, it would be entirely proper that penalties should be imposed under the Sale of Food and Drugs Acts upon any vendor of beer or any other liquid food . . . if that liquid is shown . . . to contain 1/100th of a grain or more of arsenic in the gallon; and with regard to solid food—no matter whether it is habitually consumed in large or in small quantities, or whether it is taken by itself . . . or mixed with water or other substances . . . if the substance is shown . . . to contain 1/100th grain of arsenic or more in the pound.[48]

Spray residues had been discussed by the Royal Commission during its deliberations,[49] but since arsenicals were not yet widely used in England (they had, in fact, only recently been imported from America), little concern was expressed for this source of contamination. French farmers, on the other hand, had followed American practices more closely, and the Manchester epidemic provoked a lengthy debate in the Académie de Médicine over the use of arsenicals in France.[50] During the fifth year of this discussion, one of the academicians consulted A. L. Quaintance, a respected American entomologist, with regard to the control of

American farmers' use of arsenical insecticides. Quaintance replied that "there exists, in this country, no regulation in force and no precaution is taken toward preventing accidents resulting from the use of arsenicals."[51] Such freedom was no occasion for alarm, Quaintance felt, since, in his opinion, an arsenic concentration, in or on food, of 1 part per 7,000 might be the lowest harmful level, and such large residues had never been detected on sprayed produce. Quaintance's proposed limit, however, translates into one grain per pound, exactly 100 times the British tolerance, and was suggested in 1913, ten years after the publication of the Royal Commission's *Final Report*, the most authoritative study of chronic arsenical poisoning conducted up to that time.

Quaintance's uninformed optimism was typical of entomologists' attitudes toward spray residues. Although the determination of quantities of arsenic remaining on various kinds of produce after spraying continued to be a subject of entomological interest, studies of this question invariably concluded that any residues were too small to be harmful and often enforced this conclusion with calculations of the number of barrels of apples or heads of cabbage one would have to consume in order to swallow a lethal dose of arsenic. Many of these studies, however, dating as far back as 1887, reported as safe arsenic residues comparable to and greater than the level accepted in Europe as dangerous.[52] Nevertheless, the United States Department of Agriculture published in 1922 the results of a study begun in 1915 which indicated that arsenical sprays represented no health hazard if applied only as often as advised in spraying schedules furnished by the Department.[53] Such a conclusion was, of course, both irrelevant and dangerously misleading as long as farmers were not constrained to follow Agriculture Department spraying recommendations. In fact, conclusive evidence that oversprayed produce was actually being marketed had already been brought to the Department's attention in 1919, three years before publication of its reassuring report.

The American medical profession's lack of concern for arsenical residues had continued into the 20th century, in spite of the Manchester epidemic, and was only finally dispelled by the action of another municipal health agency.[54] On the afternoon of August 18, 1919, an inspector from the Boston City Health Department happened to notice some pears, spotted with a white powder, on sale at a neighborhood fruit stand. His suspicion aroused, the inspector purchased the pears and delivered them to the Health Department's chemist, whose analysis revealed that the white powder was arsenic in the amount of as much as 0.01 grain per pear (or about 40 times the British arsenic tolerance!).[55] Apples bearing excessive arsenic were also found, and the Health Department immediately established a program of inspecting all fruit entering the Boston market and seizing any found to hold visible arsenic residues. In addition, since the objectionable fruit had been grown in California, and thus had been shipped in interstate commerce, Boston authorities notified the United States Bureau of Chemistry of its action.

The Bureau of Chemistry was the federal agency charged with the responsibility of detecting and prosecuting violations of the 1906 Food and Drug Act. Under the provisions of that Act, the Bureau was empowered to punish by fine (and for repeated offenses by imprisonment) the interstate sale of foods containing "any added poisonous or other added deleterious ingredient which may render such article injurious to health."[56] Fruit contaminated by insecticide spray residues was obviously in violation of this provision, but Bureau of Chemistry personnel nevertheless proved extremely reluctant to exercise their power against shippers of such fruit. This disinclination to act against arsenical produce, however, seems to have been due much less to uncertainty about the necessity of such action than to fear of its potential political and economic repercussions.

The realization that spray residues constituted a public health hazard unfortunately coincided with the United States' post-World War I "return to normalcy," a period characterized by both a renascent conservatism in government attitudes toward intervention in private enterprise and a growing federal concern to advance and protect the economic interests of farmers. The latter program was forwarded by the Farm Bloc, a coalition composed of congressmen from rural states and backed during its early years by Secretary of Agriculture Henry C. Wallace. Wallace's Department of Agriculture, which for years had encouraged farmers to use arsenical insecticides, was also, however, the parent agency of the Bureau of Chemistry.

Consequently, officials in charge of preventing the sale of farm products contaminated with insecticide residues found themselves in a situation in which the conscientious discharge of their duties would inevitably conflict with the political objectives of their Department chief and with the traditions and the very *raison d'être* of the Department itself. This administrative conflict of interest, reinforced by the general political-economic atmosphere of the 1920s, nearly precluded effective regulation of the spray residue problem as soon as it was recognized. The files of the Bureau of Chemistry during the 1920s, in fact, contain extensive documentation to support the charge that officials of an important public health agency continually subordinated public welfare to agricultural convenience.[57]

Thus, while the Boston Health Department quickly destroyed the fruit it had confiscated, the Bureau of Chemistry did not take its first action until more than a month later, when it convened a Washington meeting with representatives of the fruit industry and several senators from western fruit-growing states.[58] The agriculturalists attending the conference were informed of their industry's abuse of arsenical insecticides and asked to cooperate with Bureau personnel to persuade farmers to apply arsenicals with less profligacy and, when necessary, to clean fruit before packing and shipping it. The fruit growers denied they had misused arsenicals and that residues were a public health threat, but agreed to try to market fruit with lower levels of arsenic. This agreement, however, was attained only at the price of a Bureau pledge not to publicize the residue problem. Public awareness of the common presence of arsenic on produce, the fruit men feared, would severely injure sales volume, while the Bureau's acquiescence to these fears established a precedent which it was to honor throughout the ensuing decade.

The early 1920s witnessed several seizures of arsenical produce by local health departments,[59] but the Bureau of Chemistry did not make its first seizure until 1925. Even then, the Bureau acted only after New Jersey apple growers defied repeated warnings not to market their fruit until it had been cleaned, and still allowed the growers an additional three weeks to attempt to clean the fruit before it was destroyed.[60] This relaxed posture toward residue control was not finally stiffened until it was

recognized that leniency might injure the fruit industry's health. In late November, 1925, four Londoners became ill after eating American apples which, subsequent investigation revealed, had been contaminated with considerable quantites of arsenic.[61] British health officials immediately prohibited the sale of American fruit and levied fines on those who had already sold it. The British press, meanwhile, ever eager to comment on the barbarous ways into which their former colonials had degenerated, fell upon the scandal with such fervor that within two months the U.S. Department of Agriculture had collected more than 900 articles, editorials, and cartoons from British newspapers, all critical of American fruit and farmers. The scientific press was only slightly more charitable,[62] and pressure from Parliament finally forced the British Ministry of Health to threaten an embargo of American fruit unless immediate steps were taken to insure that only fruit meeting the British arsenic tolerance would be exported to Great Britain. Thus faced with the loss of a substantial portion of their export trade, American pomologists eagerly joined with the Bureau of Chemistry in a cooperative inspection and cleaning program.

Englishmen were the only beneficiaries of this cooperation, however, for the British tolerance was applied only to fruit destined for Great Britain, while produce intended for domestic consumption was permitted to carry considerably larger residues. The Food and Drug Act had failed to provide for the establishment of official tolerances for poisonous ingredients, thus placing upon the Bureau of Chemistry the onus of justifying in court any seizure of adulterated food contested by the product's shipper. Bureau officials fully appreciated the difficulty of convincing 12 laymen that very small amounts of even so infamous a poison as arsenic might prove harmful over the long term. Consequently, the "administrative tolerance" which the Bureau adopted as a guide for domestic residue control was a compromise between the level considered safe for public consumption and a figure sufficiently high to frighten a jury. The actual value of this administrative tolerance, unfortunately, is not clear, for the Bureau, forced to allow greater residues of arsenic than desirable, attempted to compensate by keeping the tolerance secret in the vain hope that farmers would fear it to be very low and thus make more serious efforts to market clean produce.[63] It is clear, however, that prior to 1927, government inspectors permitted the sale of fruit bearing arsenic equivalent to four times the British tolerance.[64] It is likewise clear that the welfare of the agricultural industry was an additional factor influencing the determination of a domestic tolerance. The Bureau's W. G. Campbell admitted in 1927 that

> heretofore, the Secretary of Agriculture, in recognition of the needs of the fruit industry and appreciating that a drastic enforcement of the 0.01 grain tolerance would result in disaster to the industry, has assumed the risk of stultifying himself before the consuming public by observing an informal tolerance considerably more liberal than is justified by the physiological facts.[65]

Farmers, understandably, were less alarmed about the possible stultification of the secretary of agriculture than they were about the confidential classification of the arsenic tolerance, an "un-American and undemocratic" procedure, as one agriculturalist saw it, comparable to the establishment of "a speed law with a secret limit which was to be known only to the traffic officers."[66] Rural discontent with the Bureau of Chemistry's domestic residue policy, fortunately, was shared by Bureau officials themselves, who finally undertook reevaluation of that policy early in 1927. On January 3 of that year, the Bureau sponsored a conference of eminent toxicologists, chaired by Harvard's Reid Hunt, to provide "the best available opinion upon the limits of lead and arsenic which shall be tolerated in human foods."[67] In its confidential report to the Bureau, this Hunt Conference recommended an arsenic tolerance approximately twice the British limit but also placed great emphasis on the danger of chronic lead poisoning from lead arsenate residues.[68] Although there had been concern for some time among Bureau officials that lead might pose a more serious threat than arsenic, nothing had been done to directly control lead residues, because analytical procedures for determining small amounts of lead in organic materials required three days to complete. Since Bureau agents needed analytical proof of excessive residues before initiating seizure actions, fruit with dangerous levels of lead could be shipped, sold, and consumed before the Bureau could complete its laboratory work. It was not until 1933 that Bureau

chemists were able to develop a rapid method of lead analysis applicable to produce, and before that date only arsenic residues could be controlled.[69]

Even the control of arsenic, however, was far from satisfactory. Shortly after the Hunt Conference, Bureau of Chemistry personnel met in Salt Lake City with representatives of the fruit industry to announce the new domestic arsenic policy.[70] For its own inscrutable reasons, though, the Bureau ignored the tolerance recommendation of the Hunt Conference and declared that, beginning with the 1928 season, the strict British arsenic tolerance would be applied to all domestic produce. To provide a period of adjustment to the new policy, furthermore, the Bureau suggested that a tolerance of 0.025 grain of arsenic per pound be enforced for the 1927 season, a proposal to which the agricultural representatives unanimously agreed. Shortly thereafter, on July 1, 1927, the Bureau of Chemistry's regulatory responsibilities were transferred to the newly formed Food and Drug Administration (FDA). The FDA was retained within the Department of Agriculture, however, so that residue control continued to be hindered by the general Department emphasis on promoting agricultural prosperity. The FDA's task was complicated still further by renewed opposition from the farmers themselves, for the spirit of accord reached at Salt Lake City had quickly soured. By the summer of 1927, fruit growers were complaining loudly that their delegates to the Salt Lake conference had misrepresented them and agreed to an unnecessary and unjust program of residue regulation.[71] Enforcement of the British tolerance was considered unnecessary because such small amounts of arsenic were obviously harmless, and numerous farmers wrote the FDA to relate their personal observations that consumption of sprayed produce did not cause death or even illness. This pragmatic attitude was expressed most succinctly, if not most eloquently, by a Colorado orchardist:

> We don't know what it is all about, but presume some professor heard that someone said another had learned someone somewhere got too much poison. The writer has lived here twenty-three years where men, women, children, cows, calves, horses, colts, and pigs eat these apples; and has never heard of a case of illness due to this nor of anyone else who has heard of a case. That's that.[72]

Unnecessary meddling with agricultural enterprise, moreover, was regarded as a grave injustice, for it imposed undue financial hardship on an already depressed segment of the economy. Farmers had, it is true, been in a distressed financial situation ever since the conclusion of the war, but the cleaning of sprayed produce does not appear to have been either so difficult or so costly[73] as to justify complaints such as the one a Washington apple grower sent his senator:

> I suppose you are aware that the Chemical Department at Washington, D.C. has ruled that N.W. apple business homeless by the ruling on arsenate of lead residue. This will make homeless, nothing to eat, nothing to clothe, 100,000 families at least. Can you comprehend the enormity of this ruling, yet no one of our Congressmen have endeavored to condemn such a ruling as far as I know. Is the Chemical Department prepared to feed this half a million souls, besides clothe and make them homes[?] Besides the ruin of much business possibly 100 cars out of a possible 40,000 carload crop might be able to pass this chemical test. Please do your best to get Washington, D.C. into action. Whatever is done must be done speedily or we are ruined.[74]

Congressmen from fruit-growing states received so many letters expressing similar sentiments, however, that an attempt was finally made to legislate an end to the FDA's residue control program. Senator W. C. Waterman of Colorado proposed an amendment to the 1928 McNary-Haugen Farm Relief bill to the effect that the provisions of the Food and Drug Act be declared inapplicable to "any fresh or natural fruit in the condition when severed from the tree, vine, or bush upon which it was grown." Waterman justified this amendment (which was included in the bill which passed the Senate) on the grounds that "it will be extremely beneficial to the fruit growers of the West and relieve them from a burden under which they have been suffering now for the last five or six years."[75] Approved by the House of Representatives as well, the Farm Relief bill was finally vetoed by the President, who regarded its attempts at price fixing of agricultural commodities as unconstitutional.[76]

The residue program survived, but opposition to it had made it clear to the FDA that residue controls could not be tightened too quickly. Thus early in 1928, leaders of the fruit industry received FDA questionnaires soliciting their opinions on the feasibility of the agreed-upon 0.01 grain per pound arsenic tolerance for 1928.[77] Predictably, the fruit growers suggested that so low a tolerance was unrealistic before 1929, and the FDA subsequently reset its 1928 tolerance at 0.02 on the condition that the British tolerance would be instituted in 1929. The folly of entrusting public health policy to the economic group responsible for the health hazard to be policed requires no comment; it is sufficient to add that similar questionnaires were employed each of the next three years, and not until 1932 did the domestic arsenic tolerance reach its long-sought level of 0.01 grain per pound.[78]

The validity of the agricultural industry's claim to be unable to meet such a low tolerance before 1932 does deserve a final comment. The 1925 altercation with British health authorities had demonstrated that impending economic loss could inspire fruit growers to solve residue problems which had appeared insurmountable before, and one suspects that their inability to meet a domestic tolerance of 0.01 grain per pound stemmed from a similar lack of inspiration. During the summer of 1931, after the fourth annual postponement of the institution of the British tolerance for non-British fruit, the secretary of the International Apple Shipper's Association notified the FDA that several European countries, including Czechoslovakia, Austria, and Poland, were objecting to excessive arsenic on American apples. In a handwritten postscript to this letter, the secretary concluded that "if this thing keeps on, you will have to go to 0.01 before next year in order to protect our foreign commerce."[79]

### III

"This thing" did not keep on. Skillful diplomacy by the Departments of Agriculture, Commerce, and State overcame the European objections, so that foreign commerce was protected and American agriculture rescued from a premature imposition of the British tolerance. This deliverance could only be temporary, however, for by the early 1930s the FDA was no longer faced simply with a frontal assault by the nation's embattled farmers but was now trapped in a crossfire laid down by critics of the Administration's leniency.

The increasing reliance by the Bureau of Chemistry and the FDA on medical scientists for toxicological advice and for testimony at residue trials[80] had alerted the medical profession to the residue hazard, and during the late 1920s physicians finally began regularly to criticize the abuse of arsenical insecticides. The leaders of this medical opposition were C. N. Myers and Binford Throne, two New York physicians who considered insecticides to be "the great menace of the decade."[81] Their colleagues tended to view the threat of spray residues in somewhat less cataclysmic terms, but Myers and Throne nevertheless attracted enough supporters[82] that by 1935 the American Public Health Association considered the residue problem important enough to deserve a symposium,[83] while the American Medical Association agreed that "spray residues must constitute an important menace to the public health."[84]

Medical critics of arsenicals were joined by the consumer champions who abounded in the 1930s and who recognized the spray residue problem as an exploitable example of the abuses which could be remedied by legislative reform of the inadequate Food and Drug Act. Through such works as the sensational best-seller *100,000,000 Guinea Pigs*,[85] the public was informed of its "steady diet of arsenic and lead" and exhorted to demand greater protection. Improved protection was finally provided by the 1938 Food, Drug and Cosmetic Act, which included a provision for the establishment of "official tolerances" for added poisonous ingredients and thus freed the FDA of the burden of winning court approval of every contested seizure.[86] In the meantime, the FDA had been responding to demands for stricter residue controls,[87] but never quickly enough to satisfy medical and consumer critics and always too quickly for entomologists and farmers. The controversy between these opponents and proponents of arsenical insecticides was nevertheless moderated by passage of the Food, Drug and Cosmetic Act and finally subsided altogether with the post-World War II introduction of the synthetic organic pesticides which promised an escape from the dangers of the old arsenicals.

## NOTES

This paper was presented in part at the 43rd annual meeting of the American Association for the History of Medicine, Birmingham, Alabama, April 3, 1970.

1  George Ordish, "150 years of crop pest control," *World Rev. Pest Control*, 1968, *7*: 204.

2  The various factors influencing the 19th-century industrialization of American agriculture are discussed by Georg Borgstrom, "Food and agriculture in the nineteenth century," in *Technology in Western Civilization*, ed. M. Kranzberg, and C. W. Pursell, Jr. (New York: Oxford Univ. Press, 1967), Vol. I, pp. 408–424; the relationship between the modernization of agriculture and the intensification of the insect problem is treated by A. J. Ihde, "Pest and disease controls," *ibid.*, Vol. II, pp. 369–385.

3  T. W. Harris, *A Treatise on Some of the Insects of New England Which Are Injurious to Vegetation* (Boston: White and Potter, 1852). The author consulted this second edition of a work originally published in 1841.

4  T. Glover, *Report of the Commissioner of Patents. Agriculture*, 1854, p. 58. Glover's first name, incidentally, is often misspelled Townsend by historians of entomology.

5  T. Glover, *Report of the Commissioner of Patents. Agriculture*, 1855, p. 66.

6  B. D. Walsh, "Introductory," *Practical Entomologist*, 1865, *1*: 4.

7  B. D. Walsh, "The new potato bug," *ibid.*, 1867, *2*: 15.

8  The earliest claim for the use of Paris green seems to be that of Byron Markham, a Michigan farmer who many years afterward recalled dusting his potato vines with the arsenical as early as 1867 ("On the first use of Paris green for the potato beetle," *Insect Life*, 1892–1893, *5*: 44).

9  "Potato bugs. Unsave advice," *Am. Agriculturalist*, 1868, *27*: 321.

10  C. V. Riley, "Paris green poisonous," *Am. Entomologist*, 1870, *2*: 92.

11  T. Glover, *U.S. Department of Agriculture Annual Report*, 1870, p. 75.

12  W. McMurtrie, *ibid.*, p. 144.

13  W. P. Headden, "Arsenical poisoning of fruit trees," *Colorado Agric. Exper. Station, Bull. 131*, 1908.

14  "The Colorado beetle and Paris green," *Am. Agriculturalist*, 1879, *38*: 292.

15  A. J. Cook, "Spraying with the arsenites," *Michigan Agric. Exper. Station, Bull. 53*, 1889.

16  Another of the consequences of the careless use of arsenicals was the poisoning of honey bees; see F. M. Webster, "The effect of arsenical insecticides upon the honey bee," *Insect Life*, 1889–1890, *2*: 84–85.

17   C. F. Fernald, "The evolution of economic entomol-
     ogy," *USDA, Bureau of Entomology, Bull. 6,* 1896, p. 8.
18   S. L. Allen, "Applying Paris green," *Country Gentle-
     man,* 1877, *42*: 168.
19   *Am. Agriculturalist,* 1877, *36*: 274–275.
20   W. McMurtrie, *U.S. Department of Agriculture Annual
     Report,* 1874, pp. 147–155; *ibid.,* 1875, pp. 141–151.
     E. Davy, "On the presence of arsenic in some arti-
     ficial manures and its absorption by plants grown
     with such manures," *Philosophical Magazine,* 1859, *18*
     (No. 4): 108–113, however, had earlier reported
     arsenic in peas, cabbages, and turnips grown in soil
     enriched by arsenically contaminated fertilizer.
21   Cited in "Does Paris green poison the potatoes?"
     *Am. Agriculturalist,* 1879, *38*: 251.
22   A. J. Cook, "Experiments with insecticides," *Proc.
     Soc. Promotion Agric. Sci.,* 1880–1882, *1*: 112–114.
23   For examples of these studies, see *U.S. Department
     of Agriculture Annual Report,* 1887, p. 103; J. Fletcher,
     "The results of an experiment to prove that apples
     are not poisoned by spraying with Paris green for
     codling moth," *Exper. Station Rec.,* 1892–1893 *4*: 437;
     L. R. Taft, "The use of poisons as fungicides and
     insecticides," *Science,* 1893, *21*: 259–260; R. C. Ked-
     zie, "Mineral residues in sprayed fruit," *Michigan
     Agric. Exper. Station, Bull. 101,* 1893; H. Garman,
     "Spraying for codling moth," *Kentucky Agric. Exper.
     Station, Bull. 53,* 1894, pp. 119–125.
24   See n. 13 above.
25   *U.S. Department of Agriculture Annual Report,* 1891, p.
     376.
26   E. G. Lodeman, *The Spraying of Plants* (Norwood,
     Mass.: MacMillan, 1896), pp. 231–232.
27   Kedzie, "Mineral residues," p. 21.
28   *J. Cutan. & Ven. Dis.,* 1886, *4*: 179, 218–220, 362–
     365, 366–367, contains a thorough discussion of the
     pros and cons of arsenical medication. Also see Isa-
     dor Dyer, "The use and abuse of arsenic in the treat-
     ment of skin diseases," *Med. News,* 1894, *65*: 227–
     230, and J. J. Putnam, "On motor paralysis and
     other symptoms of poisoning from medicinal doses
     of arsenic," *Boston Med. & Surg. J.,* 1888, *119*: 1–4.
29   That arsenical medications might cause skin can-
     cer was first suggested by Jonathan Hutchison, "Ar-
     senic cancer," *Brit. Med. J.,* 1887, *2*: 1080–1081. For
     a survey of subsequent studies on arsenic as a car-
     cinogen, see Otto Neubauer, "Arsenical cancer: a
     review," *Brit. J. Cancer,* 1947, *1*: 192–251.
30   "Arsenical preparations as cosmetics," *Med. & Surg.
     Reptr.,* 1878, *39*: 193–194. After noting the existence
     of such cosmetics, the journal's editor commented,
     "What a prospect is this for the man whose wife
     is thus absurdly immolating herself on the altar of
     vanity! What danger it intimates for the infant
     whose nurse shares in this ambition to be beauti-

fied." The supreme cynic Ambrose Bierce also took
     note of these cosmetics, defining arsenic as "a kind
     of cosmetic greatly affected by the ladies, whom it
     greatly affects in turn." *The Devil's Dictionary* (New
     York: Castle Books, 1967), p. 9.
31   As $(C_2H_5)_2H$, produced from arsenical compounds
     by certain fungi. For a discussion of the scope of
     the domestic arsenic problem, see F. C. Shattuck,
     "Some remarks on arsenical poisoning, with spe-
     cial reference to its domestic sources," *Boston Med.
     & Surg. J.,* 1893, *128*: 540–546.
32   See, for example, W. P. Headden, "Arsenical poison-
     ing of fruit trees," *J. Econ. Entomology,* 1910, *3*: 35;
     C. D. Woods, "Field experiments," *Maine Agric. Ex-
     per. Station, Bull. 224,* 1914, p. 48.
33   Medical journals occasionally observed that Paris
     green manufactured for agricultural use was an eas-
     ily obtained source of arsenic for suidical purposes,
     and the *Philadelphia Med. Times,* 1875, *5*: 806 ("Ar-
     senic in agriculture") defended the use of arsenical
     insecticides after McMurtrie's experiments had in-
     dicated them to be safe.
34   See "Arsenic eaters," *Boston Med. & Surg. J.,* 1855,
     *51*: 189–195.
35   H. E. Roscoe, "On the alleged practice of arsenic
     eating in Styria," *Edinburgh New Philos. J.,* 1861, n.s.,
     *14*: 164–165, reported witnessing a Styrian peas-
     ant swallow 4½ grains of arsenic one day, 5½ grains
     the next, and suffer no apparent ill effects.
36   Entomologists were similarly impressed with the
     benefits of arsenic-eating and even well into the
     present century defended the safety of arsenical resi-
     dues on produce, on the grounds that what is good
     for Styrians cannot be too bad for Americans (see,
     for example, O'Kane, *Hampshire Agric. Exper. Sta-
     tion, Bull. 183,* 1917). E. W. Schwartze, "The so-
     called habituation to 'arsenic.' Variation in the
     toxicity of arsenious oxide," *J. Pharmacol. & Exper.
     Therap.,* 1922, *20*: 181–203, finally demonstrated
     that the Styrians' immunity to large doses of arse-
     nic was only apparent, since they generally took the
     poison in a lump form which was not readily ab-
     sorbed from the gastro-intestinal tract.
37   "Arsenical wall papers," *Med. Rec.,* 1899, *55*: 360.
38   "The danger from arsenic," *Med. Rec.,* 1891, *39*: 600.
     The legislature and State Board of Health were in-
     deed at work upon the question, and although man-
     ufacturing interests mounted strong opposition to
     this investigation, it resulted finally, in 1900, in a
     Massachusetts statute regulating the "manufacture
     and sale of textile fabrics and papers containing ar-
     senic." The text of the act is reprinted in *Boston Med.
     & Surg. J.,* 1900, *143*: 413.
39   W. B. Hills, "Chronic arsenical poisoning," *Boston
     Med. & Surg. J.,* 1894, *131*: 454.

40 "Poisoned grapes on sale," *New York Times,* Sept. 25, 1891. Related articles appeared daily through September 29.

41 S. T. Maynard, "The amount of copper on sprayed fruit," *Massachusetts (Hatch) Agric. Exper. Station, Bull. 17,* 1892, p. 39.

42 *U.S. Department of Agriculture Annual Report,* 1891, p. 376.

43 *Ibid.,* pp. 375–376; "Spraying fruits for insect pests and fungous diseases," *USDA, Farmers' Bull. 7,* 1892; S. A. Beach and L. L. Van Slyke, "Analyses of materials used in spraying plants," *New York Agric. Exper. Station, Bull. 41,* 1892; Maynard, "The amount of copper on sprayed fruit," pp. 38–41; W. B. Alwood, "Treatment of diseases of the grape," *Virginia Agric. Exper. Station, Bull. 15,* 1892; C. M. Weed, "An agricultural revolution," *Pop. Sci. Monthly* 1892–1893, *42*: 638–647.

44 J. J. Putnam, "The character of the evidence as to the injuriousness of arsenic as a domestic poison," *Boston Med. & Surg. J.,* 1891, *124*: 623–626.

45 E. G. Packard, "Spray, o spray," *Entomological News,* 1906, *17*: 256.

46 Not all insecticides, it should be noted, were arsenical. There were several other spray mixtures, such as kerosene emulsion for the San Jose scale, which did not leave potentially harmful residues, but arsenicals remained the most widely used insecticides.

47 A. L. Melander, "Filling the calyx cup," *J. Econ. Entomology,* 1908, *1*: 219.

48 Great Britain, *Royal Commission on Arsenical Poisoning. Final Report* (London: H. M. Stationery Office, 1903), p. 50. The term *arsenic,* as used by the Royal Commission and by myself throughout this paper, refers to arsenic trioxide, $As_2O_3$. The Commission's proposed tolerance of 0.01 grain of arsenic per pound or gallon of food was unofficially adopted by the British government and received recognition from so many other European nations that it became known as the "world tolerance" for arsenic. For a history of the British arsenic tolerance, see H. Martin, "Present safeguards in Great Britain against pesticide residues and hazards," *Residue Rev.,* 1963, *4*: 17–32.

49 *Ibid.,* p. 251; also, Great Britain, *Royal Commission on Arsenical Poisoning. First Report* (London: H. M. Stationery Office, 1901), pp. 90, 280.

50 The question of arsenical spray residues was brought to the Académie's attention by P. Cazeneuve, "Sur les dangers de l'emploi des insecticides à base arsenicale en agriculture au point de vue de l'hygiène publique,:" *Bull. Acad. de méd.,* 1908, *59*: 133–154. Discussion of this question was carried on in the pages of subsequent volumes of the *Bulletin* for several years.

51 Quoted in *Bull. Acad. de méd.,* 1913, *70*: 375.

52 Examples of studies indicating excessive arsenic residues are *U.S. Department of Agriculture Annual Report,* 1887, p. 103; Taft, "The use of poisons. . . ,"; S. A. Forbes, "Spraying apples for the plum curculio," *Illinois Agric. Exper. Station, Bull. 108,* 1906; Woods, "Field experiments," p. 48; O'Kane, *Hampshire Agric. Exper. Station, Bull. 183.*

53 W. D. Lynch and others, "Poisonous metals on sprayed fruits and vegetables," *USDA, Bull. 1027,* 1922.

54 Apparently the only notable exception to this generalization about medical indifference to arsenic was A. J. Carlson's 1913 criticism of arsenic and lead residues, quoted in O'Kane, *New Hampshire Agric. Exper. Station, Bull. 183,* pp. 27–28, and even Carlson was moved to speak out only after his opinion had been solicited by O'Kane.

55 Information of the Boston episode is taken from the record on the Conference on "Arsenic on Apples and Pears, caused by Spraying," Washington, D.C., Sept. 30, 1919, Records of the Food and Drug Administration, General Spray Residue File, 1919, Dec. 31, 1925, National Records Center, Record Group 88.

56 *U.S. Statutes at Large,* 1907, *34*: 770.

57 The government records cited are contained in the Records of the Food and Drug Administration, Record Group 88, National Records Center, Suitland, Maryland, and in the Records of the Office of the Secretary of Agriculture, Record Group 16, National Archives, Washington, D.C.

58 This was the previously cited Conference on "Arsenic on Apples, etc."

59 The Boston City Health Department again seized apples and pears from western states during the fall of 1920, and again in 1921. Also in 1921, the Los Angeles Board of Health took separate actions against celery and apples contaminated with arsenic.

60 The New Jersey affair was discussed in an "anonymous address to New Jersey Horticultural Society, by member of Bureau of Chemistry"; also see *U.S. Department of Agriculture, Bureau of Chemistry, Service and Regulatory Announcements,* 1926, Notice of Judgement 13936 (p. 485). In contrast to the Bureau of Chemistry's leniency, Pennsylvania health officials prosecuted fruit dealers who attempted to sell the New Jersey fruit in Philadelphia (anonymous address to New Jersey Horticultural Society, p. 10).

61 Discussion of the British episode is based on information contained in Special Cable to *New York Times,* Nov. 25, 1925; speech by R. G. Phillips, secretary, International Apple Shippers' Association, Salt Lake City Spray Conference, Feb. 21,

1927; statement by P. B. Dunbar, Conference on Arsenical and Lead Spray Residues, Philadelphia, Dec. 29, 1926. It is interesting that the British had objected to American fruit before 1925, complaining as early as 1892 that imported fruit often was covered with arsenic (see "Arsenic in American apples," *Brit. Med. J.,* 1892, *1*: 471).

62  See, for instance, "Parliamentary intelligence," *Lancet,* 1925, 103, 2: 1295.

63  The Bureau's domestic residue policy was explained in a letter from C. L. Alsberg, chief, Bureau of Chemistry, to W. C. Woodward, health commissioner of Boston, May 14, 1921.

64  Statement by P. B. Dunbar, Conference on Arsenical and Lead Spray Residues.

65  Speech by W. G. Campbell, Salt Lake City Spray Conference.

66  Letter to W. M. Jardine, secretary of agriculture, December 17, 1926.

67  Memorandum from C. A. Browne, chief, Bureau of Chemistry, to W. M. Jardine, secretary of agriculture, Dec. 4, 1926.

68  Report of Conference at Bureau of Chemistry, Jan. 3, 1927.

69  The problem of the analysis of lead residues is discussed in Report, "Method for Determination of Arsenic and Lead on Fruits and Vegetables," by J. H. Wichmann and C. W. Murray, May 27, 1933.

70  See record of Salt Lake City Spray Conference, Feb. 21, 1927.

71  Letter from G. J. Morton, chief, San Francisco Station, FDA, to J. W. Herbert, chief, Western District, FDA, Mar. 5, 1928, relates that Washington orchardists felt they had been betrayed by their representatives at the Salt Lake City Conference; many farmers also claimed never to have been informed of the Salt Lake agreement (letter from L. D. Elliot, chief, Denver Station, FDA, to P. L. Smithers, county extension agent, Cañon City, Colorado, July 18, 1927).

72  Market Letter Number 5, The Associated Fruit Company, Delta, Colorado, Sept. 29, 1927.

73  There were available by the mid-20s effective and inexpensive methods of removing residue from fruit with 1 percent hydrochloric acid and other solutions. For a discussion of cleaning techniques, see H. C. Diehl and others, "Removal of spray residue from apples and pears in the Pacific Northwest," *USDA Circular 59,* 1929.

74  Letter to Senator W. C. Jones, Sept. 10, 1926.

75  *Congressional Record,* 1928, Vol. 69, p. 6166.

76  *Ibid.,* pp. 9524–9531.

77  Questionnaire from W. G. Campbell, Feb. 24, 1928.

78  The intermediate tolerances were: 1929 − 0.017; 1930 − 0.015; 1931 − 0.012.

79  Letter from R. G. Phillips to W. G. Campbell, July 16, 1931.

80  The first trial at which the Bureau of Chemistry was challenged to prove that the residue on confiscated produce was sufficient to endanger health resulted from a 1926 seizure of apples and pears from Suncrest Orchards, Medford, Oregon. Although the Bureau won this case, others soon followed, and the verdicts were not always favorable to the government.

81  C. N. Myers and Binford Throne, "Health hazards from the ingestion of small amounts of metals," *N.Y. St. J. Med.,* 1929, *29*: 1258.

82  For example, W. D. Sheldon and others, "Neuritis from arsenic and lead," *Arch. Neurol. & Psychiat.,* 1932, *27*: 322-332; Samuel Ayres, Jr., and N. P. Anderson, "Cutaneous manifestations of arsenic poisoning," *Arch. Dermatology & Syphilis,* 1934, *30*: 33-43.

83  Papers presented at the symposium are published in *Am. J. Public Hlth.,* 1935, *26*: 369-389.

84  "Report of the Federal Food and Drug Administration," *J.A.M.A.,* 1935, *104*: 220.

85  A. Kallett and F. J. Schlink, *100,000,000 Guinea Pigs* (New York: Vanguard Press, 1933). The authors devoted their third chapter ("A Steady Diet of Arsenic and Lead," pp. 47-60) to the problem of spray residues; other works treating this subject include Ruth Lamb, *American Chamber of Horrors* (New York: Faraar and Rinehart, Inc., 1936); and R. L. Palmer and I. M. Alpher, *40,000,000 Guinea Pig Children* (New York: Vanguard Press, 1937).

86  *U.S. Statutes at Large,* 1938, *52*: 1040-1059. See especially section 406 (a), p. 1049, which applies to the setting of tolerances.

87  The arsenic tolerance was maintained at 0.01 grain per pound throughout the 1930s. A lead tolerance was finally set in 1933, being placed at 0.025 grain per pound, lowered for a few weeks to 0.014, then raised again to 0.020. The FDA expressed an intention of eventually lowering the lead tolerance to 0.014, but agricultural opposition prevented lowering it beyond 0.018. When fluorine-containing insecticides came into use during the 1930s, the FDA at first decided to set a zero tolerance on fluorine (letter from W. G. Campbell to Chiefs of FDA Districts, Mar. 9, 1933), but agricultural complaints again moved the Administration to adopt a more lenient standard, setting the fluorine tolerance at 0.01 grain per pound until 1938, when it was doubled to 0.02.

# Changing Public Health Concerns

With the advent of the bacteriological era, public health activities underwent significant changes. While many 19th-century problems remained, the knowledge gained through the germ theory suggested new solutions. Public health workers spent more time tracking down and trying to destroy specific bacteria and less time on general urban cleanups.

Institutions developed in the 19th century to meet the health needs of urban populations underwent transformation in the 20th. As the popularity of the dispensary for treating the poor declined in the early 20th century, the neighborhood health center arose to take its place. This new institution, which George Rosen defines as "an organization which provides, promotes and coordinates needed medical service and related social service for a specified district," flourished until the late 1930s. Following a three-decade hiatus, it reappeared in the mid-1960s as part of President Lyndon B. Johnson's "war on poverty." Funded by the Office of Economic Opportunity and the Public Health Service, comprehensive health centers provided medical care and advice to millions of poor Americans from Watts in Los Angeles to Mound Bayou, Mississippi, often with startling results. In some primarily black southern communities such centers helped to reduce infant mortality by nearly 40 percent in only four years. Nevertheless, the problem of providing adequate medical care for the poor, both rural and urban, remains a pressing national concern.

The public health movement generally failed to reduce infant mortality until the early 20th century, when deaths of infants under one year old, particularly from infectious diseases, decreased. Maternal mortality declined more slowly. As Joyce Antler and Daniel M. Fox point out, childbirth remained dangerous for mothers until the 1940s. The successful movement to make maternity safe illustrates how 20th-century reformers dealt with a major health problem.

Little progress occurred in the area of occupational health until the 20th century. David Rosner and Gerald Markowitz describe the early movement for occupational safety and health and analyze the composition of 20th-century reforms. The occupational health movement represented a coalition of interest groups: workers, reformers, journalists, politicians, business interests, and professionals — of all political ideologies — joined together to bring about changes that were in the public interest. The authors agree that "many aspects of this movement were paternalistic," but they conclude that nonetheless the plight of industrial workers became a political and medical issue because of the success in building a broad coalition.

In the late 20th century we are still plagued with public health problems. Some of the lessons learned in the early years of the century about effecting change by combining public and private sectors and involving a wide range of interest groups may continue to find application today. Public health remains a national concern.

# 34

## The First Neighborhood Health Center Movement: Its Rise and Fall

### GEORGE ROSEN

## INTRODUCTION

Among aspects of urban life in modern times which have been regarded as conducive to social disease and decay, the connection between poverty and ill-health has long been recognized as a major focus of community concern and action. Awareness of the widespread prevalence of disease among the poor and of the inadequacy of the health care available to them has at various times motivated efforts to improve their health by providing more effective medical care. Historically, such concern has expressed itself in the creation of programs and facilities ranging from the dispensaries of the 18th century to the current neighborhood health centers.

Indeed, the latter grew out of a recognition that existing arrangements and programs in the United States were not satisfactorily meeting the complex health needs of the poor.[1] As a result, the neighborhood health center has been developed to remedy this situation by providing "a one-door facility, in which virtually all ambulatory health services are available; close coordination with other community resources; professional staff of high quality; and intensive participation by and involvement of the population to be served."[2] In these terms, the current wave of neighborhood health centers has been viewed by some as having brought forth a new institutional form. Yet neither the concept of providing health services on a local basis, nor the creation of facilities to deliver such care, nor the stated objectives of the neighborhood center are essentially new. The concept of a community health center providing service on a neighborhood basis, and its embodiment in organizational forms provided the core for a widespread movement which developed in the United States during the second and third decades of this century, reached its peak during the 30s, and then declined. Since the circumstances out of which this movement grew, the objectives at which it aimed, and the organizational forms it assumed are not unlike those characteristic of the neighborhood health center movement, an examination of the earlier movement may perhaps throw some light on the future possibilities of current trends.

## URBANISM, IMMIGRATION, AND HEALTH

The roots of the health center movement, which began around 1910, are to be found in the changes which occurred in American society during the preceding decades. From 1860 to 1910 the urban portion of the population rose from 19 to 45 percent of the total, due in large measure to a flood of immigrants which poured into the cities and industrial towns where workers were in demand.[3] From about 1880 the majority of the immigrants came from southern and eastern Europe where they had left the backward, wretched circumstances of countryside and hamlet to seek a better life in the New World.[4] Some were skilled workers and craftsmen, a category which was largest among Jewish immigrants, of whom thousands entered the needle trades. A certain number of Italian immigrants also possessed skills adaptable to urban conditions, and some, particularly women, took jobs

GEORGE ROSEN (1910–1977), distinguished pioneer in the social history of medicine, was Professor of the History of Medicine and of Epidemiology and Public Health, Yale University.

Reprinted with permission from the *American Journal of Public Health,* 1971, *61*: 1620–1635.

in the garment industry. Others entered service occupations or set up as shopkeepers or peddlers. As early as 1890, for example, most fruit peddlers and bootblacks in New York City were Italian, and not much later Italians were already heavily represented among waiters, barbers and shoemakers. Most immigrants, however, were unskilled and had to accept poorly paid jobs performing heavy manual work. But even those who were skilled worked excessively long hours for low wages under unhealthful conditions. Frequently they worked for their compatriots, often converting their dwellings into sweatshops.

Separated from the native Americans by language and custom, the immigrants crowded together in segregated neighborhoods where mutual aid and understanding were available. These neighborhoods were a geographic expression of the immigrants' endeavor to maintain their identity by living within a cultural environment in which they had roots, and from which they might make contact with and learn about the unfamiliar American world in which they found themselves. To the native American, however, the areas where these impoverished aliens congregated were loathsome, sickening slums whose denizens challenged and threatened the fabric of his social and psychological order. As early as 1883 Henry George, anticipating the end of the public domain, viewed the flooding immigrant tide with alarm and asked "What in a few years are we to do for a dumping ground? Will it make our difficulties the less that our human garbage can vote?"[5] George was not alone in his opinion, which was echoed with numerous variations in succeeding decades. Robert A. Woods, a leading Boston social worker of the period, recoiled from the "unspeakable degraded standard of life" of the immigrants, while his collaborator Joseph Lee was amazed that this "human rubbish" produced a "number of physically, mentally and morally efficient citizens."[6]

The revulsion and dismay expressed in such statements are related to two reactions to the immigrants which clashed in principle but in practice tended to blend in various, sometimes ambiguous ways. One was a reaction to the differing lifestyles and values of the immigrants, comprising feelings of contempt, distrust and fear, as well as a sense that the alien masses were inferior and a menace. General antiforeign attitudes, views of foreigners

as unruly and dangerous were refracted through specific ethnic or national stereotypes to which unfavorable characteristics and qualities were attributed.[7] This attitude found its more unsophisticated expression in the tendency to single out "wops," "sheenies," "polacks," "bohunks" or some other group as inherently criminal, avaricious or subversive.

But even those Americans who were sympathetic to the foreign-born were not completely exempt from the influence of the current stereotypes. In the early 1900s, the distinguished physician, Richard Cabot, examining his reactions to foreign-born patients at the Massachusetts General Hospital, noted that "the chances are ten to one that I shall look out of my eyes and see, *not* Abraham Cohen, but *a Jew* . . . I do not see *this* man at all. I merge him in the hazy background of the average Jew. But," he went on, "if I am a little less blind than usual to-day . . . I may notice something in the way his hand lies on his knee, something that is queer, unexpected. That hand . . . it's a muscular hand, it's a prehensile hand; and whoever saw a Salem Street Jew with a muscular hand before? . . . I saw *him.* Yet he was no more real than the thousands of others whom I had seen and forgotten, — forgotten because I never saw *them,* but only their ghostly outline, their generic type, the racial background out of which they emerged."[8]

Cabot's self-analysis is an aspect of the other reaction to the immigrants, an aspect of an endeavor to come into close enough contact with them to learn about them as people, to begin to understand the stresses and strains to which they were exposed in an alien environment. This tendency appeared most prominently with the establishment of social settlements in the 1890s in the poorest sections of Chicago, New York, and other cities. Since these sections, the slums, were also overwhelmingly the foreign quarters, most of those with whom settlement dwellers worked were immigrants. The settlement workers soon became aware of the deep gulf which separated the poor immigrants from the larger society in which they lived, but to which they did not belong. Recognizing the need for social integration of the newer immigration with the older America, they set themselves the task, as Lillian Wald put it, of "fusing these people who come to us from the Old World Civilization into . . . a real brotherhood among men."[9]

For the most part, the settlements approached this task in practical, concrete terms. Recognizing that the influences to which the immigrants were subjected, and the treatment which they received after arrival, resulted in exploitation and neglect, they endeavored to prevent or repair the damage by turning to social action and dealing with specific problems such as economic exploitation, overcrowded and decrepit housing, destitution, broken homes, crime, alcoholism, prostitution and ill-health. The settlement dwellers worked largely on a local basis, directing their efforts and programs specifically at immigrant needs, at the needs of an oppressed minority. In so doing, they planted the seeds of a national social welfare program but their immediate concern was the neighborhood. This positive interest in the welfare of the immigrant poor went hand-in-hand with a desire to work with them, as well as for them, and also with a growing awareness that by accepting the cultural heritage and enhancing their self-respect, the slum dwellers were more likely to become involved in solving or ameliorating the problems of their group and their neighborhood.[10]

The great importance of health problems within this complex context was well-recognized. In 1909, Edward T. Devine,[11] a leading social worker, noted not only that "ill health is perhaps the most constant of the attendants of poverty," but he went on to emphasize that "An inquiry into the physical condition of the members of the families that ask for aid . . . clearly indicates that whether it be the first cause or merely a complication from the effect of other causes, physical disability is at any rate a very serious disabling condition at the time of application in three-fourths . . . of all the families that come under the care of the Charity Organization Society, who are probably in no degree exceptional among families in need of charitable aid."[12]

Activities in New York and Chicago also are indicative of the importance attached to health work among the poor immigrants. In 1893, Lillian D. Wald and Mary Brewster opened the Nurses' Settlement on Henry Street in New York in order to bring the benefits of public health nursing to an entire neighborhood. The Henry Street Settlement developed an organized community service intended to prevent disease, as well as to help the sick. As its program grew, involvement in studies

of health and social welfare extended the influence of Henry Street far beyond the locality.[13]

Also in 1893, four years after Jane Addams opened Hull House, a public dispensary was organized at the settlement in Chicago. It was open every day from three to four in the afternoon and from seven to eight in the evening. There was also a physician in residence at Hull House, and another doctor who lived nearby helped out. A nurse from the Visiting Nurses' Association was stationed at the settlement, and received her orders there. In addition, various studies and programs were undertaken to improve health conditions in the neighborhood where the settlement was located. These involved improvement of housing and garbage collection, combatting cocaine addiction among minors, regulation of midwifery, studies of tuberculosis in relation to overcrowding, and of typhoid fever and poor sanitation.[14]

Thus, throughout the last decades of the 19th century and the early years of this century, the growing cities of the United States were increasingly confronted by the problems of poverty, crime, disease, and other attendant ills of the slums, problems most often associated with immigration.[15] The inescapable fact of these urban problems, plus a growing conviction of the need for social change led to a broad movement of reform dedicated to the eradication of demonstrable social ills and the realization of conditions for a better life through planned social action. From this standpoint campaigns were mounted to deal with a wide range of problems: poverty and dependency, tenement house reform, sweatshops, prostitution, juvenile delinquency, and others among which ill health was prominent as a cause or a consequence.[16]

## COORDINATING HEALTH WORK

While these changes were taking place, the work of Pasteur, Koch, and their contemporaries had been answering some of the pertinent questions concerning the causation and prevention of communicable diseases, and this knowledge was being applied in public health programs. As a result, by the end of the first decade of this century, there was a solid basis for the control of a number of infectious diseases and throughout succeeding decades advances along this line continued.[17] Alongside these trends, a shift was beginning to take place in the concept and orientation of community health action, a shift of attention from the environment to the individual. As health authorities and others became aware of noxious influences, other than those emanating from the physical environment, as activities in connection with maternal and child health, industrial hygiene, tuberculosis, venereal disease, and mental ill-health developed, public health expanded. As new areas of concern became a part of public health, new programs developed and new personnel were trained to execute them.[18] Increasing expansion of the scope of community health work created problems for official and voluntary health agencies. As more and more special programs, operated by separate personnel and often through special agencies, came into being, it also became increasingly clear that better ways of organizing and administering health work were needed.[19] It was recognized that there was a need for the coordination of hitherto separated agencies, facilities and services, many of which were concerned with the same population. Even within a single agency (such as a large urban health department), duplication of effort and lack of coordination among its constituent units were found both wasteful, inefficient and irritating to the people who needed the services. In 1914, S. S. Goldwater, the Health Commissioner of New York City, observed that "Various bureaus send their representatives into the same house, which results in undue expenditure of time and energy and in annoyance to the individual citizens."[20] A similar point of view was expressed by Charles F. Wilinsky in Boston. ". . . Gaps in the programs," he said, "duplication and consequent waste, frequent inefficiencies and misunderstandings, could not help but lead to the conclusion that there was a great need for better coordination and correlation, more efficient organization, and more harmonious understanding between those agencies concerned with the public health and with the amelioration of human suffering." He went on to add "that the fault of public health administration in large cities particularly was due to the fact that it was too far removed from the people it attempted to serve."[21]

Wilinsky's last remark touches on another factor which reinforced the tendency to develop local health work, namely, recognition that effective application of health programs, especially among the poor and the foreign-born, required an approach to the people on their own ground, in their neighborhood. By locating a service in the section where they lived, one avoided the necessity of drawing these people away from familiar streets and landmarks. Strangeness and distance, as well as language barriers and long waiting periods, were serious limiting factors in the use of health facilities such as dispensaries and hospitals.[22] As Michael M. Davis pointed out, long waits were particularly important for mothers, "when children must either be brought along or left at home in the care of a busy neighbor, or of children too young to take the responsibility."[23] Moreover, "the mother in her home, seldom, if ever, getting out to gatherings of any sort, is the hardest member of the immigrant group to reach, and often the slowest to give up her racial habits; yet in her position as homekeeper she has most to do with the health of her family. Taking our health work into her neighborhood is the surest way to get acquainted with her."[24]

Nevertheless, even such a localization of health and social services was not enough as long as the prospective users, the consumers, confronted a multiplicity of uncoordinated agencies in a situation where they were Alices in a Wonderland of confusing community resources. About the time of World War I, in East Harlem, in New York City, for example, there were many clinics, dispensaries, and district offices of welfare agencies, but the ordinary citizen had only the vaguest idea of what they did, what services they provided. Nor did he have any more precise notion of the service he needed. "He might be in trouble of some kind," wrote Homer Folks, "his health failing, or one of the children backward at school, or running afoul of the police, or the family just could not make ends meet. He needed assistance badly, somewhere, from somebody, but just what sort of help, or where to go to find it, or whether it could be had, were vague uncertainties. . . . Possibly he remembered having seen a sign somewhere in the locality or someone had told him that somebody had said that someone had been helped from an office on the north side of 116th Street near First Avenue. If of an optimistic and pioneering type, he bravely started on a voyage of discovery of what we call the social resources of the community.

"If his courage were strong, and his health not too bad, the needy person might persevere and by making the rounds, calling on one office and clinic after another, and being referred from one agency to another, he might finally arrive at the place where he should have gone in the first instance for real help for his particular trouble." The consequences of this situation were frequently deplorable; ". . . the fact of not knowing just what was needed, nor just where to go, resulted on the part of the less enterprising, in not going anywhere. And, going nowhere and doing nothing meant that things went from bad to worse."[25]

An implicit consequence of this statement is that health and welfare agencies should, as far as possible, be brought together, perhaps under one roof. As settlement workers had already recognized, the problems for which poor people needed help were usually neither simple nor single and had no easy solutions. More often than not their health and social problems were closely linked, so that those endeavoring to solve them had to establish the closest possible collaboration. This point was explicitly underscored by Robert A. Woods. "The local health center," he wrote, "gathers under one head a group of services which in greater or lesser degree have been undertaken in the past by the settlement. In all their technical phases the settlement clearly and unquestionably must be ready to pass them over to the health center. It is however, equally clear — and this the promoters of the health centers do not always appreciate — that all the values of acquaintance and influence which the settlement has in its various organizations — must continue to be of indispensable importance to any sort of comprehensive local health campaign."[26] With this comment Woods touched upon another important dimension, the sociopsychological. Unless geographic localization and administrative coordination were complemented by social organization of the neighborhood with active participation of the population served, the fullest benefits of localized services would not be achieved. What was needed was a democratic educational process involving local people on an organized basis.

This aspect was most fully developed by Wilbur C. Phillips and his wife Elsie Cole Phillips.[27] The initial source for his idea of a community health plan was his experience as secretary of the New York Milk Committee established in 1907 by the Association for Improving the Condition of the Poor.[28] The objective of the committee was to reduce infant mortality in New York City by improving its milk supply, and seeing that babies received clean milk. Phillips undertook to achieve this aim by establishing infant milk depots throughout the city. This in itself was not new; the philanthropist Nathan Strauss had begun to establish a system of milk stations in 1893.[29] However, Phillips soon recognized that distribution of milk was not enough. Stimulated by the work of Pierre Budin, Professor of Obstetrics at Paris who, in 1892, established a system of infant consultation centers, and based on his own experience, by 1909, Phillips had developed a concept of the milk depot as a "centre of influence for child life" where babies could receive medical examinations, where mothers could be taught how to keep their babies well, and from which would "radiate the influences of education and social betterment."[30]

## THE FIRST HEALTH CENTERS, 1910–1919

In 1911, this idea was expanded by Phillips in a Polish district of Milwaukee into a demonstration center for maternal and child care on a broad democratic basis using a so-called "block plan."[31] After resigning from the New York Milk Committee in 1910, he left for Milwaukee where implementation of his idea appeared feasible. Milwaukee had a high infant mortality, and seemed ready to deal with such problems in terms of basic social change, since it had recently elected a Socialist administration to office, the first large American city to do so. Phillips was then a member of the Socialist Party, having joined because as he says, "I knew at that time no other way of registering my opinion that poverty could and should be abolished — and that it could not be abolished through charity. But first, as the Socialists preached, came education — getting wider and wider numbers of people to understand the root causes of poverty and the way to remove them."[32]

In May 1911, at the instigation of Phillips, a nonpartisan Child Welfare Commission was appointed of which he became secretary. Its objective was to investigate the causes of infant mortality, and to formulate and carry out a plan of child welfare work from the standpoint of the entire community. By the end of the year the studies had been completed and a child health program based on a system of preventive health centers was proposed. This program was to be carried out by the municipality through its health department which would direct the work of social organization, promotion and education that was regarded as absolutely essential for the development of the child health program, and which the Phillipses had been doing. As a demonstration, they set up a child health station in a Polish area, comprising 33 city blocks with a population of 16,000 people and between 350 to 400 mothers and babies. The medical staff to provide the preventive consultations was selected by the physicians of the district, who also agreed on a fixed fee of two dollars to be paid each doctor for his period at the clinic. Cooperation of midwives and other local people was obtained. An unprecedented degree of support was obtained from the mothers by the creation of block committees headed by a block worker for each of the blocks in the demonstration area. This was the germ of the social unit idea which Phillips was then to try to implement in Cincinnati.

This was in the spring of 1912, but by June of that year, Wilbur Phillips and his wife were on their way to New York. Their activities had been upset by a change in the municipal administration. The Child Welfare Commission was terminated, and the child health program was limited to its purely medical aspects as part of a health department activity. But the idea of an "Educational Health Center" had been formulated, an idea which was to provide the basis for the Social Unit Organization, which in 1917 took form under Phillips' leadership in the Mohawk-Brighton district of Cincinnati. This was undertaken as a demonstration of the National Social Unit Organization created by Phillips in 1916, with headquarters in New York City. The purpose of this group was "to promote the type of democratic community organization through which the citizenship as a whole can participate directly in the control of community affairs, while at the same time making constant use of the highest technical skill available."[33]

After some deliberation, the Mohawk-Brighton district of Cincinnati was chosen for the purpose of carrying out a "social unit" community experiment on a large scale, and funds were made available by the national organization for a period of three years, with a certain proportion of the budget to be raised in Cincinnati. This city was chosen

in large measure because Courtenay Dinwiddie, secretary of the Cincinnati Anti-Tuberculosis League (realizing the importance of community organization) worked hard to have the demonstration there. The league had developed plans in 1917 for a neighborhood health center through which its aims might be attained, and now felt that the Social Unit Plan was capable of achieving even more than their initial goals.

The demonstration was carried out in a neighborhood of some 15,000 inhabitants, of whom between 5 and 10 percent were recent immigrants.[34] The areas was divided into 31 "blocks" of approximately 500 people each, and in each block, the residents over 18 years of age elected a council. This council elected a block worker who represented the residents of the block on the Citizens' Council of the unit. Her duties were to visit the families in her section, keep them in touch with the unit, and to bring specific problems they had to the proper department of the organization. The block worker was paid four dollars a week for the time lost from her household activities. Just as the Citizens' Council represented the people of the district, an Occupational Council secured the interest and cooperation of the various occupational and professional groups in the district, while the doctors, nurses, and social workers had their groups for the consideration of problems involved in their work. The Occupational Council was a neigborhood planning body working with other groups in the city. No new activities were undertaken until they had been endorsed by the people of the district through their representatives on the various councils. Most of the health and welfare agencies in Cincinnati, not only the Anti-Tuberculosis League, but also the Associated Charities, the Better Housing League and the Humane Society, cooperated with the Social Unit Organization.

The Cincinnati Social Unit demonstration was an experiment in applied democracy with health as its focal point. The health activities carried on included antepartum care, well child care for infants and preschool children, antituberculosis work, dental examination of school children, nursing service, medical care during the influenza epidemic of 1918, and periodic examination of adults. In short, beginning with health as a field of activity, Phillips and his coworkers endeavored to develop a consciously self-governing local unit in the midst of a large city. This enterprise was one of the most seminal experiments in social organization for health in the United States. If offered a vision of a community in which citizens working together as members of a vitally cooperating group sought the common welfare rationally and intelligently. It also raised profound political and social questions which are still unresolved. Can such a vision be realized in the heart of a large urban center? Can its inhabitants become truly conscious of mutual interests and be, in some degree, self-governing? Do such aims require a stable population, and how can such stability be maintained?

The Cincinnati experiment answered some but not all the questions. Opposition to it developed from the Director of Public Welfare, the newly elected mayor, a local medical society and various conservatives who charged that the Social Unit demonstration was a Red plot, a not uncommon occurrence in the supercharged patriotic atmosphere at the end of World War I. Although an investigation of the charges showed that they were unfounded, and a referendum within the Mohawk-Brighton district revealed a strong sentiment for the demonstration, the municipal administration withdrew its support, the funds that had been pledged were not forthcoming, and by 1920 the Social Unit demonstration was over. Without political and economic leverage, the inhabitants of the district could hardly make their wants felt. Phillips had not adequately established a financial base nor had there been adequate time to create a political power base. The demonstration raised questions but provided only partial or ambiguous answers.

Meanwhile, efforts had been made elsewhere to provide health services to a definite population on a local basis. In 1912, William C. White, a physician and medical director of the Tuberculosis League of Pittsburgh, tried such an approach to tuberculosis control. As his model, he took the district system of the public schools. "In the educational field," he said, "there has gradually developed a knowledge of the equipment necessary for a given population, and this equipment has been apportioned so as to be readily accessible to those whom it is to serve. The management of these units is centered in a legally constituted governing body which also controls the expenditure of funds collected by taxation. The same form of control is applicable to tuberculosis and other health problems."[35] However, White's scheme lasted only six months. That year also saw an effort in Philadelphia by Samuel M. Hamill, a physician, to apply the same idea to child health work creating a basis for a growing program. Broader and more enduring efforts were also undertaken in New York, Boston, and Buffalo.

In 1913, the New York Milk Committee established a health center on the lower West Side of Manhattan to serve a district populated largely by Syrians and Irish-Americans, where housing was poor and medical resources were limited.[36] The Bowling Green Neighborhood Association composed of local residents and outside specialists was formed to administer the center which provided chiefly antepartum and infant care. Neighborhood associations composed of voluntary groups of citizens were not new in New York City and many of them had worked with the Health Department in one way or another.[37]

S. S. Goldwater, Health Commissioner of New York, was aware of these developments and in September 1914 formulated a plan to apply the principle of localization to health administration in order to see how far the work of the department could "be improved by the substitution of a system of local or district administration for the present purely functional administrations."[38] To answer this question an experimental health district was established by January 1915 on the lower East Side of Manhattan in an area populated almost entirely by Jews.[39] The district comprised a highly congested area of 21 blocks housing 25,000 people. The staff comprised a part-time district health officer in full charge of local administration, a part-time medical inspector who was responsible for medical inspection of preschool and school children as well as the infants' milk station, three nurses and one nurses' assistant, a food inspector and a sanitary inspector, both part-time. The basic principles underlying district work were coordination of health department functions, local administration in terms of local needs, and establishment of a community spirit. In accordance with the latter point, the health officer of the district was a Jewish physician who understood the people, their language, backgrounds and characteristics.

The experiment proved so satisfactory that on May 1, 1916, it was extended by Haven Emerson

(Health Commissioner from 1915 to 1917) to Queens, where four health districts were opened (Long Island City, Flushing, Ridgewood, and Jamaica). In 1916, there was also created within the Health Department a Division of Health Districts under the Deputy Commissioner of Health, and in 1917 the district health officers were placed on a full-time basis.[40] Unfortunately, at this time, there was a change in the city government, and the new administration slipped smoothly back into the established rut of the *status quo ante*. Among other actions, it halted the plans to extend district health administration to other parts of the city, and it was not until more than 12 years later that district health centers were established on a more solid basis in New York. Nevertheless, experience had been gained for such a program, and some advantages to be derived from decentralized public health administration were demonstrated. For example, as a consequence of the coordination of services, it was possible to serve families more efficiently, with all services rendered to a family provided by a single nurse. This led to the introduction of a Family Record Card which contained a continuous history of the family as far as Health Department services were concerned. However, this abortive attempt to apply the principle of local administration to health work in New York City brought forth a problem which was to plague the revived district system in 1930s, namely, the division of responsibility and the relationships between the district health officers and the chiefs of the central functional bureaus of the department.

During this period, health departments and private health and welfare agencies in a number of American cities and towns undertook to coordinate their activities on a localized basis and to develop neighborhood health centers and programs. In 1916, on the initiative of Charles F. Wilinsky, Deputy Health Commissioner of Boston (who has been referred to above), the Blossom Street Health Unit was opened in the West End, one of the most congested sections of the city.[41] The objective was to provide a local center from which agencies engaged in health and welfare work could serve a geographically defined population. Among the agencies included in the center were the Consumptives Hospital Department, the Instructive District Nursing Association, the Milk and Baby Hygiene Association, the visiting physician of the Boston

Dispensary, and the Hebrew Federated Charities. Later additions were clinics for dental care and mental health counseling. Eventually, Boston had eight centers, each serving a population of 50,000. This expansion was assisted by a bequest by George Robert White of six million dollars to the city of Boston for this purpose.

Similar developments occurred in other large cities. Beginning with one experimental station in 1914, Buffalo developed a citywide system of district services. By 1920 there were seven districts of 26,000 to 91,000 population (average about 75,000) with a center in each. The system represented a cooperative arrangement between the Department of Health and the Department of Hospitals and Dispensaries. Arrangements and proceedings were also worked out to govern the relationships with private medical and social agencies. Basically this system was intended for the poor people of the city, and the districts were correlated with the existing tracts covered by the Charity Organization Society.[42]

## HEALTH CENTERS SPREAD

As C.-E. A. Winslow noted in 1919, "The most striking and typical development of the public health movement of the present day is the health center."[43] World War I had emphasized the possibilities of coordinated effort in achieving results, as well as the importance of health, and these lessons were not lost on community leaders. When the war ended, health centers and demonstrations financed by foundations, voluntary health agencies, or other social welfare organizations, as well as by local governments were established in many parts of the United States. A decision by the American Red Cross at the end of the war to further the establishment of health centers gave additional impetus to this trend.[44] Local chapters undertook to create health centers, and more generally such facilities became the fashion in community health work.

The scope of this development is evident from the following figures obtained by the Red Cross during the latter part of 1919 in a survey of existing and planned health centers.[45] The report showed that as of January 1, 1920, there were 72 centers in 49 communities, of which seven cities had more than one center. In addition to the existing centers, 33 centers were being proposed or planned in 28 other communities. An analysis of the existing and proposed centers showed that at the time of the report, 33 were administered entirely by public authorities, 27 were under private control, and 16 were under combined public and private control. The Red Cross was involved in 19 instances. There was considerable variation in the work and aims of the existing health centers. In 40 communities with health centers in operation, 37 contained clinics of some type, 34 carried on visiting nursing, 29 did child welfare work, and 27 did anti-tuberculosis work. Twenty-two had venereal disease clinics, 14 had dental clinics, and 11 had eye, ear, nose and throat clinics. Only 10 had laboratories, and 9 had milk stations.

The succeeding decades witnessed a further development of health centers and districting of health services. In 1930, a subcommittee on health centers collected information for the White House Conference on Child Health and Protection. It obtained data for 1,511 major and minor health centers throughout the United States. Eighty percent had been established since 1910. Of the total number, 725 were operated by private agencies, 729 by county or municipal health departments, and a small number by the Red Cross, hospitals, tuberculosis associations, case-work agencies and the like. In nearly half these centers, the principal support came from public funds, while supplementary aid came through community chests, or from private funds.

As is not infrequently the case when a professional development or trend is in "fashion," the name by which it is designated acquires an aura of approval, and is used to describe activities and enterprises that differ widely, so that they may share some of the aura. This was also the fate of the health center concept, and is in part responsible for its decline. As one observer put it in 1921, "We find it used as a name for child welfare stations, tuberculosis dispensaries, venereal disease clinics, out-patient departments of hospitals, settlement houses, and substations of local health departments."[46] The Red Cross concept of a health center was that of an institution which could be locally operated with a minimum of outside direction and with an emphasis on its function as an educational, informational facility. "Functionally, the health center is an institution through which the community may get in touch with all health

promoting agencies and with the health problems of local and of national importance."[47] Administratively, however, the Red Cross view was that the health center should be under the combined guidance and control of all the local health agencies.

Michael M. Davis, writing in 1927, defined the health center more definitely and related it more specifically to health care, both preventive and curative. "Observation of a large number of health centers," he said, "leads to an indication of two factors which all those studied appeared to present: first, the selection of a definite district, or of a population unit, with the aim of serving all therein who need the services offered; second, coordination of services within this area, embracing both the facilities furnished by the health center itself and those provided by other agencies. A definition might therefore be stated as follows: A health center is an organization which provides, promotes and coordinates needed medical service and related social service for a specified district."[48] Davis also emphasized that there were still many unanswered questions concerning policy, objectives, organization, administration and evaluation of health centers. For example, he asked, "How far is organization of the people of a district themselves a practical means of promoting the services at the center, and of advancing health education throughout the district? Experience shows great value in a loose local organization of agencies interested in medical or health work, in education, especially public and parochial schools, and neighborhood and recreational bodies. On the other hand, the attempt to organize the people of a district into a local council, with or without block workers, has generally yielded little result in proportion to the effort expended. The reasons for this difficulty lie deep in the characteristics of American neighborhood life, whether among native or foreign born."[49]

Meanwhile, significant district health programs were created and developed in a number of American communities. It is obviously impossible to discuss those developments in detail, but several selected examples can indicate some of their characteristics. In New York City a program of district health administration was developed after 1929, and a group of health centers was opened beginning with one in rented quarters in central Harlem. Actually, this program grew out of two demonstrations in the 1920s. The East Harlem Health

Center was initiated in 1920 by the New York County chapter of the Red Cross, and was opened in November 1921. The demonstration was planned as a three-year project involving the cooperation of the Health Department and 21 voluntary agencies, and was described as a "department store of health and welfare,"[50] where clients could find under one roof almost all the health and welfare services needed. Throughout the decade the Health Center continued to develop, and eventually became one of the municipal district health units. While East Harlem was the first general health center, the Bellevue-Yorkville Health Demonstration, organized in 1924 and opened to the public in 1926, led eventually to the adoption by New York City of the principle of district health administration.[51] Financed by the Milbank Memorial Fund and the Health Department, the demonstration was carried on for ten years in cooperation with a very large number of participating official and voluntary agencies.[52] With the example of two health centers in operation, and under pressure from leaders in the private health and welfare field, the Health Department developed a citywide plan of district administration, with a health center building in each district serving as a local headquarters for both private health and welfare agencies and for the field activities of the department. In 1934, under the administration of Fiorello H. La Guardia, the city embarked on a program of districting which has had its ups and downs over the years—but is still in existence at present. Owing to changing policies and intramural conflicts the potential of this system was never fully realized.

Plans initially started by William H. Welch in Baltimore in the 20s eventuated in 1932 in the establishment of the Eastern Health District as a cooperative endeavor of the Baltimore City Health Department, the Johns Hopkins School of Hygiene and Public Health, as well as several voluntary agencies. This district has made possible the intensive study of public health problems and has provided a field laboratory for the testing of new administrative procedures and for the training of personnel. A second district was organized in 1935.

The district health center, coordinating hitherto separated clinics and services, was inaugurated to replace centralized control of particular services. Generally, the health center has been a branch or unit of a local health department or some other official health agency. Except for such diseases as tuberculosis, venereal diseases and a few other conditions considered as public health problems, most medical care concerned with diagnosis and therapy remained outside the sphere of activity of health centers, which emphasized prevention. Farsighted leaders in the health field realized that the health center concept might be employed to improve the organization and provision of medical care, issues which had come to the forefront of public attention at the same time as the health center. The Social Unit experiment in Cincinnati had touched on this problem, as did J. L. Pomeroy, the County Health Officer of Los Angeles, in his ambitious program undertaken in 1919.[53] In his centers, Pomeroy originally included clinics staffed by physicians, nurses and social workers to provide preventive and curative services on an ambulatory basis. The clinics were available to the poor whose eligibility was established by a means test. Due largely to the complaints of physicians that medical care was being given to patients who should go to private practitioners, by 1935 this work had, for the most part, been turned over to the Welfare Department and the county general hospital. This attempt foundered on the slogan that undeserving individuals were abusing the service intended only for the indigent, a theme which has been played with variations for about one hundred years.[54]

The most imaginative approach was made by Hermann Biggs in 1920 when he endeavored to deal with health service for rural areas in New York State.[55] As Commissioner of Health, he proposed the establishment of local health centers to include one or more of the following elements: hospital, clinics (for tuberculosis, venereal diseases, prenatal and child care, mental illness, dental care, and general medical care), laboratories, public health nursing, and district health administration. Such centers could be established in any county with the approval of the State Health Commissioner. The proposal was permissive and not mandatory in any of its details. In addition to coordinating public health services, these centers were intended "to encourage and provide facilities for an annual medical examination to detect physical defects and disease"; and "to provide for the residents of rural districts, for industrial workers and all others in need of such service, scientific medical and surgical treatment, hospital and dispensary facilities and nursing care at a cost within their means or, if necessary, free." State aid in the form of 50 percent cash grants for buildings, a cash allowance for the treatment of patients unable to pay, together with certain allowances toward maintenance, were to be furnished to all communities fulfilling the requirements of the State Health Department. While a large number of community organizations supported these proposals, the Sage-Machold Bill which embodied this health center program, was defeated in the New York legislature. The whole concept was ahead of public opinion, and especially of opinion in the medical profession.

Biggs had realized that the next step in the development of community health services required a coalescence of preventive and curative medicine. Since 1920, this seminal concept has evolved in several directions. Among these the idea of comprehensive group practice coupled with prepayment, as exemplified by the Kaiser-Permanente Foundation and the Health Insurance Plan of Greater New York, has been demonstrated as practicable. Another approach was promoted by Joseph W. Mountin, of the U.S. Public Health Service, based on his belief that hospitals and health departments must eventually combine or coordinate their facilities and resources to provide a comprehensive health service for the communities they serve. As part of such a plan, he proposed to correlate the health center with the general hospital in the community.

After 1946, following the passage of the Hill-Burton Act, there was a renewal of the earlier interest in the role of the health center. A proponent of the idea who tied it to regionalization was John B. Grant of the Rockefeller Foundation. In fact, in 1949, he pointed out that the health center of the future had not yet been established.[56] Nevertheless, such centers did not really take hold after the 1940s.

## WHY DID THE HEALTH CENTER MOVEMENT DECLINE?

The concept of a local health center had developed largely in response to the circumstances and the needs of the urban poor, particularly the immigrants. From the time of World War I, however, these elements were changing, especially during the decades of the 20s and the 30s. Consequently, the time setting in which the movement for local health centers emerged and became institutionalized is important for understanding its further development.

The cessation of immigration during the war years and the restrictive legislation of 1921 and 1924 were undoubtedly important factors in changing the circumstances of the foreign-born. As the flow of new immigrants was cut down to a trickle, the foreign-born and even more so their children adapted to American life under the influence of economic and educational factors.[57] As they moved up the economic ladder, there was an increasing tendency to move out of the areas of initial settlement and toward the periphery of the community. Between 1920 and 1930 there appeared to be a growing trend toward less clustering of the foreign-born in ethnic neighborhoods. Movements within the cities and towards suburbs scattered members of these groups in areas that were mixed. Many of those involved in this process were younger persons of the second generation, largely native-born, with a greater earning capacity than their parents or older families with few children below working age. Hand-in-hand with these changes went higher levels of schooling among the children of the foreign-born and a wider use of English by their parents, changes clearly reflected in the foreign language press of the period.

As this potential clientele for local health centers changed its character, it turned more and more to the use of private health care. This tendency was reinforced by the limited nature of the services provided in most local health centers. Thus, there was practically no integration of preventive and curative services. As Michael Davis saw in 1921, "curative work furnishes the best approach to preventive" service. "In the field of preventive medical and health work," he said, "there is particular need for emphasizing . . . that the study of people must run parallel to the study of technique. As a corollary to this, curative work must be connected with preventive work, so that the service which the people seek of their own initiative can be supplemented by the service which we believe the larger interests of all require."[58] Therapeutic services were provided only to a limited degree, for the most part to patients with tuberculosis and venereal disease. At the same time medical practice was changing. Immunization, antepartum care and well child care were incorporated into the work of the private practitioner, and this was to happen later with the treatment of tuberculosis and venereal disease when the antibiotics became available.

The Depression of the 1930s retarded these tendencies, but they were reinforced indirectly as the attention of many concerned with the provision of medical care and its costs turned to the problem of organizing the financing of such care on a compulsory or voluntary basis. The improvement of economic conditions toward the end of the decade coincident with the outbreak of World War II made it financially possible for more people to seek private medical care, especially when labor-management negotiations provided varying forms of health insurance. Thus, the local health centers tended to lose one part of the rationale for their creation.

The same period also saw the erosion of another part of the theoretical underpinning of the health center movement. Need for coordination of health and welfare services had been adduced as a reason for bringing them together under one roof or at least in close contiguity. However, the role of social agencies changed greatly during the Depression as government, particularly on the federal level, assumed a larger and more active part in welfare, specifically in its financial aspects. At the same time social work was beginning to move away from an interest in social problems and reform. Case work became the dominant facet of social work, and in turn social work focused on the individual, on his personal strengths and weaknesses, and on individual psychological mechanisms, with psychoanalysis providing a theoretical rationale for this orientation.[59] Along this line of development, social agencies withdrew from health centers to other locations where they could centralize their therapeutic services and utilize them more efficiently.

In addition to the factors discussed above, there were a number of others that hindered the development of health centers and led to the decline of the movement. Thus, despite the often expressed aim of involving the local population in the neighborhood health program, this goal was hardly realized and remained more of a pious intention. Although Bellevue-Yorkville in New York City may have been envisaged as an experiment to crystal-lize community consciousness around health as a center, the demonstration was actually run by a group of voluntary health and welfare agencies, financed by a foundation in collaboration with the municipal health department.[60] In the New Haven Health Center Demonstration (1920–1923), efforts to develop active participation by local people were admittedly unsuccessful, mainly because the necessary rapport was not established with the largely Italian population.[61]

Another negative factor was the resistance by political forces in the broadest sense. The ability of government (municipal or state) to hinder or to facilitate the creation and development of health center programs is evident from the examples of Milwaukee, Cincinnati, and New York. Antagonism of professional groups such as physicians or welfare agencies was significant in some cases. Administrative infighting within the municipal health department was a factor in weakening the New York City health center program, and such a factor may have been operative elsewhere. Finally, one should note that the health center movement participated in the general pattern of development of public health during this period. In the late 1930s public health was beginning to approach the end of a period of development that had begun around the first decade of the century. World War II was an interlude in this transition which is still in process. By that time, however, the health center movement had run out of steam.

## QUESTIONS

Analysis of the earlier health center movement raises certain questions about the current neighborhood health centers. These too have come into being to provide for the needs of the urban poor, of people who have migrated to the city and who live under circumstances highly adverse to health. These centers clearly fill an immediate need, and no doubt fulfill their purpose better than did the earlier centers.[62] Today they are located in impoverished areas. But what should happen if and when the economic status of the population changes? One aim of the centers is job training, which implies a change in economic condition. Is it not possible that improved economic circumstances may lead to a shift of population, and thus to a loss of health center clientele? Or is there an unexpressed assumption that the poor will always be with us and a separate system is needed for them? Furthermore, should neighborhood centers remain purely local, or should they become part of a larger system of health care toward which we appear to be moving? Should they become part of a national health insurance system and of a larger health-care delivery system? Obviously, such questions have no immediate answer, but they do arise from a consideration of the earlier local health center movement.

## NOTES

On April 14, 1971, this paper was presented to the John Shaw Billings History of Medicine Society, Indiana University School of Medicine, Indianapolis, Indiana. This paper is also based in part on the author's experience as a clinic diagnostician in the Bureau of Tuberculosis, as a district health officer and borough health officer in the Office of District Health Administration, and as the director of the Bureau of Health Education in the New York City Department of Health (1940–1943, 1946–1950).

1  Sar A. Levitan, *The Great Society's Poor Law. A New Approach to Poverty* (Baltimore: Johns Hopkins Press, 1969), pp. 191–197.

2  Lisbeth Bamberger, "Health care and poverty: what are the dimensions of the problem from the community's point of view?" *Bull. N.Y. Acad. Med.*, 1966, *42*: 1140.

3  U.S. Bureau of the Census, *Historical Statistics of the United States: Colonial Times to 1957* (Washington, D.C.: Government Printing Office, 1960).

4  For the following see Moses Rischin, *The Promised City: New York's Jews, 1870–1914* (Cambridge, Mass.: Harvard Univ. Press, 1962); Hutchins Hapgood, *The Spirit of the Ghetto* (Cambridge, Mass.: Belknap-Harvard Univ. Press, 1967); Giuseppe Prezzolini, *I Trappiantati* (Milan: Longanesi, 1963), pp. 401–430; Phyllis H. Williams, *South Italian Folkways in Europe and America* (New Haven: Yale Univ. Press, 1938); Robert E. Park and Herbert A. Miller, *Old World Traits Transplanted* (New York: Harper & Bros., 1921). The literature on this theme is large and the above references are simply illustrative.

5  Henry George, *Social Problems* (New York, 1886), pp. 40–46, 161–162.

6  Barbara M. Solomon, *Ancestors and Immigrants. A Changing New England Tradition* (Cambridge, Mass.: Harvard Univ. Press, 1956). Quotation is from the edition published by John Wiley & Sons, 1965, pp. 140–141.

7  John Higham, *Strangers in the Land. Patterns of American Nativism, 1860–1925* (1955) (New York: Atheneum, 1963), pp. 88–94.

8  Richard C. Cabot, *Social Service and the Art of Healing* (1909) (New York: Dodd, Mead & Co., 1931), pp. 4–7.

9  R. L. Duffus, *Lillian Wald: Neighbor and Crusader* (New York, 1939), p. 147.

10  Jane Addams, "Hull House: an effort toward social democracy," *Forum*, 1892, *14*: 226; Jane Addams et al., *Philanthropy and Social Progress: Seven Essays* (New York, 1893), pp. 2–3, 15–16, 35–38; Lillian D. Wald, *The House on Henry Street* (New York: Henry Holt & Co., 1915), pp. 66, 184, 290, 310; Frank J. Bruno, *Trends in Social Work . . . 1874–1946* (New York, 1948).

11  Edward Thomas Devine (1867–1948) was General Secretary of the Charity Organization Society in New York City, 1896–1912, and Secretary until 1917; Director of the New York School of Philanthropy, 1904–1907, 1912–1917, and from 1905 to 1919 Professor of Social Economy at Columbia University.

12  Edward Thomas Devine, *Misery and Its Causes* (New York: Macmillan Company, 1910), p. 55. See the section on ill health in this book, pp. 53–112.

13  Wald, *The House on Henry Street*; Lillian D. Wald, *Windows on Henry Street* (Boston: Little, Brown & Co., 1934).

14  *Hull House Maps and Papers. A Presentation of Nationalities and Wages in a Congested District of Chicago, together with Comments and Essays on Problems Growing Out of the Social Conditions by Residents of Hull House* (New York and Boston: Thomas Y. Crowell, 1895), p. 228; Jane Addams, *Twenty Years at Hull House* (New York: Macmillan, 1910), pp. 342–358.

15  Kate H. Claghorn, "The foreign immigrant in New York City." In *United States Industrial Commission: Reports on Immigration* (Washington, D.C., 1901), XV, 449 ff.; see also *Harper's Weekly*, Jan. 12, 1895, pp. 42, 60–62, and June 22, 1895, pp. 586–587.

16  George Rosen, *A History of Public Health* (New York: MD Publications, 1958), pp. 344–349.

17  *Ibid.*, pp. 319–343.

18  "Health and national efficiency," *Modern Med.*, 1919, *1*: 2–3; H. W. Hill, "The new public health," *Ibid.*, 1919, *1*: 57–58.

19  Michael M. Davis, *Immigrant Health and the Community* (New York: Harper & Brothers, 1921), pp. 406–407.

20  *Annual Report of the Department of Health of the City of New York for the Calendar Year 1914* (New York,

1915), p. 25. *The House that Health Built. A Report of the First Three Years' Work of the East Harlem Health Center Demonstration,* prepared under the Direction of Kenneth D. Widdemer (New York, 1925), p. 4.

21   *The Health Units of Boston, 1924–1933* (City of Boston Printing Department, 1933), quoted in I. V. Hiscock, "The development of neighborhood health services in the United States," *Milbank Mem. Fund Quart. Bull.,* 1935, *13*: 30–51, p. 35.

22   Davis, *Immigrant Health,* p. 299.

23   *Ibid.,* p. 329.

24   *Ibid.,* p. 299.

25   Homer Folks, Preface, *House that Health Built,* p. 3.

26   Robert A. Woods, *The Neighborhood in Nation-Building* (Boston and New York: Houghton Mifflin Co., 1923), p. 279.

27   Wilbur C. Phillips, *Adventuring for Democracy* (New York: Social Unit Press, 1940). Unfortunately, Phillips rarely dates the events he describes so that the evolution of his activities and ideas has had to be reconstructed from other sources indicated below.

28   Charles E. North, "Milk and its relation to public health," in *A Half Century of Public Health,* ed. Mazyck P. Ravenel (New York: American Public Health Association, 1921), pp. 279–280; William H. Allen, "Health needs and civic action," in *The Public Health Movement* (Philadelphia: American Academy of Political and Social Science, 1911), pp. 3–12, see p. 7.

29   Rosen, *History of Public Health,* pp. 354–355.

30   Wilbur C. Phillips, "The achievements and future possibilities of the New York Milk Committee," *Proceedings of the Child Conference for Research and Welfare, 1909, Clark University, Worcester, Mass., July 6–10, 1909* (New York: G. E. Stechert & Co., 1910), pp. 189–192.

31   Wilbur C. Phillips, "The trend of medico-social effort in child welfare work," *Am. J. Public Hlth.,* 1912, *2*: 875–882, see pp. 881–882; Phillips, *Adventuring for Democracy,* pp. 46–47, 55–56, 63–114.

32   Phillips, *Adventuring for Democracy,* pp. 59–60.

33   A. C. Burnham, *The Community Health Problem* (New York: Macmillan Co., 1920), p. 108.

34   N. A. Nelson, "Neighborhood organization vs. tuberculosis," *Modern Med.,* 1919, *1*: 515–521; Courtenay Dinwiddie and A. G. Kreidler, "A community self-organized for preventive health work," *Modern Med.,* 1919, *1*: 26–31; Wilbur C. Phillips, "Democracy and the unit plan," *Proceedings of the National Conference of Social Work, Atlantic City, New Jersey, June 1–8, 1919* (National Conference of Social Work, 1920), p. 562.

35   William C. White, "The official responsibility of the state in the tuberculosis problem," *J.A.M.A.,* 1915, *65*: 512–514.

36   Davis, *Immigrant Health,* p. 381.

37   Shirley W. Wynne, "Neighborhood health development in the City of New York," *Milbank Mem. Fund Quart. Bull.,* 1931, *9*: 37–45.

38   *Annual Report of the Department of Health of the City of New York for the Calendar Year 1914* (New York, 1915), p. 25.

39   Davis, *Immigrant Health,* pp. 381–384. According to Herbert Kaufman, *The New York City Health Centers* (Inter-University Case Program #9) (Indianapolis: Bobbs-Merrill Co., 1959), the population was 35,000.

40   *Annual Report of the Department of Health of the City of New York for the Calendar Year 1916* (New York, 1917), pp. 23, 31; *Annual Report of the Department of Health of the City of New York for the Calendar Year 1917* (n.p., n.d.), pp. 12–13; Hiscock, "Development of neighborhood health services in the United States," pp. 38–39.

41   Charles F. Wilinsky, "The Blossom Street health unit," *Nation's Hlth.,* 1924, *6*: 397–398; Charles F. Wilinsky, "The health center," *Am. J. Public Hlth.,* 1927, *17*: 677–682.

42   Michael M. Davis, *Clinics, Hospitals and Health Centers* (New York: Harper & Brothers, 1927), pp. 354–355; Hiscock, "Development of neighborhood health services," p. 48.

43   [C.-E. A. Winslow], "The health center movement," *Modern Med.,* 1919, *1*: 327.

44   Burnham, *Community Health Problem,* pp. 99–100; E. A. Peterson and W. H. Brown, "The American Red Cross and health," *Nation's Hlth.,* 1921, *3*: 73–80.

45   James A. Tobey, "The health center movement in the United States," *Modern Hosp.,* 1920, *14*: 212–214.

46   Peterson and Brown, "American Red Cross," p. 79.

47   E. A. Peterson, "What is a health center?" *Nation's Hlth.,* 1921, *3*: 272–274.

48   Michael M. Davis, "Goal-post and yardsticks in health center work," *Am. J. Public Hlth.,* 1927, *17*: 433–440, p. 434.

49   *Ibid.,* p. 439.

50   *House that Health Built,* p. 4; *A Decade of District Health Center Pioneering: A Report of Ten Years Work of the East Harlem Center* (New York City, 1932), p. 23; George R. Bedinger, "Cooperative Health Plan in New York County," *Nation's Hlth.,* 1921, *3*: 486–489.

51   C.-E. A. Winslow and Savel Zimand, *Health Under the "El"* (New York & London: Harper & Brothers, 1937).

52   The exact number seems uncertain, but was probably close to 70. According to Hiscock there were 85, according to Kaufman about 65.

53   J. L. Pomeroy, "County health administration in Los Angeles," *Am. J. Public Hlth.,* 1921, *11*: 796–800; J. L. Pomeroy, "Health center development in

Los Angeles County," *J.A.M.A.*, 1929, *93*: 1546–1550.

54  George Rosen, The impact of the hospital on the patient, the physician and the community," *Hosp. Admin.*, 1964, *9*: 15–33.

55  Milton Terris, "Hermann Biggs' contribution to the modern concept of health centers," *Bull. Hist. Med.*, 1946, *20*: 387–412; B. R. Rickards, "What New York State has done in health centers," *Am. J. Public Hlth.*, 1921, *11*: 214–216.

56  John B. Grant, "Health care for the community," *Selected Papers,* ed. Conrad Seipp (Baltimore: Johns Hopkins Press, 1963), pp. 5–6, 21–24, and *passim.*

57  *Recent Social Trends in the United States. Report of the President's Research Committee on Social Trends* (New York: McGraw-Hill, 1933), pp. 469, 560, 563–564,

582; John C. Gebhart, *The Health of a Neighborhood. A Social Study of the Mulberry District* (New York Association for Improving the Condition of the Poor, 1924), pp. 5–7.

58  Davis, *Immigrant Health,* p. 419.

59  George Rosen, *Madness in Society. Chapters in the Historical Sociology of Mental Illness* (Chicago: Univ. of Chicago Press, 1968), pp. 310–312.

60  Winslow and Zimand, *Health Under the "El,"* pp. 11–13, 38–48.

61  Philip S. Platt, *Report on New Haven Health Center Demonstration July 1920–June 1923* (n.p., n.d.), pp. 21–23, 98.

62  Gerald Sparer, "Evaluation of OEO neighborhood health centers," *Am. J. Public Hlth.*, 1971, *61*: 931–942.

# 35

## The Movement toward a Safe Maternity:
## Physician Accountability in New York City, 1915–1940

JOYCE ANTLER AND DANIEL M. FOX

Until the 1940s, childbirth was, for most American women, a time of great danger and apprehension. Each year during the two decades after 1915, approximately 15,000 women perished from causes related to childbirth. Only tuberculosis accounted for more deaths among women in the childbearing years. The number of puerperal deaths, moreover, merely suggested the total loss of life in childbirth, for the deaths of many women with preexisting chronic conditions were frequently assigned not to puerperal causes but to the diseases that preceded their pregnancies. "As far as her chance of living through childbirth is concerned," wrote Dr. Josephine Baker, an authority in maternal and child health, the United States was near being "the most unsafe country in the world for the pregnant woman."[1] Many thousands of other women survived pregnancy with severe disability and lowered health status.

Although the issue of maternal mortality was the subject of many studies, conferences, and papers after 1915, it was not until the middle 30s, with the publication of a report on maternal mortality by the New York Academy of Medicine, that an effective strategy for its reduction came to be widely adopted. As we shall see, the startling facts produced by that report, together with the academy's unusual tactic of seeking maximum publicity in the lay press for its findings, galvanized the medical

JOYCE ANTLER is Assistant Professor of American Studies and Chair of the Women's Studies Program, Brandeis University, Waltham, Massachusetts.
DANIEL M. FOX is Professor of Humanities in Medicine, Health Sciences Center, State University of New York at Stony Brook.

Reprinted with permission from the *Bulletin of the History of Medicine*, 1976, *50*: 569–595.

profession into action, and led to widespread reform of obstetric practice in New York and other cities. The report has consequently been regarded as an important contributory factor in the marked decline of maternal mortality rates that occurred throughout the nation after 1935.

By the 1920s, the high rates of puerperal mortality in the United States attracted urgent attention. Because maternal death threatened family stability, it was seen as an even greater social loss than infant mortality, a problem to which health professionals had much earlier directed their attention. Saving mothers' lives, furthermore, was an issue which cut across the birth control controversy of the time, uniting conservative and liberal physicians and lay reformers. Safeguarding pregnancy rather than avoiding it became a central motive in the campaign to reduce the risk of childbirth.

While puerperal mortality rates in the United States remained stationary over a long period of time, mortality from most other diseases had shown marked decline. Spectacular improvements in medical science and technology, particularly in the field of prevention, occurred in the last decade of the 19th century and the first decades of the 20th. From 1890 to 1915, deaths per 100,000 in the U.S. Death Registration Area were reduced from 252 to 148.8 in tuberculosis, from 186.9 to 82.9 in pneumonia, from 97.8 to 15.7 in diphtheria and croup, and from 46.3 to 12.4 in typhoid fever.[2] The death rate from causes incidental to bearing children, however, showed no improvement. In 1890, the maternal death rate per 100,000 population was 15.3; in 1915, it was 15.2, while a year later it had risen to 16.3.[3] In spite of the introduction of prenatal supervision, wider dissemination of aseptic technique, and the increasing incidence of hospitalization for delivery, little progress was made in reducing the maternal death rate after 1915. Maternal mortality in the U.S. Registration Area never went below 61 per 10,000 births, the 1915 figure, prior to 1936.[4] In contrast, after 1915 infant mortality from practically every cause was reduced by 40 percent, from 99.9 per 10,000 live births in 1915 to 60.1 in 1934.[5]

No matter what statistical procedure was used, the United States maintained a high rate in comparison with other nations. In 1930, it ranked last out of 25 nations, its rate more than double that of Sweden, Denmark, Finland, Holland, Italy, Japan, and Uruguay.[6] Though mortality rates were not absolutely comparable among the various nations, studies showed that differences in statistical procedures or in methods of assigning causes to deaths did not explain the United States' exceedingly high rate.[7]

The stable rates of puerperal mortality threatened medical self-esteem. Physicians acknowledged that approximately one-half to three-quarters of puerperal deaths were caused by infection, toxemia, and hemorrhage, diseases considered controllable through adequate supervision during pregnancy and appropriate technique in labor and delivery.[8]

The failure to reduce maternal mortality rates produced lively debates within the medical community. Indeed, the problem of maternal mortality was amongst the most controversial public health problems of the day, generating heated arguments concerning the nature and conduct of obstetrics. Yet, in spite of the recognition of the problem, no clear consensus on the reasons for the high death rates emerged. Speculations involved a wide range of causes, including the lack of adequate prenatal care, pernicious midwifery, incompetence of general practitioners, poor obstetrical training of medical students and nurses, the low status and fee scale of obstetrics in contrast to general medicine and surgery, the expansion of indications for operative interference together with the more regular use of anesthesia, the absence of clinical material for training and lack of scientific interest in obstetrics, as well as its separation from gynecology, abortion and illegitimacy, falling birth rates, and finally, modern feminism, with its demand for technical-medical aids to achieve quick and painless labor.[9] Running through the debate was a fundamental

question whose resolution would be decisive in shaping the future pattern of obstetric practice: Should childbirth be viewed mainly as a natural, physiological process, usually resulting in spontaneous delivery and which, under appropriate supervision, could be managed by nonphysician attendants? Or was the more useful perception that it was a dangerous, and sometimes pathological, condition, frequently necessitating radical operative intervention, which required the attendance of skilled physician practitioners throughout?

## I

Medical interest in maternal health had been relatively slow to develop.[10] The prevention and control of illness and death of mothers and children was the most neglected of all public health services, Grace Abbott, director of the U.S. Children's Bureau, once commented.[11] Public responsibility for the securing of maternal and child health services in the U.S. lagged behind European initiatives. New York City in 1908 became the first governmental unit at any level to establish a division of child hygiene concerned solely with maternal and child health; ten years later, similar bureaus existed in only a handful of states.

The publication of mortality statistics by the U.S. Census Bureau in 1906 had first called attention to the prevailing high infant and maternal mortality. Over the next decade, health reformers interested in maternal and child welfare centered their efforts on the eradication of infant mortality. Services to childbearing mothers consisted primarily of limited, sporadic antepartum care for pregnant women, provided in an attempt to reduce the high infant death rate.

A 1917 report by Dr. Grace Meigs of the Children's Bureau, the first of its several studies of maternal mortality, was credited by several physicians with awakening the medical profession to an awareness of the severity of the problem of puerperal death.[12] The Meigs report characterized childbirth in the United States as suffering from an "unconscious neglect due to age-long ignorance and fatalism," and emphasized, assembling relevant statistics, that thousands of women died in childbirth from preventable causes.[13] The road to improvement, the report declared, was for women themselves to demand better care.

The passage of the Maternity and Infancy Act of 1921 (Sheppard-Towner Act), which marked the definite recognition of maternal mortality as a public health problem, was largely the work of a national woman's lobby. The legislation, drawn up by the Children's Bureau as a direct response to conditions revealed in its study of infant and maternal deaths, provided federal grants to states for fostering health services to mothers and children. The organization of state maternal and child health units followed. Thousands of prenatal and infant care programs initiated under these state divisions were developed.[14] While the Sheppard-Towner Act had little effect on maternal mortality rates before it lapsed in 1929, it aroused great public interest in maternity, enabling many women to learn what to ask and expect of their physicians, and alerting the medical profession to their demands.

By the 1920s, largely because of the impetus provided by the Sheppard-Towner program, prenatal care had become the favorite strategy of health reformers (though not of the medical profession generally) interested in maternal welfare.[15] But a minority of obstetricians, including the influential George Kosmak, editor of the *American Journal of Obstetrics and Gynecology*, began to question commonly held assumptions about the effectiveness of prenatal care in reducing maternal mortality.[16] They believed that while antepartum care helped diminish such accidents of pregnancy as toxemia, the leading cause of puerperal death — infection — occurred during and shortly after labor, and was more closely related to obstetric practice at these times than to the care of the expectant mother.

The definition of good obstetrics was, however, in contention. For many years, the untrained, poorly regulated midwife had borne the brunt of complaints about the low level of American obstetrics. Midwives delivered a significant proportion of American babies in 1915, approximately 40 percent nationwide (30 percent in New York City). In 1930, the nation's 47,000 midwives were responsible for 15 percent of births, though in some states, primarily in the South, they delivered 40–50 percent of babies.[17] Though they were required to register with local health departments in the majority of states, only a few states required licensing as a prerequisite for registration, and even these had minimum educational qualifications for licensure. Many unlicensed, unregistered midwives practiced without supervision of any kind. Educational opportunities for midwives were almost totally lacking: in the United States, there were only two schools, one in New York and one in Philadelphia, that trained midwives.[18]

According to widely held medical opinion, the use of incompetent midwives by low-income families was responsible for the high rates of maternal mortality. By the 1920s, however, the declining number of midwives in large cities threatened the easy correlation of puerperal mortality with their attendance. Moreover, the lowest mortality rates were frequently found in cities with the highest percentage of births attended by midwives.[19] In states where childbirth was completely in physician hands, like New Hampshire, Vermont, and Oregon, maternal death rates were as high as the national average.[20] Finally, maternal mortality was lower in all European countries (except Scotland) than in the United States, although at least one-half and usually more than 80 percent of births in these nations were attended by midwives, as compared to only 15 percent in the United States (in 1930).[21]

Many medical observers considered the general practitioner the great danger in obstetrics.[22] According to this view, the G.P. took on obstetric work as a loss leader to acquire the medical practice of the patient's family, but gave it as little time and attention as possible because fees for obstetric cases were low. Hurried and under great pressure, the young practitioner would frequently resort to techniques he had little skill in performing in the interest of hastening labor. While it was usually agreed that general practitioners were suitable attendants for normal confinements, the absence of specified standards for obstetric specialization permitted them free access to more complicated cases of abnormal labor, despite their lack of training and experience. Furthermore, the G.P.'s constant contact with infectious diseases treated in his routine practice increased the chances of puerperal sepsis. "Obstetrics," it was said, "is the general practitioner's specialty."[23]

Part of the problem lay in the low status accorded to obstetrics among medical specialties. Obstetrics was considered the least appreciated branch — the "Cinderella" or "stepdaughter" — of medicine. Practitioners did not receive as complete a training in obstetrics as they did in medicine and surgery. Medical students were given at least twice and often five times as many hours in general surgery as in obstetrics, although most general practitioners spent twice as much time in obstetric care as surgery. Because childbirth had historically been seen as a natural function, the public at large thought the obstetrician's accomplishments less than those of his surgical colleagues in gynecology. Since females originally practiced it, obstetrics was conceived of as "hardly a man's job," which could apparently be mastered by inspiration after the observation of a small number of cases.[24] Even the leading figure in early 20th-century American obstetrics, J. Whitridge Williams of Johns Hopkins, annually apologized to medical students for the long association of his discipline with ignorant midwives.[25] That maternal mortality was lowest, however, in countries in which medical schools gave the longest and most complete undergraduate training in obstetrics did not fail to attract attention, and most reformers concluded that any improvement in obstetrics would have to follow curriculum revision directed toward securing more hours of obstetrical training.

The great increase in radical, or operative, obstetrics after 1915 appeared to be a primary cause of rising puerperal mortality, counterbalancing lives saved as the result of the introduction of asepsis and improved prenatal care. Forceps delivery, previously uncommon, was now practiced routinely for fetal as well as maternal indications. Caesarian sections, performed in the past only for definite indications like contracted pelvis and obstructed birth canal, had been extended to almost all complications of pregnancy and labor, including patient convenience. In many hospitals, one-quarter to one-half of all deliveries were performed by forceps, Caesarian sections, or version, a trend no doubt accelerated because surgical deliveries commanded fees twice those for spontaneous births. Economic factors also prevented the physician from spending time waiting for women to deliver spontaneously, another reason for the upsurge in surgical delivery. Experts believed, nevertheless, that 90–95 percent of all pregnancies were capable of being delivered by normal means. They pointed out that the lowest maternal death rates in the world were those of Holland, Sweden, and Denmark where at least 95 percent of births were spontaneous.[26]

The great increase in hospitalization of parturient women and the easy accessibility of anesthesia were cited as factors leading to increased, rather than decreased, maternal mortality, because they fostered surgical intervention. In the early 1930s, 56–85 percent of all live births in the ten largest U.S. cities took place in hospitals. Though hospitalization had advantages for the pregnant woman, it exposed her to infections and led, said some observers, to the "often false feeling of security of the operating room" and thus to unnecessary and dangerous operations.[27] The popularity of in-hospital surgical interventions, moreover, influenced the training of interns, so that while artificial deliveries were stressed, the importance of the physiology of labor and of conservative obstetrics was ignored.

The departure from the traditional "watchful expectancy" of obstetrics in favor of routine surgical delivery was based on a conception of labor as "decidedly pathologic" and the idea that the modern woman, a "neurasthenic product of civilization," stood suffering with less fortitude than her forebears, demanding anesthesia and even Caesarian section to escape its dangers and pains. The patient herself was regarded as a cause for the high puerperal death rates almost as frequently as were midwives and G.P.'s. Her self-indulgent demands for a quick and painless labor—a result, it was said, of modern life-styles, education, and magazine publicity—forced physicians against their will into a "reign of operative terror," where anesthesia inhibited the normal contractions of labor and made intervention imperative.[28] "American obstetrics," said one critic to a convention of the American Medical Association in 1936, "seems to be becoming a competitive practice to please American women in accordance with what they read in lay magazines."[29]

Although some women physicians supported the use of anesthesia to relieve childbirth suffering, they generally opposed routine surgical delivery. Many believed that the solution to the problem of maternal mortality lay in the assumption of obstetric practice by female doctors, who, they believed, were more sensitive to the needs of patients during childbirth, a position rigorously denied in the male-dominated discussion of maternal mortality. The superiority of female doctors in childbirth, they believed, was clearly indicated by the low maternal death rates of women's hospitals staffed by female physicians.[30]

Abortion and birth control, finally, were recognized as causes of increased maternal mortality. The desire to limit family size or to terminate growing numbers of unwanted out-of-wedlock pregnancies, some physicians claimed, resulted in large numbers of maternal deaths from intentional abortions, neutralizing gains made from improved obstetric practice.[31] Falling birth rates, furthermore, meant an increasing number of older primiparas who were less resistant to puerperal accidents, and hence, greater maternal mortality.[32] Birth control advocates, on the other hand, recognized that abortion deaths contributed to maternal mortality, but modified the argument. According to their view, the chief reason for the high death rates was the unwillingness of many women of impaired health or desperate economic circumstances to bear children, and their consequent resort to illegal abortion, frequently ending in death.[33]

## II

New York City had long maintained a tradition of leadership in obstetrics and child welfare. The first effort to regulate midwife practice in the United States was undertaken in New York City in 1906; the following year, the first organized attempt to provide prenatal services to mothers began when the New York Association for Improving the Condition of the Poor engaged several nurses to visit mothers in tenement homes to instruct them in infant hygiene and "prevent infant deaths by caring for the mothers before the babies were born."[34] In 1908, the nation's first Bureau of Child Hygiene was established in the New York City Department of Health, and in 1911, the first school for midwives opened at Bellevue.

New York City had just begun to reorganize its system of maternal and obstetric care in 1915 following a study by a committee of New York physicians appointed by the then Health Commissioner, Dr. Haven Emerson, to analyze the conditions of childbirth in Manhattan, and their relation to the deaths of infants under one month of age. The committee, finding that many such deaths were caused by lack of prenatal care and poor care at the time of delivery, recommended that the city be divided into zones, in each of which would be established a maternity center where mothers could come for prenatal care. As a result of the study, the first maternity center in the United States was formed by the Women's City Club of New York in 1917, its work later taken over by the Maternity Center Association, founded the following year, which organized 30 prenatal clinics throughout the city. Later the association discontinued sponsorship of the prenatal clinics in favor of complete and intensive care for all phases of the maternity cycle at one model center. More than any other single agency, the Maternity Center Association developed and demonstrated a model for a community maternity service, and through its institutes for public health nurses and other educational work, stimulated other communities to establish similar services.[35]

Despite its superior health services and record of accomplishment in obstetrics and child health, New York City's puerperal death rate in 1930 was barely a percentage point lower than the national average. While the city's infant mortality rate had declined from 85.4 deaths per 1,000 live births in 1920 to 50.9 in 1933, its rate of maternal mortality had in fact increased from 5.33 per 1,000 live births in 1921 to 5.98 in 1932. The Public Health Relations Committee of the New York Academy of Medicine had been aware of the city's high puerperal death rate since 1917, when at the urging of Dr. George Kosmak, a subcommittee was appointed to gather data on maternal mortality in New York. When this study, based on hospital questionnaires, as well as a successive study which utilized Health Department statistics, failed to produce accurate results, a new plan to study the public health problems of obstetrics in New York was suggested by Drs. Kosmak and Ralph W. Lobenstine at the request of the Public Health Relations Committee. The committee then appointed a Subcommittee on Maternal Mortality, consisting of Dr. Frederic E. Sondern, chairman, and Drs. Philip Van Ingen, Benjamin P. Watson, and Ransom S. Hooker. The subcommittee decided to undertake a survey based on a direct, personal inquiry of puerperal deaths, to begin January 1, 1930, and continue for three years, running concurrently with the deaths. An Obstetrical Advisory Committee, chaired by Dr. Watson, and with Kosmak, John O. Polak, and Harry Aranow as members, was appointed. Ransom Hooker was chosen director of the study. The work of gathering and tabulating the material was performed by two women physicians, Dr. Marynia Farnham and Dr. Elizabeth Arnstein, and several registered nurses. Dr. Farnham, along with Kosmak, wrote much of the final report. The New York Obstetrical Society provided an initial loan, and the Commonwealth Fund provided funds for the completion of the study.[36]

Kosmak and Watson, both prominent New York obstetricians deeply concerned about the problem of maternal mortality, were active and influential members of the Obstetrical Advisory Committee. Kosmak was president, in 1930, of the New York Obstetrical Society, and in 1932, of the New York County Medical Society, and edited the *American Journal of Obstetrics and Gynecology*. His long-standing interest in the problem of maternal mortality was related to his vigorous, orthodox Catholic opposition to birth control and the belief that, to maintain the birth rate, pregnancy had to be made desirable through elimination of the fear of childbirth. A medical as well as social conservative, Kosmak questioned trends toward hospitalization of all confinements, routine surgical delivery and anesthesia, and the widespread promotion of prenatal care as the remedy for maternal mortality. After a 1927 trip to Scandinavia, which impressed him with the excellent results obtained from carefully supervised midwife practice, he retreated from his former antipathy to midwifery, and began to consider the trained midwife as a possible participant in a reformed system of obstetric care.[37]

Watson, Professor of Obstetrics and Gynecology at Columbia University, had trained in Scotland, taught and practised in Canada, and participated in a survey of maternal mortality in Scotland in 1925. His account of an outbreak of puerperal infection at Sloane Hospital in 1927 received national publicity, although it discomforted many in the profession. Like Kosmak, he espoused a conservative obstetrics, questioning the routine hospitalization of obstetric patients. However, he was more definitive in recommending a system of trained nurse-midwives as part of a professional hospital team to handle normal deliveries, a decidedly minority opinion in the medical profession.[38] A third member of the Advisory Committee, John O. Polak of the Long Island College Hospital, was an exponent of the value of home deliveries.

The methodology employed in the New York in-

vestigation was adopted from a Children's Bureau study of maternal mortality in 15 states in 1927–1928 (published in 1933), the first thorough clinical study of large numbers of maternal deaths, and involved an analysis of individual case records supplemented by a personal interview with the attending physician. Each week during the period of the survey, the New York City Health Department forwarded to investigators copies of all death certificates which named a puerperal condition as primary or contributory, or which stated the existence of pregnancy. Within one month of each death, while circumstances were fresh in the minds of attendants, interviews were conducted with everyone who attended the patient at any time during pregnancy, delivery, or the puerperium. Investigators had access to all written hospital records.

The Obstetric Advisory Committee, in consultation with investigators, then examined each case to determine the true cause of death and whether the death was preventable, using as the criterion for an avoidable death whether the "best possible skill in diagnosis and treatment which the community could make available" had been applied. Responsibility for a preventable death was assigned either to the attendant — physician or midwife — or to the patient herself. If every possible precaution had been taken by the patient and attendant, and if the delivery had been properly carried out, the death was considered nonpreventable. Accounts of the quality of care were correlated to the patient's economic status, which was determined from housing data; and information on hospital procedures, standards and personnel was gathered by questionnaire.[39]

The benefit of clinical methodology was demonstrated by the finding that the usual reporting methods which relied on vital statistics routinely filed with departments of health resulted in a high margin of error, 17.8 percent. In the case of abortion, the disparity between the actual and reported cause of death was 34.7 percent, and for septicemia, 29.2 percent.[40]

The outstanding finding of the study was that in the total series (2,041 deaths) nearly two-thirds (65.8 percent) of all deaths were judged to be preventable had the patient received proper care. By cause, 77.1 percent of deaths from induced abortions, 75.1 percent of deaths from septicemia, 76.1 percent of deaths from hemorrhage, and 87.1 percent of deaths following accidents of labor were considered avoidable. For all the preventable deaths, responsibility lay with the physician in 61.1 percent of cases, with the patient in 36.7 percent, and with midwives in only 2.2 percent. Following operative delivery, 76.8 percent of deaths were considered avoidable, a higher percentage than in the total series, with responsibility assigned to the physicians 86.8 percent of the time. Physician responsibility for preventable deaths was divided almost equally between faults of technique, 50.9 percent, and errors of judgment, 49.1 percent, suggesting a "surprisingly high degree of actual technical incompetence" and "a lack of respect for operative undertakings."[41]

By cause, the largest proportion of deaths (25.0 percent) was due to septicemia; next in importance were deaths from abortion (17.5 percent).[42] Almost half the deaths in the entire series (45 percent) had followed operative delivery. The mortality rate for operative delivery was found to be five times that for spontaneous delivery (10.5 to 2.0). Caesarian sections, although they represented only 2.2 percent of total deliveries in the series, constituted a remarkable 19.8 percent of total deaths (excluding deaths from abortions and extrauterine pregnancies).[43] Anesthesia was the direct cause of death in 20 cases, but was administered to 87.7 percent of patients whose death was attributed to operative shock. (Noting the close association between anesthesia and operative delivery, the report warned against the casual use of anesthesia for the "mere alleviation or the entire elimination of pain."[44])

For hospital deliveries, the death rate was more than two times that for deliveries in homes (4.5 to 1.9), where about 30 percent of all births took place, leading the committee to suggest a reexamination of attitudes toward home confinement.[45] There was no difference in the result of home deliveries by physicians or by midwives, even though only one-third of the midwives interviewed were found to be truly competent. The death rate for deliveries by midwives who had contact with 5.4 percent of patients in the series was, at 1.6 per 1,000 live births, 64 percent lower than the general series rate of 4.5 per 1,000 live births.[46]

Data on hospital practice throughout the city, collected by questionnaire, showed that the proportion of preventable deaths was significantly lower in municipal (34.2 percent) than in either voluntary (49.1 percent) or obstetric (51.4 percent) hospitals, a finding the committee attributed to the fact that the percentage of Caesarian sections performed in municipal hospitals was less than one-half that in obstetric hospitals and little more than one-half that for voluntary hospitals. The report concluded that no adequate control of voluntary or proprietary hospitals was maintained in the city.[47]

Finally, the risk of death in pregnancy was found to be highly correlated with economic status, race, and nativity. The highest puerperal death rate was found among the least-favored group, the lowest among the most privileged, although the white-collar class showed a higher rate than the less well-off artisan group, which relied on free care provided by municipal and voluntary hospitals.[48] For Negro women and foreign-born women, the data, however disturbing, followed customary curves: the death rate for black women was twice as great as for white women; the rate for foreign-born women from all puerperal causes greatly exceeded that for native-born women.[49]

From these statistical findings, the committee concluded that the death rate of women in childbirth in New York was unnecessarily high because of the following reasons: (1) *Inadequate and improper prenatal care*. In almost 60 percent of the cases examined, the patient failed to seek prenatal care, and where it was sought, the attendant frequently failed to provide it. (2) *High incidence of operative interference during labor*. Frequently operations were performed for the wrong indications, at improper times, and without an appropriately trained attendant. (3) *The attendants' incapacity in judgment or skill*. Here, errors included the failure to provide proper prenatal care, frequently incorrect prognosis and improper conduct of delivery, the lack of consultation, and the failure to maintain proper asepsis. (4) *Inadequate hospital standards*. These included improper physical equipment; lack of appropriate labor and delivery facilities; failure to carry out isolation; use of operating rooms as delivery rooms; the performance of major operative procedures by unsupervised residents or junior members of attending staffs without consultation with chiefs; the failure of many proprietary hospitals to exercise staff supervision. (5) *Midwife incompetence*. The training of midwives, many of them elderly, illiterate, foreign-born women, was frequently insufficient, and there was no attempt to evaluate qualifications for licensure.[50]

The committee's recommendations for changes in methods of obstetric practice included: education for the public as to the necessity of prenatal care, the dangers of operative delivery, and the relative safety of home delivery, with the more active participation by physician organizations in lay education through press, radio, and publications; improved training of medical students, including prolonged graduate study for specialization, and of hospital interns; the confinement of nonspecialist practitioners to normal cases, requiring frequent and early consultations with highly trained specialists; improved hospital facilities and supervision of staff, including stricter control of proprietary hospitals, the appointment of qualified obstetricians as staff directors, the maintenance of separate obstetric delivery rooms, the observation of rules for asepsis, especially masking, and stringent isolation; and finally, improved training and supervision of better qualified midwives.[51]

While the committee had found many midwives poorly trained, it concluded that, since the results of their practice were as good as those obtained by physicians under comparable circumstances, the midwife was an "acceptable attendant for properly selected cases of labor and delivery" and should have a position in any scheme for providing for maternity care. "In face of the pressing problem of assuring proper care for all women at an outlay that is not prohibitive," it reported, "she has proven her value." The medical profession must accept the midwife as "one of its adjuncts," an "ally" in reducing childbirth morbidity and mortality. "There must be a readiness to cooperate with her."[52]

The report left no doubt as to the major source of the high puerperal death rate:

> Sixty percent of all deaths which could have been avoided have been brought about by some incapacity in the attendant. . . . Most are plainly the results of incompetence. Prevention in this field will mean increasing the respect of the physician for the gravity of obstetrical operations and educating him to a greater caution in attacking problems which are properly the field only of the highly trained obstetrician. . . .
>
> The hazards of childbirth in New York City are greater than they need be. Responsibility for reducing them rests with the medical profession.[53]

Despite its greater detail and more elaborate methodology, the conclusions of the New York study were similar to those of recent surveys elsewhere in the United States and abroad. Studies of maternal deaths in Britain and Scotland, a study of puerperal mortality in Massachusetts and one in Cleveland, the 15-state Children's Bureau study and reports presented to the White House Conference on Child Health and Protection called by President Hoover pointed to the conclusion that maternal mortality was preventable, and was related to such factors as lack of prenatal care, operative interference by incompetent attendants, inadequate and improperly supervised institutional facilities, poorly trained, unregulated midwives, as well as contributing negligence of patients and their families.[54] The remedies, too, were similar: education, standards, and obstetrical restraint. What distinguished the academy report from other studies were: a precise and detailed clinical methodology which provided indisputable evidence about preventability; the undisguised attribution of blame for preventable deaths to the medical profession; and an acceptance of trained midwives and home delivery in normal obstetrical cases, contrary to general medical opinion. Most important, the academy deliberately and effectively publicized its findings through an unusual media release that was designed to attract attention and precipitate controversy within the medical profession.

The report received wide medical and lay attention. Before the report, published by the Commonwealth Fund in November 1933, was reviewed in any medical journal, the Medical Information Bureau of the academy released to the lay press a carefully worded summary of it entitled, *Why Women Die in Childbirth*.[55] The findings, especially the responsibility assigned to physicians for many preventable deaths, were given prominent attention in more than 300 newspapers in 30 states. "When a doctor attacks another doctor," the *Nation* editorialized, "it is time for the general public to take notice."[56]

Despite the committee's matter-of-fact approach, the assignment of responsibility to the medical community was controversial. The New York Obstetrical Society, an original sponsor of the study, filed a formal complaint with the academy, whose council had approved the committee report by a unanimous vote, protesting this publicity.[57]

The medical societies of Queens, Bronx, and Albany counties also protested the method of publicity.[58] Many physicians, as was customary when the profession was embarrassed, suggested sinister motives.

A subcommittee of the academy's Public Health Relations Committee, composed of two former academy presidents, Dr. S. W. Lambert and Dr. J. S. Hartwell, was appointed to report on the press release and the Obstetrical Society's protest against it. The committee concluded that the abstract had been released by the Medical Information Bureau in accordance with academy bylaws, and that much criticism of the method of publicity arose from the decision to postpone reviewing the report in the medical press until after publication of the book and lay articles about it. It found that the release did provide an accurate summary of the report's findings, and that its much-criticized caption, *Why Women Die in Childbirth*, described the study appropriately. The committee defended the deliberate publicity, concluding that the saving of even one mother's life was more important than medical prestige. Unfavorable criticism arose, the academy spokesmen declared, from the "startling nature of the facts" themselves, which provoked fear that the revelations would do harm to physicians. Minimizing the seriousness of the situation would, they countered, open the profession to the charge of shielding itself from attack.[59]

The Obstetrical Society counterattacked, appointing its own committee to report on the academy abstract. While the target ostensibly was the manner of publicity, in fact the society committee attacked the major interpretations of the report itself. It argued, first, that preventability was an imprecise concept (the obstetricians preferred the term "controllable"), which might result in unfair lawsuits for malpractice. Secondly, it argued that the report distorted the facts in assigning midwives only 2.2 percent of preventable deaths, since midwives attended a small proportion of deliveries out of the total series. (The true percentage of preventable mortality, it suggested, was 75 percent in midwife-attended cases compared to 68 percent for the physician group.) Licensing any additional midwives was opposed, for as long as the midwife was permitted to practice, "obstetrics will never be elevated to the position it rightly deserves." Home delivery, furthermore, was not safer than delivery in well-organized hospitals. Surgical interventions when performed under proper indications by skilled personnel were "merciful" and "life-saving." Caesarian section was one of the "greatest blessings" to modern women. Proper administration of anesthesia was "essential," "valuable," and "humane."[60]

At its April meeting, the Obstetrical Society endorsed the committee's report, and authorized its immediate release to the lay press in an abstract titled *How Childbirth May Be Made Safe*.[61] Dr. Benjamin Watson, chairman of the Obstetrical Advisory Committee to the academy study, promptly resigned his office as first vice-president of the Obstetrical Society in protest.[62] Kosmak also resigned from the society's council, and refused to publish either the society's transactions concerning the academy study, or its abstract, in the *American Journal of Obstetrics and Gynecology*. The issue was purely a local one, he wrote the society's secretary, for which there would be no national audience.[63]

The academy strategy of maximum publicity achieved the intended political effect. Medical associations in cooperation with the Health Department acted with unaccustomed speed to eliminate obstetric mismanagement and carry out the recommendations of the report. The New York Obstetrical Society offered the services of its newly formed Maternal Advisory Committee to the city Health Commissioner, and most of the county medical societies appointed their own subcommittees on maternal welfare.[64] An Advisory Obstetric Council to the Departments of Health and Hospitals, with Kosmak as general secretary, was appointed to make a citywide survey of obstetric facilities, methods and personnel, and submit recommendations. As a consultant to the Bureau of Child Hygiene, Kosmak also assisted in the development of a prenatal program for the city.[65] By 1938, Dr. Watson, who had resigned as vice-president of the Obstetrical Society during the controversy, became its president.

Several months after the report was published, Kosmak presented the political analysis which justified the deliberate publicity to a meeting of the Obstetrical Society itself.[66] The failures revealed by the study, "were the shortcomings of medical men" which could be corrected only by the profession. The report did not threaten the 70 obstetric specialists who were society members, but rather, the 4,000 practitioners of medicine in New York who necessarily performed the bulk of its obstetrics. The most important task in correcting the situation was to restrict the G.P. The society should therefore present a united front in support of the academy report, and not allow its criticisms of it to be used by G.P.'s against it. As for the midwife, "like it or not" she was "an institution and we simply must make the best of it and must provide for improvement" until a substitute could be found. Trained midwives, Kosmak asserted, were superior in skills and ability to the student nurses to whom hurried doctors regularly entrusted the care of their hospitalized maternity patients.

Some weeks later, Kosmak addressed a special meeting called by the New York Academy of Medicine to discuss "the constructive aspects" of its report.[67] He spoke of the problem of the general practitioner and of the poorly supervised intern and junior staff member, who, because of the absence of standards, "could do things in obstetrics which he would not be tempted to do in other fields of medicine." Kosmak admitted that the imposition of restraints through "self-imposed regulations" of medical agencies might be interpreted as "interference with the legal rights of a licensed physician" but he believed such action would do much to reestablish public confidence and "thus react favorably rather than otherwise" on medical practice.

Kosmak endeavored to enlist wide community and lay support of mortality review in the belief that the securing of a safe motherhood was a collective responsibility to be carried out at the local level. The strategy of maximum exposure undertaken by the academy to publicize its report reflected this view. Physicians were to provide leadership through the establishment of committees to survey and evaluate local data, Kosmak explained, but a wide segment of the community—nurses' groups, women's clubs, and allied professions and agencies—had to be actively engaged in order to act upon the data. Only through intense community involvement ("community control," as Kosmak phrased it) could the tide of maternal mortality be reversed and an "obstetric conscience" created. Self-regulation at the local level, furthermore, could prevent the introduction of some degree of federal control of medical practice, a possibility which Kosmak, a staunch opponent of state intervention in medicine, greatly feared.[68]

The methods expounded by Kosmak produced successful results in a short period of time. Maternal mortality in New York City declined by 45 percent in the five years following publication of the report.[69] While several factors may have contributed to the reduction, New York City's positive experience helped establish mortality review as an important preventive tool in curbing puerperal death.

## III

The analysis of maternal deaths proceeded in several other cities, where, as in New York, initial studies led to the establishment of permanent committees mandated to conduct continuous reviews of obstetric practice. The results of the New York study were publicized extensively by agencies like the Maternity Center Association of New York. Many cities and counties began to study their maternal deaths and to formulate inclusive plans for the care of mothers and babies. Along with the New York model, Philadelphia's maternal mortality committee became a prototype for a mortality review mechanism widely adopted across the country. In 1930, the Philadelphia County Medical Society appointed a maternal welfare committee, under the chairmanship of Dr. Philip Williams, to investigate obstetric conditions in the city. Patterning its three-year survey directly after the New York Academy study in an attempt to determine causes of death, whether preventable, and where responsibility lay, its conclusion—that the major blame for the city's high death rate rested primarily with the medical profession, with midwives a negligible factor—repeated the New York findings.[70]

After the completion of the study, the Philadelphia committee decided to continue its analysis of maternal deaths through a cooperative program developed between hospital obstetric staffs and the County Medical Society. The committee expanded its membership to include representatives from maternity departments of all Philadelphia hospitals as well as interns, residents, social workers, and other interested parties. Under Dr. Williams' guidance, and without fear of malpractice suits, maternal deaths were carefully analyzed in an "open monthly forum" to assess responsibility for blame.

The monthly seminars revealed the practice of

"much bad obstetrics," according to Dr. Williams, and corrective measures, particularly to prevent unnecessary obstetric surgery by unqualified staff, were taken. Hospitals accepted new rules specifying obligatory consultations before Caesarian section as well as techniques in labor, delivery room, and nursery, and redefined staff privileges.[71]

As a result of the monthly review meetings, an "obstetric conscience" was created in Philadelphia. An excellent description of how the committee achieved this result was provided by Dr. Thaddeus Montgomery, a participant in the Philadelphia committee. "At first," he wrote,

> no very noticeable effect upon maternal mortality was observed, but as the years passed and the activities of the Committee became more widely recognized, a subtle change of attitude took place. Hospital staffs became zealous in the analysis of their own obstetric fatalities. . . . The occurrence of a maternal death became a calamity to be carefully studied by the institution in which it occurred. . . . Gradually physicians began to feel that in the conduct of obstetric delivery they were not free agents to act as they would, but that the medical opinion of the city was looking over their shoulders to see that they gave to each patient the best that modern obstetric practice had to offer. Consultation in different situations was expected, and "acrobatic" obstetrics became taboo — no longer to be tolerated.[72]

The work of this committee resulted in a dramatic decline in maternal deaths, a result which Williams believed preceded improvement caused by the widespread use of antibiotics, sulfa drugs, and blood banks. From 1931 to 1940, the rate of maternal mortality in Philadelphia dropped by almost two-thirds (from 68 per 10,000 live births to 23).[73] So highly successful was its work, in fact, that the Obstetrical Society established similar mortality review committees to investigate problems of stillbirths, fetal deaths, and premature births, where further problems of obstetric mismanagement had been revealed. Similar gains took place in other large cities, and in fact, throughout the United States as a whole, although it seemed that the rate of maternal mortality decreased more quickly and substantially in states like New York, Pennsylvania, Connecticut, Rhode Island, and New Jersey, where cooperation and self-criticism reached its peak.

By the end of the 30s, many more maternal mortality review committees had been formed by state and county medical societies in cooperation with hospitals and health departments. Their establishment stimulated healthy rivalry among communities jealous of their progress in the field, each vying with the others to show lower mortality figures from year to year. Following the procedure developed in New York and Philadelphia, each maternal death was carefully studied and analyzed, in open meetings, to determine how the death might have been prevented and who was at fault. The process deterred unnecessary and dangerous procedures by unqualified attendants, and by case discussion reinforced the need for expert obstetric consultation when problems arose. Descendants of these committees, in most states and many local areas, are today major participants in peer review in cases of maternal mortality and morbidity.[74]

IV

The establishment of maternal mortality review committees was one aspect of a vast expansion in maternal welfare work that took place in the 1930s. By the end of the decade, many communities had active maternal welfare agencies engaged in a wide variety of educational, preventive, and regulatory work, including mortality review. Many experts correlated the rapid reduction of maternal mortality after 1935 with these activities.[75] Our data suggest, however, that cause and effect are more complicated.

After remaining stationary for so many decades, the puerperal death rate had begun to fall in the early 30s, though rather slowly. After 1936, the decline accelerated. From 1930 to 1936, the United States maternal mortality rate fell 15 percent (from 6.7 to 5.7 per 1,000 live births), or approximately 3 percent a year. In the years 1936–1938, the rates fell 12 percent annually (from 5.7 to 4.2). The comparative rate of decrease was 14 percent in the years 1930–1935, 35 percent in 1935–1940, and in the 1940s, 74 percent.[76]

During the decade after 1933, when the New York Academy's report was published, the maternal death rate in the United States declined by 60 percent, almost double the rate of reduction for infant mortality, which decreased 31 percent.[77] The decline in maternal mortality rates, moreover, was not paralleled by decreases in rates of other important causes of death. By 1949, the maternal mortality rate for the entire United States was less than one maternal death per 1,000 live births, comparing favorably with the lowest rates obtainable abroad. The change had occurred in every part of the country—in 1949, even the highest state rate (2.4) was about one-half the lowest rate in 1933 (4.3 per 1,000 live births)—and had affected rates from every cause of puerperal mortality.[78] Maternal mortality was no longer a serious nationwide problem, even if rates remained relatively high in particular areas.

Although the decline in maternal mortality rates in the 1930s appears to have been most dramatic in places like New York and Philadelphia where the greatest medical and civic activity to control obstetric practice occurred, the reduction in maternal mortality in the United States was so widespread that it cannot be comfortably accounted for by increased maternal welfare services and improved obstetric care alone. Moreover, maternal mortality rates fell sharply in the same period of time throughout the world. Beginning about 1936, maternal mortality dropped sharply in the United States, Switzerland, the Union of South Africa, Mexico, Scotland, New Zealand, the Irish Free State, Australia, Canada, England, and Wales. Within seven to eight years, the rate had been reduced by half in many of these nations.[79]

There is at present no satisfactory explanation for the change occurring with such apparent uniformity among countries so obviously disparate, and with such varying levels of medical care and services.[80] For the United States, several contributory causes can be suggested.

Advances in medical knowledge and techniques were of major importance, particularly the development and use, after 1933, of antibiotics, sulfonamides, and blood and blood substitutes. The beginning of the sharpest declines in maternal mortality rates coincided with the wider adoption of these measures, although rates had started to fall even earlier. Furthermore, the reduction in puerperal mortality was not limited to deaths due to infection and to hemorrhage, shock, and trauma, those causes most affected by use of the new drugs and blood substitutes.

Better training and the institutionalization of ob-

stetrics as a specialty improved obstetric practice. Beginning in 1930, when the American Board of Obstetrics and Gynecology was established, there was a considerable expansion of educational and training programs in obstetrics for general practitioners and explicit standards for certification of specialists. Other notable educational efforts were those of the American Committee on Maternal Welfare, and in midwifery, the Maternity Center Association of New York, and the Frontier Nursing Service in Kentucky.

Improved hospital facilities for obstetric care governed by published and increasingly well-enforced standards and an expansion of prenatal services reduced the risks of puerperal death. Minimum standards established by the American College of Surgeons and by the American Hospital Association helped promote better hospital regulations for asepsis, stricter supervision of house staff, and the isolation of obstetric departments. Hospitalization for confinement increased more than 100 percent in the ten years after 1933 (from approximately 35 percent to 72 percent of all births), and for the first time was not associated with higher rates of puerperal death. Expansion of prenatal care facilities, aided by funds provided in the Social Security Act of 1935, helped create improved antepartum services throughout the country.

Increased public awareness of pregnancy and childbirth also helped foster a safer maternity. During the 1930s, long-standing taboos against public discussion of pregnancy and childbirth were broken. The Maternity Center Association's national campaign of public information played a crucial role in this development: it conducted institutes for 15,000 public health nurses throughout the United States on pregnancy and childbirth, and sponsored exhibits at the Chicago and New York World Fairs which were seen by hundreds of thousands. The landmark film "Birth of a Baby," produced under the auspices of the American Committee on Maternal Health, was widely shown. The educational work of thousands of local health departments also helped foster a greater knowledge of the need for adequate prenatal, intranatal, and postnatal care for mothers.

Although it is impossible to measure their comparative contributions with any degree of precision, all of these factors played some role in reducing the high level of maternal deaths to a fraction of their previous toll. A major econometric study of maternal mortality conducted in 1950 concluded that for the first time in history a large nation like the United States had pushed its puerperal death rate slightly under the apparently irreducible minimum of one maternal death per 1,000 live births. Seeking an explanation for this finding, the authors compared maternal deaths by cause in 1933 and 1948, assigning three major reasons for the decline — better prenatal care, introduction of antibiotics and other drugs, and improved medical care of pregnant women (intra- and post-natal), involving more adequate physician training and skills. The reduction in mortality rates, they concluded, indicated that the "improved training and the increased skill of the physician are by far the most important factors."[81] Improved physician ability, which affected all classes of puerperal death, each of which had shown reduction, was thus the key variable in the decline of puerperal mortality.

Better training and physician skills were, to an extent which is unfortunately unmeasurable, effected by education and peer review. Many leading physicians were persuaded that maternal mortality review played a major role in improving physician skill and maintaining accountability during these years. One participant, in a comment typical of many others, observed that he "learned more obstetrics by sitting on the Maternal Welfare Committee in Chicago" than in all his other efforts in 40 years of medicine.[82] Dr. Philip Williams of Philadelphia also commented on the efficacy of continuing year-round obstetric mortality review, as opposed, for example, to institutes and seminars conducted by county medical societies, as a method of extramural graduate education for local physicians and general practitioners.[83]

## V

Much of the credit for institutionalizing the review committee as a self-regulatory device goes to the landmark report of the New York Academy of Medicine, whose competent and thorough fact-finding served as an indictment and challenge to physicians, stimulated other investigations across the nation, and demonstrated a viable strategy for self-regulation within the profession.[84]

While the academy report succeeded in providing a mechanism for reform and regulation in obstetrics, its own prescriptions for the direction of change were largely avoided. Although conservatism in obstetrics was a by-product of the report and the many maternal mortality reviews it engendered, the Committee's cautious endorsement of a maternity scheme based on home confinements of normal pregnancies under the care of trained midwives as well as physicians became almost immediately irrelevant. In the five years after publication of the report, hospitalization of maternity patients in New York City increased by 30 percent to 91 percent of all births. Accompanying this change was a decline in the number of midwives in the city from 863 to 280, and a decrease in midwife-attended births from 10 percent in 1933 to 2 percent in 1938, a product of stricter regulation by the Department of Health and the closing of the Bellevue School of Midwifery.[85] Similar changes were taking place on the national level.[86]

The possibility of a basic shift towards a system based on the assumption that birth was not pathologic no longer existed. The 1930s represented a transition period in American obstetrics. By the end of the decade, childbirth had been made safer, but it had advanced irrevocably toward a technological focus. Potentially dangerous medical and surgical practices continued, today affecting infants more often than mothers, though under conditions of greater physician accountability. The New York Academy of Medicine's report on maternal mortality marked a point in time when another option seemed available. The immediate problem — the waste of women's lives in childbirth — was solved. The underlying issue remained.

## NOTES

Presented to the 50th anniversary meeting of the American Association for the History of Medicine, Philadelphia, Pennsylvania, May 2, 1975.

1   Josephine Baker, "Maternal mortality in the United States," *J.A.M.A.*, 1927, *89*, 2016.

2   Society of the Lying-In Hospital of the City of New York, *Maternity: An Educational Survey of a National Problem* (New York, 1923), p. 6.

3   *Ibid.*

4   The urban rate, moreover, was consistently higher

than the rural, not being less than 64 since 1915, or less than 70 since 1917, with a peak of 96 in 1918 and a rate of 74 in 1932. For nonwhite women, maternal mortality in 1915 was 106. In 1932 it was 98, the only year in which the 1915 rate improved. Fred L. Adair, "Maternal, fetal and neonatal morbidity and mortality," *Am. J. Obst. & Gynec.,* 1935, *29*: 389.

5   Robert M. Woodbury, "Infant mortality in the United States," *Ann. Am. Acad. Polit. & Soc. Sci.,* 1936, *188*: 96.

6   In infant mortality, however, the U.S. ranked seventh, both in 1919-1921, with a rate of 82.3, and in 1929-1931, with rate of 64.6. Jacob Yerushalmy, "Infant and maternal mortality in the modern world," *Ann. Am. Acad. Polit. & Soc. Sci.,* 1945, *237*: 134-141.

7   Elizabeth C. Tandy, *Comparability of Maternal Mortality Rates in the United States and Certain Foreign Countries,* U.S. Children's Bureau Pub. 229 (Washington, D.C.: Government Printing Office, 1935).

8   See, for example, White House Conference on Child Health and Protection, *Obstetric Education* (New York: The Century Co., 1932), p. 49.

9   Significant works on maternal mortality during this period include Grace L. Meigs, *Maternal Mortality —from All Conditions Connected with Childbirth in the United States and Certain Other Countries,* U.S. Children's Bureau Pub. 19 (Washington, D.C.: Government Printing Office, 1917); George Clark Mosher, "Maternity morbidity and mortality in the United States," *Am. J. Obst. & Gynec.,* 1924, *7*: 294-298, discussion, 326-330; Austin Flint, "Responsibility of the medical profession in further reducing maternal mortality," *Am. J. Obst. & Gynec.,* 1925, *9*: 864-866; Susan Coffin et al., "Maternal mortality in Massachusetts," *J.A.M.A.,* 1926, *86*: 408-413; Robert Morse Woodbury, *Maternal Mortality: The Risk of Death in Childbirth and from All Diseases Caused by Pregnancy and Confinement,* U.S. Children's Bureau Pub. 158 (Washington, D.C.: Government Printing Office, 1926); Lee K. Frankel, "The present status of maternal and infant hygiene in the United States," *Am. J. Public Hlth.,* 1927, *12*: 1209-1217, discussion, pp. 1217-1220; Henry Jellett, *The Causes and Prevention of Maternal Mortality* (London: J. & A. Churchill, 1929); J. V. De Porte, *Maternal Mortality and Stillbirths in New York State, 1915–1925* (Albany: New York State Department of Health, 1928); Matthias Nicoll, Jr., "Maternity as a public health problem," *Am. J. Public Hlth.,* 1929, *19*: 961-968; Louis I. Dublin, "Mortality among women from causes incidental to childbearing," *Am. J. Obst. & Dis. Women & Children,* 1918, *78*: 20-37; "The risks of childbirth," *Forum,* 1932, *87*: 250-284; White House Conference on Child Health and Protection, *Fetal, Newborn and Maternal Morbidity and Mortality* (New York: D. Appleton-Century Co., 1933); Edward S. Brackett, "Observations on the problem of maternal mortality," *New Eng. J. Med.,* 1934, *210*: 845-51.

10   On the development of maternal and child health services in the United States, see John Blake, *Origins of Maternal and Child Health Programs* (New Haven: Department of Public Health, Yale Univ. School of Medicine, 1953); and William M. Schmidt, "The development of health services for mothers and children in the United States," *Am. J. Public Hlth.,* 1973, *63*: 419-427.

11   Cited in George Clark Mosher, "The problem of mother and child," *Med. Woman's J.,* 1927, *34*: 217.

12   See, for example, Robert de Normandie, "Medical men and maternal mortality," *Woman Citizen,* December 1926, pp. 20-22.

13   Meigs, *Maternal Mortality,* p. 5.

14   For a representative description of maternity education programs established during the Sheppard-Towner period, see Florence McKay, "What New York State is doing to reduce maternal mortality," *Am. J. Obst. & Gynec.,* 1925, *9*: 704-708. Also see J. Stanley Lemons, "The Sheppard-Towner Act: progressivism in the 1920s," *J. Am. Hist.,* 1969, *55*: 776-786.

15   The importance of prenatal care as a factor in maternal health was established in a landmark study by John Whitridge Williams of Johns Hopkins in 1915 (J. Whitridge Williams, "The limitations and possibilities of prenatal care," *J.A.M.A.,* 1915, *64*: 95-101). Williams understood, as many of his contemporaries did not, the close connection between prenatal care and good obstetric care in hospital settings.

16   Kosmak testified before the Committee on Interstate and Foreign Commerce of the 70th Congress that Sheppard-Towner activities concentrated unnecessarily on prenatal care. See Nicoll, "Maternity as a public health problem," p. 965. This view was confirmed some years later in a clinical study conducted at Yale University Medical School under the auspices of the American Public Health Association. The study concluded that "quality of delivery service is probably a greater factor than any other, including prenatal care, in the improvement of the outcome of maternity and the lessening of maternal mortality." See Margaret Tyler, J. H. Watkins, and H. H. Walker, *Report on the Evaluation of Prenatal Care* (New Haven: Institute of Human Relations, Yale Univ. School of Medicine, 1934).

17   Palmer Findley, *The Story of Childbirth* (Garden City, N.Y.: Doubleday Doran, 1933), p. 127, and *Obstetric Education,* p. 204.

18   Woodbury, *Maternal Mortality*, p. 78.

19   Dr. Julius Levy of New Jersey's Bureau of Child Hygiene showed for example that, in 1921, four of the largest cities, Newark, New York, Baltimore, and Cleveland, each with more than 25 percent of births attended by midwives, had lower rates of maternal mortality than Boston, with a highly organized medical system, a well-educated general public, and only 2.5 percent of births delivered by midwives. Julius Levy, "Maternal mortality and mortality in the first month of life in relation to attendant at birth," *Am. J. Public Hlth.*, 1923, *13*: 89.

20   Baker, "Maternal mortality in the U.S.," p. 2017.

21   *Obstetric Education*, p. 96. European midwives, however, particularly in the Scandinavian countries, received lengthy and intensive training in obstetrics.

22   See, for example, comments by Drs. Davis, Speidel, Polak, and Lanford, in Mosher, "Maternal morbidity and mortality," pp. 295, 326; Dublin, "The risks of childbirth," p. 281; and Findley, *The Story of Childbirth*, p. 325.

23   George Gray Ward, "Our obstetric and gynecologic responsibilities," *J.A.M.A.*, 1926, *87*: 1.

24   On the status of obstetrics, see B. P. Watson, "Can our methods of obstetric practice be improved?" *Bull. N.Y. Acad. Med.*, 1930, *6*: 647-663; Mosher, "Maternal morbidity and mortality," pp. 295-296; and Nicoll, "Maternity as a public health problem," p. 966.

25   *Dr. Williams' Obstetrics, 1897-1898*; Rufus I. Cole MSS (Health Sciences Library, State University of New York at Stony Brook).

26   See the report of E. D. Plass, "Forceps and Cesarean section," in *Fetal, Newborn, and Maternal Morbidity and Mortality*, pp. 215-247. Also see J. Whitridge Williams, "A criticism of certain tendencies in American obstetrics," *N.Y. St. J. Med.*, 1922, *22*: 493-499; Rudolf W. Holmes, "The fads and fancies of obstetrics: a comment on the pseudoscientific trend of modern obstetrics," *Am. J. Obst. & Gynec.*, 1921, *2*: 225-237, and discussion, pp. 297-397; Ward, "Our obstetric and gynecologic responsibilities," pp. 1-3; Watson, "Can our methods of obstetric practice be improved?" p. 655; and Flint, "Responsibility of the medical profession on further reducing maternal mortality," p. 866.

27   *Obstetric Education*, p. 18.

28   Examples of this attitude are found in Joseph de Lee, "Obstetrics vs. midwifery," *J.A.M.A.*, 1934, *103*: 308; Findley, *Story of Childbirth*, pp. 53-54, 196-197; George Clark Mosher, "Ten years of painless childbirth," *Am. J. Obst. & Gynec.*, 1932, *3*: 142-143. Also see the comments of Dr. Ray Lyman Wilbur, quoted in Helene Huntington Smith, "The case for anesthesia," *Delineator*, 1932, *125*: 50.

29   The critic was Dr. Buford Garvin, cited in "Pains of childbirth," *Time*, May 25, 1936, 36.

30   See, for example, the statement of Dr. Bertha Van Hoosen, head of the Department of Obstetrics at Loyola University, quoted in Rosine Wistein, "Maternal mortality: a comparative study," *Med. Woman's J.*, 1932, *39*: 29, and "Maternal mortality" (editorial), *ibid.*, p. 66. On the low puerperal death rates of women's hospitals, see Maude Glasgow, *The Subjection of Woman and the Traditions of Men* (New York: Maude Glasgow, 1940), 232-233.

31   Adair, "Maternal, fetal, and neonatal morbidity and mortality," p. 387.

32   "Maternal mortality," *Med. Times & Long Island Med. J.*, May 1934, 157.

33   Lydia Allen de Vilbiss, "A proposed method for reducing the maternal mortality rate," *Med. J. & Rec.*, 1930, *132*: 391-392; and Helen Miller, "Contraception as a means of conserving maternal health," *Birth Control Rev.*, 1929, *13*: 281-282.

34   Iago Galdston, *Maternal Deaths — the Ways to Prevention* (New York: The Commonwealth Fund, 1937), p. 7.

35   Maternity Center Association, *Annual Report, April 1918-Dec. 31, 1921* (New York, 1921), pp. 13, 20-21, 24; *45th Annual Report & Log 1915—1963 of the Maternity Center Association* (New York, 1964), *11*: 1-7.

36   New York Academy of Medicine Committee on Public Health Relations, *Maternal Mortality in New York City: A Study of All Puerperal Deaths, 1930-1932* (New York: The Commonwealth Fund, 1933), pp. ix-xii. Dr. Polak died while the study was in progress, and was replaced by Dr. Charles A. Gordon.

37   George W. Kosmak, "Sensible standards for proper obstetric care," *J. Med. Soc. N.J.*, 1930, *27*: 331-335; "Results of supervised midwife practice in certain European countries," *J.A.M.A.*, 1927, *89*: 2009-2012; "Community responsibilities for safeguarding motherhood," *Public Health & Nursing*, 1932, *26*: 292-299; B. P. Watson, "In memoriam: George William Kosmak," *Tr. Am. Gynec. Soc.*, 1955, *78*: 233-234; and Howard C. Taylor, Jr., "Memorial for Dr. George W. Kosmak," New York Obstetrical Society MSS (New York Academy of Medicine). Collection hereafter referred to as N.Y.O.S. MSS.

38   Watson, "Can our method of obstetric practice be improved?" pp. 656-663.

39   On methodology, see N.Y.A.M., *Maternal Mortality in New York City*, pp. 11-13.

40   *Ibid.*, p. 17.

41   *Ibid.*, p. 32-38.

42   *Ibid.*, p. 54, and Ransom S. Hooker, "Maternal mortality in New York," *The Health Examiner*, 1933, *3*: 13.

43  N.Y.A.M., *Maternal Mortality in New York City,* pp. 126, 130, 137.

44  *Ibid.,* pp. 115–116.

45  *Ibid.,* pp. 139–140.

46  *Ibid.,* pp. 195–198.

47  *Ibid.,* pp. 181–182.

48  *Ibid.,* pp. 151–152.

49  *Ibid.,* pp. 163–167. Caesarian section as a cause of death, however, was more frequent among white women (20.5 percent), than Negro women (14.7 percent). *Ibid.,* p. 131.

50  *Ibid.,* pp. 213–216.

51  *Ibid.,* pp. 216–221.

52  *Ibid.,* pp. 209–212.

53  *Ibid.,* pp. 49, 222.

54  See U.S. Department of Labor, Children's Bureau Pub. 223, *Maternal Mortality in Fifteen States* (Washington, D.C.: Government Printing Office, 1934); Robert Bolt, "Maternal mortality study for Cleveland, Ohio," *Am. J. Obst. & Gynec.,* 1934, *27:* 309–313; J. Parlane Kinloch, *Maternal Mortality: Report on Maternal Mortality in Aberdeen, 1918–1927* (Edinburgh: Scottish Board of Health, 1928); as well as studies by Coffin et al. and the White House Conference on Child Health and Protection. Also see James Young, "Maternal mortality studies," *Am. J. Obst. & Gynec.,* 1936, *31:* 198–212.

55  N.Y.A.M., Medical Information Bureau, "Why women die in childbirth," Nov. 20, 1933.

56  "Hazards of childbirth," *Nation,* 1933, *137:* 612.

57  Draft of letter from New York Obstetrical Society to Dr. Bernard Sachs, president, N.Y.A.M., Dec. 4, 1933, N.Y.O.S. MSS.

58  Philip Van Ingen, *The New York Academy of Medicine* (New York: Columbia Univ. Press, 1949), p. 445.

59  *Report of Subcommittee on Publicity of Maternal Mortality Report* (New York: N.Y.A.M., Public Health Relations Committee, 1934).

60  *Report of the New York Obstetrical Society to Review the Maternal Mortality Report of the Public Health Relations Committee of the New York Academy of Medicine* (New York: N.Y.O.S., 1934).

61  *How Childbirth May Be Made Safe* (New York: N.Y.O.S., 1934).

62  Benjamin P. Watson, Sect. New York Obstetrical Society, to Hervey Williamson, April 11, 1934, N.Y.O.S. MSS.

63  George W. Kosmak to Hervey Williamson, April 12, 1934, and June 15, 1934, N.Y.O.S. MSS.

64  Hervey Williamson to John L. Rice, N.Y.C. Commissioner of Health, March 14, 1934, N.Y.O.S. MSS.

65  John L. Rice, *Guarding the Health of the People of New York City, Preliminary Reports for 1934–1936* (New York: N.Y.C. Department of Health, 1936), p. 36; *50 Years of Better Health for New York's Mothers and Babies, 1908–1958* (New York: N.Y.C. Department of Health, 1958), p. 16.

66  N.Y.O.S., *Transactions of Proceedings,* Feb. 13, 1934, pp. 41–45, N.Y.O.S. MSS.

67  *Constructive Aspects of the Maternal Mortality Report of the New York Academy of Medicine* (New York: N.Y.A.M., 1934), pp. 1–9.

68  Kosmak, "Community responsibilities for safeguarding motherhood," pp. 292–299; and "Editorial comment: the trend of modern obstetrics," *Am. J. Obst. & Gynec.,* 1938, *36:* 315.

69  See Alfred Hellman, "Better obstetrics and the Subcommittee on Maternal Welfare," *New York Medical Week,* July 22, 1939, *18:* 4; and Benjamin P. Watson, "Problems of maternity," in *Preventive Medicine in Modern Practice,* ed. James Alexander Miller et al. (New York: P. B. Hoeber, 1942), p. 176.

70  One difference between the New York and Philadelphia reports lay in the definition of preventable deaths. A death was preventable according to the New York definition, if the "best" possible skill of the community had been available, while preventability, to the Philadelphians, referred to a "reasonable" degree of physician skill. The Philadelphia study summarized four major causes of maternal mortality: self-induced, criminal abortions; errors of judgment on the part of the medical profession; lack of appreciation of the need of prenatal care by lay people; and failure of hospitals, organized medicine, and allied agencies to grasp their responsibilities. Abortions, with resulting septicemia, were the largest single cause of puerperal death in Philadelphia. In its report, the committee spoke of the "overwhelming" evidence of the advisability of abortion legalization, based on the example of the Soviet experience, and called for an impartial analysis to be made of the question. Philadelphia County Medical Society, *Maternal Mortality in Philadelphia, 1931–1933* (Philadelphia, 1934), pp. 127–133; Philip Williams, "The preventive aspects of maternal mortality," *J. Mich. St. Med. Soc.,* 1943, *42:* 25–26.

71  Philip Williams, "Graduate education in obstetrics," *Am. J. Obst. & Gynec.,* 1942, *43:* 529; and P. Williams, "The responsibility of the hospital obstetric staff conference in maternal welfare," *Med. Ann. District of Columbia,* 1942, *11:* 298.

72  Thaddeus L. Montgomery, "The maternal welfare program in Philadelphia," *Proceedings of the First American Congress on Obstetrics and Gynecology, 1938,* p. 542.

73  "After office hours: a visit with Dr. Philip F. Williams," *Obst. & Gynec.,* 1956, *8:* 121–122; and Williams, "The preventive aspects of maternal mortality," p. 30.

74  Jose G. Marmol, Alan L. Scriggins, and Rudolph F. Wollman, "After office hours: history of the maternal mortality study committees in the United States," *Obst. & Gynec.,* 1969, *34*: 126.

75  See, for example, James Knight Quigley, "Maternal welfare, what are its fruits?" *Am. J. Obst. & Gynec.,* 1940, *39*: 349–353; Williams, "The preventive aspects of maternal mortality," p. 25; and Watson, "Problems of maternity."

76  Quigley, "Maternal welfare, what are its fruits?" p. 351; Sam Shapiro, Edward R. Schlesinger, and Robert E. L. Nesbitt, *Infant, Perinatal, Maternal and Childhood Mortality in the United States* (Cambridge, Mass.: Harvard Univ. Press, 1968), pp. 145–146.

77  Marjorie Gooch, "Ten years of progress in reducing maternal and infant mortality," *The Child,* 1945, *10*: 77–81.

78  Frank G. Dickinson and Everett L. Welker, "Maternal mortality in the United States in 1949," *J.A.M.A.,* 1950, *144*: 1395–1400.

79  Yerushalmy, "Infant and maternal mortality in the modern world," p. 139.

80  Reasons for the decline in maternal mortality after 1933 are suggested in Quigley, "Maternal welfare, what are its fruits?" p. 350; Gooch, "Ten years of progress in reducing maternal and infant mortality," p. 80; Dickinson and Welker, "Maternal mortality," p. 1398; Shapiro et al., *Infant, Perinatal, Maternal and Childhood Mortality in the U.S.,* pp. 145–146; and in Nicholas Eastman and Louis M. Hellman, *Williams' Obstetrics,* 13th ed. (New York: Appleton-Century Crofts, 1966), pp. 8–9.

81  Dickinson and Welker, "Maternal mortality," p. 1399.

82  Cited in Marmol et al., "History of the maternal mortality study committees," p. 133.

83  Williams, "Graduate education in obstetrics," pp. 528, 532.

84  The role of the academy report in lowering mortality rates throughout the nation was commented upon in 1974 by Dr. George Baehr, president of the New York Academy of Medicine. Baehr noted that corrective action taken by communities after release of the New York study resulted in a 66 percent decline in maternal mortality rates throughout the country (from 6.6 deaths per 1,000 live births in 1931 to 2.2 deaths in 1946), thus, by the way, achieving the academy goal that two-thirds of maternal deaths were preventable. The fact that the decline in New York City, where rates fell 80 percent over the same period of time (from 6.0–6.2 deaths per 1,000 live births in 1930–32 to 1.4 deaths in 1946), far exceeded that in other cities indicated to Baehr the catalytic role of the academy report in effecting obstetric improvement. George Baehr, *Maternal Death: A Problem in Preventive Medicine, The New York Academy of Medicine's Study of Fifteen Years Ago* (New York: N.Y.A.M., 1947).

85  Katherine Fayville, "Maternity care in New York City from the public health point of view," *Proceedings of the First American Congress on Obstetrics and Gynecology, 1939,* pp. 533–534. However, in 1931, the Maternity Center Association, a private organization, initiated a home delivery service and nurse-midwifery school, the Lobenstine Midwifery Clinic. Over the next decades, the school trained a small but growing number of public health nurses from many different states in midwifery. Three of the school's original incorporators, Drs. George Kosmak, Benjamin Watson, and John O. Polak, were members of the Obstetric Advisory Committee to the New York Academy of Medicine's study of maternal mortality. Dr. Kosmak became chairman of the Medical Board of the Maternity Center Association in 1931, serving in this capacity until his death.

86  During the next decade, the distribution of live births, according to persons in attendance, increased only for in-hospital deliveries by physicians (from 36.9 percent of births in 1935 to 84.8 percent in 1947), and declined significantly for out-of-hospital births attended by physicians (from 50.6 percent of births in 1935, to 10.1 percent in 1947). *Vital Statistics,* Special Reports, Feb. 8, 1949, *31* (1), cited by Richard Bolt, "Maternal infant and preschool health," in *Nelson New Loose Leaf Medicine,* 1941, *7*: 762.

# 36

## The Early Movement for Occupational Safety and Health, 1900–1917

### DAVID ROSNER AND GERALD MARKOWITZ

One of the most important aspects of the history of Progressivism and American labor was the struggle from the turn of the century to World War I to achieve a safe and healthful work environment. During these years a broad-based movement to reform working conditions arose; it succeeded in achieving some major legislative victories at the state and federal levels and heightened consciousness about workplace hazards among the population at large.

Unfortunately, the significance of this movement has been obscured for historians and those working in safety and health today, for we have concentrated on only one aspect of the effort to control work conditions: the political battles surrounding the passage of workers' compensation laws in the years 1908–1914. In this article we will analyze the broader movement for safety and health at the turn of the century. This early movement was successful in developing a multiclass and multi-interest constituency that succeeded in bringing workers' safety and health issues to the consciousness of millions of Americans. The movement built on existing state factory-inspection programs and efforts in the 1880s and 1890s to enact protective legislation for women and children. It reached its peak during the first two decades of the 20th century and garnered support among reformers working in public health, conservation, housing, and labor legislation, especially legislation aimed at protecting children and women. Contemporary discussion of occupational safety and health was wedded to broader social concerns regarding workers' hous-

ing, sanitation, and general living conditions. "In one aspect," reflected one observer, the early 20th-century movement was "a chapter in the general health movement . . . next of kin to the crusade against tuberculosis, infant mortality, hookworm, and typhoid." But, "in another aspect it is part and parcel of the movement for labor legislation, being intermingled with the program of child labor reform, factory legislation, and factory inspection, and standing as a counterpart of measures for the compensation of industrial accidents."[1] Workers, social workers, housing reformers, journalists, politicians, big business representatives, social scientists, professionals, socialists, wobblies, and charity workers, who rarely agreed on much of anything, found themselves in alliance to stop the slaughter of workers in American industry.

It is important to recognize, however, the serious limitations of this movement. Because it was a broad-based coalition, it brought together radical and conservative groups. There was always a tension between the goals of socialist leaders such as Crystal Eastman and business groups such as United States Steel. By 1914, the movement lost its radical edge and became a vehicle for voluntaristic and management-sponsored approaches to reform. The movement's energy became focused on state workers' compensation laws, thus channeling the broader environmental and political concerns into narrow legalistic and administrative efforts. Management itself began to set the agenda for improving working conditions through its sponsorship and domination of the National Safety Council. It was able to redefine the issue to be one of safety rather than health and to take the issue out of the political sphere and place it in the technical and engineering arena.

DAVID ROSNER is Associate Professor of History, Baruch College, Graduate Center, City University of New York.
GERALD MARKOWITZ is Professor of History at John Jay College, City University of New York.

I

The growing concern over safety and health issues in the first decade of the 20th century arose in the wake of the revolutionary social and economic changes that America had just undergone. In little more than three decades Americans had witnessed the virtual explosion of urban and manufacturing centers. This was shocking to Americans reared in rural settings. Before the Civil War, most Americans lived on farms or in small towns; the few factories that existed were scatttered in mill towns and villages in the Northeast. With the growth of the transcontinental railroads, however, the development of national markets, increased exploitation of natural resources such as coal and iron, and the massive immigration of labor from rural Europe to the cities of the East and Midwest, conditions of work changed dramatically. America moved from being a fourth-rate industrial power to the leading industrial producer in the world. But work for the vast majority of laborers deteriorated. Speed-ups, monotonous tasks, exposure to chemical toxins, metallic and organic dusts, and unprotected machinery made the American workplace among the most dangerous in the world. In mining, for instance, England, Germany, and France experienced death rates of fewer than 1.5 per 1,000 workers during the first years of this century. In the United States more than 3 miners in every 1,000 could expect to die while working in a mine during any given year.[2]

The enormous wealth produced by the new industrial plants was achieved at an inordinate social cost. "To unprecedented prosperity . . . there is a seemy side of which little is said," reported one observer in 1907. "Thousands of wage earners, men, women and children, [are] caught in the machinery of our record breaking production and turned out cripples. Other thousands [are] killed outright," he reported. "How many there [are] none can say exactly, for we [are] too busy making our record breaking production to count the dead."[3] In a theme that would repeatedly appear, reformers compared the toll of industrial accidents to an undeclared war. As early as 1904 *The Outlook*, a mass-circulation magazine, commented on the horrendous social effects of industrialization. "The frightful increase in the number of casualties of all kinds in this country during the last two or three

years is becoming a matter of the first importance. A greater number of people are killed every year by so-called accidents than are killed in many wars of considerable magnitude," it pointed out. "It is becoming as perilous to live in the United States as to participate in actual warfare." The editorial demanded that the state document the extent of industrial accidents "in order that the people of the United States may face the situation and understand how cheap human life has become under American conditions."[4]

The power of the early 20th-century movement depended on the widespread publicity provided by a group of journalists and writers. These "muckrakers" exposed the horrible conditions of work to millions of Americans through magazine articles, pamphlets and books. Their primary aim was to arouse the public through a widespread propaganda campaign aimed at forcing reform legislation through Congress and especially state legislatures. They also sought to force particularly dangerous industries to clean up their workplaces. William Hard was one such muckraker. His 1904 article, "Making Steel and Killing Men," in *Everybody's Magazine* detailed the horrible work conditions in the south Chicago plant of the United States Steel Corporation. Hard described the dangerous conditions that led to the deaths of 46 workers and the permanent disablement of 386 others in just one year. He accused the company of endangering workers' lives by failing to provide a variety of safeguards near the blast furnaces and cauldrons into which the molten metal was cast for steel rails and girders. In vivid detail he described how men dropped into vats of molten metal or were showered with steel by sudden explosions in the furnace. The article created a tremendous stir among the 3 million readers of *Everybody's* and forced the company to provide elementary safeguards for its workers. Looking back just three years after its publication, John Fitch, another popular writer, noted that Hard's article spurred the company to begin a safety campaign. Subsequently, U.S. Steel would boast of its impressive safety record without acknowledging the role that popular pressure played in forcing improvements.[5]

As bad as conditions are today for American workers, we often forget how much worse they were just a few decades ago. During the first part of the century, stories of the plight of workers were reported daily in popular magazines and newspapers. These stories attest to the pervasiveness of industrial hazards and to the heightened consciousness that then existed. Reports of severe accidents on the railroads, in the mines, and in the factories reminded Americans that industrialism was taking an enormous toll.

*The Survey, Everybody's Magazine*, and *The Outlook* served as the outlets through which muckrakers and others exposed conditions in the dangerous trades. In their pages authors detailed "the death roll of industry" and documented how workers died in the mines, on the railroads, and in the factories. In an article on the dangers of various trades, one author charged that industrialists sent "to the hospital or the graveyard one worker every minute of the year."[6] Others noted that "the price we pay in human lives for our industrial progress is . . . appalling. For nearly every floor of every skyscraper that goes to make up Manhattan's picturesque skyline a man gives up his life."[7] One of the most graphic popular descriptions of the dangers of the meat packing industry was Upton Sinclair's *The Jungle*.

The publishers of these magazines and books were not printing this material as a public service. Rather, they recognized that it could sell magazines, and they were therefore willing to devote space, time, and money to a variety of occupational safety and health issues. "We spent a great deal of money in getting the material for *Everybody's Magazine*," noted the owner, "but we want to go further. We want it to count in the industrial life of this nation. Our hope is that after reading it you will enroll yourself with those who feel that nothing which concerns man should be a matter of indifference to any man."[8]

Publicity for labor's plight was also provided by an extraordinary group of social activists, academics, and professionals such as Alice Hamilton, Paul Kellogg, and John R. Commons, who, as doctors, writers, lawyers, and social workers, were instrumental in popularizing this issue. They lectured, wrote articles, exposés, and books, sponsored meetings, and conducted independent investigations of conditions of Pennsylvania coal miners, Birmingham and Pittsburgh steel workers, New York City garment workers, Massachusetts textile workers, Minnesota iron miners, and numerous other industries. Their work was of the highest academic

standards, but they were not embarrassed to express their concern for workers and their commitment to reform. For instance, Dr. Alice Hamilton, a pioneer in the occupational safety and health movement, is remembered today for her important pathbreaking scientific investigations into conditions of work in a variety of industries, most notably lead. But she also saw herself as an advocate of reform. Presaging her later work around lead poisoning and other industrial toxins, she noted the terrible mortality from accidents and diseases that slowly ate away at the body and soul of the workforce.[9] Along with others such as Frances Perkins and Eleanor Roosevelt, who would later be instrumental in shaping labor legislation during the New Deal, Hamilton developed political skill and experience during the early movement for occupational safety and health.

What is especially exciting about the early 20th-century movement is that it gained strength from its heterogeneous constituency. "The most important economic movement underway in America today is the movement for the conservation of the human resources of the country," said Earl Mayo in an article entitled "The Work That Kills." This movement "has its humanitarian as well as its commercial side . . . it is a many-sided movement and its ultimate possibilities have not yet begun to be appreciated."[10] Thus, the movement was a multiclass effort that united groups of widely different interests. In the following pages, we will discuss four different themes that dominated the thinking and concerns of the various groups. First, we will outline the different ideological strands that made up this broad coalition. Second, we will look at their very different notion of occupational safety and health that helped give unity to the movement. All groups recognized that workers' health could be maintained only by improvements in both the home and work environments. Third, we will examine how different actors interpreted the obvious suffering that affected industrial workers. All parties were acutely aware that the extraordinary number of workers maimed and killed exacerbated the conflict between labor and capital. Fourth, we will outline the growing consensus that it was necessary to provide the working class some minimal protection. All parties came to recognize that workers' health could be safeguarded only through the intervention of the state.

## II

The movement for occupational safety and health was made up of two major ideological strands. Most of the reformers used concepts and language borrowed from the lexicon of business when analyzing the problems of death, disability, and disease created at the workplace. Others, however, including socialists and moralists rejected a worldview that saw workers as machines or the raw materials for industry.

Those reformers that worked within a capitalist ideological framework used words such as *costs*, *efficiency*, *resources*, and *breakdowns* to describe the problem that accidents and disease posed for the society. Injured workers were compared to broken-down machines in need of repair, and workers killed on the job were seen as "wasted resources."

The most blatant statement of this ideology was provided by big business itself. Big business saw human conservation purely in terms of the long-term financial benefits of company stockholders. "A careful businessman sees that his property is maintained in excellent condition," said one propagandist for the International Harvester Company in 1912. "His buildings are kept in good repair and fully insured against loss from fire. His machinery is always maintained at a high point of efficiency, no rust is allowed to accumulate. . . . In short, every dollar he invests in his business is guarded and nursed so that it brings forth its full and legitimate earning power." Conserving the workforce "is simply applying the same business principles to his workers that he applies to the rest of his business."[11]

More important than the big-business view itself was the acceptance by many reformers of the underlying economic rationale for the protection of workers. In an article subtitled "Human Life as a National Asset," one physician noted that "all economists today agree that the greatest asset of any country is the vital efficiency of its citizens." Others asked, "What, in dollars and cents, may be roughly figured as a man's worth to the community." Still others noted that industrial accidents meant "incalculable loss of time and energy in business."[12] Clearly, reformers thought that it was the almighty dollar that would capture the public's imagination in a dynamic capitalist economy. One author suggested: "Starting on the lowest level let us formulate our initial axiom in terms of dollars. A sound man can do more than a sick man. Therefore, he can make more money." Similarly, "a sound city can do more work than a sick city. Therefore, in the long run, it can accumulate more wealth."[13] Propagandists used the rhetoric of business to justify their positions, because they knew that few reforms could be achieved without a strong commercial rationale. In a period dominated by the new corporate giants even the most basic human values had to be justified in terms of their price tags.

Others completely rejected the view of a worker's life as a commodity and distrusted the motives of corporate welfare programs. "Businessmen would rather risk their neighbor's lives than their own money," was the underlying philosophy of many. Ultimately, these critics believed that business would abandon its safety efforts and forsake the workforce. "Greed feels nothing, knows nothing, cares for nothing but profit. It fears nothing but the loss of dollars. . . . There is no . . . reason to suppose [employers] are distressed by the sight of human beings crushed under falling walls or leaping all aflame from tenth story windows."[14] Left-wing unions raised even more fundamental objections to the values of business civilization. "The average person is never tired of boasting about the wonderful achievements of modern civilization," noted a writer in *The Glass Worker* in 1908. "The huge factories dot the earth everywhere, polluting the landscape with their unsightly vomitings, but the question arises, are these mighty achievements worth the price that humanity is paying for them. To everyone who is inclined to draw his conclusions from the facts," the writer continued, "it is well known that the vast majority of the people in all civilized countries lead lives of arduous and ill-paid toil that cannot fail to result in physical and moral degeneration. . . . Driven as they are to the limit of human endurance in the factory, mill and sweat shop, . . . forced to crowd into narrow quarters, subsist upon a scanty supply of food of the cheapest and most inferior quality, the healthy physical and moral development of these urchins of modern industry is out of the question." *The Glass Worker* condemned modern capitalist industry and turned business rhetoric against itself: "The facts stand glaringly forth that social health and welfare are not being conserved. It is being forced into physical and moral bankruptcy because of the fearful price it has to pay for those achievements of which the average man is so boastful."[15]

It was not only the labor radicals who objected to the treatment of life as a commodity. Some middle-class reformers also defined such a view as innately immoral. "Products that are made . . . by hours longer than health endurance are anti-social and immoral products and express a ruinous social cost no matter what the selling cost may be," said Margaret Dreier Robbins in her presidential address to the Women's Trade Union League. "In shop and factory and mill all over our country women are working under conditions that weaken vitality and sap moral fiber—conditions that are destructive alike to physical health and moral development."[16]

Others agreed that "people are a natural resource," but rejected a purely commercial definition of that term. William Ludlow Chenery of Chicago's Hull House wrote: "Society . . . which has begun to feel with the great force of an elemental emotion the necessity for conserving the trees, the rivers, the lands and the mineral deposits of the nation hitherto has given but small thought to the protection of the people. . . . It is a kind of commentary on the American conception of things that no one thought of investigating these things until about three years ago. We were too busy to think about the human factor of industry, the thing, the product was the end and object." Chenery concluded that he hoped "the national emphasis [would] be shifted from the integrity of property to the welfare of people."[17]

Another group, frightened by industrialization itself, had little faith that industry's excesses could be contained by government or labor. Using moral and religious rhetoric, they longed for a return to a more bucolic past. "Surely our modern industrial civilization resembles a Frankenstein," noted Josiah Strong, a leader in the Social Gospel Movement. "And unless something is done to check the monster it is creating he will grow ever more murderous."[18]

For most religious and moral leaders the impetus for their concern was a fundamentalist fear that science and technology posed a threat to a spiritual life. This resistance to technological change led them to support efforts that reasserted human and spiritual values over materialistic ones. For in-

stance, they were ardent supporters of a six-day week. The Reverend George W. Grannis, general secretary of the Lord's Day Alliance of the United States, appeared before a New York State commission to advocate a shortened work week. Similarly, William P. Swartz of the New York Sabbath Committee testified that "thousands and thousands are robbed of the privilege and opportunity for that higher development of character[,] . . . one of the staple elements of our country and necessary for its existence, by the fact that they don't have . . . time . . . for the home or family ties, for the conditions that surround and make sound and elevate the manhood underlying and making the nation." Swartz pressed the commission to enact reforms and to "do everything we can to take off . . . the seven days yoke."[19] While these leaders were romantics and often religious fundamentalists in their beliefs, the logic of their views drove them to radical stances on a variety of labor issues. Their desire to limit the effects of industrialization, by initiating shorter hours and work weeks, put them in an alliance with radical elements of the trade union movement who were pushing for the eight-hour day.

One of the first and most important ways that muckrakers and other reformers sought to awaken the public to the horrible costs of industrialism was through popular discussion of the plight of women and children in mines, mills, and factories. Beginning in the late 19th century, magazines carried lurid stories of children awakening at dawn to toil at the looms, and women leaving their loved ones to work in the factory. By the early years of this century, there was hardly a journal that did not have articles such as the "Slavery of Childhood" or "Women's Factory Work." By 1900 over 1.7 million children worked for wages, many of them for 10 to 14 hours a day. Edwin Markham, a popular writer of the period, told of the little boys and girls who "sicken and faint" from "the heat and the odors . . . in the fancy box and candy factories." He also described how children in glass factories toiled in front of "red hot furnaces becoming numb and blistered."[20] Others described sickly women toiling in the bakeries and cracker factories. "Girl workers in the excessive heat, with the smell of dough, staring at the trays which pass slowly, continuously beneath their eyes, become light-headed and ill."[21]

The depiction of the plight of women and children served both progressive as well as reactionary ends. For some, the publicity was meant to force industries to improve working conditions by spurring unionization of women workers. For others, the publicity was seen as a means of securing for women protective legislation that could serve as an opening wedge to improve conditions for all workers. But others sought to use the issue of women's safety and health to force women to abandon work and return to the home.

The Women's Trade Union League, made up of union women and middle-class reformers, sought to organize women workers. In one pamphlet, it asked its readers, "Perhaps you have complained about the chemicals used in the washing of your clothes, which cause them to wear out quickly, but what do you suppose is the effect of these chemicals upon the workers?" The pamphlet detailed the long hours, intense heat, and bad air that these women workers faced every day and suggested that it was inevitable "that these workers became physical wrecks in a very short time, just because you and I never count the cost." What was the "way out" according to the league?—"The Laundry Workers Union" because "the great school of the Working People [is] the Trade Union." Margaret Dreier Robbins, the president, maintained that other unions, such as the United Textile Workers, had "never ceased in its demands for better sanitary conditions . . . ."[22]

Few reformers were willing to place the hope for women's salvation in the hands of a trade union, and instead put their faith in protective legislation which sought to limit the number of hours and night work, and to prohibit women entirely from certain trades. While we recognize today that this effort resulted in the displacement of women from industry, and especially from the higher paying jobs, some reformers had hoped for a different result. They believed that if shorter hours were required for women, if special requirements were enacted for women's employment, it would redound to the benefit of both men and women. William Hard and Rheta Childe Dorr argued that "legislative concern for women leads unavoidably to legislative concern for men." They continued, "We cannot debar women from Industry. We must make Industry fit for women. And when it is fit for them not many years will pass before it will

become fit for men. Industry, the bachelor, needs in his bachelor quarters the touch, the effect, of feminine occupancy before he can really cease to be but masculine, before he can really become completely human."[23]

But Hard and Dorr still accepted that there were innate differences which made women the weaker sex. They suggested that women couldn't stand as long as men, they were not as strong, and a "woman's nervous system is more unstable than man's and more easily shaken from its equilibrium." They believed that women should be excluded from a few jobs involving "hideously severe, de-sexing physical toil."[24] Others seized upon the alleged inferiority of women to seek to exclude women from many fields of endeavor and to return them to the home or at least to the lowest paying jobs. *The Glass Worker*, a union publication radical on most issues, was outraged that women were employed in traditional male roles in some foundries. They used as an excuse for their stance the physical nature of the work. They claimed the work was unfeminine: "Their faces and hands are begrimed with black dust and grease, and were they not required to wash themselves before leaving the plant they would present an unseemly appearance on the streets."[25]

The major complaint against women working was that it caused irreparable harm to their ability to bear healthy children. The Woman's Label League, an organization of women formed to support the mostly male trade union movement, featured a report by the New York Department of Charities that said the increased number of "feebleminded children is a direct result" of women's work in factories. The *Woman's Label League Journal* said, "Ten years of the work . . . unfits women for the duties and responsibilities of motherhood."[26] The National Child Labor Committee issued a flyer (see Fig. 1) which suggested that mothers who worked outside the home became a burden on both husbands and children, and were a direct cause of child labor. This, in turn, resulted in children who suffered from "impaired health, illiteracy, inefficiency, delinquency, (and) dependence." The reformers sought to "set it right" by taking working mothers "who neglect home and children" and making them into homemakers who could "enhance the efficiency of father and children."[27]

The focus on women and children was a double-edged sword. It could be used to arouse the country to the dangers that all workers faced; it was also used to exclude female workers by asserting that it was wrong to subject the weaker sex to horrible working conditions.

## III

Underlying much of the agitation for reform was the belief that the high human costs of industrialism were producing severe class antagonisms. Social workers felt that the worker, especially the immigrant worker, might never become fully integrated into the fabric of American life if subjected to undue physical strain or intolerable conditions on the job. Settlement workers were fearful that industrialism and its attendant hardships were creating a generation of disaffected and dangerous classes. Graham Taylor, a leading social worker, warned, "Nothing is more dangerous in a democracy than to allow a sense of detachment to divide a class from the mass, a craft or individual from the community of interest, . . . personal and private instincts and ideals from public welfare."[28]

To many at the turn of the century, worker safety and health was a primary source of conflict between workers and owners. Some labor and socialist groups maintained that the extraordinary number of deaths and accidents that workers suffered was proof that capitalism was unable to serve workers' interests. But others, primarily from the middle and upper classes, argued that reform was possible, indeed necessary to restore the harmony of interests between workers and capitalists. All agreed with the findings of the United States Commission on Industrial Relations: dangerous and unhealthy working conditions were a crucial source of conflict and dissatisfaction in American industry. The commission found that labor was especially upset that "the rapid pace of modern industry . . . results in accidents and premature old age," and that there was a "lack of attention to sickness and accidents" as well as "difficulty and delay [in] securing compensation for accidents." The commission also reported a widespread "fear . . . of being driven to poverty by sickness, accident or involuntary loss of employment."[29]

The American Association for Labor Legisla-

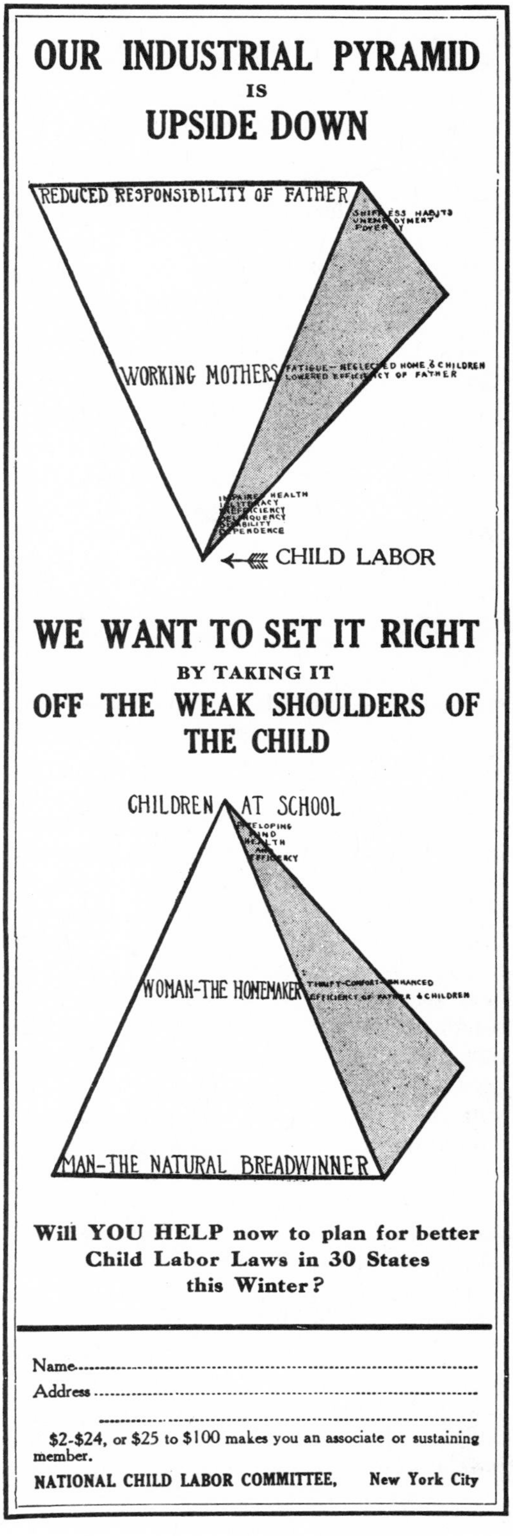

Fig. 1: From *The Survey*, Jan. 18, 1913, *29*: 534.

OUR INDUSTRIAL PYRAMID
IS
UPSIDE DOWN

REDUCED RESPONSIBILITY OF FATHER

WORKING MOTHERS

← CHILD LABOR

WE WANT TO SET IT RIGHT
BY TAKING IT
OFF THE WEAK SHOULDERS OF
THE CHILD

CHILDREN AT SCHOOL

WOMAN-THE HOMEMAKER

MAN-THE NATURAL BREADWINNER

Will YOU HELP now to plan for better
Child Labor Laws in 30 States
this Winter?

Name
Address

$2-$24, or $25 to $100 makes you an associate or sustaining member.
NATIONAL CHILD LABOR COMMITTEE,    New York City

tion (A.A.L.L.) was one of the foremost organizations dedicated to reform. The members of the association were prominent labor leaders, corporate liberals, social reformers, and academics of the day, including Jane Addams, Samuel Gompers, John Mitchell, Robert Hunter, Florence Kelley, and Everit Macy. The A.A.L.L., funded by some of the biggest capitalists of the era, sought to find a model of change that would reconcile labor and capital.[30] In 1909 Henry W. Farnum, the president of the A.A.L.L., described the problem that his organization sought to address. "Some, exaggerating the incidental evils of progress, decry all efforts of betterment, and long for the good old times when there were no reformers," he noted in his presidential address. "Others, realizing strongly the evils which grow up without regulation, think that reform has not been carried far enough and advocate some extreme remedies such as Socialism." The A.A.L.L. sought to avoid both of these courses. Farnum wondered "if there is no principle based upon experience which will enable us to steer the Ship of State so as to avoid the Scylla of conservatism and the Charybdis of radicalism."[31] Its fears of the two extremes made it adopt as its slogan, "Social Justice Is the Best Insurance Against Social Unrest."[32]

The A.A.L.L. was active in organizing conferences on industrial work conditions, workers' compensation, various forms of tenement and social legislation, unemployment, and compulsory health insurance. It organized the first annual conferences on the growing problems of industrial diseases. True to its desire to build a consensus, the A.A.L.L. sought to "bring physicians, employees and employers together in a united effort to lessen the ravages of occupational diseases," and to instill them with the "zeal and enthusiasm of social workers." In addition to labor and capital the conferences were attended by insurance experts, efficiency engineers, state and federal public health officials, doctors, and settlement house workers.[33]

Occupational safety and health was the major focus of the association. In an article entitled "An Immediate Labor Program," the A.A.L.L. called for eight legislative initiatives, seven of which addressed workers' safety and health: protection from lead poisoning, a uniform system of reporting accidents and diseases, systematic investigations of industrial hygiene and safety, factory inspection

and labor law enforcement, revision of the Federal Employees Compensation Act, better state workers' compensation legislation, and one day's rest in seven. John B. Andrews, secretary of the association (and its major spokesperson), summarized the importance of occupational safety and health to the A.A.L.L.: "Since its organization in February 1906, the Association has regarded the prevention of industrial accidents, and the enactment of a just plan of compensation for industrial injuries, as the most pressing immediate problem in labor legislation."[34]

The association organized the National Commission on Industrial Hygiene in 1908, and a year later an A.A.L.L. representative gave a major address on industrial diseases and occupational standards at the National Conference on Charities and Correction. The association also published an influential investigation of phosphorus poisoning in the match industry which led to federal legislation eliminating the use of deadly white phosphorus in matches. This was the first federal action that proved effective in controlling an occupationally caused disease.

Middle-class Progressives and enlightened capitalists believed that it was possible to reform and improve dangerous working conditions. But others, most notably socialists, saw such conditions as an inevitable product of capitalist production. For them, the only way the workplace could be made safe was if the workers took over the management of the factory. At a mass meeting of the cloak makers union called by the New York Socialist party, Morris Hillquit proclaimed, "We protest against the wanton and ceaseless murder of our sons and daughters in factories, mines, and mills and we declare that if the capitalist class cannot conduct the industries of the country without murder the workers will assume management of the industries and conduct them with safety to the employees and for the good of the community."[35] Others suggested that workers could protect themselves only through political organization. In order to make their plants safe, they "should join the Socialist Party and help to abolish capitalism and introduce socialism."[36]

The horrible conditions that many workers faced every day led some socialists to call for revolution. "When I read . . . such records as this: 'Helper— flooring factory—age 19—clothing caught by setscrews in shafting; both arms and legs torn off;

death ensued in five hours,' my spirit revolts," declared Crystal Eastman, the famous socialist spokeswoman in 1911. "And when the dead bodies of girls are found piled up against locked doors . . . after a factory fire[,] . . . who wants to hear about a great relief fund? What we want is to start a revolution."[37] Eastman and other socialists saw industrial accidents as one sign of the war that management waged against the working class in industrializing America.

For many socialists the revolution was not necessarily one fought out with guns. Rather, what was needed was a radical redirection in its uses of science, technology, and spirit. Among some impassioned advocates of reform were many who had a fervent belief in the power of knowledge and information in the struggle to attain safe workplace conditions. "We must pause and consider what are the essential weapons in our campaign," Eastman said. Rather than guns, the "first thing we need is information, complete and accurate information about the accidents that are happening. It seems a tame thing to drop so suddenly from talk of revolutions to talk of statistics," she acknowledged, "but I believe in statistics just as firmly as I believe in revolutions. . . . And what is more, I believe statistics are good stuff to start a revolution with."[38] The passion with which Eastman called for accurate statistics reflected the fervent belief among this generation that information itself was an integral tool in the battle for social justice.

Labor's anger at such conditions was frequently expressed in strikes at unhealthy and dangerous shops. One long and dramatic example of the discord created by dangerous health conditions was the nine-week general strike of cloak makers in New York City. The strike was called because of the "unsanitary condition in a large number of shops." The settlement, reached after the bitter and acrimonious picketing and public pressure, included the creation of a Joint Board of Sanitary Control. This body, composed of employers and employees, sought to establish sanitary standards for the industry.[39] In one year the cloak makers union called 28 successful "sanitary" strikes in New York, and set the stage for the public outcry that followed the tragic deaths of 140 young women in New York's infamous Triangle Shirt Waist Fire in 1911.[40]

The shock of the Triangle fire prompted many to indict industrial capitalists for their callousness and

their greed (see Fig. 2). After a march and rally of 50,000 trade unionists, Rose Schneiderman, vice president of the Women's Trade Union League, argued, "I would be a traitor to these poor burned bodies if I came here to talk of good fellowship. The old Inquisition had its rack and thumb screws and its instruments of torture with iron teeth. We know what these things are today," she continued. "The iron teeth are the necessities, the thumb screws the high powered and swift machinery close to which we must work, and the rack is here in the fire-trap structures that will destroy us the minute they will catch fire."[41]

## IV

The need to ameliorate the threat of class conflict and the nature of the problems that workers faced led to a broad conception of occupational safety and health. In the early years of the century labor joined with middle-class reformers to argue for a new definition of the intimate relationship between the health of workers and the health of the general community.

Social workers were some of the earliest and most articulate advocates of this broader vision. Their first-hand experience with the immigrant poor made them sensitive to the relationship between poverty, illness, and work. They knew that most workers lived in neighborhoods that bordered or surrounded the factories. The crowded conditions in the home, the lack of light and ventilation in the slum streets, and the horrible working conditions combined to produce unhealthy environments for workers and their families. Thus, social workers recognized that to improve the health of immigrant workers it was necessary to go beyond industrial hygiene and include housing conditions, diet, and individual morality.

The most important example of this view of disease causation was contemporary discussion of tuberculosis, the devastating lung disease which ravaged working-class families, incapacitating children and grown-ups alike. In 1904, *Charities*, the journal of the Charity Organization Society, noted that tuberculosis, one of the worst scourges of the working classes, went hand-in-hand with industrialism. It maintained that any effective program aimed at controlling the disease would have to acknowledge the relationship between homelife, neighborhood, and workplace. Social workers and other professionals believed that tuberculosis struck those weakened by overwork, poor nutrition, or crowded living conditions. When these conditions were combined with a dusty work environment, a worker's health was almost sure to be impaired. An effective program, therefore, to control consumption required close attention to all aspects of a worker's life. Consumption "must be checked by public sanitary preventive measures in street and shop and home." It could "be eradicated only by a movement democratic enough to reach intimately all three."[42]

For charity workers the issue of consumption illustrated the environmental, rather than the individual, roots of illness and dependence. "I would like to speak of the importance to the Charity Organization Society of health and safety conditions for labor," said Frederick Almy, secretary of Buf-

falo's chapter of the organization. "I think one-third or perhaps one-half of our work would disappear if labor conditions were all they might be. I mean if employers took as good care of their men as they do of their machinery." Almy continued by rejecting explanations that blamed the workers themselves for their poor health. It was obvious "that sickness [was] due to the housing and working conditions. . . ."[43] In contrast to the 19th-century charity notion that illness was a reflection of the personal worthiness of the sufferer, social workers in the Progressive Era recognized that social conditions were far more important determinants of health and illness.

Reflecting this broader ecological notion, Graham Taylor argued that there was no clear demarcation between occupational safety and health and other social and environmental problems. He said that the activities of social workers were "those

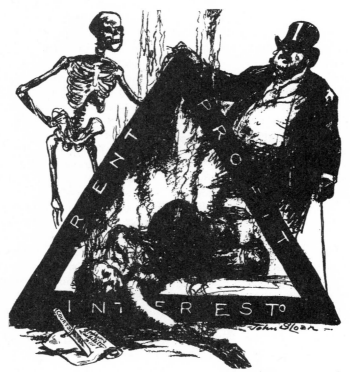

*Sloan in New York Call.*

"HERE IS THE REAL TRIANGLE."

Fig.2: Cartoon in the New York socialist daily newspaper, *The Call,* was designed to invoke the Triangle Waist Company. The mutilated employers' liability bill in the foreground was a comment on a New York State Court of Appeals decision that workers were not constitutionally protected from the economic losses incurred in the 1911 fire. From *The Survey,* April 8, 1911, *26:* 81.

increasingly discerned, but illy defined connections between industrial conditions and relationships and the social, moral and civic interests of our times." He went on to note that "industrial casualties [were] among the deepest taproots of dependency."[44]

Social workers, forced by their experiences in the nation's growing slums, formed a *de facto* alliance with labor and turned to it for information and support. At the 25th Annual Convention of the American Federation of Labor in 1906, for instance, the delegates identified tuberculosis as one of its most pressing problems. In a dramatic chart showing the death rate from consumption in 53 occupations the A.F. of L. pointed out that marble and stone cutters, cigar makers and plasterers, printers and servants all had death rates well above 4 per 1,000, while bankers, brokers, and officials had the lowest death rates, below 1 per 1,000. (It is unclear whether the A.F. of L. accurately identified tuberculosis, or if they grouped other lung disorders such as silicosis, byssinosis, or other pneumonoconioses together.) In an address before the convention one speaker spelled out the connection between work, wages, living conditions, and tuberculosis: "All this means, really, the regulation of factory conditions, the regulation of housing, and the passage of child labor laws" was essential for battling the "Great White Plague." Like the social workers, the convention demanded improved public accommodations and play areas as well as more traditional demands for shorter hours and better pay. They called for the "development of playgrounds adjacent to all public schools" and "large open 'breathing spaces' interspersed in all cities." This was in addition to their advocacy of the elimination of sweatshops, "rigid inspection of mines, mills, factories and workshops," and the "incorporation in trade agreements in collective bargaining, covering working conditions, for suitable sanitation and ventilation." Significantly, the A.F. of L. claimed that health was a direct reflection of the success of the trade union movement. "In the same degree that the trade union movement becomes powerful will it establish such improved conditions that will check and eliminate the ravages of consumption."[45] In the following years unions became more active in fighting tuberculosis. They recognized that it was particularly prevalent among the working class, and

as *The Glass Worker*'s editor noted, "At least one-third of the deaths during the chief working period of life are caused by pulmonary tuberculosis. . . . In some trades . . . from 35 to 50% of all deaths are caused by tuberculosis." The editorial noted that "no movement" that ignores the industrial workplace can mount an effective "campaign against tuberculosis."[46]

Union campaigns to make shop conditions more sanitary were linked to broader public health issues, most important, the battle against infectious disease. Cleaning up the workplace and keeping the workforce healthy were seen as benefits to both the worker and the public. In 1910 the greater New York local of the International Union of Bakers and Confectionary Workers conducted a successful strike to demand more sanitary working conditions. "Perhaps no phase of the trade union movement has ever affected the public so directly as the agitation for sanitary conditions in the bake shops," commented one leading periodical. In May of 1909, 3,000 Jewish bakers struck, and less than a year later 4,000 German workers followed suit.[47] The union identified unsanitary workshops and the spread of infectious disease with nonunion bakeries. They insisted "on proper ventilation and sanitary conditions" and demanded "the great bread eating public of this country should see to it that the bread they eat bears the bakers' union label."[48] Their ability to link unsanitary working conditions to the health of the public gave their strike a tremendous appeal and power.

The very prevalence of contagious diseases, such as diphtheria, influenza, tuberculosis, and typhoid, within the working class spurred consumer groups to take up the issue of health conditions on the job and in the home. In part the appeal was based on fear, to make sure the middle class and wealthy would not be infected by goods tainted by sick workers. In the growing garment industry of New York, many dresses, shirts, and trousers were sewn on a piece-work basis in tenement slums, raising the spectre that the same diseases infecting those in tenements would be transmitted to the men, women, and children of the middle class. It was this terror that led the National Consumers League to become active in tenement reform and anti-tuberculosis campaigns. Its label on goods came to represent the mark of clothing manufactured under hygienic conditions. The league became involved in a wide variety of labor-related issues, including fire safety, workers' compensation, and occupational disease legislation.[49]

The concern with public health also led the National Consumers League to confront the issue of piece work in tenements. It was felt that work at home led to "long hours of uncontrolled labor for women and little children—often under far worse conditions than those of regulated factories." This in turn undermined the "health and strength" of the workforce and, therefore, spurred the spread of contagious diseases.[50] Frances Perkins, who had served for two years as secretary of the New York City Consumers League as well as at Greenwich House, also condemned the system of home work as "the most practical example which we have of the ability of industry to enslave its workers." But she also noted that this work also had a deleterious effect on public health: "One of the things which I noticed in regard to the system of this home work is that it is a menace to the health of the community and the health of the worker."[51]

The special social conditions surrounding work at the turn of the century led to the broad conception of the meaning of occupational safety and health. The rapid unregulated growth of industry, the enormous immigration of foreign workers, the growing strength of the Socialist party, the fear of social unrest, and the terror engendered by infectious disease gave the movement a special appeal. Occupational safety and health was part and parcel of a larger movement to reform American society.

## V

The movement to control workplace hazards was widespread, encompassing a variety of different groups. Among these groups were radicals such as Crystal Eastman and Morris Hillquit. At the other end of the political spectrum were "enlightened" owners of corporations such as International Harvester and United States Steel that sought to undermine the movement through voluntary welfare and safety programs. Between these two extremes were a wide variety of middle-class reformers and conservative labor representatives who recognized that uncontrolled capitalism was killing and maiming so many workers that it was undermining the legitimacy of capitalism itself. The conflicts this generated were so severe that a program of reform was essential.

The movement was most successful in making occupational safety and health a national issue. For almost a decade, exposés of inhumane working conditions and demands for reform were regular features in newspapers and magazines across the country. The outcry against the hazards that workers faced on the job raised the public's consciousness to a level that was not to be reached again until the 1970s. In its early years, socialists and labor representatives enunciated a new program for reforming the workplace. They insisted that occupational health issues, especially the control of lead, phosphorus, and other industrial poisons, be an integral part of the movement's agenda. They recognized that a broad environmental approach had to be adopted if workers' health was really to be protected. Finally, they demanded that government play the decisive regulatory role in protecting the well-being of labor. After 1914, however, business groups came to dominate this movement through organizations such as the National Safety Council. Their approach was entirely different. They narrowed the concern to safety rather than health and turned to engineers and technicians rather than to labor and government. They relied on voluntary action by industry itself to improve safety conditions and emphasized the responsibility of the worker for many accidents and the need for workers to avoid carelessness on the job.

On a concrete level the movement was successful in achieving some legislative reform. Several states had already acted in the late 19th century to initiate state factory-inspection bureaus to control workplace hazards. But it must be remembered that there was hardly any federal involvement in this area in the 19th century.

Before the Progressive Era, the dominant *laissez-faire* ideology defined government's role extremely narrowly: most officials saw themselves merely as passive facilitators of trade and industrial development. By 1900 the boundaries of government had expanded to include such activities as the regulation of interstate commerce. But it was only exceptional public officials who openly supported workers in their dealings with management.

During the first two decades of this century, however, a number of public officials began to challenge this older 19th-century notion of government's passive role. Especially in the larger industrial states of the East and the Midwest, legislators and administrators such as Senators Robert Wagner and Robert LaFollette and President Teddy Roosevelt pressed for a more activist stance for government. Labor relations was one of their major foci, and they sought to reconcile the divergent views of labor and capital.

Underlying the efforts of progressive leaders was a new conception of the state, a state that regulated for the common good. Robert Wagner summarized this view: "No government is properly performing when it permits the working people within its bounds to be employed under unsanitary conditions, when it fails to protect them from preventable diseases and accidents, when it permits the premature employment of its young children, and the excessive toil of its women." For reformers the new industrial system demanded a different conception of the state. The new industrial system, dependent as it was on the harmonious relationship between labor and capital, demanded a healthy workforce. The role of the state was to protect this "most precious asset, the workers within its bounds."[52]

Industrial accidents and diseases proved to be an attractive issue for progressives interested in expanding the role of the state. The rapid increase in the industrial labor force and the social disorder that accompanied urban growth, immigration, and industrialization made workers' health and living conditions a natural concern for government. One official writing in the Department of Labor *Bulletin* in 1903 pointed to the link between industrial conditions and America's health: "The miserable hygienic conditions existing in the working places . . . are unjust to the working classes, and sometimes react with frightful results upon the public. . . . With the multiplication of factories the improvement in the lot of the laboring man has become a vital question of the day. . . . The health of society in general is both directly and indirectly menaced by insanitary conditions in any industry."[53]

From the modern perspective, the efforts by reformers to establish a governmental role in workplace regulation may seem trivial or even conservative. But at the time these efforts were supported by many radicals as significant reforms. In little more than two decades, we saw the establishment

of a meaningful federal Department of Labor, active women's and children's bureaus, the reinforcement and subsidization of state factory-inspection systems through state departments of labor, and the beginnings of a role in occupational safety and health within local health departments. We also saw the passage of the first significant child and women's labor legislation and a host of specific state acts regulating working conditions in tanneries, bakeries, foundries, and numerous other industries. Also, for the first time, there was a serious attempt to organize a more reliable method for collecting statistics on occupational injuries and deaths. Finally, it must be pointed out that in 1900 no state in the Union had a workers' compensation law. By 1915 every highly industrialized state had passed an act for some form of compensation.

On the federal level, the reform movement was successful in passing a number of significant pieces of legislation. The railroad workers' compensation act in 1907 and a broader federal employees' compensation act were two of the landmark legislative efforts. But other attempts at outlawing certain special hazards also were important milestones in this early period of governmental activity. The passage of the Esch Phosphorus bill, an act placing a prohibitive tax on kitchen matches that used deadly white phosphorus, was a dramatic victory of the early reform movement, even if it was later than European actions.[54]

The movement forced politicians to pay attention to certain elemental safety and health issues. In 1912, the yearly Conference of Charities and Correction issued a "Platform of Industrial Minimums" in anticipation of the upcoming presidential elections. Included among them were the traditional demands for "a living wage," an eight-hour day, and a six-day work week. But added to the list was a set of demands that had never appeared before. The conference called for mandatory governmental investigations of all industries "with a view to establishing standards of sanitation and safety and a basis for establishing compensation for injury." Also among these standards was a call to prohibit "the manufacture or sale of poisonous articles, dangerous to the life of the worker and his family" and a law that required the mandatory reporting of all "deaths, injuries and diseases due to industrial operations." The conference also called for workers to have a right to a "safe and sanitary home."[55]

The platform developed by the national conference received wide publicity and was used as the model for the industrial platform of Teddy Roosevelt's Progressive party in 1912: "The supreme duty of the national government is the conservation of human resources through an enlarged measure of social and industrial justice. . . ." They called for "effective legislation looking to the prevention of industrial accidents, occupational disease, over work, involuntary unemployment, and other injurious effects incident to modern industry."[56]

Despite the very real differences in emphasis and approach, the various elements of this movement were able to unite around a few legislative and programmatic goals. Workers' compensation was one especially important reform goal that has received a great deal of attention. But a host of other efforts also characterized the movement and, taken together, these efforts force us to reevaluate the meaning of the movement. A look at its impact on the consciousness of the American population gives it an exceedingly radical appearance.

On one level, the importance of the movement was reflected in the profound effect that propagandistic efforts had on the thinking of the majority of Americans. During the 19th century job-related injury and death were often seen as necessary byproducts of industrialization. Personal health and safety were believed to be the responsibility of the workers themselves. Legal doctrines such as the "fellow servant" rule and the notion of "assumed risk" spoke to the prevailing 19th-century belief that the burden of responsibility for occupational injury and disease resided with the workforce rather than with management. The efforts of reformers altered the prevailing assumptions of many Americans. The notion that workers assumed the risks of work by taking the job in the first place was largely discredited. But workers continue to be maimed, poisoned, and killed at their workplaces. However limited the success in reforming the workplace, the true legacy of the early movement is the principle that workers have a right to a safe workplace, and it is the responsibility of society to guarantee that right.

## NOTES

1  Paul S. Pierce, "Industrial diseases," *North Am. Rev.,* Oct. 1911, *194*: 530.
2  Arthur B. Reeve, "The death roll of industry," *Charities and the Commons,* 1907, *17*: 791.
3  *Ibid.*
4  Editorial, "Slaughter by accident," *The Outlook,* Oct. 8, 1904, *78*: 359.
5  William Hard, "Making steel and killing men," *Everybody's Magazine,* Nov. 1907, *17*: 579–592; John Fitch, "The human side of large outputs," *The Survey,* Nov. 4, 1911, *27*: 1149.
6  Reeve, "Death roll of industry," p. 807.
7  "The price, in blood, for industrial progress," *Current Literature,* Dec. 1911, *51*: 629.
8  William Hard and others, *Injured in the Course of Duty,* pamphlet (n.p., n.d.).
9  Alice Hamilton, *Exploring the Dangerous Trades: the Autobiography of Alice Hamilton* (Boston, 1943).
10  Earl Mayo, "The work that kills," *The Outlook,* Sept. 23, 1911, *99*: 203.
11  *International Harvester Company and Its Employees,* pamphlet (Chicago, 1912), pp. 3, 4.
12  Thomas F. Harrington, "Prevention of disease versus cost of living," *Scient. Am. Suppl.,* June 28, 1913, *75*: 402–403; Arthur B. Reeve, "Our industrial jug-

gernaut," *Everybody's Magazine,* Feb. 1907, *16*: 149; William Hard, *Injured in the Course of Business* (n.p., n.d.).
13  Paul S. Pierce, "Industrial diseases," *North Am. Rev.,* Oct. 1911, *194*: 530.
14  Editorial, "Business and manslaughter," *The Independent,* May 2, 1919, *72*: 964–965.
15  "Is it worth the price?" *The Glass Worker,* June 1908, 5.
16  Margaret Dreier Robbins, The President's Report, *Third Biennial Convention of the National Women's Trade Union League of America* (Boston, 1911).
17  William Ludlow Chenery, "Occupational diseases," *The Independent,* Feb. 9, 1911, *70*: 306–309.
18  Josiah Strong, "Our industrial juggernaut," *North Am. Rev.,* Nov. 16, 1906, *183*: 1034. See also Strong's commitment to changing work conditions in his founding and assuming the presidency of the American Museum of Safety Devices and Industrial Hygiene in 1907/1908: "Apparently little is done in this country for the protection of working men and women." Josiah Strong to Miss E. L. M. Tate, Feb. 25, 1908, American Association for Labor Legislation (A.A.L.L.) manuscript, Labor-Management Documentation Center, New York State School of

Industrial and Labor Relations, Cornell University, Microfilm R 2390.

19  New York, *Second Report of the Factory Investigating Commission*, 1913, Vol. IV, pp. 1361, 1364.

20  Quoted in Nora Gause, "The slavery of childhood," *The Woman's Label League Journal*, May 1907: 15.

21  Elizabeth Beardsley Butler, "The cracker industry in Pittsburgh," *Charities and the Commons*, Sept. 5, 1908, *20*: 648–655.

22  Margaret Dreier Robbins, "Foreward for the Women's Trade Union League," *The National Women's Trade Union League* (n.p., n.d.).

23  William Hard with Rheta Childe Dorr as collaborator, "The woman's invasion," *Everybody's Magazine*, 1910, *21*: 372–385.

24  *Ibid.*

25  *The Glass Worker*, Apr. 1912, *9*.

26  *The Woman's Label League Journal*, Oct. 1913, *11*: 1.

27  *The Survey*, Jan. 18, 1913, *29*: 534. For Hull House's commitment to occupational safety and health, see Jane Addams to John Commons, Mar. 5, 1908, and Irene Osgood to Charles Henderson, Oct. 8, 1908, A.A.L.L. manuscript, Microfilm R 2390.

28  Graham Taylor, "Industrial basis for social interpretation," *The Survey*, Apr. 3, 1909, *22*: 10.

29  U.S. Commission on Industrial Relations, Preliminary Report, *The Survey*, Dec. 12, 1914, *33*: 288.

30  See Domhoff, *The Higher Circles* (New York, 1965) and Irwin Yellowitz, *New York and the Progressive Movement* (New York, 1968).

31  Henry W. Farnum, "Labor legislation and economic progress," address by the president at the annual meeting, Dec. 28, 1909, Columbia Univ., Butler Library.

32  See letterhead of A.A.L.L. correspondence.

33  Shelby M. Harrison, "2nd National Conference on Industrial Diseases," *The Survey*, June 15, 1912, *28*: 448–450. See also, the A.A.L.L.'s pamphlet, *The Menace of Lead* [c. 1911]: "What the absence of state sanitary control means to workers" is that "thousands of workers are daily exposed to [lead's] influence and thereby run the risk, not only of disability, but even of death." A.A.L.L. manuscript, Microfilm R 2453.

34  John B. Andrews, "Report of work, 1910," *Am. Labor Legis. Rev.*, 1911: 95.

35  "The responsibility is on all citizens," *The Survey*, Apr. 8, 1911, *26*: 85.

36  John M. Work, "Give us justice not charity," *The Glass Worker*, Aug. 1911, *9*: 6.

37  Crystal Eastman, "The three essentials for accident prevention," *Annals*, June 1911, *38*: 98–99.

38  *Ibid.*

39  "Joint sanitary standards in the cloak, suit and skirt industry," *The Survey*, Aug. 19, 1911, *26*: 734.

40  "Strikes for good health," *The Survey*, Jan. 20, 1912, *27*: 1592.

41  "Responsibility is on all citizens," p. 84.

42  "The tuberculosis fight in an industrial city," *Charities*, Dec. 17, 1904: 279.

43  Frederick Almy, "Transcript of Proceedings, New York," *Second Report of the New York Factory Investigating Commission*, 1913, Vol. IV, pp. 1831–1832.

44  Graham Taylor, "Industrial basis for social interpretation," p. 9.

45  "How to prevent consumption," *The International Woodworker*, May 1906, *16*: 137–139; "Paul Kennaday on tuberculosis," *ibid.*, pp. 139–140.

46  "Labor is against tuberculosis," *The Glass Worker*, Apr. 1909, *6*: 6.

47  "A strike for clean bread," *The Survey*, June 18, 1910, *24*: 483–488.

48  "Investigations have disclosed the fact that unhealthy and poisonous bread is made in non-union bake shops," *The Woman's Label League Journal*, June 1913: 13.

49  Charles Swan, "Enterprise liability for industrial injuries," *Ann. Am. Acad. Polit. & Soc. Sci.*, July 1911, *38*: 262–263; "The Consumers League label and its offspring," *The Survey*, Aug. 8, 1914, *32*: 478.

50  Mary H. Loines, chairman of the Brooklyn Auxiliary of the Consumers League of the City of New York, to Hon. Robert F. Wagner, Dec. 12, 1912, New York, *Second Report of the New York Factory Investigating Commission*, 1913, Vol. II, 1330–1331.

51  *Ibid.*, Vol. IV, 1576–1577.

52  Quoted in Paul Kennaday, "The Reorganization Bill," *The Survey*, Feb. 22, 1913, *29*: 727–728.

53  C. F. W. Doehring, "Factory sanitation and labor protection," U.S. Department of Labor *Bulletin*, Jan. 1903, *44*: 12.

54  Gordon Thayer, "Matches or men?," *Everybody's Magazine*, Apr. 1912, *26*: 490–498.

55  "A platform of industrial minimums," *The Survey*, July 6, 1912, *28*: 517–518.

56  Paul U. Kellogg, "The industrial platform of a new party," *The Survey*, Aug. 24, 1912, *28*: 668.

# Reference Material

# A Guide to Further Reading

Books and articles in this Guide are arranged under the following headings: *General, Allied Professions, Diseases, Domestic and Folk Medicine, Education, Faith Healing and Quackery, Hospitals, Hygiene, Image and Income, Mental Health, Military, Minority Medicine, Practice, Public Health: Colonial, Public Health Since 1776, Research, Sanitation, Sectarians, and Women.*

## GENERAL

Brieger, Gert H., ed. *Medical America in the Nineteenth Century: Readings from the Literature.* Baltimore: Johns Hopkins Press, 1972.

Cassedy, James H. *American Medicine and Statistical Thinking, 1800–1860.* Cambridge: Harvard University Press, 1984.

Duffy, John. *The Healers: The Rise of the Medical Establishment.* New York: McGraw-Hill Book Co., 1976.

Grob, Gerald. "The social history of medicine and disease in America: problems and possibilities." *Journal of Social History* 10 (1977): 391–409.

Haller, John S., Jr. *American Medicine in Transition, 1840–1910.* Urbana: University of Illinois Press, 1981.

Kaufman, Martin, Stuart Galishoff, and Todd L. Savitt, eds. *Dictionary of American Medical Biography.* 2 vols. Westport, Conn.: Greenwood Press, 1984.

Kett, Joseph F. *The Formation of the American Medical Profession: The Role of Institutions, 1780–1860.* New Haven: Yale University Press, 1968.

King, Lester S. *American Medicine Comes of Age, 1840–1920.* [Chicago]: American Medical Association, 1984.

Lerner, Monroe, and Odin W. Anderson. *Health Progress in the United States, 1900–1960.* Chicago: University of Chicago Press, 1963.

McKeown, Thomas. *The Modern Rise of Population.* New York: Academic Press, 1976.

Numbers, Ronald L. "The history of American medicine: A field in ferment." *Reviews in American History* 10 (1982): 245–263.

Reverby, Susan, and David Rosner, eds. *Health Care in America: Essays in Social History.* Philadelphia: Temple University Press, 1979.

Rosen, George. *Preventive Medicine in the United States, 1900–1975: Trends and Interpretations.* New York: Prodist, 1976.

Rothstein, William G. *American Physicians in the 19th Century: From Sects to Science.* Baltimore: Johns Hopkins University Press, 1972.

Shryock, Richard Harrison. *Medicine and Society in America, 1660–1860.* New York: New York University Press, 1960.

Shryock, Richard Harrison. *Medicine in America: Historical Essays.* Baltimore: Johns Hopkins Press, 1966.

Starr, Paul. *The Social Transformation of American Medicine.* New York: Basic Books, 1982.

Stevens, Rosemary. *American Medicine and the Public Interest.* New Haven: Yale University Press, 1971.

Vogel, Morris J., and Charles E. Rosenberg, eds. *The Therapeutic Revolution: Essays in the Social History of American Medicine.* Philadelphia: University of Pennsylvania Press, 1979.

## ALLIED PROFESSIONS

Ashley, JoAnn. *Hospitals, Paternalism and the Role of the Nurse.* New York: Teachers College Press, 1976.

Burnham, John C. "The struggle between physicians and paramedical personnel in American psychiatry, 1917–41." *Journal of the History of Medicine and Allied Sciences* 29 (1974): 93–106.

Donegan, Jane B. *Women and Men Midwives: Medicine, Morality and Misogyny in Early America.* Westport, Conn.: Greenwood Press, 1978.

Kalisch, Philip A., and Beatrice J. Kalisch. *The Advance of American Nursing*. Boston: Little, Brown and Company, 1978.

Lagemann, Ellen Condliffe, ed. *Nursing History: New Perspectives, New Possibilities*. New York: Teachers College Press, 1983.

Litoff, Judy Barrett. *American Midwives: 1860 to the Present*. Westport, Conn.: Greenwood Press, 1978.

McCluggage, Robert W. *A History of the American Dental Association: A Century of Health Service*. Chicago: American Dental Association, 1959.

Marshall, Helen E. *Mary Adelaide Nutting: Pioneer of Modern Nursing*. Baltimore: Johns Hopkins University Press, 1972.

Melosh, Barbara. *"The Physician's Hand": Work Culture and Conflict in American Nursing*. Philadelphia: Temple University Press, 1982.

Mottus, Jane E. *New York Nightingales: The Emergence of the Nursing Profession at Bellevue and New York Hospital 1850–1920*. Ann Arbor, Mich.: UMI Research Press, 1980.

Safier, Gwendolyn. *Contemporary American Leaders in Nursing: An Oral History*. New York: McGraw-Hill, 1977.

Schwartz, L. Laszlo. "The historical relations of American dentistry and medicine." *Bulletin of the History of Medicine* 28 (1954): 542–549.

Shryock, Richard Harrison. "Nursing emerges as a profession: The American experience." *Clio Medica* 3 (1968): 131–147.

Sonnedecker, Glenn. *Kremers and Urdang's History of Pharmacy*. 4th ed. Philadelphia: J. B. Lippincott Co., 1976.

## DISEASES

Ackerknecht, Erwin H. "Anticontagionism between 1821 and 1867." *Bulletin of the History of Medicine* 22 (1948): 569–593.

Ackerknecht, Erwin H. *Malaria in the Upper Mississippi Valley*. Baltimore: Johns Hopkins Press, 1945.

Blake, John B. *Benjamin Waterhouse and the Introduction of Vaccination: A Reappraisal*. Philadelphia: University of Pennsylvania Press, 1957.

Brandt, Allan M. *No Magic Bullet: A Social History of Venereal Disease in the United States since 1880*. New York: Oxford University Press, 1985.

Caulfield, Ernest. *A True History of the Terrible Epidemic Vulgarly Called the Throat Distemper which Occurred between the Years 1735 and 1740*. New Haven: Beaumont Medical Club, 1939.

Courtwright, David T. *Dark Paradise: Opiate Addiction in America before 1940*. Cambridge: Harvard University Press, 1982.

Crosby, Alfred W., Jr. *Epidemic and Peace, 1918*. Westport, Conn.: Greenwood Publishing, 1976.

Dowling, Harry F. *Fighting Infection: Conquests of the Twentieth Century*. Cambridge: Harvard University Press, 1977.

Duffy, John. *Sword of Pestilence: The New Orleans Yellow Fever Epidemic of 1853*. Baton Rouge: Louisiana State University Press, 1966.

Etheridge, Elizabeth. *The Butterfly Caste: A Social History of Pellagra in the South*. Westport, Conn.: Greenwood Publishing, 1972.

Fox, Daniel M., and Judith F. Stone. "Black lung: Miners' militancy and medical uncertainty, 1968–1972." *Bulletin of the History of Medicine* 54 (1980): 43–63.

Kaufman, Martin. "The American antivaccinationists and their arguments." *Bulletin of the History of Medicine* 41 (1967): 463–478.

Musto, David F. *The American Disease: Origins of Narcotic Control*. New Haven: Yale University Press, 1973.

Powell, J. H. *Bring Out Your Dead: The Great Plague of Yellow Fever in Philadelphia in 1793*. Philadelphia: University of Pennsylvania Press, 1949.

Rosenberg, Charles E. *The Cholera Years: The United States in 1832, 1849, and 1866*. Chicago: University of Chicago Press, 1962.

Shryock, Richard Harrison. *National Tuberculosis Association, 1904–1954*. New York: National Tuberculosis Association, 1957.

Smith, Dale C. "Gerhard's distinction between typhoid and typhus and its reception in America, 1833–1860." *Bulletin of the History of Medicine* 54 (1980): 368–385.

Smith, Dale C. "The rise and fall of typhomalarial fever." *Journal of the History of Medicine and Allied Sciences* 37 (1982): 182–220, 287–321.

## DOMESTIC AND FOLK MEDICINE

Fellman, Anita Clair, and Michael Fellman. *Making Sense of Self: Medical Advice Literature in Late*

*Nineteenth Century America.* Philadelphia: University of Pennsylvania Press, 1981.

Hand, Wayland, D., ed. *American Folk Medicine: A Symposium.* Berkeley: University of California Press, 1976.

Risse, Guenter B., Ronald L. Numbers, and Judith Walzer Leavitt, eds. *Medicine without Doctors: Home Health Care in American History.* New York: Science History Publications, 1977.

Stage, Sarah. *Female Complaints: Lydia Pinkham and the Business of Women's Medicine.* New York: W. W. Norton, 1979.

Young, James Harvey. *American Self-Dosage Medicines: An Historical Perspective.* Lawrence, Kans.: Coronado Press, 1974.

## EDUCATION

Bell, Whitfield J., Jr. *John Morgan: Continental Doctor.* Philadelphia: University of Pennsylvania Press, 1965.

Blake, John B. "Women and medicine in antebellum America." *Bulletin of the History of Medicine* 39 (1965): 99–123.

Bonner, Thomas Neville. *American Doctors and German Universities: A Chapter in International Intellectual Relations, 1870–1914.* Lincoln: University of Nebraska Press, 1963.

Fleming, Donald. *William H. Welch and the Rise of Modern Medicine.* Boston: Little, Brown and Company, 1954.

Flexner, Abraham. *Medical Education in the United States and Canada.* New York: Carnegie Foundation, 1910.

Fox, Daniel M. "Abraham Flexner's unpublished report: foundations and medical education, 1909–1928." *Bulletin of the History of Medicine* 54 (1980): 475–496.

Jones, Russell M. "American doctors and the Parisian medical world, 1830–1840." *Bulletin of the History of Medicine* 47 (1973): 40–65, 177–204.

Kaufman, Martin. *American Medical Education: The Formative Years, 1765–1910.* Westport, Conn.: Greenwood Press, 1976.

Kohler, Robert. *From Medical Chemistry to Biochemistry: The Making of a Biomedical Discipline.* Cambridge: Cambridge University Press, 1982.

Lippard, Vernon W. *A Half-Century of American Education: 1920–1970.* New York: Josiah Macy, Jr., Foundation, 1974.

Ludmerer, Kenneth M. "Reform at Harvard Medical School, 1869–1909." *Bulletin of the History of Medicine* 55 (1981): 343–370.

Ludmerer, Kenneth M. "The rise of the teaching hospital in America." *Journal of the History of Medicine and Allied Sciences* 38 (1983): 389–414.

Norwood, William Frederick. *Medical Education in the United States before the Civil War.* Philadelphia: University of Pennsylvania Press, 1944.

Numbers, Ronald L., ed. *The Education of American Physicians.* Berkeley: University of California Press, 1979.

Savitt, Todd L. "Lincoln University Medical Department—A forgotten 19th century black medical school." *Journal of the History of Medicine and Allied Sciences* 40 (January 1985): 42–65.

Stevens, Rosemary. "Trends in medical specialization in the United States." *Inquiry* 8 (1971): 9–19.

Walsh, Mary Roth. *"Doctors Wanted: No Women Need Apply": Sexual Barriers in the Medical Profession, 1835–1975.* New Haven: Yale University Press, 1977.

Warner, John Harley. "A southern medical reform: The meaning of the antebellum argument for southern medical education." *Bulletin of the History of Medicine* 57 (1983): 364–381.

## FAITH HEALING AND QUACKERY

Cunningham, Raymond J. "The Emmanuel movement: A variety of American religious experience." *American Quarterly* 14 (1962): 48–63.

Cunningham, Raymond J. "From holiness to healing: The faith cure in America, 1872–1892." *Church History* 43 (1974): 499–513.

Harrell, David Edwin, Jr. *All Things Are Possible: The Healing and Charismatic Revivals in Modern America.* Bloomington: Indiana University Press, 1975.

Ward, Patricia Spain. "'Who will bell the cat?' Andrew C. Ivy and Krebiozen." *Bulletin of the History of Medicine* 58 (1984): 28–52.

Young, James Harvey. "Laetrile in historical perspective." In *Politics, Science, and Cancer: The Laetrile Phenomenon,* ed. Gerald E. Markle and James C. Petersen (Boulder, Colo.: Westview Press, 1980), pp. 11–60.

Young, James Harvey. *The Medical Messiahs: A Social History of Health Quackery in Twentieth-*

*Century America.* Princeton: Princeton University Press, 1967.

Young, James Harvey. *The Toadstool Millionaires: A Social History of Patent Medicines in America before Federal Regulation.* Princeton: Princeton University Press, 1961.

## HOSPITALS

Dowling, Harry F. *City Hospitals: The Undercare of the Underprivileged.* Cambridge: Harvard University Press, 1982.

Drachman, Virginia G. *Hospital with a Heart: Women Doctors and the Paradox of Separatism at the New England Hospital, 1862–1969.* Ithaca: Cornell University Press, 1984.

Eaton, Leonard K. *New England's Hospitals, 1790–1833.* Ann Arbor: University of Michigan Press, 1957.

Rosenberg, Charles E. "And heal the sick: The hospital and the patient in 19th century America." *Journal of Social History* 10 (1977): 428–447.

Rosenberg, Charles E. "Inward vision and outward glance: The shaping of the American hospital, 1880–1914." *Bulletin of the History of Medicine* 53 (1979): 346–391.

Rosner, David. *A Once Charitable Enterprise: Hospitals and Health Care in Brooklyn and New York, 1885–1915.* Cambridge: Cambridge University Press, 1982.

Vogel, Morris J. *The Invention of the Modern Hospital: Boston, 1870–1930.* Chicago: University of Chicago Press, 1980.

Williams, William H. *America's First Hospital: The Pennsylvania Hospital, 1751–1841.* Wayne, Pa.: Haverford House, 1976.

## HYGIENE

Blake, John B. "Health reform." In *The Rise of Adventism: Religion and Society in Mid-Nineteenth-Century America,* ed. Edwin S. Gaustad (New York: Harper and Row, 1974), pp. 30–49.

Blake, John B. "Mary Gove Nichols: Prophetess of health." *Proceedings of the American Philosophical Society* 106 (1962): 219–234.

Cummings, Richard Osborn. *The American and His Food: A History of Food Habits in the United States.* Chicago: University of Chicago Press, 1941.

Glassburg, David. "The public bath movement

in America." *American Studies* 20 (Fall 1979): 5–20.

Kirkland, Edward C. "'Scientific Eating': New Englanders prepare and promote a reform, 1873–1907." *Proceedings of the Massachusetts Historical Society* 86 (1974): 28–52.

Nissenbaum, Stephen. *Sex, Diet, and Debility in Jacksonian America: Sylvester Graham and Health Reform.* Westport, Conn.: Greenwood Press, 1980.

Numbers, Ronald L. *Prophetess of Health: A Study of Ellen G. White.* New York: Harper and Row, 1976.

Whorton, James C. *Crusaders for Fitness: The History of American Health Reformers.* Princeton: Princeton University Press, 1982.

Williams, Marilyn Thornton. "New York City's public baths: A case study in urban progressive reform." *Journal of Urban History* 7 (1980): 49–81.

## IMAGE AND INCOME

Anderson, Odin W. *The Uneasy Equilibrium; Private and Public Financing of Health Services in the United States, 1875–1965.* New Haven: College and University Press, 1968.

Baker, Samuel L. "Physician licensure laws in the United States, 1865–1915." *Journal of the History of Medicine and Allied Sciences* 39 (1984): 173–197.

Berlant, Jeffrey Lionel. *Profession and Monopoly: A Study of Medicine in the United States and Great Britain.* Berkeley: University of California Press, 1975.

Brown, E. Richard. *Rockefeller Medicine Men: Medicine and Capitalism in America.* Berkeley and Los Angeles: University of California Press, 1979.

Burns, Chester R. "Malpractice suits in American medicine before the Civil War." *Bulletin of the History of Medicine* 43 (1969): 41–56.

Burrow, James G. *AMA: Voice of American Medicine.* Baltimore: Johns Hopkins Press, 1963.

Burrow, James G. *Organized Medicine in the Progressive Era: The Move Toward Monopoly.* Baltimore: Johns Hopkins University Press, 1977.

Duffy, John. "The changing image of the American physician." *Journal of the American Medical Association* 200 (1967): 136–140.

Hirshfield, Daniel S. *The Lost Reform: The Campaign*

for Compulsory Health Insurance in the United States from 1932 to 1943. Cambridge: Harvard University Press, 1970.

Numbers, Ronald L. Almost Persuaded: American Physicians and Compulsory Health Insurance, 1912–1920. Baltimore: Johns Hopkins University Press, 1978.

Numbers, Ronald L., ed. Compulsory Health Insurance: The Continuing American Debate. Westport, Conn.: Greenwood Press, 1982.

Poen, Monte M. Harry S. Truman Versus the Medical Lobby: The Genesis of Medicare. Columbia: University of Missouri Press, 1979.

Rosen, George. Fees and Fee Bills: Some Economic Aspects of Medical Practice in Nineteenth Century America. Baltimore: Johns Hopkins Press, 1947.

Shryock, Richard H. Medical Licensing in America, 1650–1965. Baltimore: Johns Hopkins Press, 1967.

Stevens, Robert, and Rosemary Stevens. Welfare Medicine in America: A Case Study of Medicaid. New York: Free Press, 1974.

## MENTAL HEALTH

Bell, Leland V. Treating the Mentally Ill: From Colonial Times to the Present. New York: Praeger, 1980.

Burnham, John Chynoweth. Psychoanalysis and American Medicine, 1894–1918: Medicine, Science, and Culture. New York: International Universities Press, 1967.

Caplan, Ruth B. Psychiatry and the Community in Nineteenth Century America: The Recurring Concern with the Environment in the Prevention and Treatment of Mental Illness. New York: Basic Books, 1969.

Dain, Norman. Clifford W. Beers: Advocate for the Insane. Pittsburgh: University of Pittsburgh Press, 1980.

Dain, Norman. Concepts of Insanity in the United States, 1789–1865. New Brunswick: Rutgers University Press, 1964.

Deutsch, Albert. The Mentally Ill in America: A History of Their Care and Treatment from Colonial Times. 2d ed. New York: Columbia University Press, 1949.

Fox, Richard T. So Far Disordered in Mind: Insanity in California, 1870–1930. Berkeley and Los Angeles: University of California Press, 1978.

Grob, Gerald N. Edward Jarvis and the Medical World of Nineteenth-Century America. Knoxville: University of Tennessee Press, 1978.

Grob, Gerald N. Mental Illness and American Society, 1875–1940. Princeton: Princeton University Press, 1983.

Grob, Gerald N. Mental Institutions in America: Social Policy to 1875. New York: Free Press, 1973.

Grob, Gerald N. The State and the Mentally Ill: A History of Worcester State Hospital in Massachusetts, 1830–1920. Chapel Hill: University of North Carolina Press, 1966.

Hale, Nathan G., Jr. Freud and the Americans: The Beginnings of Psychoanalysis in the United States, 1876–1917. New York: Oxford University Press, 1971.

Numbers, Ronald L., and Janet S. Numbers. "Millerism and madness: A study of 'religious insanity' in nineteenth-century America." Bulletin of the Menninger Clinic 49 (1985): 289–320.

Rosenberg, Charles E. The Trial of the Assassin Guiteau: Psychiatry and Law in the Gilded Age. Chicago: University of Chicago Press, 1968.

Rosenkrantz, Barbara G., and Maris A. Vinovskis. "The invisible lunatics: Old age and insanity in mid-nineteenth century Massachusetts." In Aging and the Elderly: Humanistic Perspectives in Gerontology, ed. Stuart F. Spicker, Kathleen M. Woodward, and David D. Van Tassel (Atlantic Highlands, N.J.: Humanities Press, 1978), pp. 95–125.

Rothman, David J. Conscience and Convenience: The Asylum and Its Alternatives in Progressive America. Boston: Little, Brown and Company, 1980.

Rothman, David J. The Discovery of the Asylum: Social Order and Disorder in the New Republic. Boston: Little, Brown and Company, 1971.

Scull, Andrew, ed. Madhouses, Mad-Doctors, and Madmen: The Social History of Psychiatry in the Victorian Era. Philadelphia: University of Pennsylvania Press, 1981.

Sicherman, Barbara. The Quest for Mental Health in America, 1880–1917. New York: Arno Press, 1980.

Tomes, Nancy. A Generous Confidence: Thomas Story Kirkbride and the Art of Asylum-keeping, 1840–1883. Cambridge: Cambridge University Press, 1984.

Tyor, Peter L., and Leland V. Bell. Caring for the

*Retarded in America: A History.* Westport, Conn.: Greenwood Press, 1984.

Tyor, Peter. "Denied the power to choose the good: Sexuality and mental defect in American medical practice 1850–1920." *Journal of Social History* 10 (1977): 472–489.

## MILITARY

Adams, George Worthington. *Doctors in Blue: The Medical History of the Union Army in the Civil War.* New York: Henry Schuman, 1952.

Breeden, James O. *Joseph Jones, M.D.: Scientist of the Old South.* Lexington: University Press of Kentucky, 1975.

Breeden, James O. "Military and naval medicine." In *A Guide to the Sources of United States Military History,* ed. Robin Higham (Hamden, Conn.: Archon Books, 1975), pp. 317–343.

Cash, Philip. *Medical Men at the Siege of Boston, April, 1775–April, 1776: Problems of the Massachusetts and Continental Armies.* Philadelphia: American Philosophical Society, 1973.

Cunningham, H. H. *Doctors in Gray: The Confederate Medical Service.* Baton Rouge: Louisiana State University Press, 1958.

Gillett, Mary C. *The Army Medical Department, 1775–1818.* Washington: Center of Military History, 1981.

Shryock, Richard H. "A medical perspective on the Civil War." *American Quarterly* 14 (1962): 161–173.

## MINORITY MEDICINE

Beardsley, E. H. "Making separate, equal: Black physicians and the problems of medical segregation in pre-World War II South." *Bulletin of the History of Medicine* 57 (1983): 382–396.

Galishoff, Stuart. "Germs know no color line: Black health and public policy in Atlanta, 1900–1918." *Journal of the History of Medicine and Allied Sciences* 40 (January 1985): 22–41.

Haller, John S. "The negro and the southern physician: A study of medical and racial attitudes, 1800–1860." *Medical History* 16 (1972): 238–253.

Jones, James H. *Bad Blood: The Tuskegee Syphilis Experiment.* New York: Free Press, 1981.

Kiple, Kenneth F., and Virginia Himmelsteib King. *Another Dimension to the Black Diaspora: Diet, Disease, and Racism.* Cambridge: Cambridge University Press, 1981.

Postell, William Dosite. *The Health of Slaves on Southern Plantations.* Baton Rouge: Louisiana State University Press, 1951.

Savitt, Todd L. *Medicine and Slavery: The Diseases and Health Care of Blacks in Antebellum Virginia.* Urbana: University of Illinois Press, 1978.

Savitt, Todd L. "The use of blacks for medical experimentation and demonstration in the Old South." *Journal of Southern History* 48 (1982): 331–348.

Summerville, James. *Educating Black Doctors: A History of Meharry Medical College.* University: University of Alabama Press, 1983.

Torchia, Marion M. "Tuberculosis among American Negroes: Medical research on a racial disease, 1830–1950." *Journal of the History of Medicine and Allied Sciences* 32 (1977): 252–279.

Vogel, Virgil. *American Indian Medicine.* Norman: University of Oklahoma Press, 1970.

## PRACTICE

Apple, Rima D. "'To be used only under the direction of a physician': commercial infant feeding and medical practice, 1870–1940." *Bulletin of the History of Medicine* 54 (1980): 402–17.

Arney, William Ray. *Power and the Profession of Obstetrics.* Chicago: University of Chicago Press, 1982.

Atwater, Edward C. "The medical profession in a new society, Rochester, New York (1811–60)." *Bulletin of the History of Medicine* 47 (1973): 221–235.

Atwater, Edward C. "The physicians of Rochester, N.Y., 1860–1910: a study in professional history, II." *Bulletin of the History of Medicine* 51 (1977): 93–106.

Bell, Whitfield J., Jr. *The Colonial Physician & Other Essays.* New York: Science History Publications, 1975.

Brieger, Gert H. "American surgery and the germ theory of disease." *Bulletin of the History of Medicine* 40 (1966): 135–145.

Brieger, Gert H. "Therapeutic conflicts and the American medical profession in the 1860's." *Bulletin of the History of Medicine* 41 (1967): 215–222.

Christianson, Eric H. "The medical practitioners of Massachusetts, 1630–1800: Patterns of change and continuity." In *Medicine in Colonial Massachusetts, 1620–1820,* ed. Philip Cash, Eric H. Christianson, and J. Worth Estes. Publications of the Colonial Society of Massachusetts, vol. 57 (Charlottesville: University of Virginia Press, 1980), pp. 49–67.

English, Peter C. *Shock, Physiological Surgery, and George Washington Crile: Medical Innovation in the Progressive Era.* Westport, Conn.: Greenwood Press, 1980.

Estes, J. Worth. *Hall Jackson and the Purple Foxglove: Medical Practice and Research in Revolutionary America, 1760–1820.* Hanover, N. H.: University Press of New England, 1979.

Pernick, Martin S. *A Calculus of Suffering: Pain, Professionalism, and Anesthesia in 19th-century America.* New York: Columbia University Press, 1985.

Reiser, Stanley Joel. *Medicine and the Reign of Technology.* Cambridge: Cambridge University Press, 1978.

Riznik, Barnes. "The professional lives of early nineteenth century New England doctors." *Journal of the History of Medicine and Allied Sciences* 19 (1964): 1–16.

Rosen, George. *The Structure of American Medical Practice, 1875–1941.* Philadelphia: University of Pennsylvania Press, 1983.

Rosenberg, Charles E. "The practice of medicine in New York a century ago." *Bulletin of the History of Medicine* 41 (1967): 223–253.

Ward, Patricia Spain. "The American reception of Salvarsan." *Journal of the History of Medicine and Allied Sciences* 36 (1981): 44–62.

Warner, John Harley. "'The nature-trusting heresy': American physicians and the concept of the healing power of nature in the 1850's and 1860's." *Perspectives in American History* 11 (1977–78): 291–324.

Warner, John Harley. *The Therapeutic Perspective: Medical Practice, Knowledge, and Professional Identity in America, 1820–1885.* Cambridge: Harvard University Press, 1986.

## PUBLIC HEALTH: COLONIAL

Beall, Otho T., Jr., and Richard H. Shryock. *Cotton Mather: First Significant Figure in American Medicine.* Baltimore: Johns Hopkins Press, 1954.

Blake, John B. *Public Health in the Town of Boston, 1630–1822.* Cambridge: Harvard University Press, 1959.

Blake, John B. "Yellow fever in eighteenth century America." *Bulletin of the New York Academy of Medicine* 44 (1968): 673–686.

Cassedy, James H. "Church Record-keeping and Public Health in Early New England." In *Medicine in Colonial Massachusetts, 1620–1820,* ed. Philip Cash, Eric H. Christianson, and J. Worth Estes. Publications of the Colonial Society of Massachusetts, vol. 57 (Charlottesville: University of Virginia Press, 1980), pp. 249–260.

Cassedy, James H. *Demography in Early America: Beginnings of the Statistical Mind, 1600–1800.* Cambridge: Harvard University Press, 1969.

Crosby, Alfred W., Jr. *The Columbian Exchange: Biological and Cultural Consequences of 1492.* Westport, Conn: Greenwood Publishing, 1972.

Duffy, John. *Epidemics in Colonial America.* Baton Rouge: Louisiana State University Press, 1959.

Duffy, John. "The passage to the colonies." *Mississippi Valley Historical Review* 38 (1951–52): 21–38.

Duffy, John. "Smallpox and the Indians in the American colonies." *Bulletin of the History of Medicine* 25 (1951): 324–341.

## PUBLIC HEALTH SINCE 1776

Brown, D. Clayton. "Health of Farm Children in the South, 1900–1950." *Agricultural History* 53 (1979): 170–187.

Cassedy, James H. *Charles V. Chapin and the Public Health Movement.* Cambridge: Harvard University Press, 1962.

Cassedy, James H. "The roots of American sanitary reform, 1843–1847: Seven letters from John H. Griscom to Lemuel Shattuck." *Journal of the History of Medicine and Allied Sciences* 30 (1975): 136–147.

Condran, Gretchen A., and Eileen Crimmins-Gardner. "Public health measures and mortality in U.S. cities in the late nineteenth century." *Human Ecology* 6 (1978): 27–54.

Duffy, John. *A History of Public Health in New York City.* 2 vols. New York: Russell Sage Foundation, 1968, 1974.

Dunlap, Thomas R. *DDT: Scientists, Citizens, and Public Policy.* Princeton: Princeton University Press, 1981.

Ellis, John. "Business and public health in the urban South during the nineteenth century: New Orleans, Memphis, and Atlanta." *Bulletin of the History of Medicine* 44 (1970): 197–212, 346–371.

Galishoff, Stuart. *Safeguarding the Public Health: Newark, 1895–1918.* Westport, Conn.: Greenwood Press, 1975.

Higgs, Robert, and David Booth. "Mortality differentials within large American cities in 1890." *Human Ecology* 7 (1979): 353–370.

Jordan, Philip D. *The People's Health: A History of Public Health in Minnesota to 1848.* St. Paul: Minnesota Historical Society, 1953.

Kramer, Howard. "Early municipal and state boards of health." *Bulletin of the History of Medicine* 24 (1950): 503–529.

Leavitt, Judith Walzer. *The Healthiest City: Milwaukee and the Politics of Health Reform.* Princeton: Princeton University Press, 1982.

McKinlay, John B., and Sonja A. McKinlay. "The questionable contribution of medical measures to the decline of mortality in the United States in the 20th century." *Milbank Memorial Fund Quarterly: Health and Society* 55 (1977): 405–428.

Meckel, Richard A. "Immigration, mortality, and population growth in Boston, 1840–1880." *Journal of Interdisciplinary History* 15 (1985): 393–417.

Meeker, Edward. "The social rate of return on investment in public health, 1880–1910." *Journal of Economic History* 34 (1974): 392–421.

Nugent, Angela. "Fit for work: The introduction of physical examinations in industry." *Bulletin of the History of Medicine* 57 (1983): 578–595.

Rosen, George. *From Medical Police to Social Medicine: Essays on the History of Health Care.* New York: Science History Publications, 1974.

Rosen, George. "Politics and public health in New York City." *Bulletin of the History of Medicine* 24 (1950): 441–461.

Rosenkrantz, Barbara. "Cart before horse: Theory, practice, and professional image in American public health, 1810–1920." *Journal of the History of Medicine and Allied Sciences* 29 (1974): 55–73.

Rosenkrantz, Barbara Gutmann. *Public Health and the State: Changing Views in Massachusetts, 1842–1936.* Cambridge: Harvard University Press, 1972.

Rosner, David. "Research or Advocacy: Federal Occupational Safety and Health Policies during the New Deal." *Journal of Social History* 18 (Spring 1985): 365–381.

Rosner, David. "Health Care and the 'Truly Needy,' Nineteenth century origins of the concept." *Milbank Memorial Fund Quarterly: Health and Society* 60 (1982): 355–385.

Schwartz, Joshua Ira. *Public Health: Case Studies on the Origins of Government Responsibility for Health Services in the United States.* Ithaca, N.Y.: Program in Urban and Regional Studies, 1977.

Sigerist, Henry. "The cost of illness to the City of New Orleans in 1850." *Bulletin of the History of Medicine* 15 (1944): 498–507.

Warner, Margaret Humphreys. "Local Control versus Natural Interest: The debate over Southern public health, 1878–1884." *Journal of Southern History* 50 (1984): 407–428.

Warner, Margaret Humphreys. *Public Health in the New South: Government, Medicine and Society in the Control of Yellow Fever.* Cambridge: Cambridge University Press, forthcoming.

Whorton, James. *Before Silent Spring: Pesticides and Public Health in Pre-DDT America.* Princeton: Princeton University Press, 1974.

Wolfe, Margaret Ripley. *Lucius Polk Brown and Progressive Food and Drug Control: Tennessee and New York City, 1908–1920.* Lawrence: The Regents Press of Kansas, 1978.

## RESEARCH

Atwater, Edward C. "'Squeezing Mother Nature': Experimental physiology in the United States before 1870." *Bulletin of the History of Medicine* 52 (1978): 313–335.

Benison, Saul. *Tom Rivers: Reflections on a Life in Medicine and Science.* Cambridge: M.I.T. Press, 1967.

Corner, George W. *A History of the Rockefeller Institute, 1901–1953: Origins and Growth.* New York: Rockefeller Institute Press, 1964.

Lederer, Susan Eyrich. "Hideyo Noguchi's leutin experiment and the antivivisectionists." *Isis* 76 (1985): 31–48.

Lederer, Susan Eyrich. "'The right and wrong of making experiments on human beings': Udo J. Wile and syphilis." *Bulletin of the History of Medicine* 58 (1984): 380–397.

Numbers, Ronald L. "William Beaumont and the ethics of human experimentation." *Journal of the History of Biology* 12 (1979): 113–135.

Numbers, Ronald L., and William J. Orr Jr. "William Beaumont's reception at home and abroad." *Isis* 72 (1981): 590–612.

Rosen, George. "Patterns of health research in the United States, 1900–1960." *Bulletin of the History of Medicine* 39 (1965): 201–221.

Shryock, Richard H., *American Medical Research: Past and Present*. New York: The Commonwealth Fund, 1947.

Strickland, Stephen P. *Politics, Science, and Dread Disease: A Short History of United States Medical Research Policy*. Cambridge: Harvard University Press, 1972.

Swain, Donald C. "The rise of a research empire: NIH, 1930 to 1950." *Science* 138 (1962): 1233–1237.


## SANITATION

Blake, John B. "Lemuel Shattuck and the Boston water supply." *Bulletin of the History of Medicine* 29 (1955): 554–562.

Blake, Nelson. *Water for the Cities*. Syracuse: Syracuse University Press, 1956.

Cain, Louis P. *Sanitation Strategy for a Lakefront Metropolis*. DeKalb, Ill.: Northern Illinois University Press, 1978.

Cain, Louis P. "The search for an optimum sanitation jurisdiction: The Metropolitan Sanitary District of Greater Chicago, a case study." *Essays in Public Works History* (July 1980): 1–35.

Galishoff, Stuart. "Drainage, disease, comfort and class: A history of Newark's sewers." *Societas* 6 (1976): 121–138.

Larson, Lawrence. "Nineteenth century street sanitation: A study of filth and frustration." *Wisconsin Magazine of History* 52 (1968): 239–247.

Leavitt, Judith Walzer. "The wasteland: Garbage and sanitary reform in the nineteenth-century American city." *Journal of the History of Medicine and Allied Sciences* 35 (October 1980): 431–452.

Melosi, Martin V. *Garbage in the Cities: Refuse, Reform, and the Environment, 1880–1980*. College Station, Tex.: Texas A & M University Press, 1981.

Melosi, Martin V., ed. *Pollution & Reform in American Cities, 1870–1930*. Austin: University of Texas Press, 1980.

Schultz, Stanley K., and Clay McShane. "To engineer the metropolis: Sewers, sanitation, and city planning in late-19th century America." *Journal of American History* 65 (1978): 389–411.

Tarr, Joel. "Urban pollution—Many long years ago." *American Heritage* 22 (1971): 65–69ff.

Waserman, Manfred J. "Henry L. Coit and the certified milk movement in the development of modern pediatrics." *Bulletin of the History of Medicine* 46 (1972): 359–390.


## SECTARIANS

Berman, Alex. "Neo-Thomsonianism in the United States." *Journal of the History of Medicine and Allied Sciences* 11 (1956): 133–155.

Berman, Alex. "The Thomsonian movement and its relation to American pharmacy and medicine." *Bulletin of the History of Medicine* 25 (1951): 405–428, 519–538.

Donegan, Jane B. *Hydropathic Highway to Health: Women and Water-Cure in Antebellum America*. Westport, Conn.: Greenwood Press, 1986.

Gevitz, Norman. *The D.O.'s: Osteopathic Medicine in America*. Baltimore: Johns Hopkins University Press, 1982.

Kaufman, Martin. *Homeopathy in America: The Rise and Fall of a Medical Heresy*. Baltimore: Johns Hopkins Press, 1971.

Legan, Marshall Scott. "Hydropathy in America: A nineteenth century panacea." *Bulletin of the History of Medicine* 45 (1971): 267–280.

Numbers, Ronald L. "The making of an eclectic physician: Joseph M. McElhinney and the Eclectic Medical Institute of Cincinnati." *Bulletin of the History of Medicine* 47 (1973): 155–166.


## WOMEN

Bullough, Vern, and Martha Voght. "Women, menstruation, and nineteenth century medicine." *Bulletin of the History of Medicine* 47 (1973): 66–82.

Gordon, Linda. *Woman's Body, Woman's Right: A Social History of Birth Control in America.* New York: Grossman Publishers, 1976.

Haller, John S., and Robin M. Haller. *The Physician and Sexuality in Victorian America.* Urbana: University of Illinois Press, 1974.

Leavitt, Judith Walzer, ed. *Women and Health in America: Historical Readings.* Madison: University of Wisconsin Press, 1984.

Mohr, James C. *Abortion in America: The Origins and Evolution of National Policy.* New York: Oxford University Press, 1977.

Morantz, Regina Markell, Cynthia Stodola Pomerleau, and Carol Hansen Fenichel, eds. *In Her Own Words: Oral Histories of Women Physicians.* Westport, Conn.: Greenwood Press, 1982.

Morantz-Sanchez, Regina Markell. *"Guardians of the Race?" A History of Women Physicians in America 1848–1984.* New York: Oxford University Press, 1985.

Reed, James. *From Private Vice to Public Virtue: The Birth Control Movement and American Society Since 1830.* New York: Basic Books, 1978.

Sandelowski, Margarete. *Pain, Pleasure and American Childbirth: From the Twilight Sleep to the Read Method, 1914–1960.* Westport, Conn.: Greenwood Press, 1984.

Sicherman, Barbara. *Alice Hamilton: A Life in Letters.* Cambridge: Harvard University Press, 1984.

Sklar, Kathryn Kish. *Catharine Beecher: A Study in American Domesticity.* New Haven: Yale University Press, 1973.

Smith-Rosenberg, Carroll, and Charles E. Rosenberg. "The female animal: Medical and biological views of woman and her role in 19th century America." *Journal of American History* 60 (1973): 332–356.

Smith-Rosenberg, Carroll. "Puberty to menopause: The cycle of femininity in nineteenth-century America." *The Journal of Interdisciplinary History* 4 (1973): 25–52.

Wertz, Richard W., and Dorothy C. Wertz. *Lying-in: A History of Childbirth in America.* New York: Free Press, 1977.

# Abbreviations of Journal Titles

*Agric. Exper. Station, Bull. (Agricultural Experiment Station, Bulletin)*

*Alabama Med. J. (Alabama Medical Journal)*

*Am. Agriculturalist (American Agriculturalist)*

*Am. Architect & Bldg. News (American Architect and Building News)*

*Am. Hist. Rev. (American Historical Review)*

*Am. J. Clin. Med. (American Journal of Clinical Medicine)*

*Am. J. Dermatology & Genito-Urinary Dis. (American Journal of Dermatology and Genito-Urinary Diseases)*

*Am. J. Insanity (American Journal of Insanity)*

*Am. J. Med. Sci. (American Journal of the Medical Sciences)*

*Am. J. Nursing (American Journal of Nursing)*

*Am. J. Obst. & Dis. Women & Children (American Journal of Obstetrics and Diseases of Women and Children)*

*Am. J. Obst. & Gynec. (American Journal of Obstetrics and Gynecology)*

*Am. J. Pharm. (American Journal of Pharmacy)*

*Am. J. Psychiatry (American Journal of Psychiatry)*

*Am. J. Psychoth. (American Journal of Psychotherapy)*

*Am. J. Public Hlth. (American Journal of Public Health)*

*Am. J. Sociol. (American Journal of Sociology)*

*Am. Labor Legis. Rev. (American Labor Legislation Review)*

*Am. Law Rev. (American Law Review)*

*A.M.A. Bull. (American Medical Association Bulletin)*

*Am. Med. Monthly (American Medical Monthly)*

*Am. Med. Times (American Medical Times)*

*Am. Medico-Surg. Bull. (American Medico-Surgical Bulletin)*

*Am. Mercury (American Mercury)*

*Am. Philatelist (American Philatelist)*

*Am. Quart. (American Quarterly)*

*Am. Rev. Tuberculosis (American Review of Tuberculosis)*

*Am. Scientist (American Scientist)*

*Am. Veg. (American Vegetarian)*

*Am. Whig Rev. (American Whig Review)*

*Ann. Am. Acad. Polit. & Soc. Sci. (Annals of the American Academy of Political and Social Science)*

*Ann. chim. phys. (Annales de chimie et de physique)*

*Ann. Intern. Med. (Annals of Internal Medicine)*

*Ann. Med. Hist. (Annals of Medical History)*

*Ann. N.Y. Acad. Sci. (Annals of the New York Academy of Sciences)*

*Ann. Surg. (Annals of Surgery)*

*Antitrust Bull. (Antitrust Bulletin)*

*Arch. Dermatology & Syphilis (Archives of Dermatology and Syphilis)*

*Arch. Med. (Archives of Medicine)*

*Arch. Neurol. & Psychiat. (Archives of Neurology and Psychiatry)*

*Arch. pathol. Anat. (Archiv für pathologische Anatomie und Physiologie)*

*Arch. Pediat. (Archives of Pediatrics)*

*Arch. Sexual Behavior (Archives of Sexual Behavior)*

*Arch. Surg. (Archives of Surgery)*

*Atlanta J.-Rec. Med. (Atlanta Journal-Record of Medicine)*

*Atlanta Med. & Surg. J. (Atlanta Medical and Surgical Journal)*

*Atlanta Med. (Atlanta Medicine)*

*Berl. klin. Wohnschr. (Berliner klinische Wochenschrift)*

*Birth Control Rev. (Birth Control Review)*

*Boston J. Hlth. (Boston Journal of Health)*

*Boston Med. & Surg. J. (Boston Medical and Surgical Journal)*

*Boston Med. Magazine (Boston Medical Magazine)*

*Brit. & Foreign Med. Rev. (British and Foreign Medical Review)*

*Brit. J. Cancer (British Journal of Cancer)*

*Brit. J. Med. Psychol. (British Journal of Medical Psychology)*

*Brit. Med. J. (British Medical Journal)*

*Brooklyn Med. J. (Brooklyn Medical Journal)*

*Buffalo Med. & Surg. J. (Buffalo Medical and Surgical Journal)*

*Buffalo Med. J. & Monthly Rev. (Buffalo Medical Journal and Monthly Review)*

*Bull. A.A.M.C. (Bulletin of the Association of American Medical Colleges)*

*Bull. Acad. de méd. (Bulletin de l'Academie de médicine)*

Bull. Hist. Med. (Bulletin of the History of Medicine)

Bull. Mass. Dept. Mental Dis. (Bulletin of the Massachusetts Department of Mental Disease)

Bull. Med. Lib. Assn. (Bulletin of the Medical Library Association)

Bull. et mém. Soc. méd. hôp. Paris (Bulletin et mémoires de la Société médicale des hôpitaux de Paris)

Bull. N.Y. Acad. Med. (Bulletin of the New York Academy of Medicine)

Bull. Soc. Med. Hist. Chicago (Bulletin of the Society of Medical History [of Chicago])

Bull. Taylor Soc. (Bulletin of the Taylor Society)

Charleston Med. J. & Rev. (Charleston Medical Journal and Review)

Chicago Med. Exam. (Chicago Medical Examiner)

Chicago Med. J. (Chicago Medical Journal)

Chicago Med. J. & Exam. (Chicago Medical Journal and Examiner)

Chicago Med. Rev. (Chicago Medical Review)

Christian Exam. (Christian Examiner)

Columbia Univ. Quart. Suppl. (Columbia University Quarterly Supplement)

Columbus Med. J. (Columbus Medical Journal)

Deutsche med. Wohnschr. (Deutsche medizinische Wochenschrift)

Eclectic Med. J. (Eclectic Medical Journal)

Edinburgh Med. J. (Edinburgh Medical Journal)

Edinburgh New Philos. J. (Edinburgh New Philosophy Journal)

Edinburgh Rev. (Edinburgh Review)

Emory Univ. Quart. (Emory University Quarterly)

Exper. Station Rec. (Experiment Station Record)

Explorations Econ. Hist. (Explorations in Economic History)

Feminist Stud. (Feminist Studies)

Films Rev. (Films Review)

Galveston Med. J. (Galveston Medical Journal)

Georgia Med. & Surg. Encyc. (Georgia Medical and Surgical Encyclopedia)

Graham J. Hlth. & Long. (Graham Journal of Health and Longevity)

Harvard Med. Alumni Bull. (Harvard Medical Alumni Bulletin)

Harvard Theol. Rev. (Harvard Theological Review)

Hastings Cent. Rep. (Hastings Center Report)

Hastings Cent. Stud. (Hastings Center Studies)

Hist. & Theory (History and Theory)

Hosp. Admin. (Hospital Administration)

Iowa Med. J. (Iowa Medical Journal)

Johns Hopkins Hosp. Bull. (Johns Hopkins Hospital Bulletin)

J. Abnormal & Social Psych. (Journal of Abnormal and Social Psychology)

J.A.M.A. (Journal of the American Medical Association)

J. Am. Culture (Journal of American Culture)

J. Am. Hist. (Journal of American History)

J. Am. Med. Women's Assn. (Journal of the American Medical Women's Association)

J. Am. Pharm. Assn. (Journal of the American Pharmaceutical Association)

J. Anat. & Physiol. (Journal of Anatomy and Physiology)

J. Assn. Am. Med. Colls. (Journal of the Association of American Medical Colleges)

J. Chron. Dis. (Journal of Chronic Diseases)

J. Cutan. & Ven. Dis. (Journal of Cutaneous and Venereal Diseases)

J. Econ. Entomology (Journal of Economic Entomology)

J. Econ. Issues (Journal of Economic Issues)

J. Exper. Med. (Journal of Experimental Medicine)

J. Florida Med. Assn. (Journal of the Florida Medical Association)

J. Gynec. Soc. Boston (Journal of the Gynecological Society of Boston)

J. Hlth. Soc. Behav. (Journal of Health and Social Behavior)

J. Hist. Ideas (Journal of the History of Ideas)

J. Hist. Med. (Journal of the History of Medicine and Allied Sciences)

J. Hyg. & Herald Hlth. (Journal of Hygiene and Herald of Health)

J. Infect. Dis. (Journal of Infectious Diseases)

J. Interdisc. Hist. (Journal of Interdisciplinary History)

J. Maine Med. Assn. (Journal of the Maine Medical Association)

J. Med. Educ. (Journal of Medical Education)

J. Med. Soc. N.J. (Journal of the Medical Society of New Jersey)

J. Mental Sci. (Journal of Mental Science)

J. Mich. St. Med. Soc. (Journal of the Michigan State Medical Society)

J. Nat. Med. Assn. (Journal of the National Medical Association)

J. Nerv. & Ment. Dis. (Journal of Nervous and Mental Disease)

J. Pharmacol. & Exper. Therap. (Journal of Pharmacology and Experimental Therapeutics)

J. Polit. Econ. (Journal of Political Economy)

J. Soc. Hist. (Journal of Social History)

J. Southern Hist. (Journal of Southern History)

J. Western Soc. Engrs. (Journal of the Western Society of Engineers)

*Libr. Hlth. (Library of Health)*

*London Med. Gazette (London Medical Gazette)*

*Long Island Med. J. (Long Island Medical Journal)*

*Los Angeles J. Eclectic Med. (Los Angeles Journal of Eclectic Medicine)*

*Maryland Med. Recorder (Maryland Medical Recorder)*

*Mass. Med. J. (Massachusetts Medical Journal)*

*Med. & Surg. Reptr. (Medical and Surgical Reporter)*

*Med. Ann. District of Columbia (Medical Annals of the District of Columbia)*

*Med. Comm. Mass. Med. Soc. (Medical Communications of the Massachusetts Medical Society)*

*Med. Exam. & Rec. Med. Sci. (Medical Examiner and Record of Medical Science)*

*Medico-Legal J. (Medico-Legal Journal)*

*Med. J. & Rec. (Medical Journal and Record)*

*Med. Life (Medical Life)*

*Med. News Libr. (Medical News Library)*

*Med. News, N.Y. (Medical News [New York])*

*Med. Press & Circular (Medical Press and Circular)*

*Med. Rec. (Medical Record)*

*Med. Rec. in N.Y. (Medical Record [in New York])*

*Med. Recorder (Medical Recorder)*

*Med. Rev. Rev. (Medical Review of Reviews)*

*Med. Times & Gaz., London (Medical Times [and Hospital Gazette], London)*

*Med. Times & Long Island Med. J. (Medical Times and Long Island Medical Journal)*

*Med. Woman's J. (Medical Woman's Journal)*

*Mich. Law Rev. (Michigan Law Review)*

*Mich. Med. (Michigan Medicine)*

*Milbank Mem. Fund Quart. Bull. (Milbank Memorial Fund Quarterly Bulletin)*

*Miss. Valley Hist. Rev. (Mississippi Valley Historical Review)*

*Modern Hosp. (Modern Hospital)*

*Modern Med. (Modern Medicine)*

*Monthly Steth. & Med. Reptr. (The Monthly Stethoscope and Medical Reporter)*

*Mt. Sinai J. Med. (Mount Sinai Journal of Medicine)*

*Nashville Med. & Surg. J. (Nashville Medical and Surgical Journal)*

*Nat. Hosp. Rec. (National Hospital Record)*

*Nation's Hlth. (Nation's Health)*

*Neurol. Bull. (Neurological Bulletin)*

*New Eng. J. Med. (New England Journal of Medicine)*

*New Orleans Med. & Surg. J. (New Orleans Medical and Surgical Journal)*

*New Orleans Med. J. (New Orleans Medical Journal)*

*New Orleans Med. News & Hosp. Gaz. (New Orleans Medical News and Hospital Gazette)*

*N.Y. Hist. Soc. Quart. (New York Historical Society Quarterly)*

*N.Y. J. Gynec. & Obst. (New York Journal of Gynaecology and Obstetrics)*

*N.Y. J. Med. (New York Journal of Medicine)*

*N.Y. Med. Gaz. (New York Medical Gazette)*

*N.Y. Med. Gaz. & J. Hlth. (New York Medical Gazette and Journal of Health)*

*N.Y. Med. J. (New York Medical Journal)*

*N.Y. Med. & Phys. J. (New York Medical and Physical Journal)*

*N.Y. Rev. (New York Review)*

*N.Y. Rev. Books (New York Review of Books)*

*N.Y. St. J. Med. (New York State Journal of Medicine)*

*North Am. Arch. Med. & Soc. Sci. (North American Archives of Medical and Social Science)*

*North Am. Rev. (North American Review)*

*North Carolina Med. J. (North Carolina Medical Journal)*

*North-Western Med. & Surg. J. (North-Western Medical and Surgical Journal)*

*Obst. & Gynec. (Obstetrics and Gynecology)*

*Ohio Med. & Surg. J. (Ohio Medical and Surgical Journal)*

*Ohio State Archaeol. & Hist. Quart. (Ohio State Archaeological and Historical Quarterly)*

*Ohio State Med. J. (Ohio State Medical Journal)*

*Pacific Coast Nursing J. (Pacific Coast Nursing Journal)*

*Pacific Med. & Surg. J. (Pacific Medical and Surgical Journal)*

*Peninsular J. Med. & Collateral Sci. (Peninsular Journal of Medicine and the Collateral Sciences)*

*Penn. Hosp. Rep. (Pennsylvania Hospital Reports)*

*Penn. Mag. Hist. & Biography (Pennsylvania Magazine of History and Biography)*

*Penn. Med. J. (Pennsylvania Medical Journal)*

*Perspect. Am. Hist. (Perspectives in American History)*

*Perspect. Biol. & Med. (Perspectives in Biology and Medicine)*

*Philadelphia Bull. (Philadelphia Bulletin)*

*Philadelphia J. Med. & Phys. Sci. (Philadelphia Journal of the Medical and Physical Sciences)*

*Philadelphia Med. Exam. (Philadelphia Medical Examiner)*

*Philadelphia Med. J. (Philadelphia Medical Journal)*

*Philadelphia Med. Times (Philadelphia Medical Times)*

*Philosophy & Med. (Philosophy and Medicine)*

*Physn. & Bull. Medico-Legal Soc. (Physician and Bulletin of the Medico-Legal Society)*

*Pop. Sci. Monthly (Popular Science Monthly)*

*Population Stud. (Population Studies)*

Proc. A.A.M.C. (Proceedings of the Association of American Medical Colleges)

Proc. Am. Inst. Homoeopathy (Proceedings of the American Institute of Homoeopathy)

Proc. Am. Medico-Psychological Assn. (Proceedings of the American Medico-Psychological Association)

Proc. Am. Pharm. Assn. (Proceedings of the American Pharmaceutical Association)

Proc. Am. Phil. Soc. (Proceedings of the American Philosophical Society)

Proc. Am. Soc. Civil Engrs. (Proceedings of the American Society of Civil Engineers)

Proc. Int. Cong. Hist. Sci. (Proceedings of the International Congress of the History of Science)

Proc. Nat. Conf. Charities & Correction (Proceedings of the National Conference of Charities and Correction)

Proc. Soc. Promotion Agric. Sci. (Proceedings of the Society for the Promotion of Agricultural Science)

Public Hlth. Rep. (Public Health Reports)

Quart. Bull. Northwestern Med. School (Quarterly Bulletin of Northwestern Medical School)

Radical Hist. Rev. (Radical History Review)

Residue Rev. (Residue Review)

Richmond & Louisville Med. J. (Richmond and Louisville Medical Journal)

Rocky Mount. Social Sci. J. (Rocky Mountain Social Science Journal)

St. Louis Clin. Rec. (St. Louis Clinical Record)

St. Louis Med. & Surg. J. (St. Louis Medical and Surgical Journal)

St. Louis Med. Reptr. (St. Louis Medical Reporter)

St. Paul Med. J. (St. Paul Medical Journal)

Saturday Rev. (Saturday Review)

Savannah J. Med. (Savannah Journal of Medicine)

Sci. Digest (Science Digest)

Scient. Am. (Scientific American)

Scient. Am. Suppl. (Scientific American Supplement)

Scribner's Mag. (Scribner's Magazine)

Social Security Bull. (Social Security Bulletin)

Soc. Sci. Hist. (Social Science History)

South Atlantic Quart. (South Atlantic Quarterly)

Southern J. Med. Sci. (Southern Journal of the Medical Sciences)

Southern Med. & Surg. J. (Southern Medical and Surgical Journal)

Southern Med. J. (Southern Medical Journal)

Southern Med. Rep. (Southern Medical Reports)

Steth. & Va. Med. Gaz. (The Stethoscope and Virginia Medical Gazette)

Surg., Gynec. & Obst. (Surgery, Gynecology & Obstetrics)

Tenn. Hist. Quart. (Tennessee Historical Quarterly)

Texas Hlth. J. (Texas Health Journal)

Texas Med. News (Texas Medical News)

Texas Med. Practitioner (Texas Medical Practitioner)

Trained Nurse & Hosp. Rev. (Trained Nurse and Hospital Review)

Tr. A.M.A. (Transactions of the American Medical Association)

Tr. Am. Gynec. Soc. (Transactions of the American Gynecological Society)

Tr. Am. Hosp. Assn. (Transactions of the American Hospital Association)

Tr. Am. Laryng. Assn. (Transactions of the American Laryngological Association)

Tr. Am. Ophth. Soc. (Transactions of the American Ophthalmological Society)

Tr. Am. Soc. Civil Engrs. (Transactions of the American Society of Civil Engineers)

Tr. Cong. Am. Phys. & Surg. (Transactions of the Congress of American Physicians and Surgeons)

Transylvania J. Med. (Transylvania Journal of Medicine and the Associated Sciences)

Tr. Coll. Physicians Phila. (Transactions and Studies of the College of Physicians of Philadelphia)

Tr. Homoeopathic Med. Soc. St. N.Y. (Transactions of the Homoeopathic Medical Society of the State of New York)

Tr. Homoeopathic Med. Soc. St. Penn. (Transactions of the Homoeopathic Medical Society of the State of Pennsylvania)

Tr. Indiana St. Med. Soc. (Transactions of the Indiana State Medical Society)

Tr. La. St. Med. Soc. (Transactions of the Louisiana State Medical Society)

Tr. Med. Assn. St. Ala. (Transactions of the Medical Association of the State of Alabama)

Tr. Med. Soc. St. N.J. (Transactions of the Medical Society of the State of New Jersey)

Tr. Med. Soc. St. N.Y. (Transactions of the Medical Society of the State of New York)

Tr. Med. Soc. St. N.C. (Transactions of the Medical Society of the State of North Carolina)

Tr. Med. Soc. St. Penn. (Transactions of the Medical Society of the State of Pennsylvania)

Tr. Med. Soc. St. Va. (Transactions of the Medical Society of the State of Virginia)

Tr. Southern Surg. & Gynec. Assn. (Transactions of the Southern Surgical and Gynecological Association)

U.C.L.A. Forum Med. Sci. (University of California at Los Angeles Forum of Medical Science)

*USDA, Farmers' Bull. (U.S. Department of Agriculture, Farmers' Bulletin)*

*U.S. Mag. & Democ. Rev. (United States Magazine and Democratic Review)*

*Va. Med. Mon. (Virginia Medical Monthly)*

*Va. Med. & Surg. J. (Virginia Medical and Surgical Journal)*

*Veg. World (Vegetarian World)*

*Verhand. d. Cong. inn. med. (Verhandlungen des Congresses für innere medizin)*

*Water-Cure J. (Water-Cure Journal)*

*Western J. Med. (Western Journal of Medicine)*

*Western J. Med. & Phys. Sci. (Western Journal of the Medical and Physical Sciences)*

*Western J. Med. & Surg. (Western Journal of Medicine and Surgery)*

*Western Med. Gaz. (Western Medical Gazette)*

*Western Penn. Hist. Mag. (Western Pennsylvania Historical Magazine)*

*Wien. med. Presse (Wiener medizinische Presse)*

*William & Mary Coll. Quart. (William and Mary College Quarterly Historical Magazine)*

*Wisconsin Mag. Hist. (Wisconsin Magazine of History)*

*Wis. Med. J. (Wisconsin Medical Journal)*

*Woman's Med. J. (Woman's Medical Journal)*

*Women & Hlth. (Women and Health)*

*World Rev. Pest Control (World Review of Pest Control)*

*Yale J. Biol. & Med. (Yale Journal of Biology and Medicine)*

*Zentralbl. Bakt. (Zentralblatt für Bakteriologie)*

*Ztschr. Tiermed. (Zeitschrift für Tiermedizin)*

# INDEX

This index was prepared by Charlotte G. Borst.